Diagnostic Endosonography

Klaus Gottlieb • Gustavo Marino

Diagnostic Endosonography

A Case-based Approach

Springer

Klaus Gottlieb, MD, MS, MBA
Clinical Professor of Medicine
George Washington University School
of Medicine
Attending Physician
VA Medical Center
Washington, DC
USA

Gustavo Marino, MD
Assistant Professor of Medicine
Georgetown University School
of Medicine
Chief Gastroenterology Section
VA Medical Center
Washington, DC
USA

ISBN 978-3-642-39117-0 ISBN 978-3-642-39118-7 (eBook)
DOI 10.1007/978-3-642-39118-7
Springer Heidelberg New York Dordrecht London

Library of Congress Control Number: 2013948393

Printed on acid-free paper

Springer is part of Springer Science+Business Media (www.springer.com)

To Our Families

Preface

There are a number of good endoscopic ultrasound (EUS) textbooks already on the market. Why did we decide to write another one.

Diagnostic Endosonography – A Case Based Approach was motivated by our experience teaching gastroenterology fellows and talking to experienced colleagues. Many fellows who have access to excellent introductory textbooks still feel only partially prepared to handle the more complex and unusual cases that they will sooner or later encounter in independent practice.

We believe that using case studies, an approach not previously employed for EUS texts, engages the reader and leads to better assimilation, greater learning gains, and better retention. Throughout the book the cases connect the EUS findings with other imaging studies, clinical manifestations, management, and current literature. The book is organized by organ systems to provide a comprehensive overview of diagnostic endosonography, including the use of fine-needle aspiration biopsy, the cornerstone of diagnosis with EUS.

We shared equally in writing the chapters and each of us reviewed the work of the other. This approach leads to a greater uniformity in how the material is presented and avoids overlap or omissions.

As the title indicates, we focused almost completely on the diagnostic aspects that we could approach with greater depth than that provided by currently available EUS textbooks. *Diagnostic Endosonography* is based on cases encountered in a tertiary care referral setting, which may challenge endosonographers, especially during their first years of practice. Beyond that it contains unusual pathology, some of which has not been previously published.

In summary, we hope that this book will help beginning endosonographers, whether still in training or already practicing without supervision, enjoy EUS even more and increase their competence.

Readers are invited to leave feedback about *Diagnostic Endosonography* and communicate with us at www.eusbook.com.

Washington, DC, USA

Klaus Gottlieb, MD, MS, MBA
Gustavo Marino, MD

Contents

1 Acquiring and Improving Skills in Diagnostic Endosonography 1
1.1 Cognitive Biases 2
1.1.1 Confirmation Bias and Framing in Imaging 3
1.1.2 Image Perception Research and Field-Dependence Bias 5
1.2 Dealing with Artifacts 8
1.2.1 The Importance of Contrast Resolution in EUS 8
1.2.2 Streak Artifacts on CT Obscuring Important Pathology Discovered by EUS 12
1.2.3 The Limitations of CT Measurements (Hounsfield Units) 14
1.2.4 Reverberation Artifact 16
1.2.5 Partial Volume Artifact 18
1.3 Anatomic Landmarks 22
1.3.1 Thyroid 22
1.3.2 Esophagus and Mediastinum 24
1.3.3 Abdomen 34
1.4 Doppler Endosonography 40
1.4.1 Mediastinum 40
1.4.2 Upper Abdomen 42
1.4.3 Pelvis 54
1.5 Medical Image Retrieval and Decision Support Systems 55
1.5.1 General Image Retrieval Platforms 55
1.5.2 Radiology Centric Image Retrieval 58
1.6 Textbooks and Journals 59
1.7 Integrating Genomics into Your EUS Practice with FNA 60
1.7.1 The Problem of Pancreatic Cysts: Could Micro RNAs Be the Answer? 60
1.7.2 Personalized Tumor Therapy: Lung Cancer Now and Pancreatic Cancer in the Future 62
1.7.3 The Primacy of FNA Cytology in the Management of Pancreatic Cancers 63
1.7.4 Stroma and Tumor Cells: The Need for Specimen Enrichment and How FNA Can Do It 63
1.7.5 Specimen Handling: Know What Needs to Happen with Your Specimen 65

1.7.6 How to Participate in Translational Research Involving Cancer Molecular Pathology 66
1.8 Solution to Challenge Case 66
References 66

2 Esophagus and Mediastinum 71
2.1 General Principles 71
2.1.1 The Esophagus: A Window into the Mediastinum 71
2.1.2 The Esophagus Is Not a Pipe 72
2.1.3 Endobronchial Ultrasound 72
2.1.4 Lymph Node Maps for the Mediastinum 73
2.1.5 Mediastinal Biopsies 73
2.1.6 Examination of the Esophagus 73
2.2 Cases and Discussions 74
2.2.1 Mediastinum 74
2.2.2 Esophagus 125
References 145

3 Stomach 147
3.1 General Principles 147
3.1.1 Anatomy 147
3.1.2 EUS Probes 148
3.1.3 Technique 148
3.1.4 Preparation 149
3.2 Cases and Discussions 150
3.2.1 Gastric Cancer 150
3.2.2 Linitis Plastica of the Stomach 154
3.2.3 Linitis Plastica with Bone Metastases 156
3.2.4 Stage 1 Mucosa-Associated Lymphoid Tissue Lymphoma 159
3.2.5 MALT Lymphoma with Local and Distant Lymph Node Involvement 162
3.2.6 Subepithelial Gastric Tumors 166
3.2.7 Gastrointestinal Stromal Tumor with Central Ulceration 167
3.2.8 Metastatic Gastrointestinal Stromal Tumor 170
3.2.9 Gastrointestinal Stromal Tumors and Interstitial Cells of Cajal 172
3.2.10 An Unusual Gastrointestinal Stromal Tumor in a Patient with Situs Inversus 174
3.2.11 Gastrointestinal Stromal Tumors: Principles of Biopsy 177
3.2.12 Gastric Carcinoid 179
3.2.13 Gastric Lipoma 182
3.2.14 Thickened Gastric Folds, Gastric Varix, or Subepithelial Lesion? 184
3.2.15 Pancreatic Rest 188
3.2.16 Submucosal Gastric Pseudotumor 191
3.2.17 Perigastric Abscess 193
References 195

4 Duodenum . . . 197
4.1 General Principles . . . 197
4.1.1 Anatomy . . . 197
4.1.2 EUS Probes . . . 197
4.1.3 Technique . . . 197
4.2 Cases and Discussions . . . 198
4.2.1 Duodenal Cancer . . . 198
4.2.2 Duodenal Diverticulum . . . 201
4.2.3 Duodenal Perforation by Foreign Body . . . 203
4.2.4 Duodenal Pseudocyst . . . 207
4.2.5 Ampullary Carcinoma . . . 211
4.2.6 Familial Adenomatous Polyposis . . . 213
4.2.7 Periduodenal Collaterals . . . 215
4.2.8 Primary Duodenal Non-Hodgkin's Lymphoma . . . 218
4.2.9 Transduodenal Abscess Drainage . . . 222
4.2.10 Zollinger-Ellison Syndrome: An Imaging Odyssey . . . 230
References . . . 233

5 Gallbladder, Liver, and Bile Ducts . . . 235
5.1 General Principles . . . 235
5.2 Cases and Discussions . . . 237
5.2.1 Gallbladder . . . 237
5.2.2 Liver . . . 248
5.2.3 Bile Ducts . . . 265
References . . . 296

6 Pancreas . . . 297
6.1 General Principles . . . 298
6.1.1 Technique . . . 298
6.1.2 Endoscopic Ultrasound Probes . . . 298
6.1.3 Anatomic Considerations . . . 298
6.2 Cases and Discussions . . . 301
6.2.1 Acute Pancreatitis with an Edematous Pancreatic Head . . . 301
6.2.2 Chronic Pancreatitis . . . 306
6.2.3 Pancreatic Parenchymal Calcifications and Stone in the Pancreatic Duct . . . 308
6.2.4 Fatty Infiltration of the Pancreas . . . 311
6.2.5 Perivascular Fat Mimicking a Dilated Main Pancreatic Duct . . . 314
6.2.6 Vanishing Pancreatic Mass . . . 317
6.2.7 Pancreatic Cancer . . . 320
6.2.8 T2 Adenocarcinoma of the Pancreas . . . 323
6.2.9 Pancreatic Tail Mass . . . 326
6.2.10 Calcifications in a Hypoechoic Pancreas Tumor . . . 328
6.2.11 Chronic Pancreatitis and Pancreatic Cancer . . . 329
6.2.12 Small Pancreatic Cancer . . . 332
6.2.13 Isodense Pancreatic Cancer . . . 334
6.2.14 Large Pancreatic Head in Relation to Body . . . 338
6.2.15 Gardner's Syndrome and Pancreatic Cancer . . . 341

6.2.16 Missed Pancreatic Cancer. 344
6.2.17 Ovarian Cancer Metastatic to the Pancreas? 348
6.2.18 Characteristic Appearance of a Wallstent on EUS 351
6.2.19 FNA Biopsies Through a Wallstent 354
6.2.20 Neuroendocrine Tumors 355
6.2.21 Primary Pancreatic Lymphoma 361
6.2.22 Mycosis Fungoides Infiltrating the Pancreas 364
6.2.23 Pancreatic Cysts 367
6.2.24 Serous Cystadenoma 379
References 381

7 Adrenals and Spleen, Peritoneum, and Retroperitoneum 385
7.1 General Principles 385
7.1.1 Anatomy and Technique 385
7.2 Cases and Discussions 386
7.2.1 Adrenal Biopsy 386
7.2.2 Myelolipoma Inside an Adrenal Adenoma. 390
7.2.3 Paraganglioma 392
7.2.4 Accessory Spleen 394
7.2.5 Ascites 396
7.2.6 Omentum 398
7.2.7 Fluid in the Lesser Sac 400
7.2.8 Mesenteric Cysts 402
7.2.9 Omental Cake 405
7.2.10 Peritoneal Carcinomatosis 409
7.2.11 Retroperitoneal Carcinomatosis 411
References 414

8 Colon, Rectum, and Anus. 415
8.1 General Principles 415
8.1.1 Anatomy of the Rectal Wall and Perirectal Structures: Correlation with EUS 415
8.1.2 Endoscopic Ultrasound Probes. 419
8.1.3 Preparation 419
8.1.4 Endoscopic Ultrasound Examination Technique 419
8.2 Cases and Discussions 421
8.2.1 Progression of Rectal Cancer from T2N0 to T3N1 . . . 421
8.2.2 T3N1 Rectal Carcinoma: Response to Treatment 425
8.2.3 Colon Cancer Metastatic to Mediastinal Lymph Nodes 428
8.2.4 Large Colon Polyp 431
8.2.5 Large Villous Adenoma with High-Grade Dysplasia. . 433
8.2.6 Anal Cancer with Extensive Intramural Spread into the Rectum. 435
8.2.7 Anorectal Melanoma 438
8.2.8 Diffuse Cavernous Rectal Hemangioma. 442
8.2.9 Cystic Lymphangioma of the Colon. 445
8.2.10 Coccygeal Chordoma 449
References 452

Index. 455

1 Acquiring and Improving Skills in Diagnostic Endosonography

Contents

1.1 **Cognitive Biases** 2
1.1.1 Confirmation Bias and Framing in Imaging 3
1.1.2 Image Perception Research and Field-Dependence Bias 5
1.1.2.1 Field Dependence 5

1.2 **Dealing with Artifacts** 8
1.2.1 The Importance of Contrast Resolution in EUS 8
1.2.2 Streak Artifacts on CT Obscuring Important Pathology Discovered by EUS 12
1.2.3 The Limitations of CT Measurements (Hounsfield Units) 14
1.2.4 Reverberation Artifact 16
1.2.5 Partial Volume Artifact 18

1.3 **Anatomic Landmarks** 22
1.3.1 Thyroid 22
1.3.2 Esophagus and Mediastinum 24
1.3.2.1 Mediastinal Anatomy Is Not Set in Stone 27
1.3.2.2 Thoracic Duct 29
1.3.2.3 Azygos Vein 31
1.3.2.4 Mediastinal Lymph Nodes 33
1.3.3 Abdomen 34
1.3.3.1 Prostate 34
1.3.3.2 Seminal Vesicles 35
1.3.3.3 Vagina 37
1.3.3.4 The Uterus 39

1.4 **Doppler Endosonography** 40
1.4.1 Mediastinum 40
1.4.1.1 Azygos Vein 40
1.4.1.2 Dorsal Intercostal Arteries 41
1.4.2 Upper Abdomen 42
1.4.2.1 Hepatic Veins 42
1.4.2.2 Portal Vein 43
1.4.2.3 Splenic Vein and Splenic Artery 45
1.4.2.4 Celiac Vessels and the Superior Mesenteric Artery 47
1.4.2.5 Celiac Artery Variants 49
1.4.2.6 Celiac Ganglia 52
1.4.3 Pelvis 54

1.5 **Medical Image Retrieval and Decision Support Systems** 55
1.5.1 General Image Retrieval Platforms 55
1.5.1.1 ITSE/iMedline 55
1.5.1.2 PubMed Central 55
1.5.1.3 BioText 55
1.5.1.4 FigureSearch 56
1.5.1.5 Yale Image Finder 57
1.5.2 Radiology Centric Image Retrieval 58
1.5.2.1 ARR GoldMiner® 58
1.5.2.2 Yottalook™ 58

1.6 **Textbooks and Journals** 59

1.7 **Integrating Genomics into Your EUS Practice with FNA** 60
1.7.1 The Problem of Pancreatic Cysts: Could Micro RNAs Be the Answer? 60
1.7.2 Personalized Tumor Therapy: Lung Cancer Now and Pancreatic Cancer in the Future 62
1.7.3 The Primacy of FNA Cytology in the Management of Pancreatic Cancers 63
1.7.3.1 The Clonal Nature of Tumors in Space and Time and the Need for Directed and Repeat Biopsies 63
1.7.4 Stroma and Tumor Cells: The Need for Specimen Enrichment and How FNA Can Do It 63
1.7.5 Specimen Handling: Know What Needs to Happen with Your Specimen 65
1.7.6 How to Participate in Translational Research Involving Cancer Molecular Pathology 66

1.8 **Solution to Challenge Case** 66

References 66

K. Gottlieb, G. Marino, *Diagnostic Endosonography*,
DOI 10.1007/978-3-642-39118-7_1, © Springer-Verlag Berlin Heidelberg 2014

The premise of this book is to make the reader better at endosonographic diagnosis. This process is iterative and never stops. The inside of the colon is at first amazing to the novice endoscopist but soon routine takes over. Indeed, the number of new features or diagnostic challenges the trainee will encounter trails off fast. Not so in endosonography. There is always something new to learn, and the more you know, the more you will see. This is a spiral staircase with the following repeating steps: concrete experience, observation and reflection, formation of abstract concepts, and testing in new situations [1]. In this introductory chapter we begin with a discussion of cognitive biases, which not only lead to wrong diagnoses but also impede learning. After a look at artifacts, we briefly review anatomic features that often are neglected and then make a pitch for the better use of Doppler studies. Some regional anatomy will be reviewed in subsequent organ-specific chapters. Furthermore, we review image retrieval web sites that are useful for decision support, lectures, and publications, and identify textbooks and journals of interest. Finally, we discuss the future of fine-needle aspiration (FNA) biopsy, the cornerstone of diagnostic endosonography.

Box 1.1: Open Access Resources

- *Endoscopic Ultrasound* (an open access journal) http://www.eusjournal.com/ch/index.aspx
- *Basic Physics of Ultrasound Imaging*, published by the World Health Organization, 2005 http://books.google.com/books?id=nHnTOfxsM9cC
- *Manual of Diagnostic Ultrasound, 2nd edition* published by the World Health Organization, 2011 http://bit.ly/U4nJNR
- Radiography Wiki: Mach Bands and Other Optical Illusions http://bit.ly/11hLJfO
- *RadioGraphics*: Ultrasound Artifacts http://radiographics.rsna.org/content/29/4/1179.full
- Yale Image Finder – general purpose scientific image retrieval http://krauthammerlab.med.yale.edu/imagefinder/
- Yottalook – comprehensive radiology-centric search engine http://www.yottalook.com

1.1 Cognitive Biases

The role cognitive biases play in contributing to wrong diagnoses and medical error is increasingly being recognized [2]. Radiologists have pointed out where cognitive biases exist in radiologic reasoning [3]. Here is our subjective list of the top three selected from Croskerry [2]:

1. *Confirmation bias:* the tendency to look for confirming evidence to support a diagnosis rather than disconfirming evidence to refute it, despite the latter often being more persuasive and definitive.
2. *Premature closure:* a powerful cognitive disposition to respond, accounting for a high proportion of missed diagnoses. It is the tendency to apply premature closure to the decision-making process, accepting a diagnosis before it has been fully verified. The consequences of the bias are reflected in the maxim: "When the diagnosis is made, the thinking stops."
3. *Search satisfying:* reflects the universal tendency to call off a search once something is found. For example, comorbidities, second foreign bodies, other fractures, and co-ingestants in poisoning may all be missed. Also, if the search yields nothing, diagnosticians should satisfy themselves that they have been looking in the right place.

Fortunately, we are not entirely defenseless against these biases. We recommend these three cognitive defense strategies for endosonographers [2]:

1. *Cognitive forcing strategies:* Develop generic and specific strategies to avoid predictable bias in particular clinical situations.
2. *Metacognition:* Train for a reflective approach to problem solving, stepping back from the

immediate problem to examine and reflect on the thinking process.

3. *Consider alternatives:* Establish forced consideration of alternative possibilities, for example, the generation of and working through a differential diagnosis. Encourage routinely asking the question, What else might this be?

The following case illustrates some of these points.

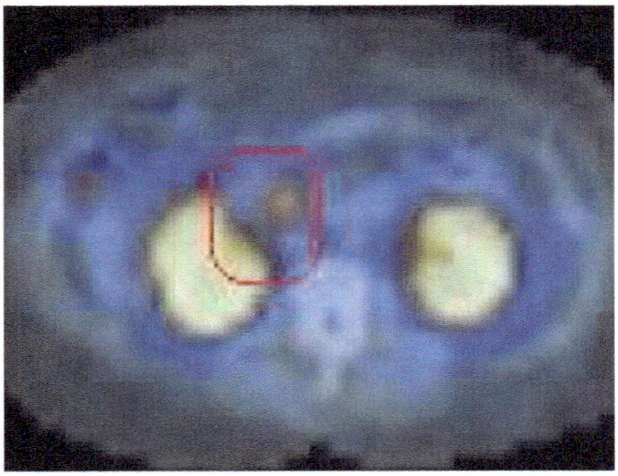

Fig. 1.1 This octreotide scan shows focally increased activity anterior and medial to the right kidney

1.1.1 Confirmation Bias and Framing in Imaging

This is a 66-year-old woman who was evaluated for a suspected gastrinoma 18 months before this presentation. An octreotide scan showed a questionable area of increased activity anterior to the right kidney. A computed tomography (CT) scan and an endoscopic ultrasound (EUS) were performed at the time and nothing was found. The patient's gastrin levels continued to rise and a second octreotide scan was performed. The report stated that the "same region of mild increased activity is seen *medial and anterior to the right kidney*."

A repeat CT scan (previously reported as negative) was read as showing a "questionable tiny focal area of soft tissue density at the medial aspect of the second portion of the duodenum which measures 1.4 cm and corresponds to the octreotide abnormality, suspicious for a small gastrinoma in the gastrinoma triangle." The corresponding slice of the CT is shown here; the arrow inserted by the radiologist can be seen.

The repeat EUS shows a lesion, which is considerably smaller (9.5 mm) and in a different

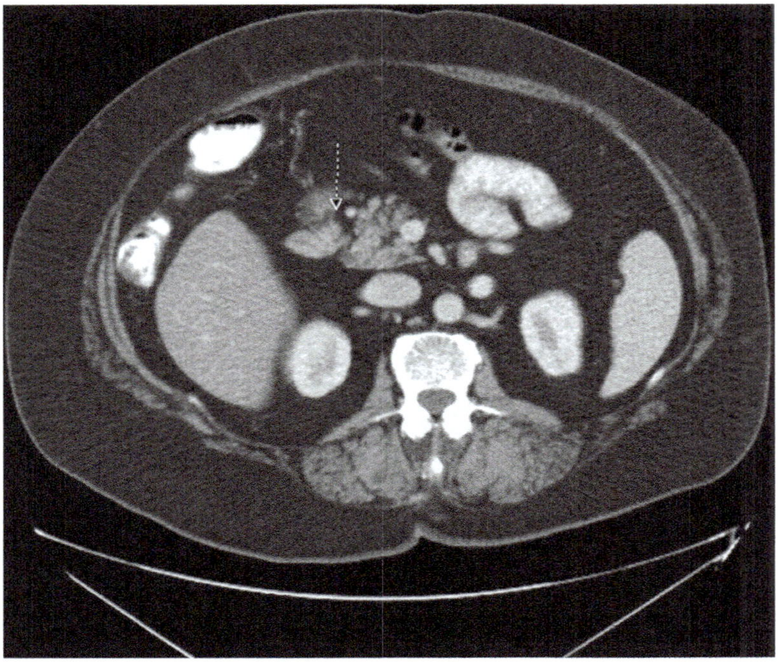

Fig. 1.2 The *arrow* (inserted by the radiologist) indicates the location of the postulated gastrinoma. Note how remote this area is from the right kidney. This is not where the gastrinoma was located. The reader of the computed tomography scan was eager to replicate the lesion seen on the octreotide scan (confirmation bias, framing)

location from what was seen on the CT scan. In fact, the lesion identified on the EUS is exactly medial and anterior to the right kidney (as would be expected based on the octreotide scan), whereas the lesion as postulated by the CT is more remote.

In retrospect, a lesion corresponding to the EUS image could also be identified on the CT, anterior and medial to the right kidney and located in the bowel wall. It appears to be slightly enhancing, as is typical for islet cell tumors [4].

Confirmation bias, or the willingness to identify abnormalities that are expected to be present but are really not, at least not where suspected, is a trap everybody can fall into. There is a blurry line between looking so hard that one starts seeing things and not looking hard enough. The next section will examine this trade-off in more detail.

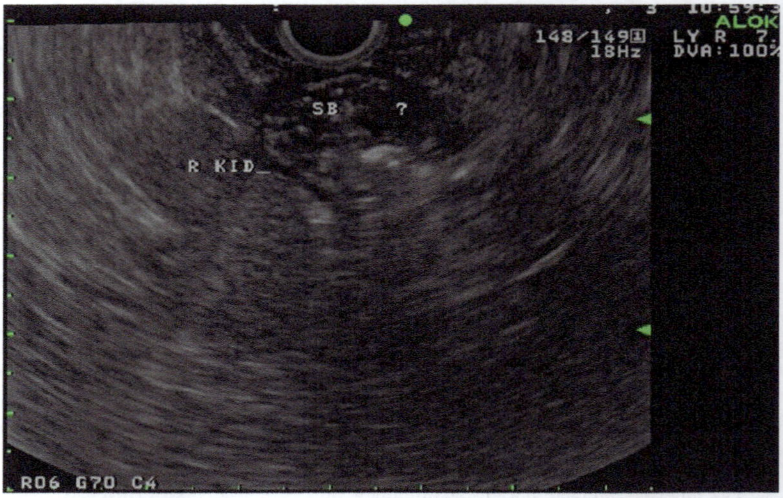

Fig. 1.3 This endoscopic ultrasound image shows a 9.5-mm-diameter hypoechoic nodule in the duodenal wall medial and anterior to the right kidney (indicated by *?*)

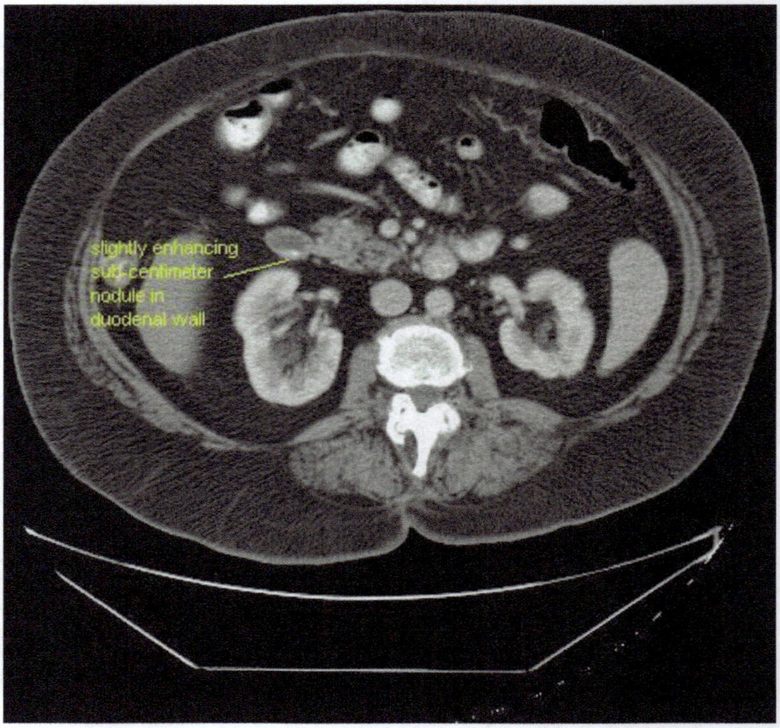

Fig. 1.4 The sub-centimeter nodule seen in the duodenal wall on the endoscopic ultrasound can also be identified (retrospectively) as a slightly enhancing duodenal wall lesion on this single-slice computed tomography (CT) scan (same CT as in Fig. 1.2). The location was confirmed during surgery

1.1.2 Image Perception Research and Field-Dependence Bias

Image perception research deals with the processes of perception and recognition of information in medical images. It is estimated that there is about a 20–30 % miss rate (false negatives) in radiology, with a 2–15 % rate of false positives [5]. Whether these numbers are really so high could be debated; let us agree, however, that they are not insignificant. Using eye position recording techniques, it has been found that false negatives can be classified into three categories based on how long they are fixated or dwelled on (visual dwell patterns) [5, 6].

- *Search errors:* Some lesions are missed because they are never looked at with high-resolution foveal vision.
- *Recognition errors:* Some lesions are looked at, but not long enough to detect or recognize any suspicious features.
- *Decision errors:* These lesions are looked at for long periods of time (often as long as lesions that are looked at and reported) but are still missed.

Decision error can be illustrated by the following case and conceptualized by the cognitive theory of field dependence. A field-dependent person has difficulty finding a geometric shape that is embedded or "hidden" in a background with similar (but not identical) lines and shapes. The conflicting patterns distract the person from identifying the given figure. A person who is field-independent can readily identify the geometric shape, regardless of the background in which it is set [7]. However, identifying hidden figures has a flip side: subjective contour formation. Subjective contour formation is a psychophysiological phenomenon in which complete "structures" are falsely constructed from minimal outlines [8].

The EUS image recognition process relies heavily on patterns that correlate with abnormalities. Lack of awareness of additional patterns or finding atypical changes may confuse the endosonographer, who could either ignore the finding or make incorrect conclusions. In these cases an open mind and awareness of unknown possibilities should be recognized. Video-recording of these findings may be useful for additional review with radiologists or other endosonographers.

1.1.2.1 Field Dependence

This case also illustrates that endoscopic ultrasound is more than an imaging technique – it is an "interrogation" technique. When suspicion is raised the endosonographer can vary transducer position, insonation angle, tissue adaptation, frequency, and other specifications to tease out more information.

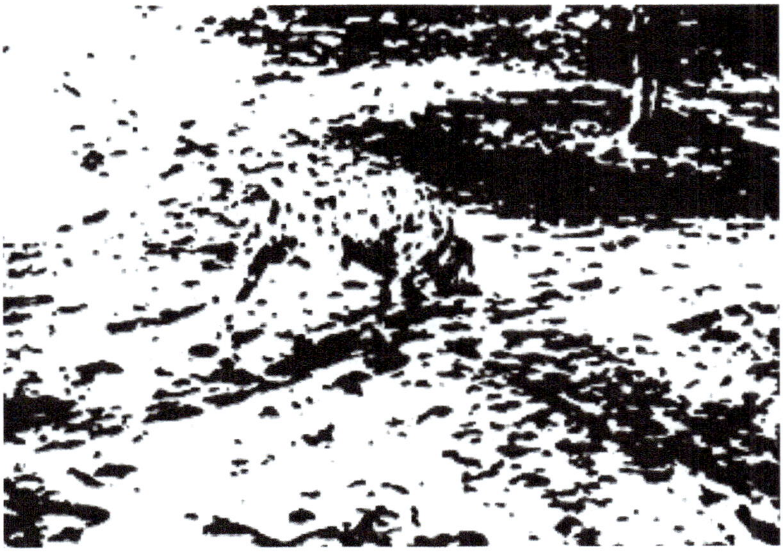

Fig. 1.5 An illustration of field independence with the hidden picture test. The concealed abject is revealed at the end of this chapter

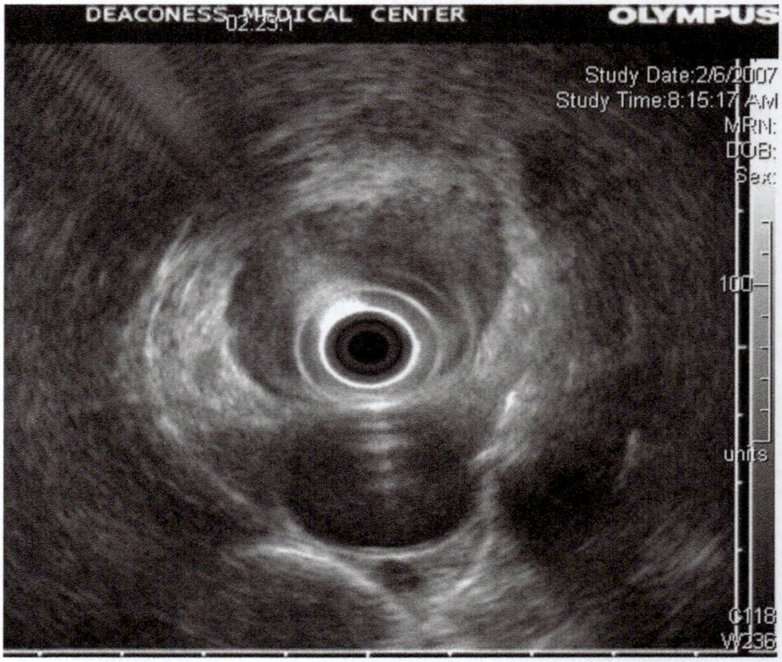

Fig. 1.6 Look closely at this image. We are in the esophagus. The aorta is at 6 o'clock. There is an almost circumferential hypoechoic mass. What is hidden?

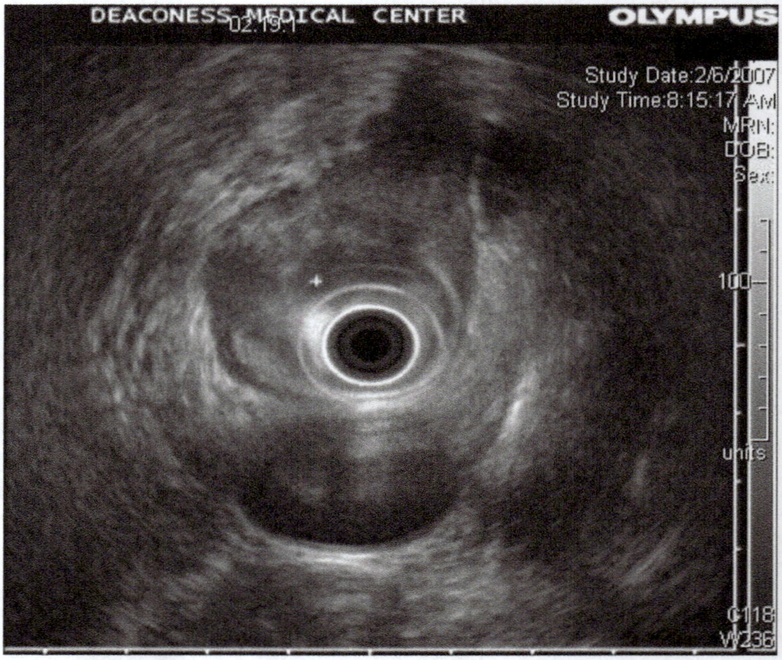

Fig. 1.7 Another view of the mass in the esophagus. Can you see it now?

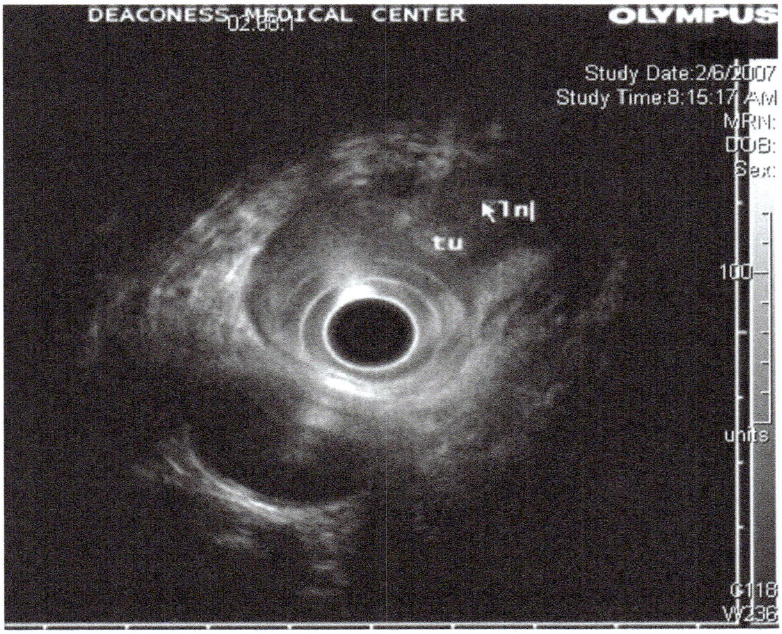

Fig. 1.8 The higher frequency clearly shows a periesophageal lymph node that at a lower frequency almost completely blended in with the tumor mass. *tu* tumor, *ln* lymph node

1.2 Dealing with Artifacts

In the context of ultrasound or imaging, an artifact is any perceived distortion, error, or addition caused by the processor and display. Artifacts can be recognized as such and then either exploited or ignored. If artifacts are not recognized but taken as "anatomic reality," diagnostic errors and procedural complications may be the consequences.

According to Kremkau and Taylor [9] there are four generic categories of ultrasound imaging artifacts:

1. *Acoustic:* error in the presentation of ultrasound information;
2. *Anatomic:* error in interpretation (often called a "pitfall" error);
3. *Optical illusion:* error in perception; and
4. *Other:* electrical noise.

This classification system mixes the technical with the cognitive and predates some of the recent interest in cognitive biases (see the earlier discussion about cognitive bias) but remains useful as long as endosonographers are aware of where the distortion occurs (before or after cortical processing).

Some of the common artifacts that occur during EUS or CT are demonstrated by the cases that follow. Obviously, artifacts also are seen with other imaging modalities. However, CT artifacts are very different from ultrasound artifacts, and this can be exploited, as Sect. 1.2.2 demonstrates.

1.2.1 The Importance of Contrast Resolution in EUS

There are three domains of image resolution: temporal, detail (axial and lateral), and contrast. Detail resolution is largely determined by image frequency and beam width. Contrast resolution, on the other hand, is generally determined by pre- and postprocessing of images [10]. Postprocessing curves can be selected on the ultrasound processor and sometimes need to be adjusted to enhance small differences in echo intensity. Some endosonographers never change their postprocessing assignments. For beginners, staying with the scheme can lead to quicker familiarization with the strange world of sonography. However, the

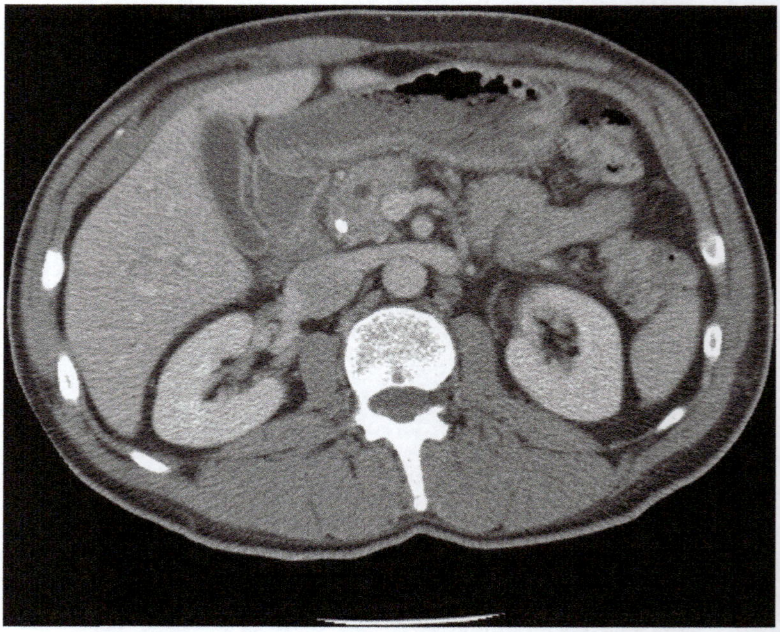

Fig. 1.9 This computed tomography scan shows a pancreatic head with biliary stent in place. A mass is not apparent

next case illustrates how not using postprocessing curve adjustments can lead to problems.

A 50-year-old man with a history of alcohol problems but no drinking for 6 years was admitted to the hospital with acute pancreatitis. He later developed jaundice. Endoscopic retrograde cholangiopancreatography (ERCP) showed a smoothly compressed bile duct. A stent was placed. CT and magnetic resonance imaging (MRI) were negative for a mass lesion. The CA 19-9 was initially elevated but this was thought to be due to the biliary obstruction and acute pancreatitis. EUS was performed; no mass was seen. Features of mild chronic pancreatitis, especially in the body and tail, were present. Three days after the first EUS the patient's repeat CA 19-9 levels came back: they had quintupled. He was brought back for a second look. Linear EUS showed the tumor and biopsies were positive for adenocarcinoma. The linear electronically switched instrument is widely believed to have an intrinsically better contrast resolution than the mechanical radial instrument, but different postprocessing settings may have revealed the tumor on the first exam.

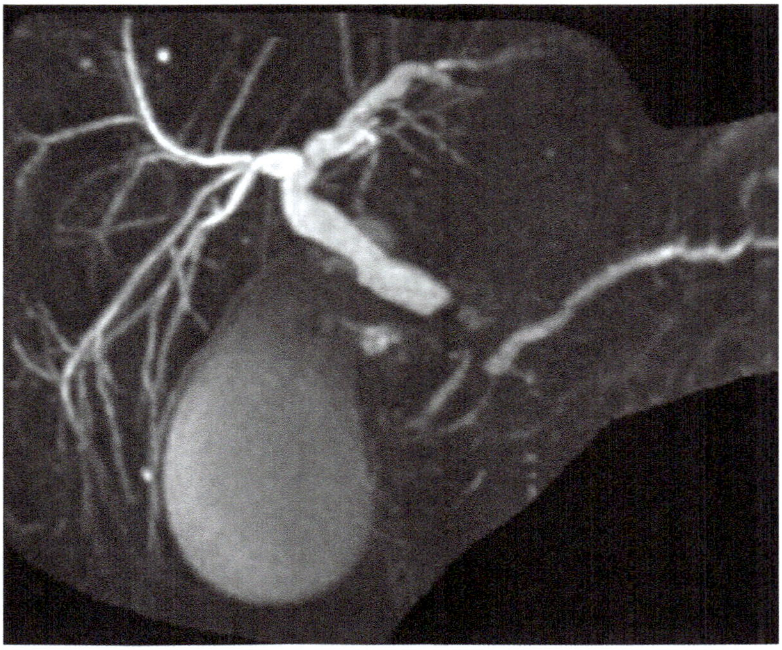

Fig. 1.10 This magnetic resonance cholangiopancreatography shows a bile duct stricture. On ERCP the stricture was described as smooth

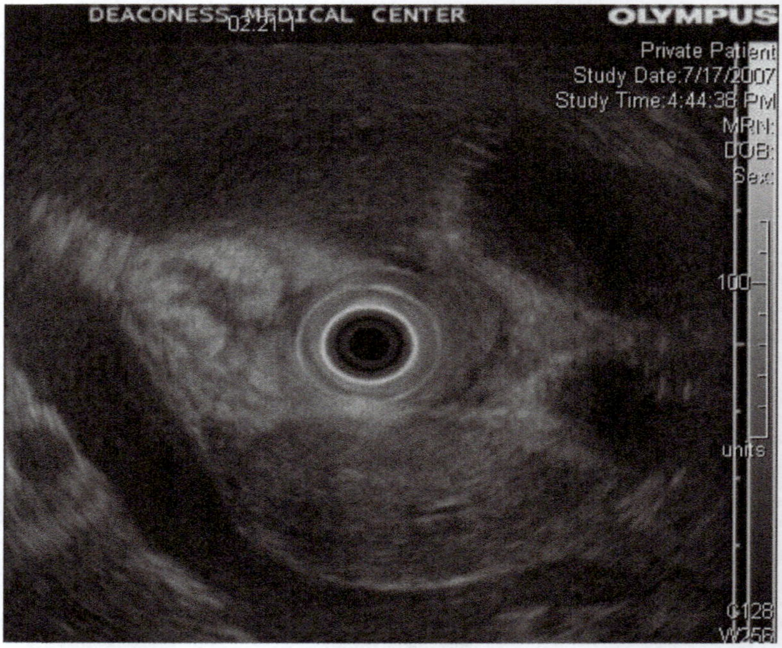

Fig. 1.11 This radial endoscopic ultrasound image shows a homogenous-appearing head of the pancreas. A mass was not appreciated at the time, but it can be seen in retrospect

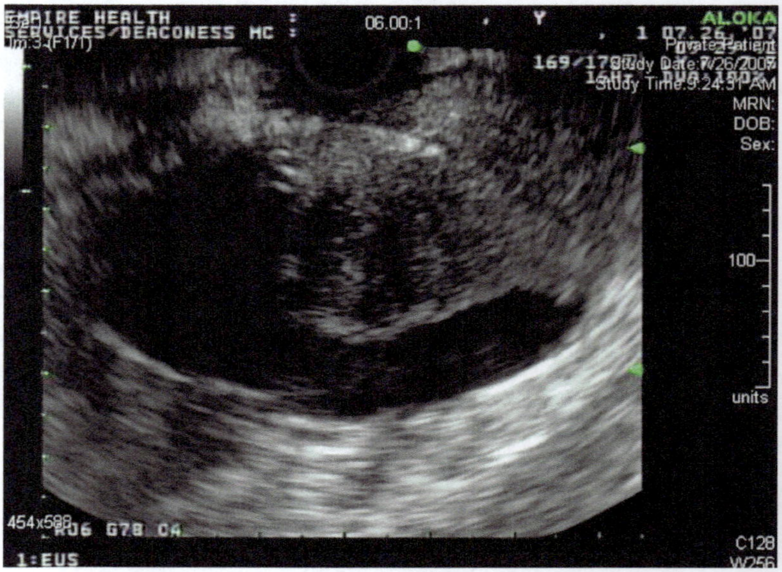

Fig. 1.12 A week later endoscopic ultrasound was performed a second time. A linear array electronically switched instrument was employed. A mass is now apparent

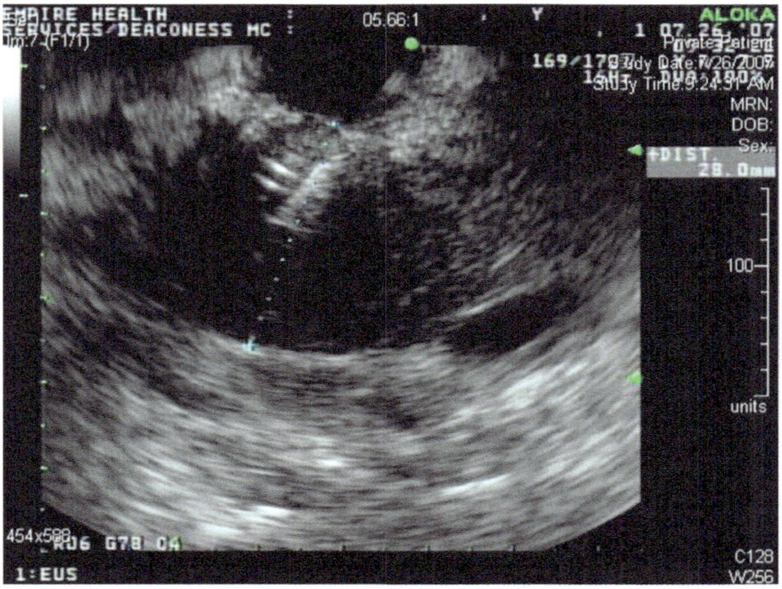

Fig. 1.13 Fine-needle aspiration biopsies of the mass showed adenocarcinoma. The needle is shown, and the bile duct stent is also visible

1.2.2 Streak Artifacts on CT Obscuring Important Pathology Discovered by EUS

This is a 73-year-old patient with generally declining health who was admitted to the hospital with a diagnosis of cholecystitis. He was considered to have poor operative risk and instead of a cholecystectomy a cholecystomy was performed. The CT scan of the abdomen showed small pancreatic cysts, and EUS evaluation was requested. The EUS showed small simple-appearing cysts, which were ignored in view of the finding of a 6-cm-diameter periesophageal lymph node mass. Biopsies revealed Hodgkin's lymphoma.

Prompted by the EUS findings, a CT scan of the chest was ordered. This CT was read as showing a 2.5-cm lymph node in the azygoesophageal recess. Interestingly, the 6-cm lymph node mass was not picked up by the reading radiologist, presumably in part because streak artifacts on the CT scan further deteriorated image quality in the region of interest.

This case illustrates two things. First, EUS is an imaging modality that looks at the same anatomy based on a reflection-based algorithm, whereas CT evaluates tissue based on its transmission characteristics. Therefore, the same pathology can be obvious on EUS and close to invisible on CT or vice versa. Second, radiologists and endosonographers need to communicate better.

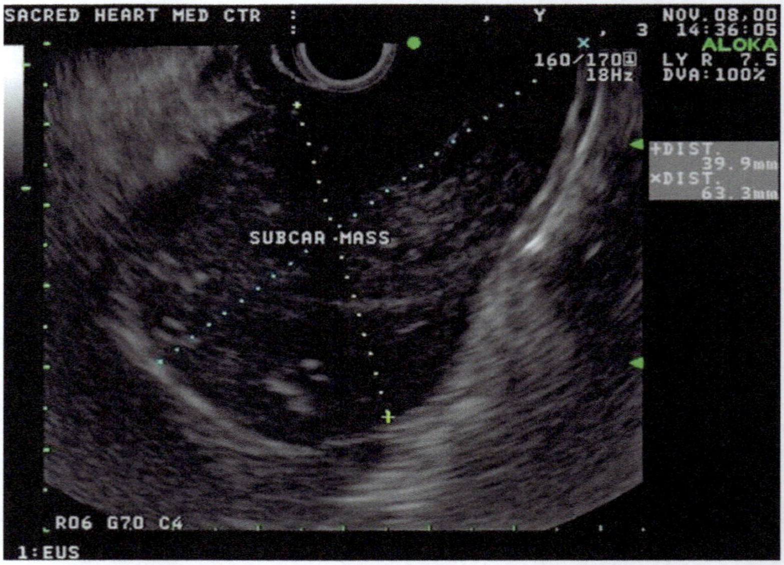

Fig. 1.14 The pancreas exam showed small simple-appearing cysts, but a screening exam of the mediastinum with linear endoscopic ultrasound unexpectedly showed a 6-cm large mass adjacent to the lower esophagus

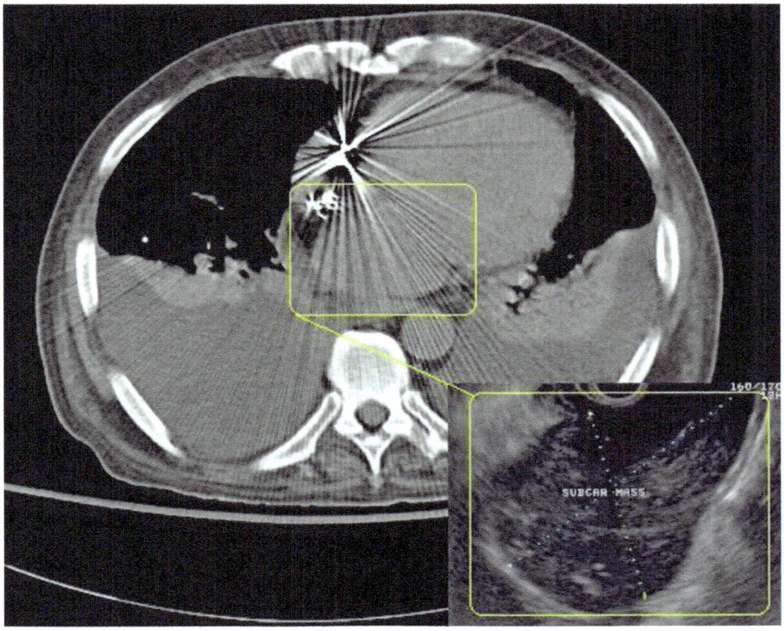

Fig. 1.15 An overlay of the endoscopic ultrasound (EUS) image on the computed tomography (CT) scan illustrates the two strikingly different appearances of the same mass, which was not recognized/reported on CT but is obvious on EUS

1.2.3 The Limitations of CT Measurements (Hounsfield Units)

Hounsfield units are a quantitative measurement of radiodensity on CT scans. Low Hounsfield units in the pancreas say little more than that the lesion is hypodense; it does not reliably distinguish between a hypodense solid tumor mass or a cyst, as this case demonstrates. Both lesions in this patient's pancreas were thought to be cysts on CT on the basis of overall impression and density measurements. EUS shows that the lesion in the head is indeed a cyst, whereas the pancreatic tail lesion is adenocarcinoma, as proven by a biopsy.

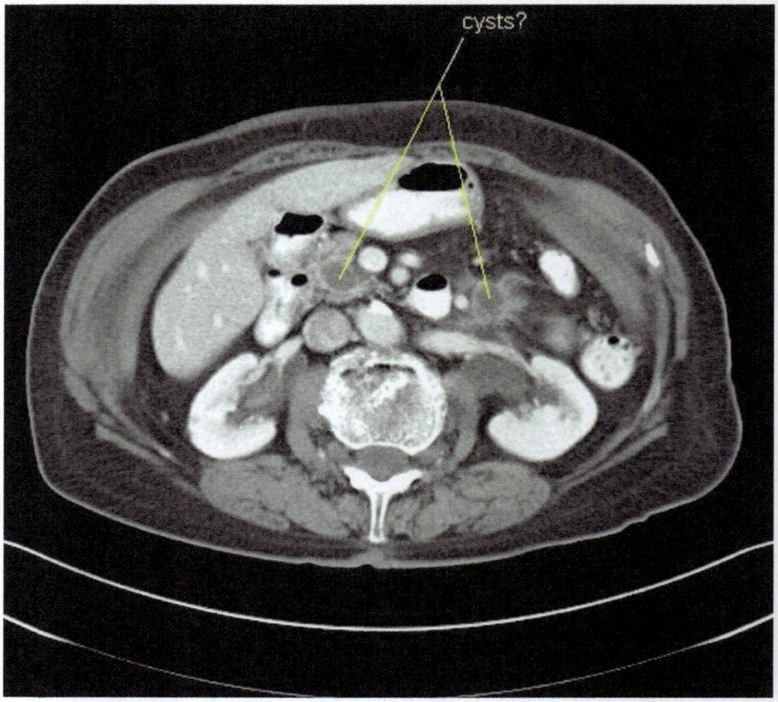

Fig. 1.16 This computed tomography scan shows hypodense lesions in the head and tail of the pancreas. Both were thought to be cysts

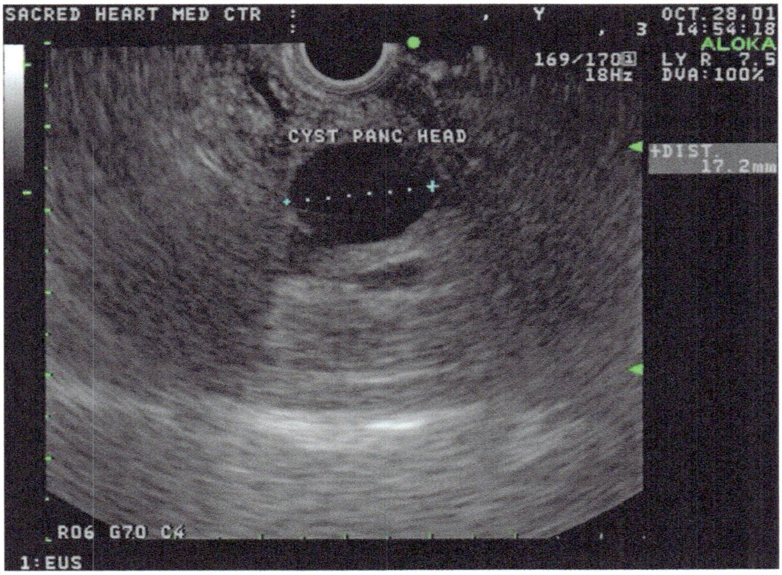

Fig. 1.17 The endoscopic ultrasound image shows that the lesion in the head of the pancreas is indeed an anechoic cyst with posterior enhancement (increased transmission), but the tail lesion is solid

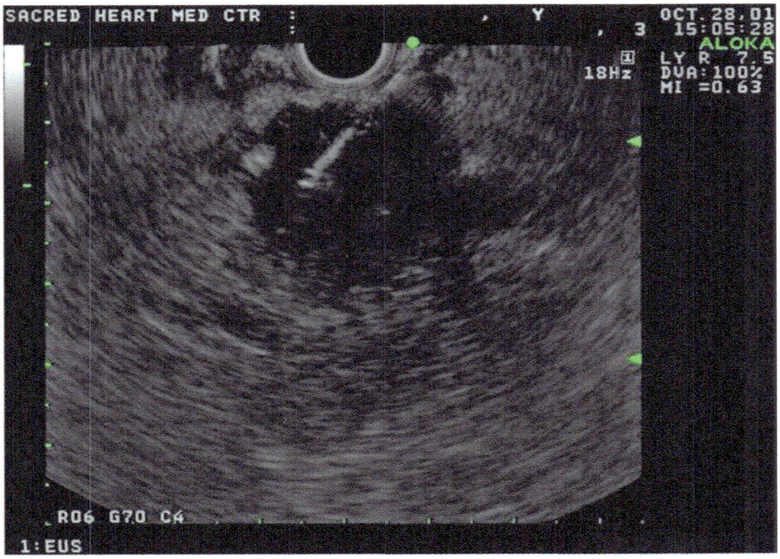

Fig. 1.18 In the tail region of the pancreas, the "cyst" seen on computed tomography is actually solid. Fine-needle aspiration biopsies revealed adenocarcinoma

1.2.4 Reverberation Artifact

Reverberation artifact in ultrasound imaging is caused by the multiple reflections of ultrasound back and forth between two closely spaced interfaces. It is commonly seen in the human body when air is trapped between tissue planes, which conduct sound well (soft tissue-to-gas interfaces). It occurs even more frequently in endosonography when the balloon around the ultrasound transducer is only partially filled with water and contains air bubbles. On the basis of its appearance, the artifact is also referred to as "ring-down artifact" and "comet tail artifact.".

This is a patient with a cholangiocarcinoma. The patient had an ERCP with placement of a stent across his common bile duct stricture 4 days before this EUS. During the EUS the gallbladder initially appeared normal; however, eventually enough air was blown from the duodenum via the stent into the gallbladder to cause the reverberation artifact shown. Chapter 2, Esophagus and Mediastinum, shows how this artifact can help detect air-filled bronchi in a consolidated lung.

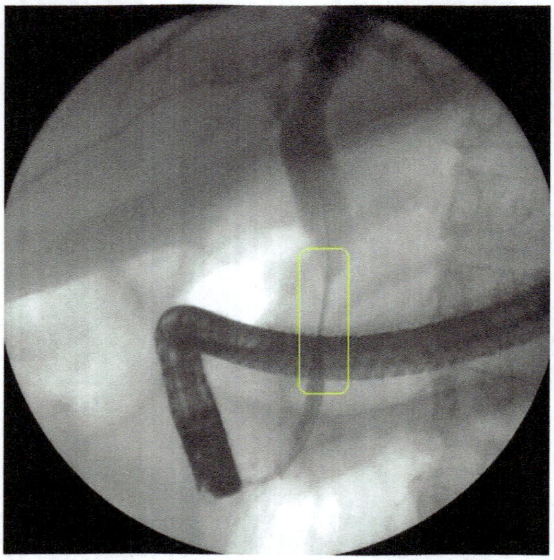

Fig. 1.19 This ERCP shows a stricture of the extrapancreatic bile duct caused by a cholangiocarcinoma

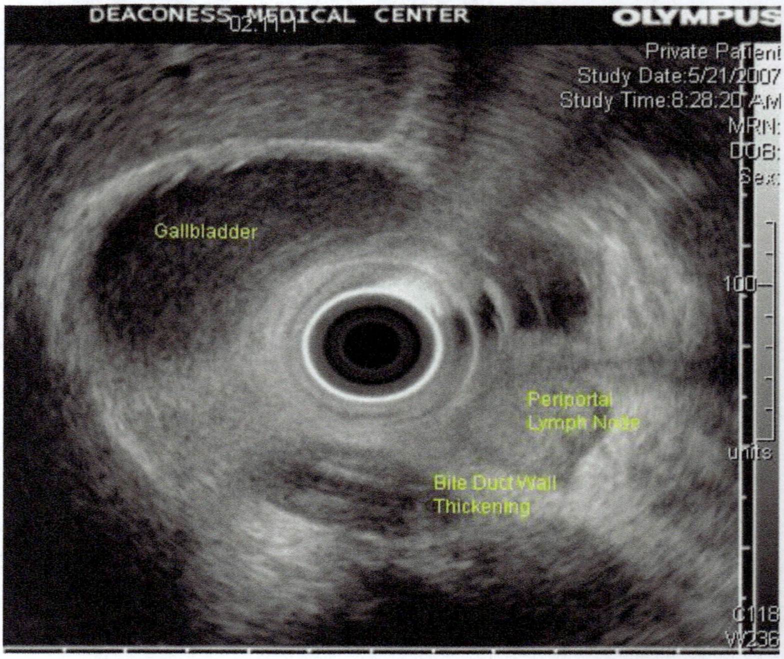

Fig. 1.20 The corresponding endoscopic ultrasound image shows marked thickening of the common bile duct wall surrounding a plastic stent. Note the enlarged periportal lymph node suspicious for nodal metastasis

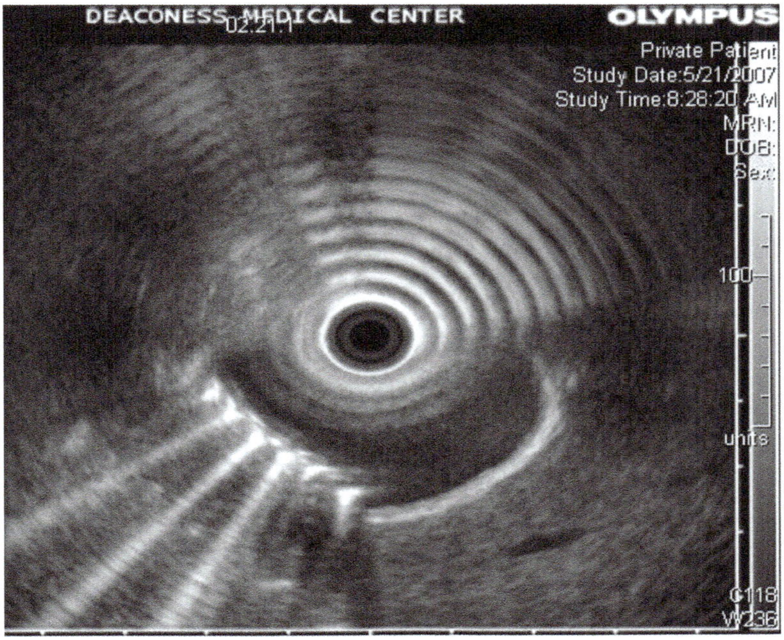

Fig. 1.21 This is a classic example of reverberation artifact. It is caused by air in the gallbladder (comet tail artifact) in the *bottom half of the image* and by air in a partially filled balloon around the transducer (ring-down artifact) in *the top half of the image*

1.2.5 Partial Volume Artifact

This is a 62-year-old man with a carcinoid of the terminal ileum metastatic to the liver. He is now being considered for debulking surgery. The CT scan showed a possible area where it seemed as if the large centrally located metastasis was invading into the portal vein. EUS evaluation was requested and did not show any such invasion. This study also illustrates the usefulness of the vascular Doppler capability of solid-state EUS scanners.

Partial volume artifacts occur with CT and MRI when a structure is only partly contained within the imaging section, voxel, or pixel. The effect is most marked in regions where two tissues with different signal intensities adjoin, such as in this case (the tumor and portal vein). In one plane this may lead to blurring, but examination of the image in another plane will often show clearly defined borders [11]. EUS is an imaging technique that creates its own artifacts (albeit of a different nature); however, when the operator suspects an artifact, the imaging plane can be adjusted and the question often resolved.

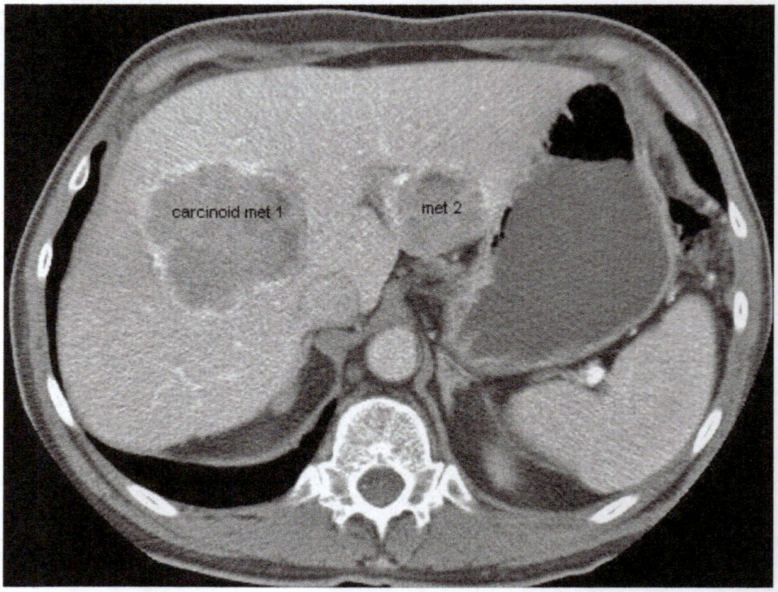

Fig. 1.22 This is a full view of the two large carcinoid metastases in the liver

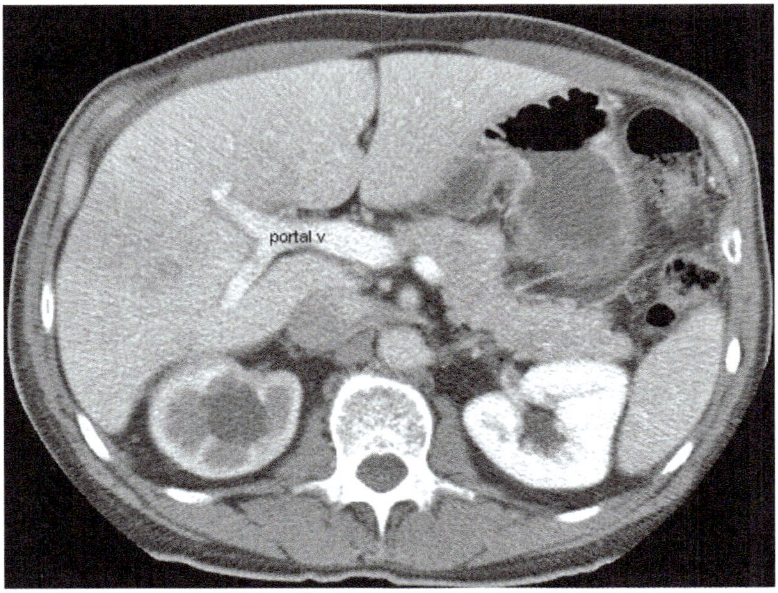

Fig. 1.23 This computed tomography scan inferior to the central metastasis shows a portal vein (*v*) and branches that appear intact

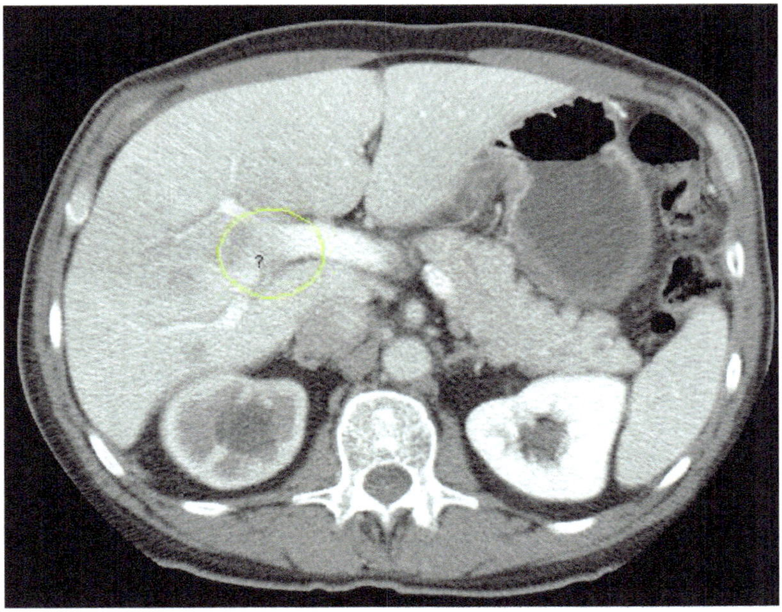

Fig. 1.24 This slice is concerning for portal vein invasion (*yellow circle*); however, volume averaging is another possible explanation

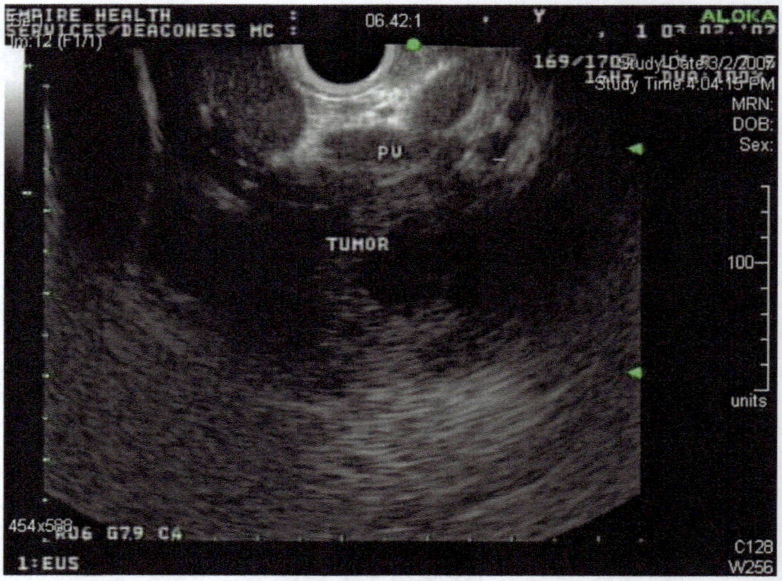

Fig. 1.25 This endoscopic ultrasound image as part of a comprehensive interrogation of the area shows a portal vein (*PV*) branch compressed by tumor but no invasion

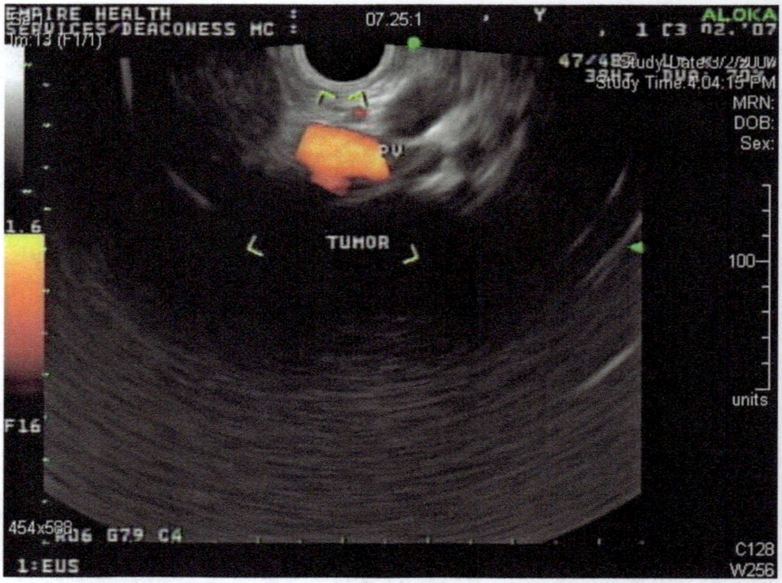

Fig. 1.26 The same area as seen in Fig 1.25 with a power Doppler signal in the portal vein (*PV*) branch

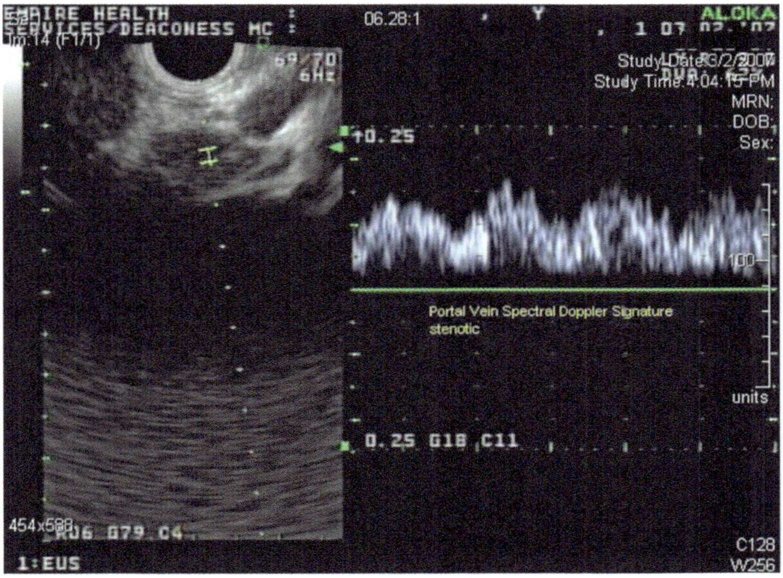

Fig. 1.27 The third image of the series of three shows that the vessel in question indeed belongs to the portal venous system and exhibits a characteristic spectral Doppler signature. No tumor invasion was seen at this level or elsewhere

1.3 Anatomic Landmarks

The following cases aim to illustrate important points without being a comprehensive review of anatomy relevant to EUS. Emphasis is placed on practical pointers and structures that endosonographers see but are not typically asked to evaluate, for example, the uterus, thyroid, and prostate.

1.3.1 Thyroid

This is a 60-year-old woman who had a plethora of complaints and was referred for EUS for the evaluation of a cyst in the pancreatic tail. Upon withdrawal of the echoendoscope through the cervical esophagus a large thyroid was incidentally noted. An evaluation of thyroid-stimulating hormone levels was ordered and came back as <0.01 uIU/ml, consistent with hyperthyroidism, in this case most likely Graves' disease. There is at least one case report where EUS was used to biopsy thyroid nodules [12], but it is unlikely that there is a role for EUS in the biopsy of thyroid masses. Percutaneous biopsies are well established, do not require sedation, and allow a view of the large portions of the thyroid, which are invisible (blocked by the trachea) to the endosonographer. Although not often tasked to evaluate the thyroid, endosonographers should be able to recognize obvious pathology. On ultrasound, thyroid tissue has a uniform solid pattern consisting of dense agglomerates of fine echoes of equal size. Compared to adjacent muscle the normal thyroid is hyperechoic. A hypoechoic appearance of the thyroid is most often due to an inflammatory process. Anteroposterior diameters of 2.0 cm or more are suspicious for pathology, and diameters exceeding 2.5 cm are clearly abnormal [13].

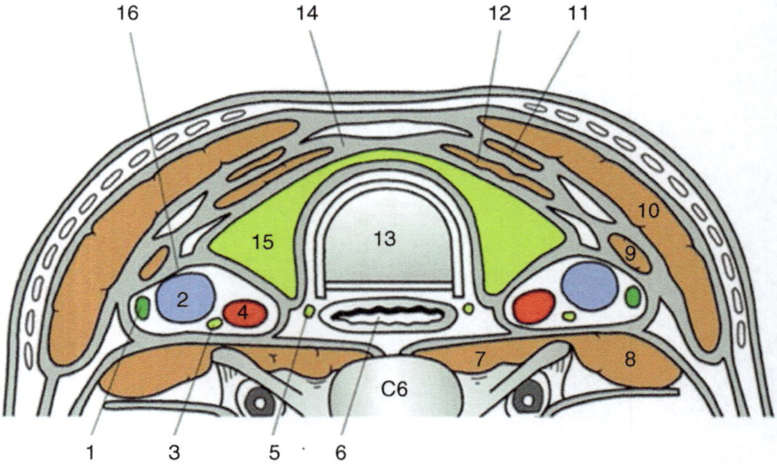

Fig. 1.28 This cross-sectional image shows the trachea, esophagus, and thyroid in relation. The transverse section at the level of C6 shows the relevant anatomy of the thyroid. *1* Cervical lymph node, *2* internal jugular vein, *3* vagus nerve, *4* common carotid artery, *5* recurrent laryngeal nerve, *6* esophagus, *7* longus colli, *8* scalenus anterior, *9* omohyoid, *10* sternocleidomastoid, *11* sternohyoid, *12* sternothyroid, *13* trachea, *14* pretracheal fascia, *15* thyroid gland, *16* carotid sheath (From Yuen et al. [14])

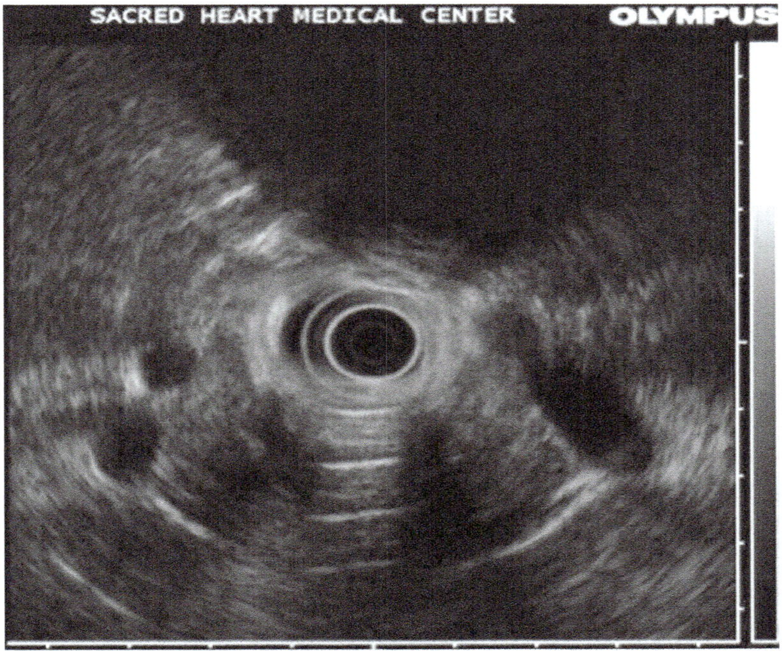

Fig. 1.29 This unlabeled endoscopic ultrasound image shows a large hypoechoic thyroid insinuating itself between the common carotid artery and internal jugular vein

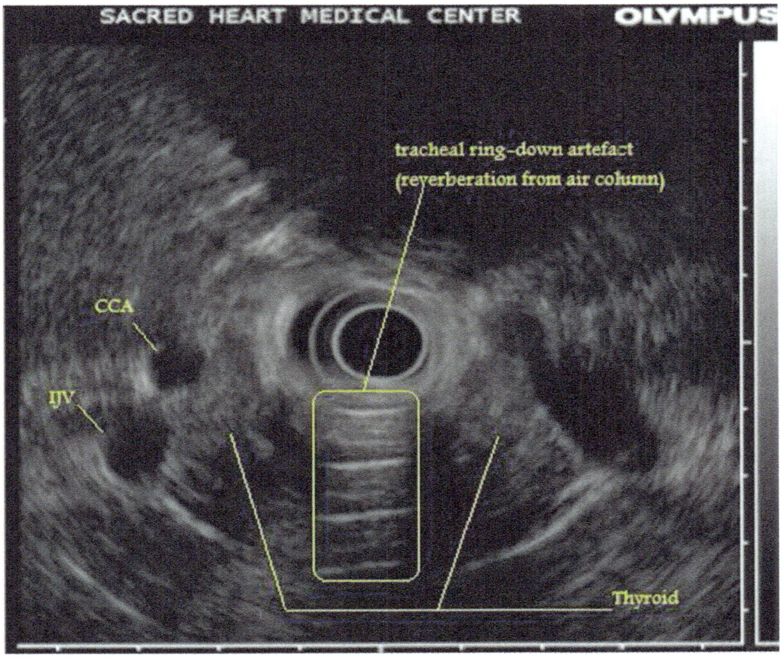

Fig. 1.30 This is a labeled version of the radial endoscopic ultrasound image in Fig. 1.29. The *shadow* on the top half of the image is caused by the vertebral body. *CCA* common carotid artery, *IJV* internal jugular vein

1.3.2 Esophagus and Mediastinum

Esophageal and mediastinal anatomy are best learned together. In fact, they are inseparable. This point is emphasized in Chap. 2, where the readers are directed to further resources. The following case illustrates that sometimes "ad hoc" landmarks need to be used to make sense of imaging findings, and this often involves the integration of several different imaging studies with EUS.

This is a 73-year-old man with a newly diagnosed left upper lobe lung nodule. Unfortunately, transthoracic biopsies revealed adenocarcinoma. The positron emission tomography–CT scan shows this nodule; it also shows another hot spot suspicious for a metastatic mediastinal lymph node on the contralateral side. This would make the patient unresectable.

The patient also has a history of a resected esophageal cancer some 12 years earlier. EUS-guided biopsies of the suspected mediastinal lymph node were requested.

A bony spur identified on EUS as causing an esophageal impression was helpful in establishing the nature of the hot spot seen on positron emission tomography.

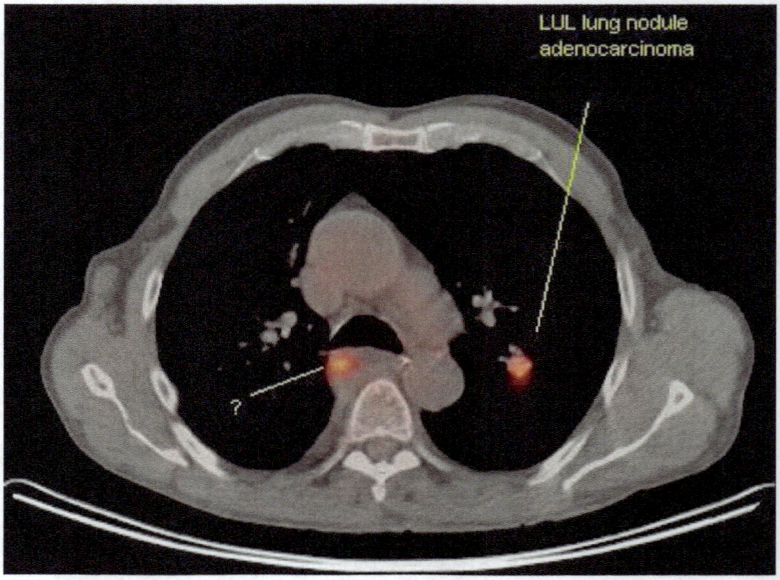

Fig. 1.31 On this positron emission tomography–computed tomography scan two hot spots (*in red*) are seen. Is this an unresectable lung cancer because there is contralateral activity? *LUL*, left upper lobe

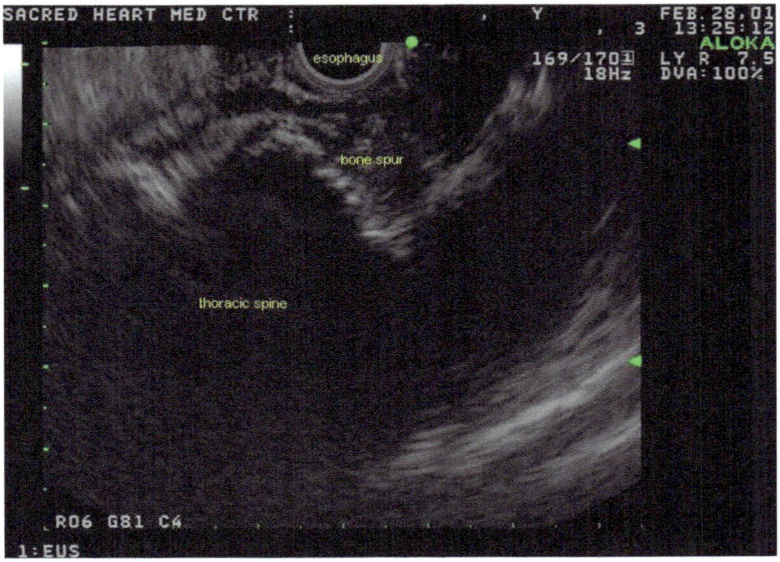

Fig. 1.32 Ultrasound reveals the presence of an esophageal impression caused by a bone spur just opposite an esophageal ulcer

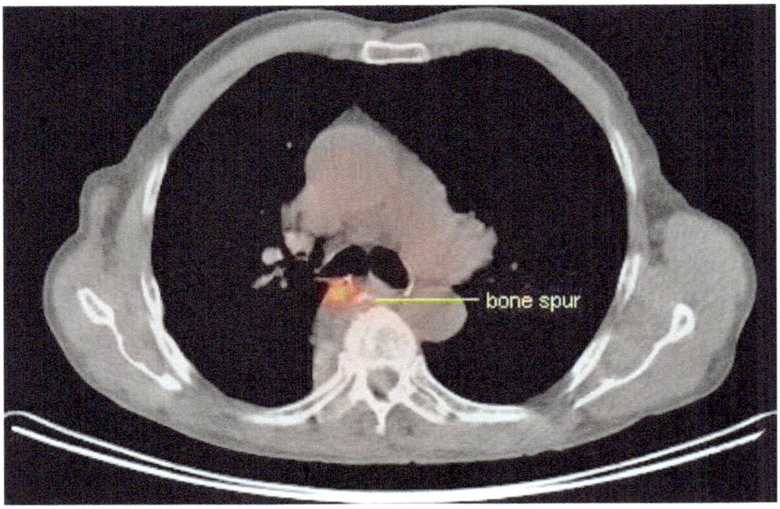

Fig. 1.33 The same PET–CT view seen in Fig. 1.31 but a cut slightly caudad to it. The left-sided lung activity is no longer visible but another abnormality has come into view: a calcified outcropping from the thoracic spine opposite the area of activity

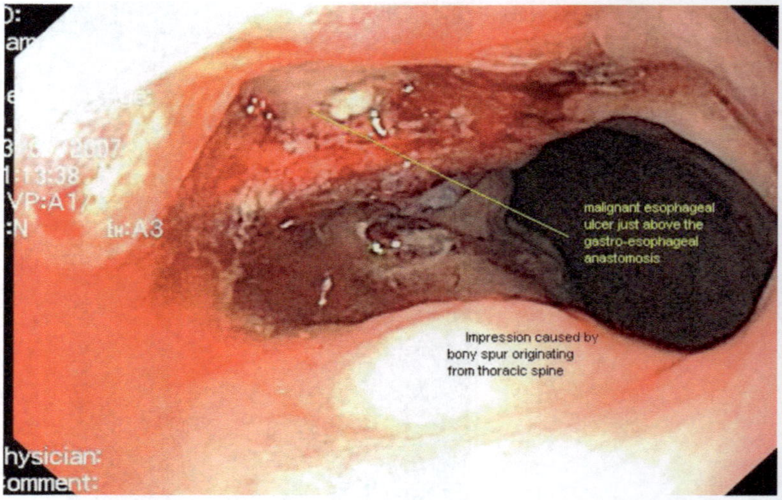

Fig. 1.34 The esophageal ulcer is opposite the bone spur on endoscopy and the bone spur is opposite the hot spot on positron emission tomography–computed tomography. The malignant esophageal ulcer causes the hot spot

1.3.2.1 Mediastinal Anatomy Is Not Set in Stone

The esophagus is not a pipe but has considerable lateral and dorsal-ventral mobility, even during normal respiration [15]. In the distal esophagus excursions of up to 9 mm were recorded during quiet respiration. More important, passive stretching of the balloon of the esophagus up to several centimeters is easily accommodated; see, for example, Larsen et al. [16]. Gentle pushing with a flexible endoscope makes remarkable excursions from the baseline possible. To our knowledge, measurements are not available, but several centimeters laterally, especially in the distal esophagus, seem probable.

The practical point is that transesophageal EUS-guided biopsies of lung masses or lymph nodes are often feasible even if it does not seem so on a CT scan. This is a 76-year-old patient who had an unsuccessful attempted bronchoscopy and was referred to us by his medical oncologist. Despite the fact that the tumor does not appear to be accessible from the esophagus, the tumor could be visualized and biopsies were easy; diagnostic material (large-cell carcinoma) was obtained.

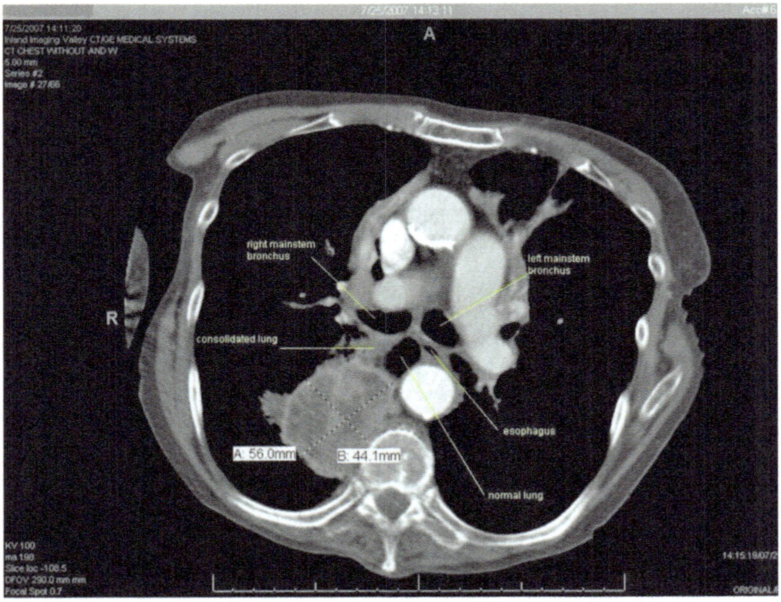

Fig. 1.35 On the basis of this computed tomography scan it does not appear that the large right lower lobe lung mass can be biopsied from the esophagus. However, the esophagus is not a rigid pipe. Instead, it accommodates gentle sideward pushing with the tip of the endoscope

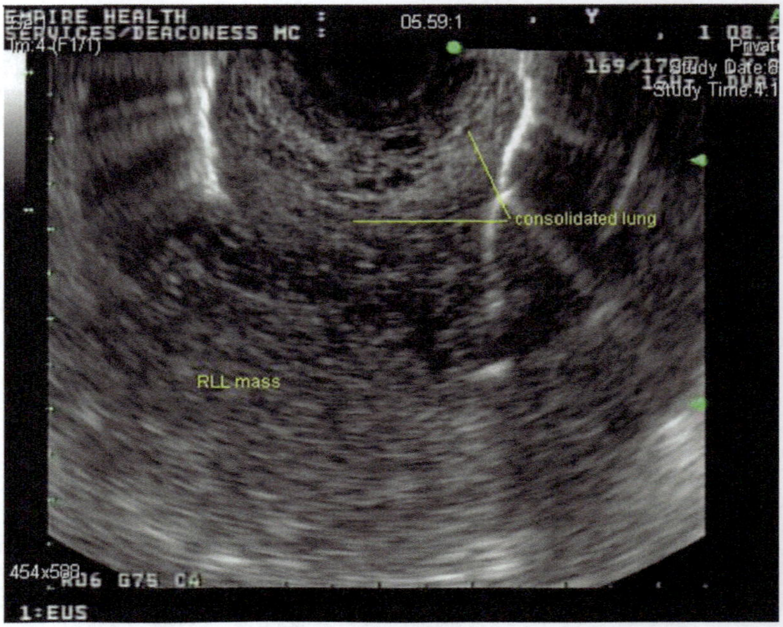

Fig. 1.36 This endoscopic ultrasound image shows the consolidated portion of the lung and the mass posterior to it. *RLL*, right lower lobe

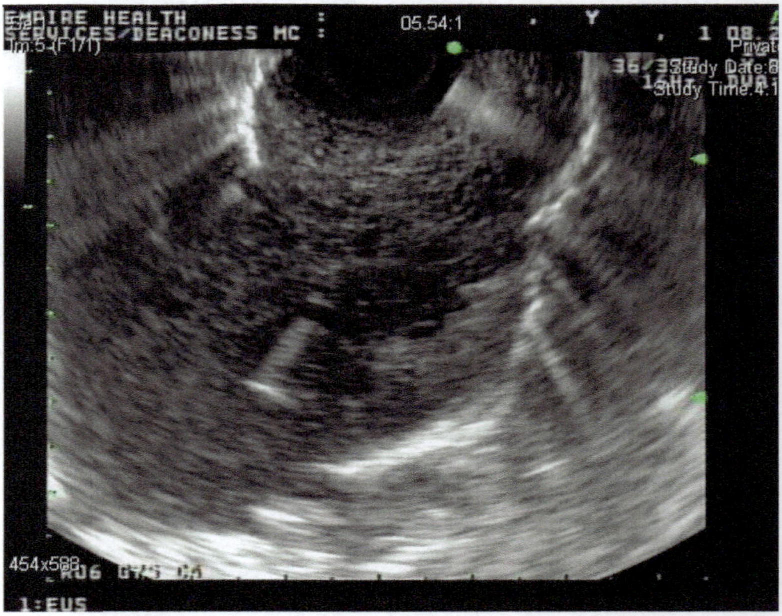

Fig. 1.37 Endoscopic ultrasound–guided fine-needle aspiration of this right lower lobe lung mass was easy and diagnostic. Note that the needle traverses the consolidated portion of the lung before it reaches the tumor mass

1.3.2.2 Thoracic Duct

In mammals, lymph vessels draining the abdominal viscera and lower half of the body converge just below the diaphragm to form the thoracic duct, a single major channel that ascends through the chest and enters the venous system on the left side of the neck. Although it is known that the lymphatic system collects plasma protein, absorbed lipid, and immunologically active cells and protein, the physiological advantage of transporting these substances from below the diaphragm through the chest to the neck is obscure [17]. Surgical ligature of the duct at any point in its course is harmless and is a means of controlling thoracic duct leaks, which can lead to chylothorax. The thoracic duct is readily identifiable on EUS [18]. It is larger than normal in patients with cirrhosis of the liver.

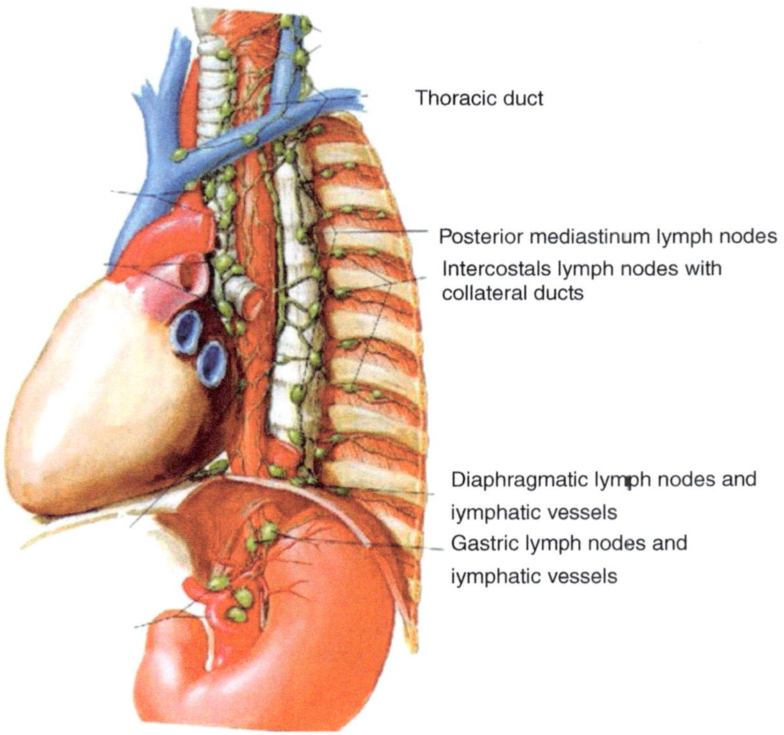

Fig. 1.38 Thoracic duct coursing between spine, esophagus, and aorta (From Casaccia et al. [19])

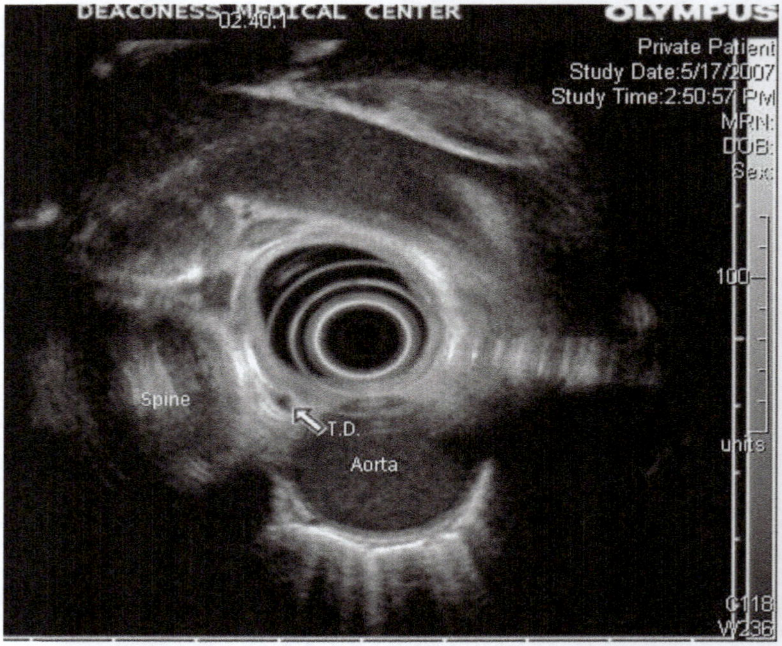

Fig. 1.39 The thoracic duct seen on endoscopic ultrasound. It is a small vessel measuring only a few millimeters in cross section and is anterior to the spine, relatively close to the aorta. In contrast, the azygos vein is much larger and located somewhat to the right from the center of the spine

1.3.2.3 Azygos Vein

The azygos vein is formed by the union of the ascending lumbar veins with the right subcostal veins at the level of the 12th thoracic vertebra, although it may be formed by a branch of the right renal vein or from the inferior vena cava (IVC). It ascends in the posterior mediastinum and arches over the root of the right lung to join the superior vena cava.

In the thorax the azygos lies on the right side of the aorta and thoracic duct and is partly covered by pleura. The azygos vein is easy to identify with radial EUS. In cirrhosis the azygos vein and thoracic duct are dilated, and in addition to esophageal or gastric varices, EUS often demonstrates thickening of the gastric mucosa and submucosa [20].

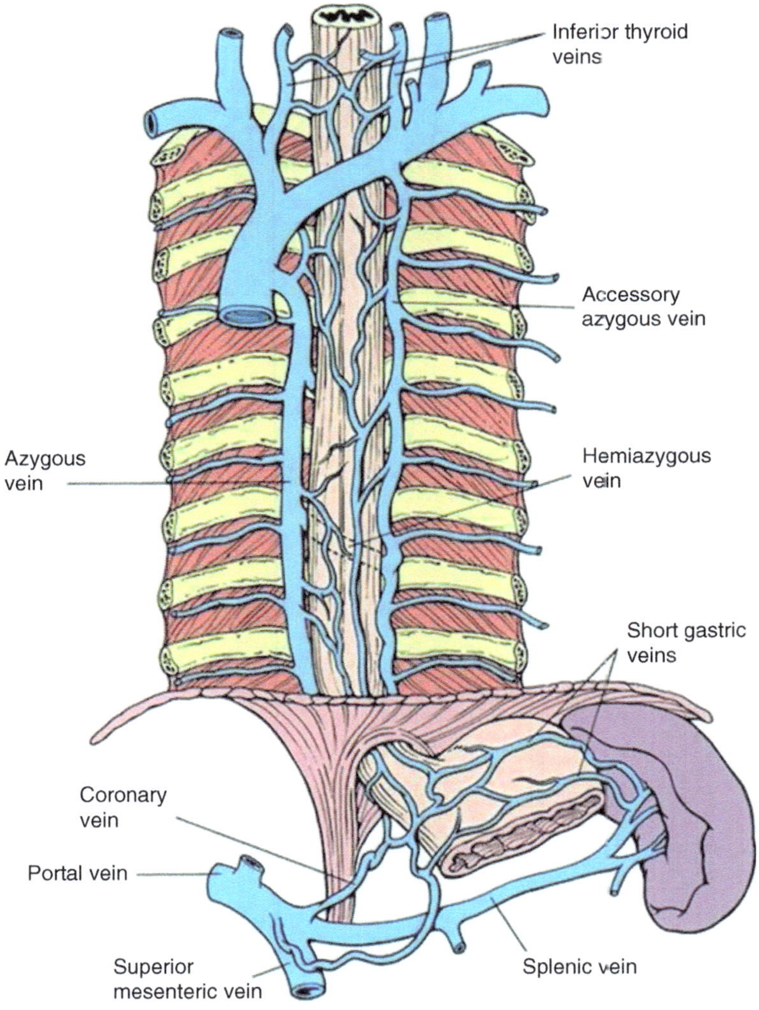

Fig. 1.40 Azygos and hemiazygos veins (From Staller and Braden Kuo [21])

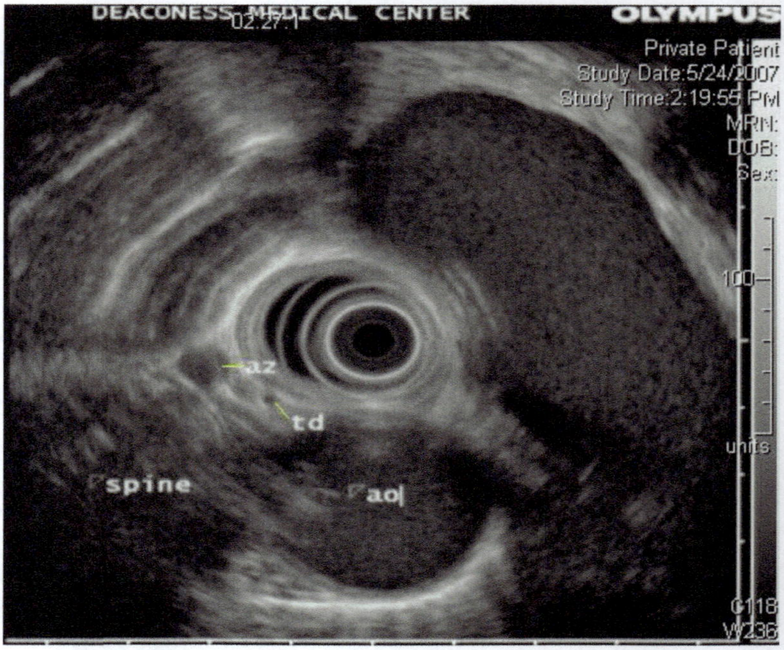

Fig. 1.41 This radial endoscopic ultrasound image shows the thoracic duct (*td*) and azygos vein (*av*). *ao* aorta

1.3.2.4 Mediastinal Lymph Nodes

In 2009 a new lung cancer lymph node map was proposed by the International Association for the Study of Lung Cancer to reconcile the differences between the Naruke and the MD-ATS maps and refine the definitions of the anatomic boundaries of each of the lymph node stations [22].

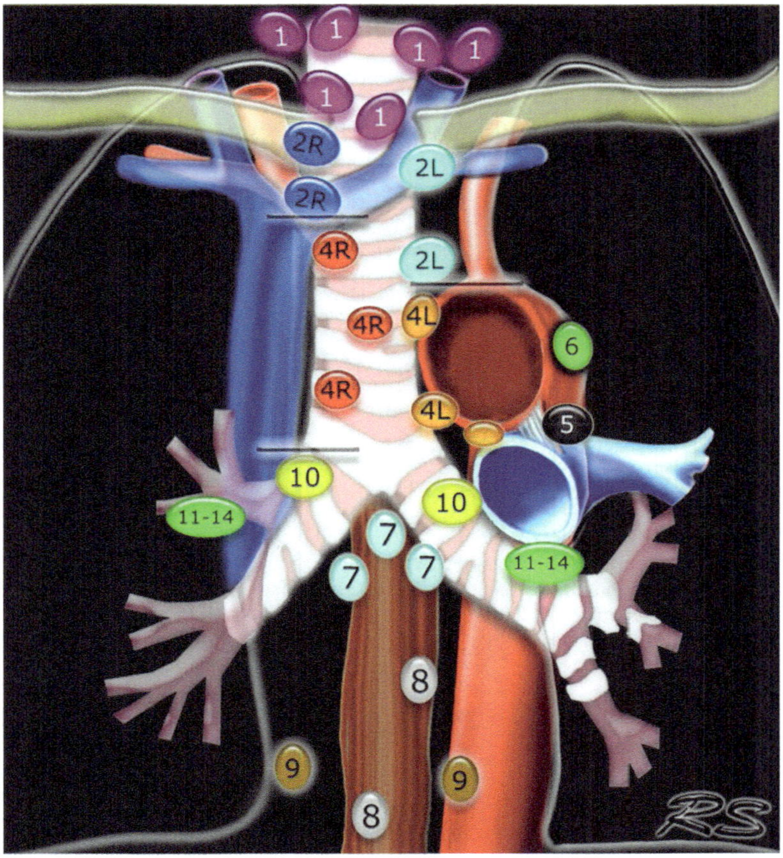

Fig. 1.42 This Mediastinal Lymph Node Map (IASLC 2009) is an excellent up-to date tool for mediastinal lymph node stations according to the International Association for the Study of Lung Cancer 2009 nomenclature. Available at: www.radiologyassistant.nl/en/p4646f1278c26f

1.3.3 Abdomen

Anatomic landmarks in the upper abdomen are reviewed in the respective organ-specific chapters. Here we review pelvic structures that are not normally the focus of the gastrointestinal endosonographer.

1.3.3.1 Prostate

Gastroenterologists or colorectal surgeons performing endorectal or transrectal ultrasound need to have a degree of familiarity with the zonal anatomy of the prostate and the likely appearance of prostate cancers on rectal ultrasound even if they cannot be expected to be experts in transrectal ultrasound of the prostate, which is used primarily to direct the biopsy needle to the desired anatomic locations to estimate the volume of the prostate and assist in sampling prostate tissue in a spatially systematic way. However, it is unreliable in differentiating normal prostate tissue from cancerous tissue [23].

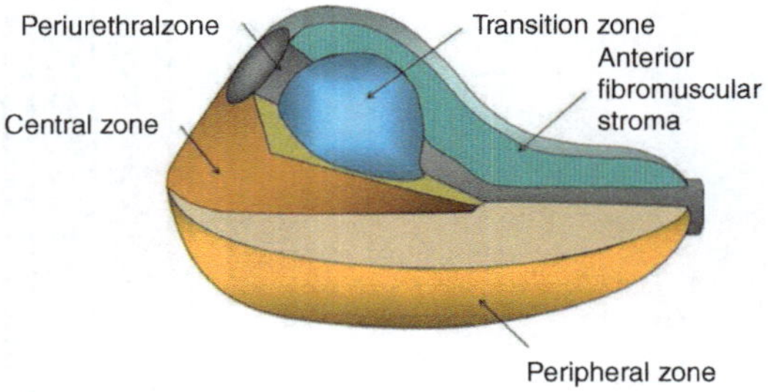

Fig. 1.43 Prostate zones. Anatomically, the gland is split into five zones: three glandular (the peripheral zone, the transition zone, and the central zone) and two nonglandular (the periurethral zone and the fibromuscular stroma) (From Kamoi and Babaian [25])

The prostate is organized in zones (Fig. 1.43). The peripheral zone forms the posteroinferior aspect of the gland and represents 70 % of the prostatic volume. It is the zone where the majority (60–70 %) of prostate cancers are found.

Most cancers of the prostate are either isoechoic or hypoechoic to the surrounding parenchyma in the outer portion of the gland. Those that are more hypoechoic or more easily visualized tend to have a higher Gleason grade [24]. Prostate cancer is frequently invisible on grayscale ultrasound; this is the rationale for sextant biopsies when prostate cancer is suspected for other reasons. The nonurologist doing transrectal ultrasound should, however, be concerned when a hypoechoic area in the peripheral zone is seen and must refer the patient appropriately.

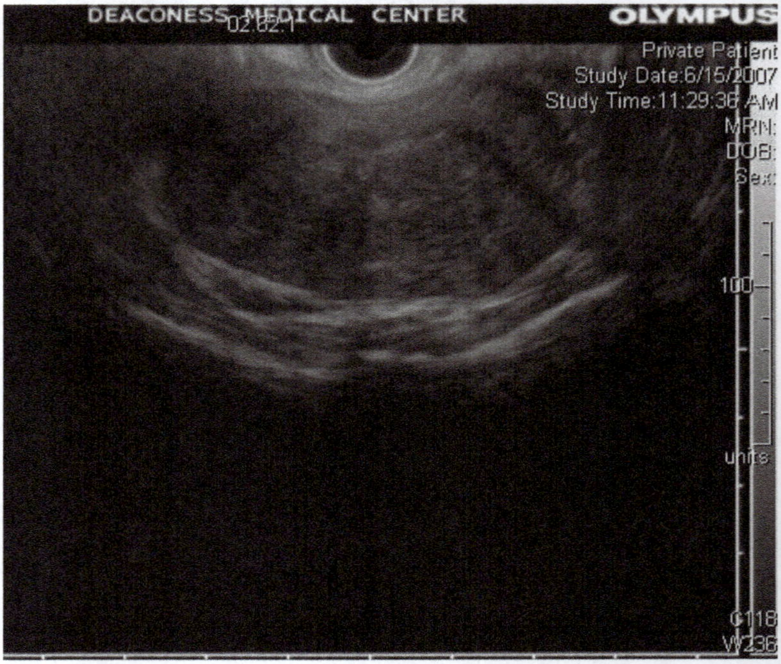

Fig. 1.44 A normal-appearing prostate imaged with a radial echoendoscope at 7.5 MHz. Most cancers of the prostate are either isoechoic or hypoechoic to the surrounding parenchyma in the outer portion of the gland

1.3.3.2 Seminal Vesicles

The seminal vesicles are useful as a landmark but are otherwise largely ignored by the endosonographer staging rectal cancers. Fortunately, malignant tumors of these glands are extremely rare. The seminal vesicles are lobulated structures, approximately 5–10 cm long and 2–5 cm wide. On transrectal ultrasound they look like handlebars. The seminal vesicles do not store sperm but produce a fructose-rich fluid. Their secretions contribute approximately 70 % of the ejaculate volume, prostatic secretions contribute 20 %, and fluid from the vas deferens containing sperm accounts for only 10 %. Andrologists use transrectal ultrasound to document ejaculatory duct obstruction. The imaging findings of pathology involving the seminal vesicles have been reviewed recently [26].

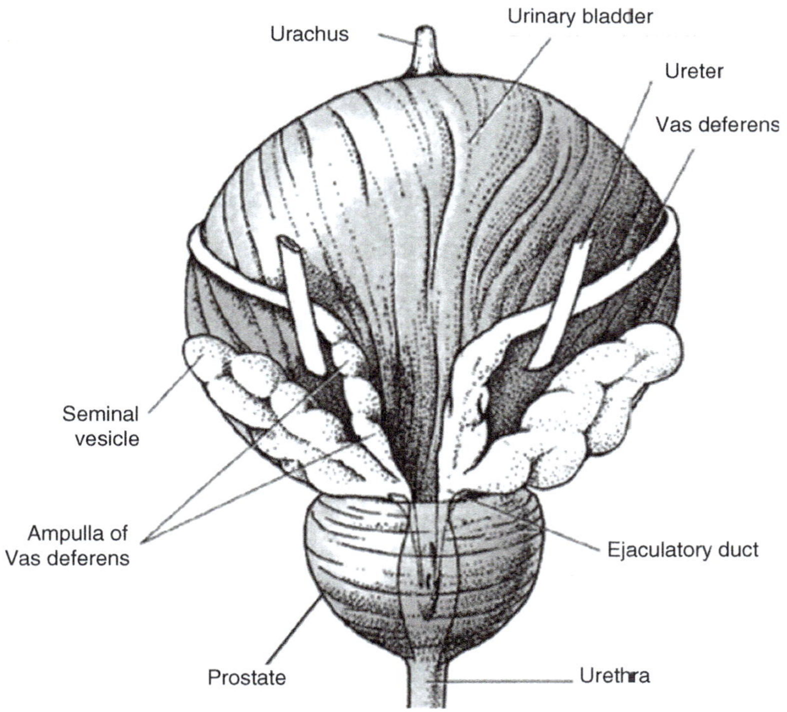

Fig. 1.45 The seminal vesicles in relation to prostate and bladder (From Wennemuth and Krause [27])

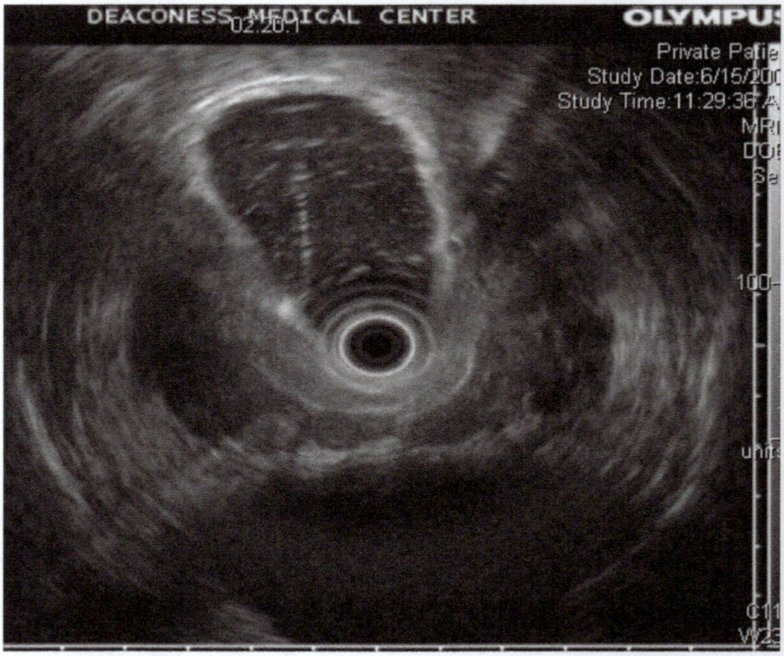

Fig. 1.46 The seminal vesicles have a typical handlebar appearance on transrectal ultrasound

1.3.3.3 Vagina

The vagina is an important landmark and is somewhat harder to recognize than the prostate. Trapped air in the vagina can give rise to reverberation artifacts.

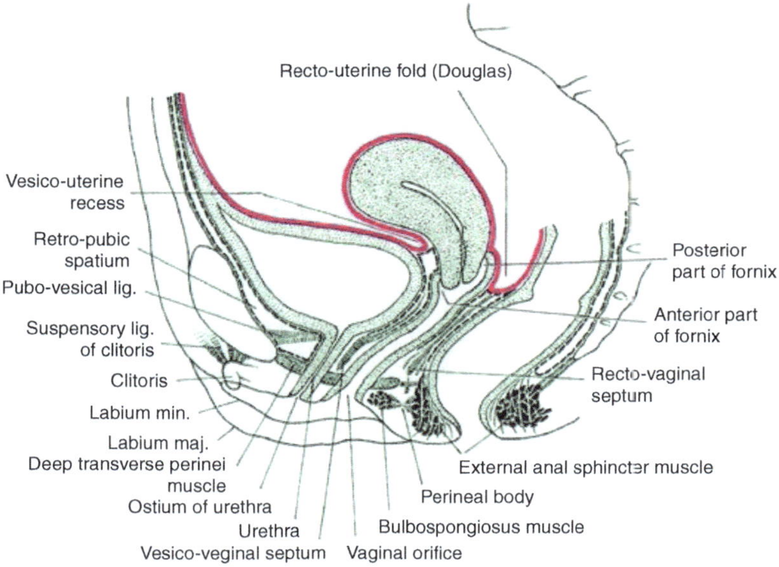

Fig. 1.47 Female pelvic anatomy (From Wennemuth and Krause [27])

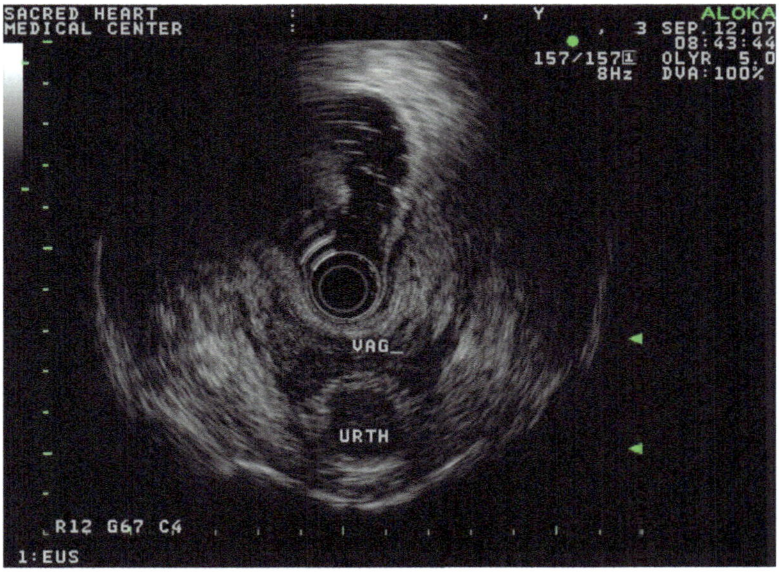

Fig. 1.48 This radial endoscopic ultrasound image shows a cross section of the urethra (*URTH*) and vagina (*VAG*)

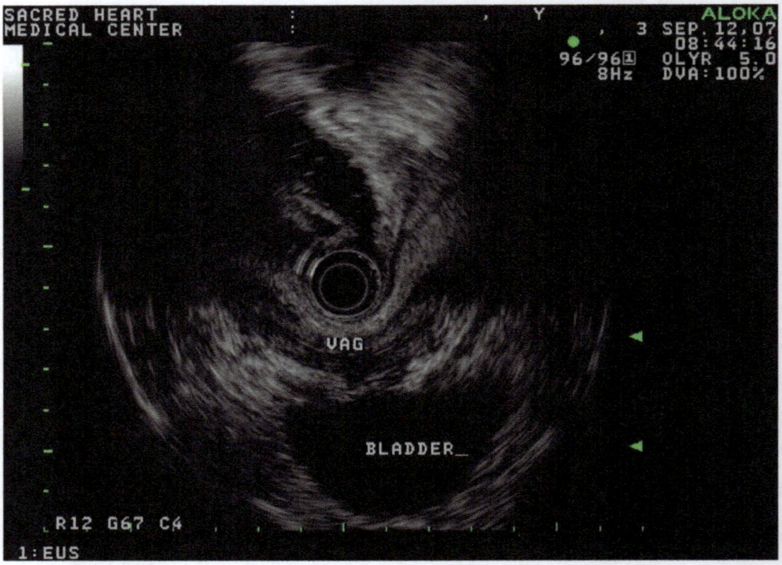

Fig. 1.49 Upon further advancement of the echoinstrument in the rectum the bladder comes into view. *VAG*, vagina

1.3.3.4 The Uterus

The uterus is normally ignored during rectal ultrasound exams performed for other reasons. However, occasionally the endosonographer will encounter a uterus that appears abnormal. During rectal ultrasound the patients are often not sedated, and a focused gynecological history can be obtained. If an abnormality is found and the patient is not currently under the care of a gynecologist, has not had a recent pelvic exam, or has symptoms, we refer the patient for pelvic and, if needed, transvaginal ultrasound.

The dimensions of the normal uterus vary with age and parity [28]. The normal myometrium is hypoechoic, homogeneous, and reasonably well demarcated from the endometrial echoes.

This is a 50-year-old woman referred for the evaluation of a submucosal nodule in the rectum, which turned out to be a gastrointestinal stromal tumor. The uterus appeared enlarged and deviated from the midline. A transvaginal ultrasound was ordered and showed normal adnexae and a mildly enlarged uterus with two 2-cm-diameter fibroids.

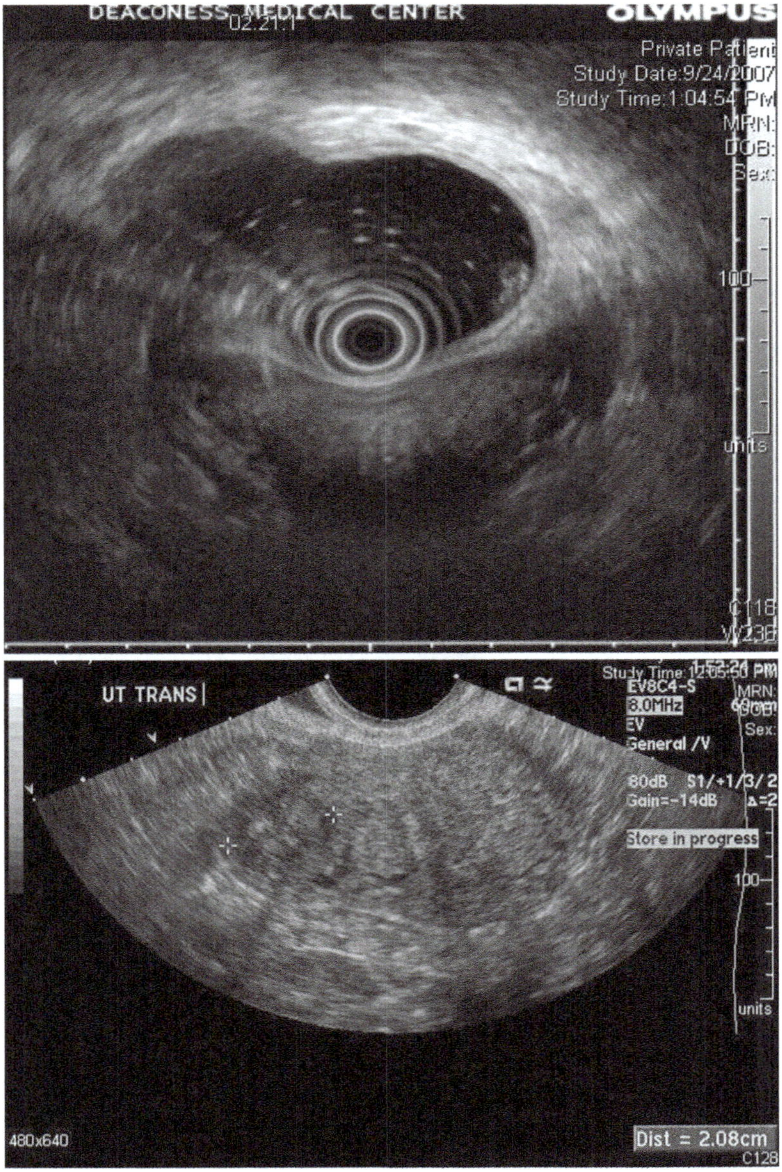

Fig. 1.50 These images were obtained transvaginally with a dedicated vaginal probe and an Acuson Sequoia 512 processor. In this image a fibroid can be seen between the *calipers* that was not recognized on the transrectal ultrasound

1.4 Doppler Endosonography

The 360° electronic radial echoendoscope allows the integration of Doppler examinations into the routine applications of radial endosonography, such as tumor staging, pancreatobiliary endosonography, and the evaluation of submucosal masses. Modern echoendoscopes provide high-resolution grayscale or color flow Doppler as well as power Doppler images at frequencies of 5, 6, 7.5, and 10 MHz. Tissue harmonic imaging helps reduce artifacts and improves resolution. This section aims to raise awareness about how routine exams can be enhanced with the Doppler capabilities of electronic radial echoendoscopes [29].

1.4.1 Mediastinum

1.4.1.1 Azygos Vein

In the thorax the azygos vein lies on the right side of the aorta and thoracic duct and is partly covered by pleura. Both structures are often enlarged to different degrees in portal hypertension, and sometimes it may be difficult to differentiate the two, especially when they are enlarged in portal hypertension [18, 20]. The azygos vein has a characteristic spectral Doppler signal.

Unfortunately, the radial echoinstrument shows the azygos vein in cross section, and a longitudinal orientation is a prerequisite for accurate measurements of azygos flow [30, 31]. Nonetheless, other authors have found that radial EUS with Doppler may enhance the evaluation of the hemodynamics of esophageal varices by showing the palisade veins and pulsatile waves more clearly [32].

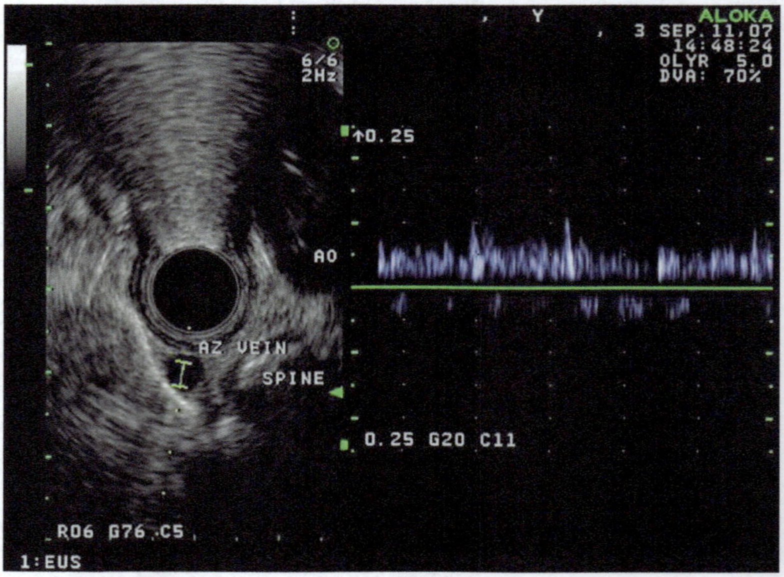

Fig. 1.51 Spectral Doppler signal in the azygos vein (*az*). *ao* aorta

1.4.1.2 Dorsal Intercostal Arteries

In our experience the dorsal intercostal arteries and some of their named branches can easily be demonstrated with radial Doppler ultrasound. These segmental arteries coming off the aorta supply blood to the anterior spinal artery via the anterior radiculomedullary arteries and often are compromised by atherosclerosis or thoracoabdominal aneurysms. A case report describes an anterior spinal cord infarction with permanent paralysis following endoscopic ultrasound celiac plexus neurolysis believed to be secondary to some solution passing via the left T12 intercostal artery, which supplies both the spinal cord via a radiculomedullary artery and the paraspinal muscles via dorsal branches [33].

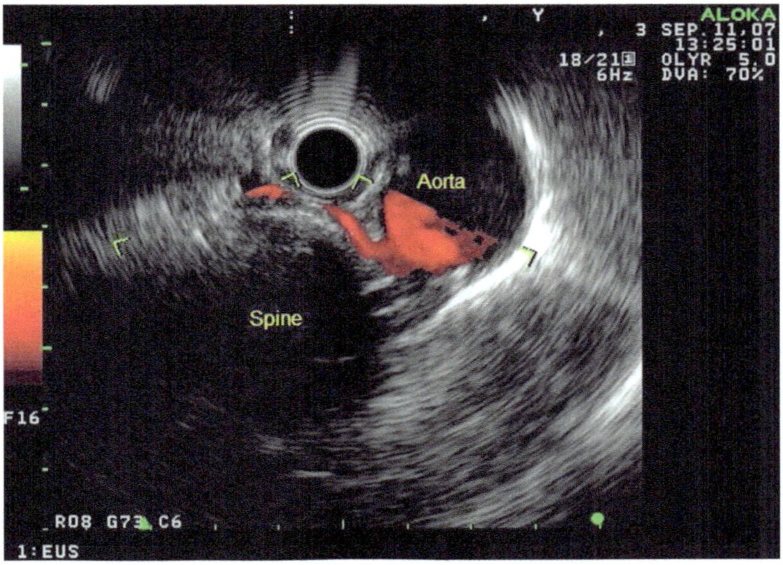

Fig. 1.52 Power Doppler image showing the dorsal intercostal arteries that give off branches to supply the spinal cord

1.4.2 Upper Abdomen

1.4.2.1 Hepatic Veins

The IVC and hepatic veins can easily be demonstrated with radial EUS. The inflow of the hepatic veins into the vena cava is an area of particular interest because it is eminently suited for evaluation by a radial Doppler-capable echoendoscope since the hepatic veins run a sagittal course and the instrument is close. Budd-Chiari syndrome (obstruction of the hepatic veins) is considered primary when obstruction of the hepatic venous outflow tract is the result of an endoluminal venous lesion (thrombosis or web) or secondary when the obstruction results from the presence in the lumen of tumor material or from extrinsic compression by a neighboring tumor [34, 35]. Despite the rarity of the syndrome it is surprising that there are, to our knowledge, no published reports of EUS evaluation of hepatic vein thrombosis.

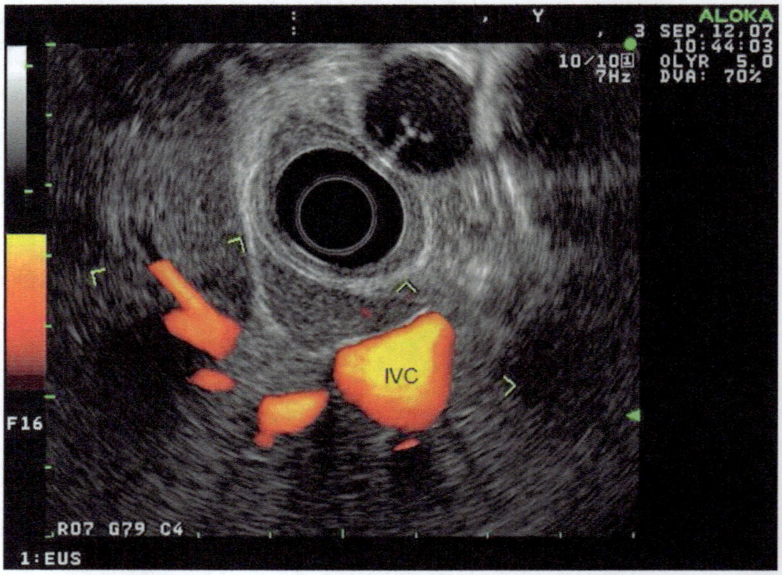

Fig. 1.53 Power Doppler image of the hepatic veins and the IVC as seen from the esophagogastric junction

1.4.2.2 Portal Vein

There are numerous articles in the general ultrasound literature dealing with portal vein hemodynamics in patients with and without liver disease, many of which come to different conclusions. For example, in a well-designed prospective study it was not possible to grade the severity of chronic liver disease by Doppler ultrasound [36], and a more recent systematic review concluded that published data on Doppler ultrasound in liver fibrosis are limited, show a lack of reproducibility, and have somewhat contradictory results [37]. Excellent pictorial reviews of portal hemodynamics are available [38, 39], and the EUS evaluation of the portal venous system also has recently been reviewed [40].

EUS can show features of portal hypertension such as dilatation of the azygos, splenic, and portal veins; increased diameter of the thoracic duct; thickening of gastric mucosa and submucosa; presence of portal hypertensive gastropathy, ascites, and rectal varices [41]; and, of course, portal vein thrombosis [42]. However, EUS does not play a major role in the monitoring of transjugular intrahepatic portosystemic shunt patency, especially since there is currently a shift to covered stents, which remain patent longer, and Doppler ultrasound is not highly accurate in predicting stent dysfunction [43]. EUS with Doppler is superb in demonstrating the presence of collateral circulation, but its precise role in the diagnosis and management of portal hypertension and esophageal varices awaits further definition [44].

Gastric varices may be difficult to differentiate from other causes of thickened gastric folds, and in these cases Doppler EUS is capable of providing a definitive answer. In addition, the patency of the splenic vein and portal vein, which is easily evaluated by EUS, should be evaluated in patients with gastric varices.

One of the main advantages of a Doppler-capable radial EUS instrument seems to be the anatomical, intuitive cross-sectional imaging of the portal vein and superior mesenteric vein to evaluate for clot or tumor invasion.

Typical ultrasound features of portal vein thrombosis are initially hypoechoic, possibly heterogeneous clots with dilatation of the affected vascular segment and decreasing amplitude of respiratory variations of the spectral Doppler signal. Clot detection by grayscale imaging can be difficult when the thrombus is hypoechoic. Color Doppler ultrasound confirms complete thrombosis by demonstrating the absence of flow or partial thrombosis by

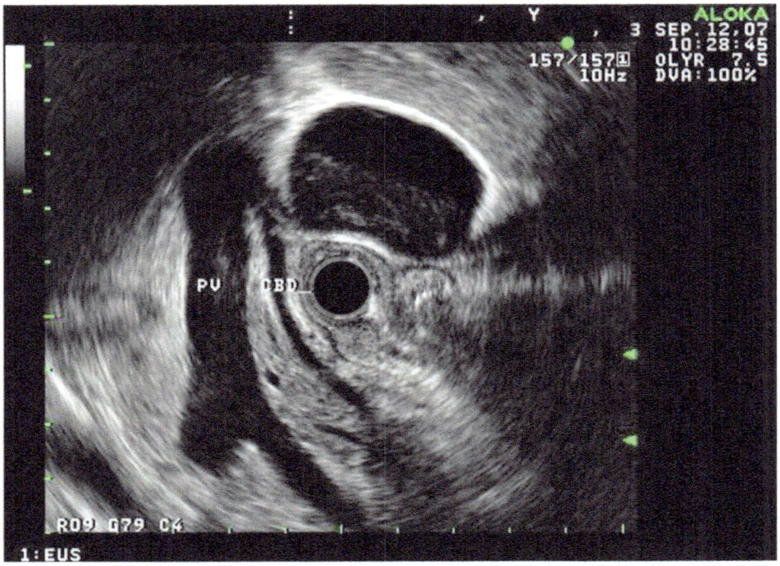

Fig. 1.54 This grayscale image shows (from *left* to *right*) the splenic vein, portal vein (*PV*), superior mesenteric vein, pancreatic duct, common bile duct (*CBD*), and gallbladder

circumferential flow. The portal vein also may be partially or completely recanalized. Cavernous transformation of the portal vein is characterized by partial recanalization and the development of periportal worm-like collaterals. A retrospective study has shown linear EUS to be a modality that can accurately detect portal venous system thrombosis [42], and this should apply to the Doppler-capable radial instruments to the same or a higher degree.

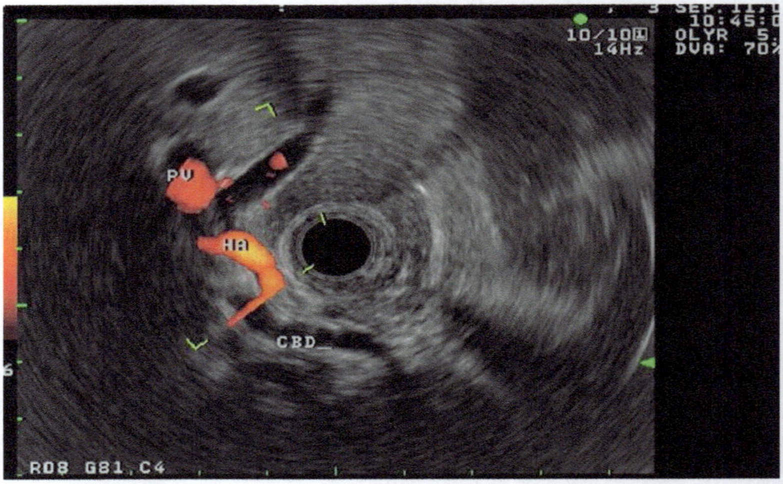

Fig. 1.55 Power Doppler image of the right and left branches of the portal vein (*PV*) and the right hepatic artery (*HA*) crossing the common bile duct (*CBD*)

1.4.2.3 Splenic Vein and Splenic Artery

Splenic vein thrombosis is generally associated with pancreatic pathology; therefore, radial EUS with Doppler may be an ideal diagnostic method to evaluate the splenic vasculature and the pancreatic parenchyma at the same time. In addition, EUS can evaluate the presence of esophageal and gastric varices [45, 46]. Chronic passive congestion due to a long-standing increase in pressure in the splenoportal venous system is a common cause of splenomegaly. Splenic blood flow rate increases because of splenomegaly and in turn causes an increase in the diameter of the splenic vein. However, the relationship between stage of cirrhosis and diameter of the splenic vein is complex and depends on the establishment of collaterals. For example, in one study using transabdominal Doppler ultrasound the splenic vein size was largest in the child A group and appeared to *decrease* in the child B and C groups [47].

Interventional radiologists increasingly perform splenic arterial embolization or endograft procedures to treat various conditions such as abdominal trauma, hypersplenism, splenic arterial aneurysm, portal hypertension, splenic arterial steal syndrome, and splenic neoplasm. These interventions may provide an alternative to open surgery, help preserve splenic function in patients with posttraumatic injuries or hypersplenism, and improve hematologic parameters in patients who otherwise would be unable to undergo high-dose chemotherapy or immunosuppressive therapy [48]. Splenic artery aneurysms can readily be demonstrated by EUS [49], but there are also interesting reports of splenic artery pseudoaneurysms secondary to pancreatitis that were successfully treated by EUS-guided interventions [50, 51].

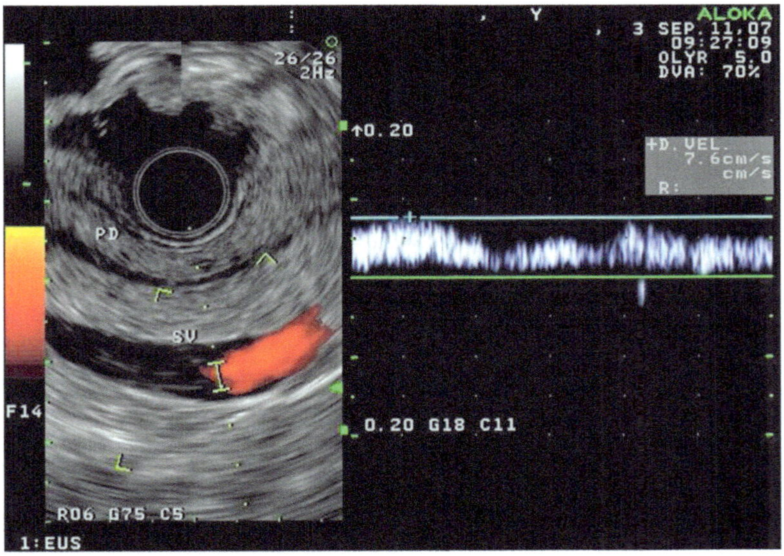

Fig. 1.56 Power Doppler image of the splenic vein on the *left* with corresponding spectral signature on the *right*. In greyscale, main pancreatic duct surrounded by parenchyma

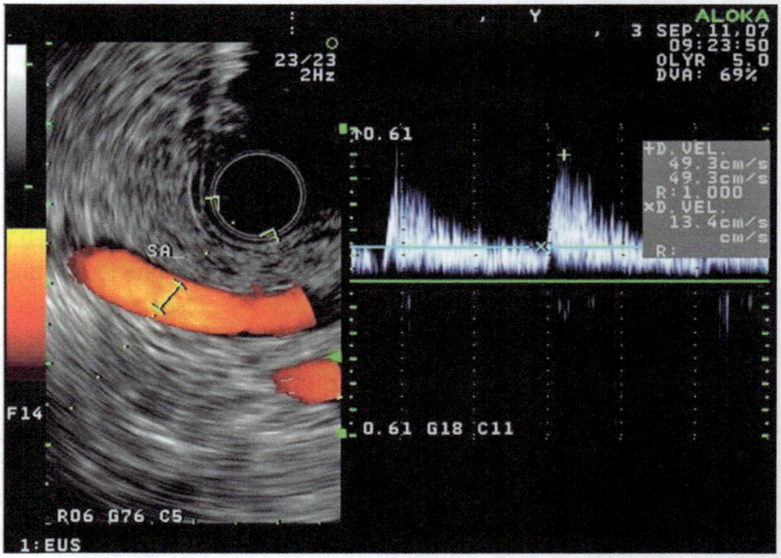

Fig. 1.57 This spectral Doppler signal (*right*) is typical for the splenic artery (*SA*) and shows a marked degree of spectral broadening (widened bandwidth of the returning signal) secondary to the tortuosity of the vessel

1.4.2.4 Celiac Vessels and the Superior Mesenteric Artery

For the endosonographer the celiac artery is a convenient landmark for celiac plexus blocks or neurolysis. Lymph nodes in this region play an important role in the locoregional staging of gastrointestinal tract and lung cancers. Beyond that the vessel has not attracted much attention in the EUS literature, which is surprising. In contrast to portal vein hemodynamics, there are relatively well-established criteria in the general ultrasound literature regarding the evaluation of stenosis of the celiac or superior mesenteric artery (SMA). A peak systolic velocity of >275 cm/s in the SMA identifies a >70 % SMA stenosis, with a sensitivity of 92 %, a positive predictive value of 80 %, and a negative predictive value of 99 %. Criteria for celiac artery stenosis are more complex, but retrograde common hepatic artery flow direction is virtually 100 % predictive of severe celiac artery stenosis or occlusion. An end-diastolic velocity of 55 cm/s or greater or no flow signal in the artery and/or a peak systolic velocity of 200 cm/s are also highly accurate [52]. Many elderly patients with abdominal pain who undergo EUS examination of the upper gastrointestinal tract for a variety of reasons might profit from an assessment of the mesenteric vasculature. Significant variations in celiac artery anatomy can be expected in approximately 10–15 % of cases [53, 54]; minor variations are much more common. In fact, the exact textbook picture occurs only infrequently [55]. This may be relevant when trying to locate the celiac ganglia.

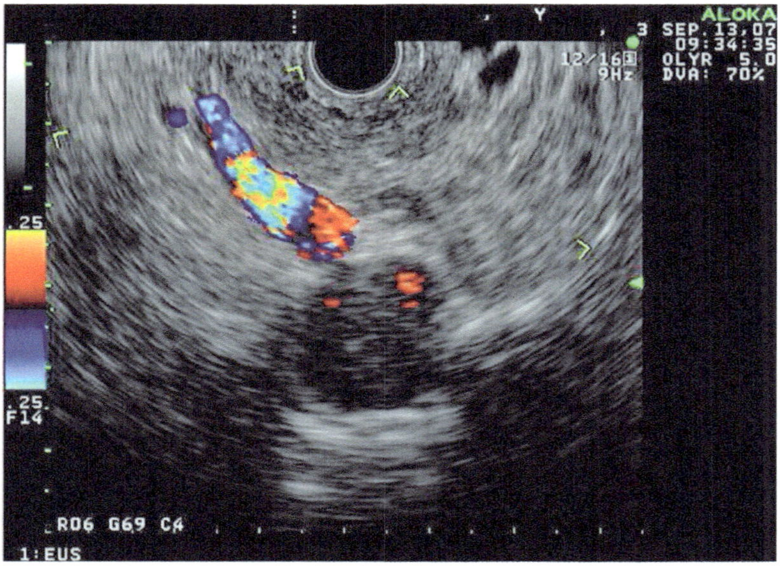

Fig. 1.58 Flow at the celiac trunk origin is often turbulent, as this color flow Doppler image shows. Flow measurements should be done more distally

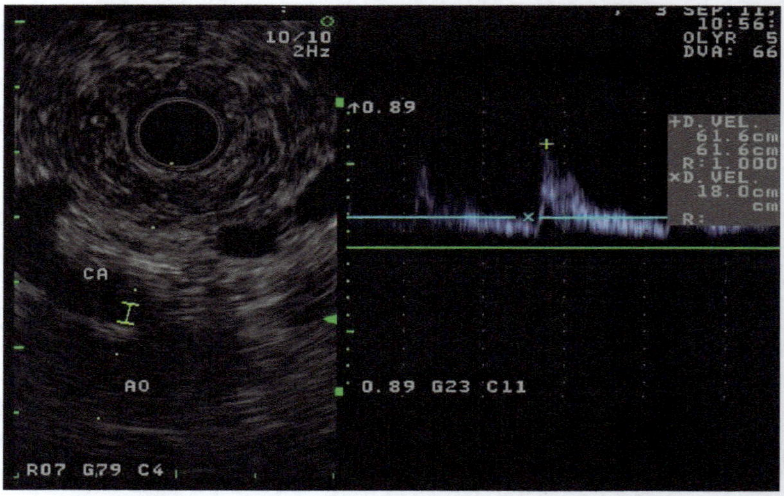

Fig. 1.59 Spectral Doppler of the celiac artery (*CA*). There is some spectral broadening (*right panel*), which is normal. Peak flows are within normal limits. *ao* aorta

1.4.2.5 Celiac Artery Variants

We have encountered a celiac trunk agenesis, an extremely rare anomaly, and a hepato-spleno-mesenteric trunk since we have started using a Doppler-capable radial echoendoscope. These anomalies could complicate identification of the area of celiac ganglion.

Absence of the Celiac Trunk

EUS of this 60-year-old patient, seen for a probably unrelated problem (pancreatitis of unknown etiology), was found to have no celiac trunk but several vessels taking off directly from the aorta. A careful analysis of the other available imaging confirmed that the left gastric artery, splenic artery, common hepatic artery, and SMA are all directly coming off the aorta. This variant is so rare that the Michels classification of celiac trunk abnormalities does not even mention it [56]. According to the Morita classification of 1935, our patient has a type 5 (typus primitivus) abnormality [57] because it resembles the embryonic situation where four primitive splanchnic branches arise from the abdominal aorta.

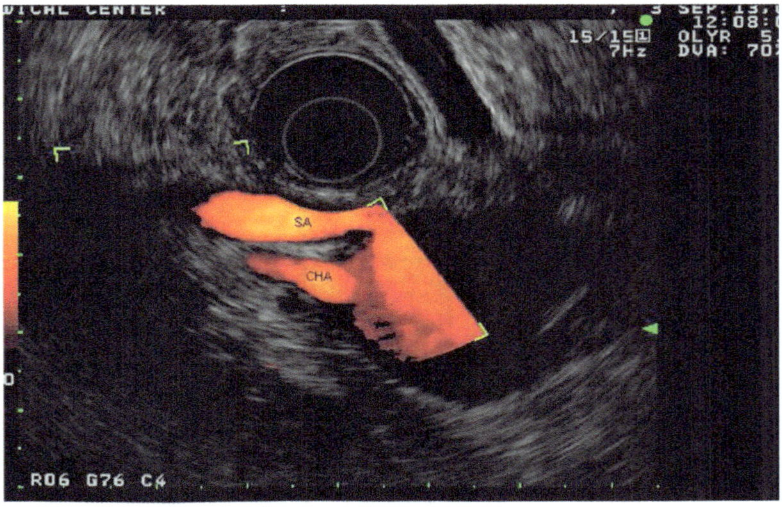

Fig. 1.60 This image shows the use of power Doppler with the GF-UE160. The vessels are the common hepatic artery (*CHA*) and the splenic artery (*SA*). A celiac trunk is not present

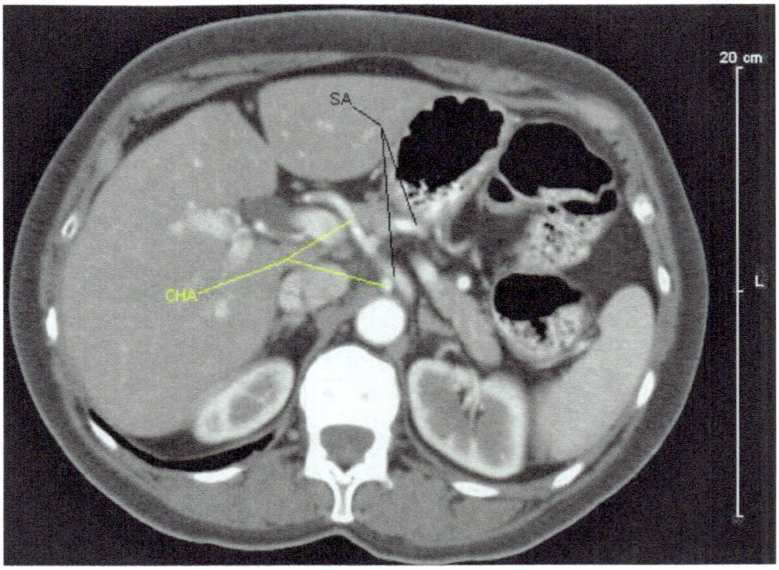

Fig. 1.61 On this cut the splenic artery (*SA*) and the common hepatic artery (*CHA*) occupy the same plane over a short stretch – the labels should help clarify the situation. Compare with the Doppler study in Fig. 1.60

Hepato-Spleno-Mesenteric Trunk

This is a 71-year-old patient who underwent a successful Whipple pancreatoduodenectomy. The surgeon noted a right hepatic artery crossing anterior to the bile duct presumably originating from the SMA. Six months after the surgery he was referred to us for an EUS-guided celiac plexus neurolysis with alcohol. EUS images showed what appeared to be a hypoplastic celiac artery and a prominent SMA. After anesthetizing the area with 3 cm^3 of 0.25 % bupivicaine, 10 cm^3 of absolute alcohol were injected above the presumed celiac artery take-off, as is customary. There was transient pain upon injection, and several days after the procedure the patient says that his abdominal pain decreased below baseline.

Reanalysis of prior CT and MRI scans revealed that the patient actually has a small left gastric artery taking off directly from his aorta while the hepatic artery and splenic artery are joined with the SMA to form a "hepatospleno-mesenteric trunk" [58].

This vessel anomaly is rare and accounted for less than 1 % of celiac trunk abnormalities in a large autopsy series. It may be underecognized on imaging. For example, this patient had two prior CT scans and one MRI and the abnormality was not commented upon. Still, injection at the level slightly above the left gastric artery seems to make the most sense in achieving an effective celiac block.

This case also highlights how reevaluating interesting cases with existing or new imaging asking slightly different questions is beneficial. Diagnosis is often not a linear but an iterative process. Premature closure (see Sect. 1.1) needs to be avoided.

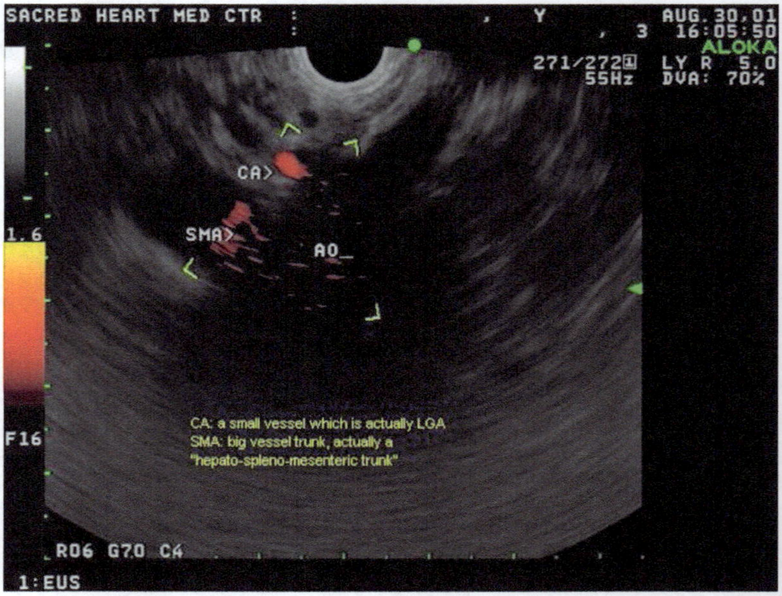

Fig. 1.62 This image shows two wrong labels: the patient actually had no celiac artery (*CA*) and no superior mesenteric artery (*SMA*) but a hepato-spleno-mesenteric trunk. *AO* aorta

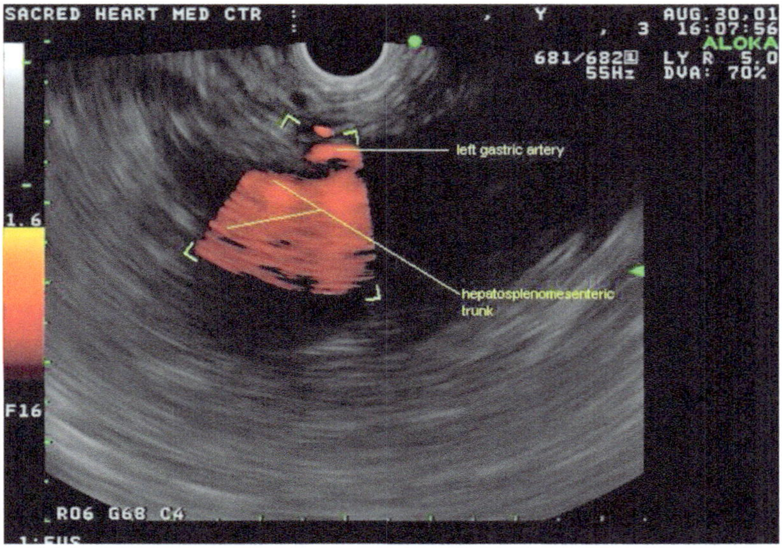

Fig. 1.63 What was labeled incorrectly as the celiac artery in Fig. 1.62 is actually a left gastric artery arising directly from the aorta. The large vessel trunk combines the hepatic, splenic, and superior mesenteric arteries

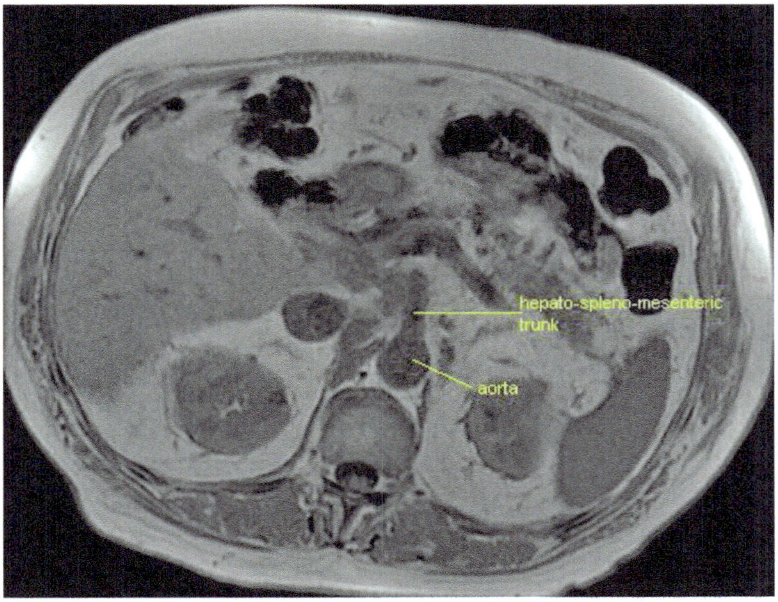

Fig. 1.64 This magnetic resonance image shows the big hepato-spleno-mesenteric trunk

1.4.2.6 Celiac Ganglia

While obviously not a vascular structure, celiac ganglia are best discussed in this context. Celiac ganglia have been seen by endosonographers for a long time but were frequently misinterpreted as small celiac lymph nodes. The distinguishing features have been described only more recently. In brief, the ganglia are hypoechoic oblong or comma-shaped structures with an irregular edge, often containing a hyperechoic focus. They are typically seen to the left of the celiac trunk and aorta, between the celiac artery and the left adrenal. They often extended inferiorly in a chain, with hypoechoic thread-like strands connecting them [59].

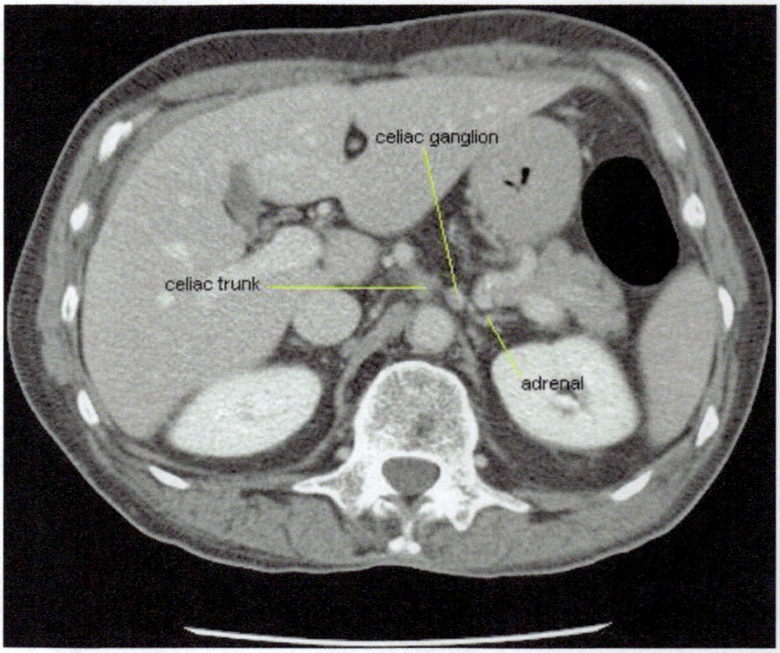

Fig. 1.65 This patient has a prominent round-appearing celiac ganglion on computed tomography

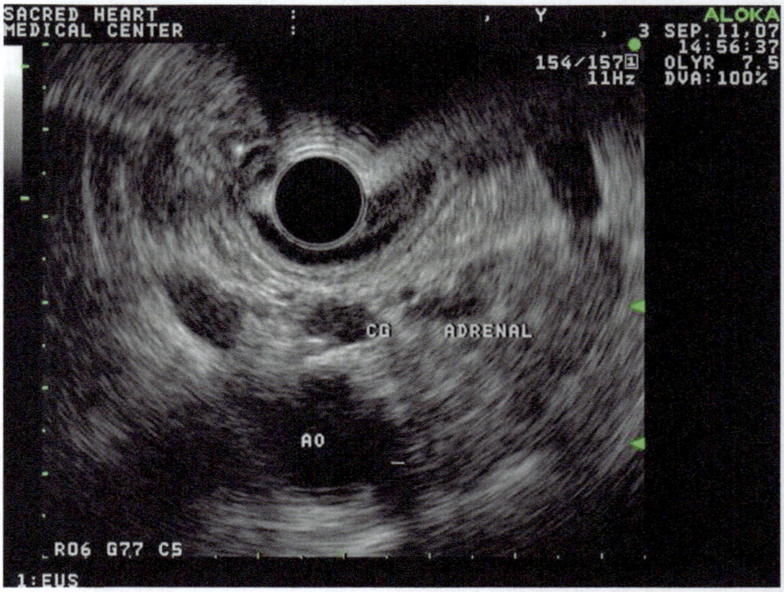

Fig. 1.66 Endoscopic ultrasound appearance of the celiac ganglion (*CG*) in the same patient as in Fig. 1.65. *ao* aorta

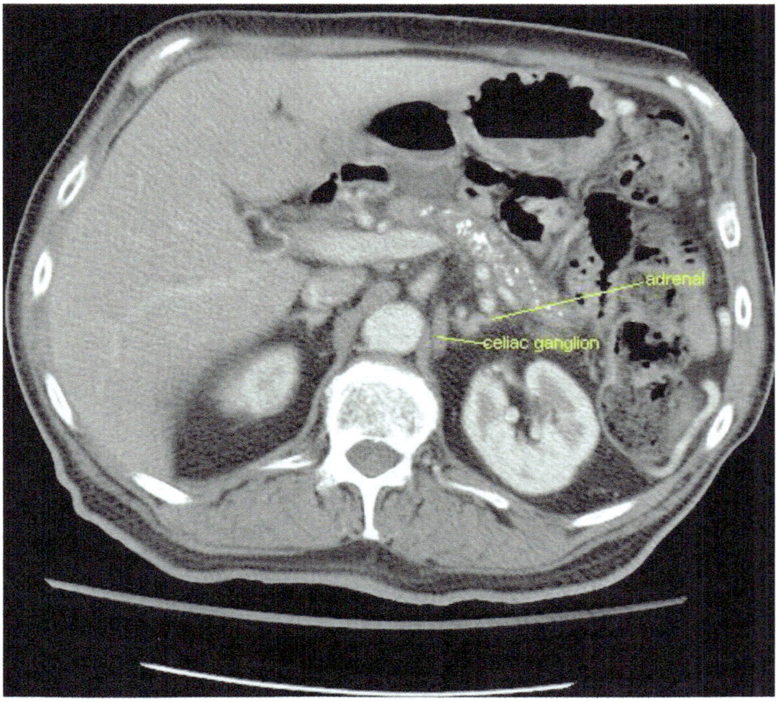

Fig. 1.67 This computed tomography scan shows a prominent disk-like left celiac ganglion

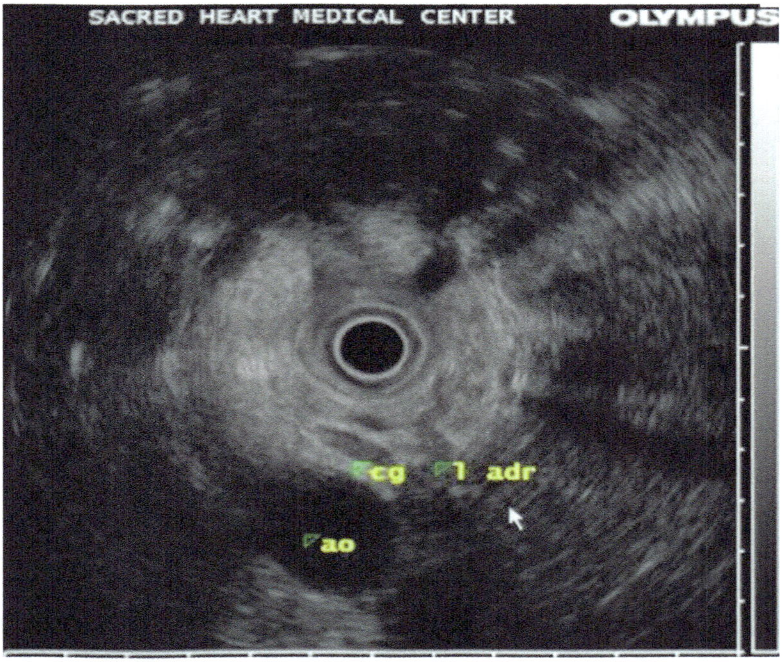

Fig. 1.68 This radial endoscopic ultrasound (GF-UM160) image with the mechanical transducer shows the celiac ganglion (*CG*) seen in computed tomography. *ao* aorta

1.4.3 Pelvis

The results of endoscopic Doppler examinations of rectal varices have been published [60]. What role, if any, hemodynamic measurements play in the treatment of rectal varices, however, remains unclear. Staging of rectal cancer with EUS is typically performed with radial echoinstruments. The evaluation of lateral pelvic lymph node involvement is important and necessary for a preoperative diagnosis and the determination of a treatment strategy. Although the iliac vessels can be seen without Doppler, the availability of the latter makes the differentiation between vein and artery much easier and should help in the identification of suspicious lateral lymph nodes, which may need to be biopsied.

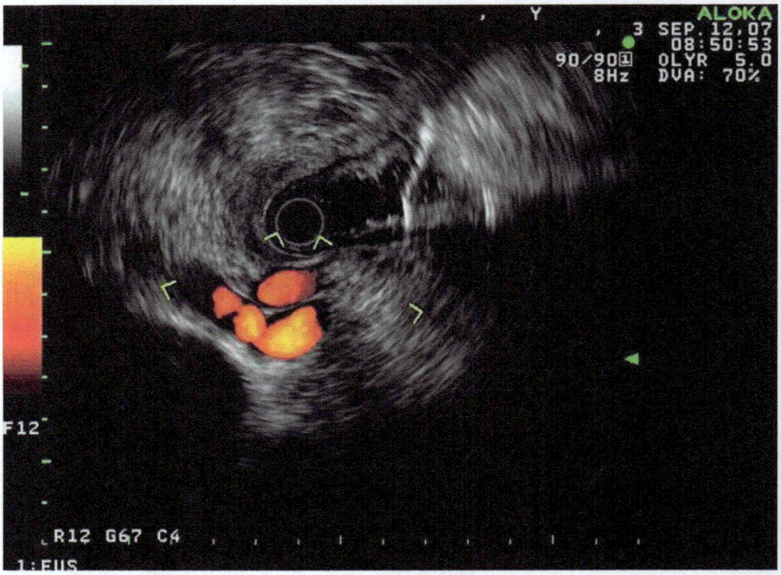

Fig. 1.69 Power Doppler image of the internal iliac artery and vein

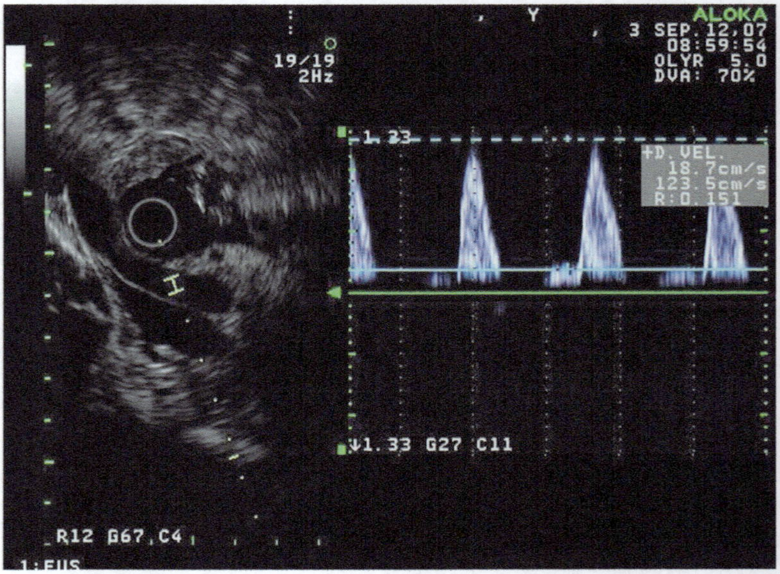

Fig. 1.70 Spectral Doppler (*right*) identifies the internal iliac artery (*left*)

1.5 Medical Image Retrieval and Decision Support Systems

Biomedical literature that is available online contains a rich source of visual information that could be used to answer ad hoc clinical questions or prepare presentations and articles. As a general purpose image search engine, Google Images is unsurpassed. However, the organization of the results is not optimized for clinical or academic purposes. There are specialized platforms for biomedical image searches that try to address these shortcomings, and most of them are not well known. Here we introduce a few of them.

To compare search engines we used a standard query term of *gastrointestinal stromal tumor EUS* as a benchmark. We evaluated the search engines subjectively and share our observations here. Ultimately readers should try them all and see which works best for their purposes. Most of these searches will return few EUS-specific images. There are several potential reasons for this: (1) Leading gastrointestinal endoscopy journals are closed access and images cannot be crawled by web spiders or indexed by search engines; they become part of the hidden web. (2) The number of EUS images in the surface web is drowned out by other cross-sectional images. (3) Some search platforms restrict their indexing to radiology journals. Nevertheless, these resources are of considerable value to the endosonographer who, once past the stage of novice, mostly has questions about other cross-sectional imaging studies rather than about EUS, and here these retrieval platforms can be quite helpful.

1.5.1 General Image Retrieval Platforms

1.5.1.1 ITSE/iMedline (archive.nlm.nih.gov/iti)

iMedline® is a multimodal search engine under development at the National Library of Medicine. It aims to retrieve images from the biomedical literature relevant to text and image queries and link evidence automatically extracted from clinical articles to patients' cases [61]. It is not limited to radiological images. Along with the traditional elements of search results display, such as titles and author names, iMedline provides captions of the retrieved images and short summaries of the retrieved abstracts. In early 2013 this project had only a prototype search engine. It was previously known as ITSE (Image and Text Search Engine). The combination of image and text retrieval is helpful for quick orientation. The current interface is clean and easy to navigate. However, the benchmark query entry resulted in the following response: "The term, gastrointestinal stromal tumor eus, must be relaxed or trimmed to find documents." After doing this the gastrointestinal stromal tumor retrieval results were visually appealing and helpful. With further development, iMedline should become one of the best biomedical image retrieval systems. The project may be incorporated into the general PubMed search when it is more mature.

1.5.1.2 PubMed Central (www.ncbi.nlm.nih.gov/pmc)

PubMed Central® (PMC) is a free archive of biomedical and life sciences journal literature that is open access at the U.S. National Institutes of Health's National Library of Medicine. In July 2011 PMC started to automatically search all image captions in the archive and retrieve images related to the topic of the search. It is not a specialized image search platform, and we like iMedline better. Our benchmark search returned ten images.

1.5.1.3 BioText (biosearch.berkeley.edu/)

The BioText literature search engine is a web-based application developed at Berkeley that allows biologists to search the contents of open access journals and see figures from the articles displayed directly in the search results [62]. It performed comparably to iMedline. In contrast to iMedline it accepted the full search query (no truncation required) but then returned only two results. The search engine was launched in 2007 and there apparently have been no significant updates since.

1.5.1.4 FigureSearch (figuresearch.askhermes.org)

FigureSearch, developed at the University of Wisconsin at Milwaukee, is part of the askHermes system. The platform retrieves images together with their respective captions. The benchmark search returned 16 highly relevant hits.

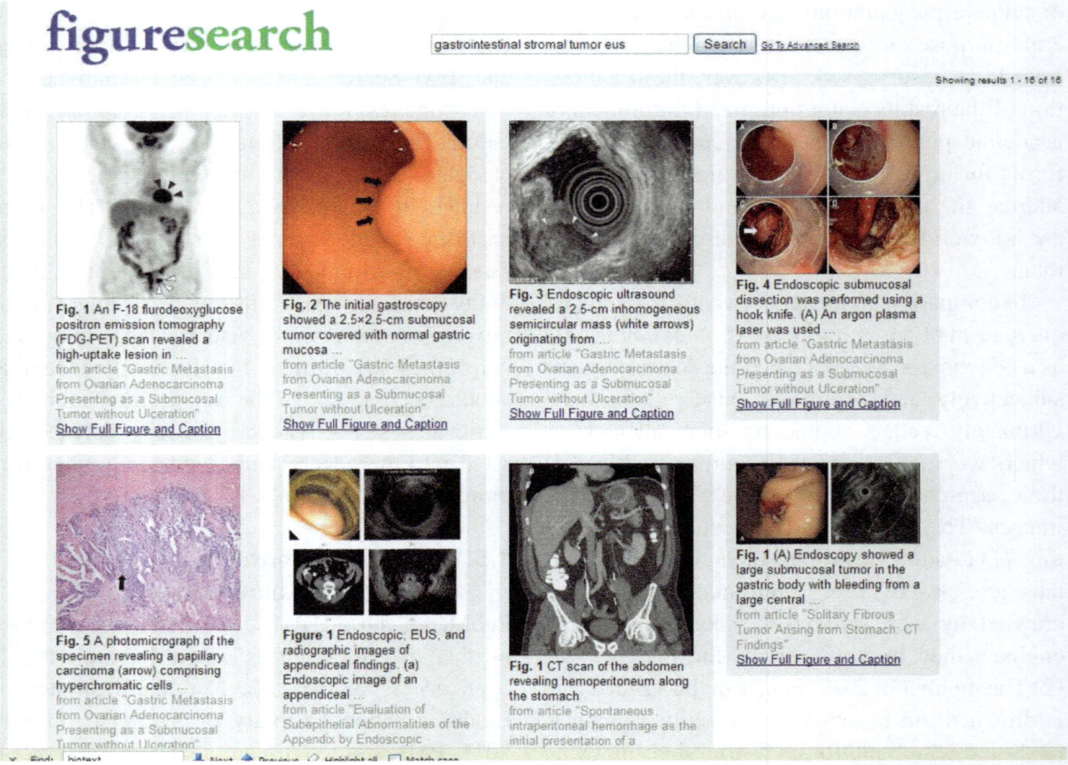

Fig. 1.71 Performing the search *gastrointestinal stromal tumor EUS* on FigureSearch returned 16 highly relevant hits

1.5.1.5 Yale Image Finder (krauthammerlab.med.yale.edu/imagefinder/)

A user provides a few search keywords and the most relevant images are returned and presented in the form of thumbnails. The visual presentation is similar to FigureSearch. Users can click on the image of interest to retrieve the high-resolution image. In addition, the search engine provides two types of related images: those that appear in the same article and those from other articles with similar image content. Retrieved images link back to their source articles, allowing users to find related articles starting with an image of interest [63]. The Yale Image Finder returned the most images in the benchmark search (199 images). However, compared to FigureSearch (which returned 16 images), many of them were not relevant.

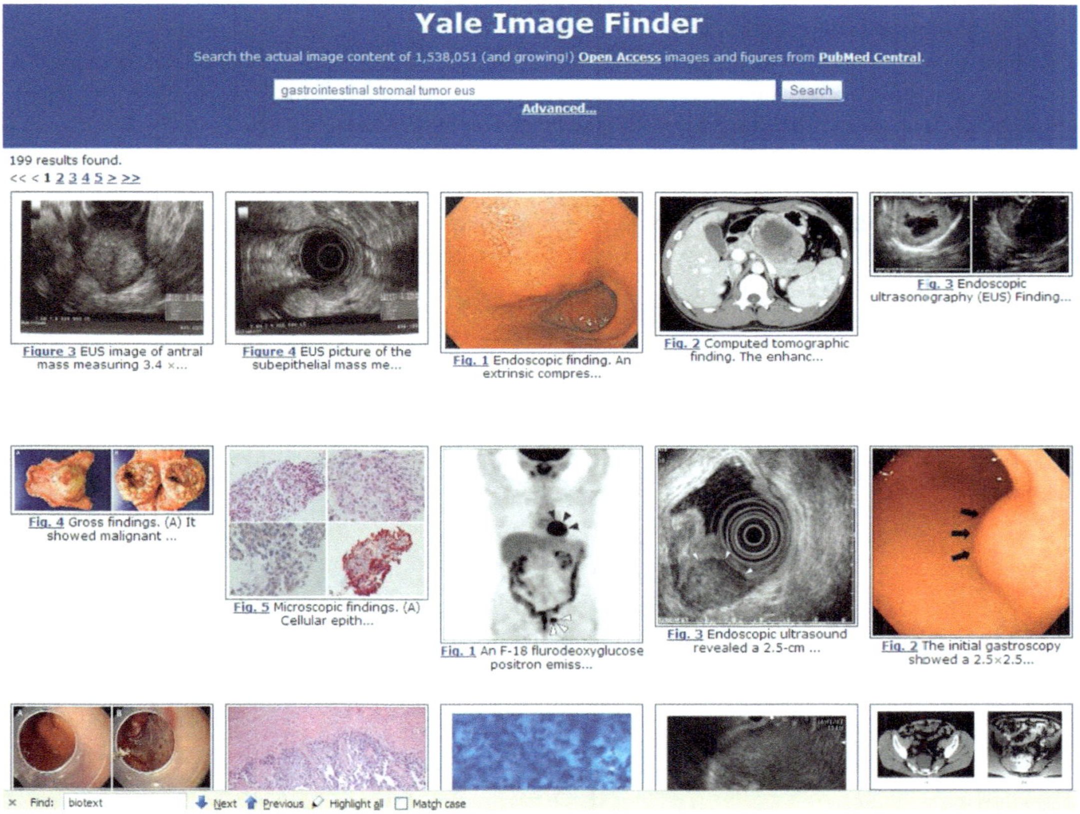

Fig. 1.72 Performing the search *gastrointestinal stromal tumor EUS* on the Yale Image Finder returned 199 hits

1.5.2 Radiology Centric Image Retrieval

1.5.2.1 ARR GoldMiner® (goldminer.arrs.org/)

The GoldMiner® is a product of the American Roentgen Ray Society. It works best for images that would be published in a radiology-specific journal since it mines peer-reviewed journal articles from the websites of the American Roentgen Ray Society, the American Society of Neuroradiology, the British Institute of Radiology, and the Radiological Society of North America. Our benchmark search returned no images. This is not to say that this site may not be helpful for EUS-related questions about other imaging modalities.

1.5.2.2 Yottalook™

In contrast to GoldMiner, Yottalook™ looks at the relevance of results to radiology and is not limited to specific journals. It has perhaps the most advanced search algorithm of all radiologic retrieval platforms discussed (for details see Ghosh et al. [61]). Results (168,000 for our benchmark search) can be further refined by area of main interest: all, X-ray, CT, MRI, ultrasound, nuclear medicine, anatomy, teaching files, journals, and .edu. A drawback is that image thumbnails are not offered on the main search page. Performing the benchmark search on the image search page showed results of questionable relevance.

In summary, biomedical image search is a rapidly developing field and at present there are several helpful platforms. Unfortunately, most have some major shortcomings. Readers should experiment with all of them and decide which are worth bookmarking. We find ourselves switching between Google Images, Yale Image Finder, and Yottalook.

1.6 Textbooks and Journals

A significant portion of training and continuing education relies on the use of journals and textbooks. EUS-related publications are predominantly found in the American journal *Gastrointestinal Endoscopy* and in the European journal *Endoscopy*. At the time of this writing both periodicals require an individual or institutional subscription. A new open access journal focused on endosonography, titled *Endoscopic Ultrasound* (www.eusjournal.com), was launched in 2012. The new publication boasts an impressive board of editors and it is hoped that it will prove a valuable addition to the publishing landscape.

There are currently a number of excellent EUS textbooks available (see Box 1.1). We feel that is difficult to recommend one over another. Given the high price of the textbooks it may be worthwhile to borrow those that are not locally available through the interlibrary loan system before making a purchase decision. Some of the books allow the purchase of individual chapters as a download.

Authors [Reference]	Title	Pages	Published	Ebook
Gress and Savides [64]	*Endoscopic Ultrasonography*, 2nd edition	216	2009	Individual chapters available http://onlinelibrary.wiley.com/book/10.1002/9781444308099
Shami and Kahaleh [65]	*Endoscopic Ultrasound*	552	2010	Individual chapters available http://link.springer.com/book/10.1007/978-1-60327-480-7/page/1
Dietrich and Allgayer [66]	*Endoscopic Ultrasound: An Introductory Manual and Atlas*, 2nd edition	554	2011	Available as an eBook but not individual chapters http://ebookstore.thieme.com/product/endoscopic-ultrasound
Hawes et al. [67]	*Endosonography*, 2nd edition	312	2011	Available as an eBook but not individual chapters http://www.us.elsevierhealth.com/product.jsp?isbn=9781437735697
Akahoshi and Bapaye [68]	*Practical Handbook of Endoscopic Ultrasonography*	314	2012	Individual chapters available http://link.springer.com/book/10.1007/978-4-431-54014-4/page/1#

1.7 Integrating Genomics into Your EUS Practice with FNA

Next-generation sequencing and other genomic technologies are rapidly entering clinical practice and will transform the way we think about tumor biology, diagnosis, and treatment. Many of the advances will have relevance for the endosonographer who obtains FNA cytology, and some of these topics will be discussed below. Molecular pathology will enter our therapeutic strategy planning, and obtaining cytology specimens that are not (or cannot be) fully interrogated will no longer be acceptable. At a minimum, endosonographers should ensure that FNA specimens can be exploited to the maximum extent necessary. This is a responsibility shared by the person who obtains the specimen, the pathologist, and the oncologist. Ideally endosonographers performing FNA should not consider themselves biopsy technicians but take an active role in translational research. This section is an introduction to the most promising advances in the field of molecular pathology.

1.7.1 The Problem of Pancreatic Cysts: Could Micro RNAs Be the Answer?

Pancreatic cystic lesions are a frequent incidental finding and many are benign, but some of them, such as mucinous cysts (intraductal papillary mucinous neoplasms [IPMN] and mucinous cystic neoplasms) have varying degrees of malignant potential. The current diagnostic evaluation of pancreatic cystic lesions often includes EUS-guided FNA for analysis of the cyst fluid. The aspirate is often clear and paucicellular and the few cells visible appear bland on microscopy; however, this frequently does not reflect the cytology of the cyst lining. While measurement of pancreatic cyst carcinoembryonic antigen (CEA) level is currently considered the most accurate means for diagnosing mucinous cysts, the recommended cutoff of 192 ng/ml represents a trade-off between sensitivity and specificity [69]. DNA oncogenes (e.g., *KRAS*, adenylate cyclase-stimulating G a protein [*GNAS*]) and loss of heterozygosity of tumor suppressor genes (e.g., tumor protein 53 [*p53*], cyclin-dependent kinase inhibitor 2A [*p16*], ring finger protein 43 [*RNF43*]) detected in cyst fluid also have been investigated for the diagnosis and determination of malignant potential [70]. Particularly promising are micro RNAs (miRNA), which are small, noncoding RNA molecules (approximately 21–30 nucleotides in length) that function in the transcriptional and posttranscriptional regulation of gene expression. It has been hypothesized that a modest number of miRNAs (200 in total) might be sufficient to classify all human cancers [71]. Tumor-derived miRNAs can be isolated from tumors as well as the bloodstream [72] and cyst fluid. A recent study of formalin-fixed paraffin-embedded (FFPE) material identified a subset of 18 miRNAs that differentiated cysts typically requiring surgery (e.g., high-grade IPMN) from less-malignant lesions that can be observed (e.g., low-grade IPMN and serous cystadenoma). A logistic regression model was then formulated using 9 miRNAs and predicted cyst pathology treated with resection versus observation with a sensitivity of 89 % and a specificity of 100 % [73]. Similar work was conducted with intraductal papillary mucinous neoplasms of the pancreas, with equally encouraging results [74], but clinical validation studies have not yet been conducted.

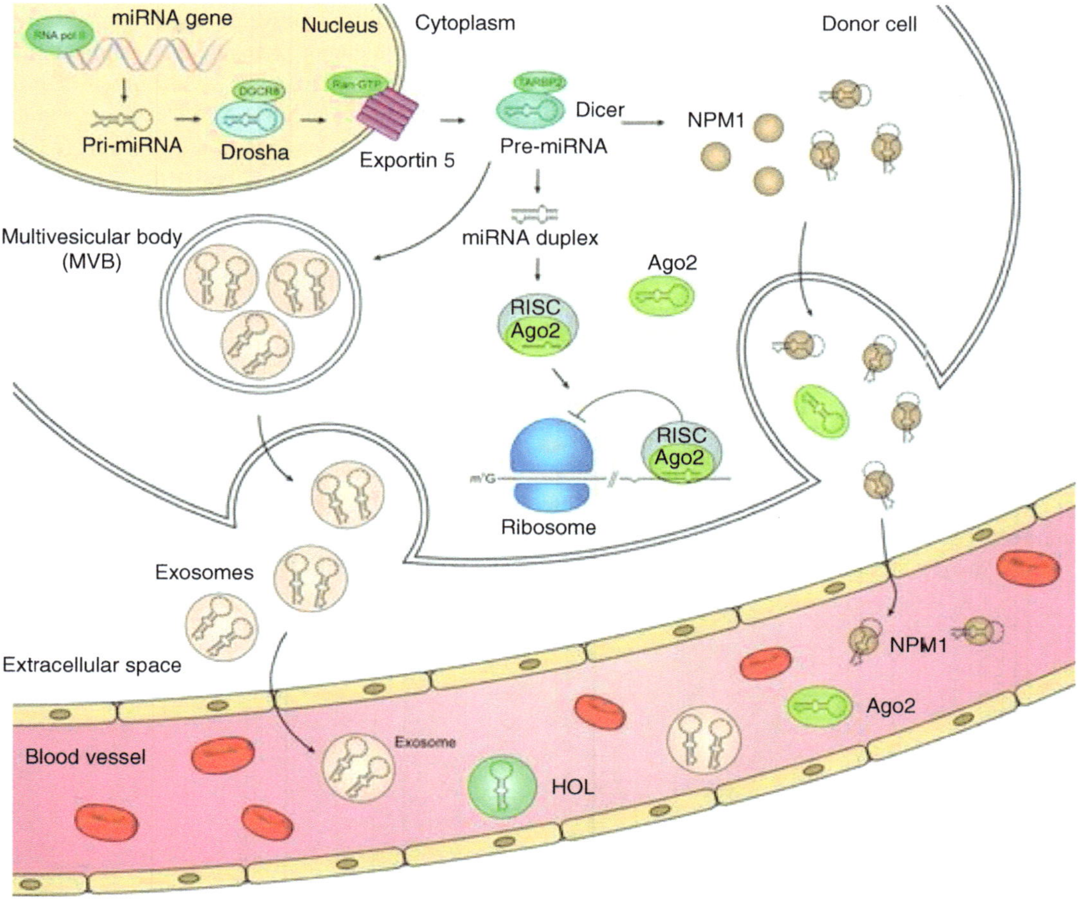

Fig. 1.73 Biogenesis and origin of circulating micro RNAs (*miRNAs*). Primary miRNA (*pri-miRNA*) transcripts are generated in the nucleus and processed to precursor miRNAs (*pre-miRNAs*). After export to the cytoplasm, the pre-miRNA is recognized and processed to a small, double-stranded RNA (dsRNA) structure of about 22 nucleotides. The dsRNA structure is recognized and unwound by the RNA-induced silencing complex (*RISC*) complex. Subsequently, the mature, single-stranded miRNA is carried to complementary miRNA target sites within messenger RNAs to regulate gene expression. Alternatively, pre-miRNAs can be transported in body fluids as circulating miRNAs (From Sørensen et al. [75])

1.7.2 Personalized Tumor Therapy: Lung Cancer Now and Pancreatic Cancer in the Future

The traditional distinction between small-cell lung cancer and non–small-cell lung cancer (NSCLC) is no longer sufficient for treatment planning. Evaluation for epidermal growth factor receptor (EGFR) mutations and anaplastic lymphoma kinase (ALK) rearrangements are now considered by many to be the standard of care for advanced-stage pulmonary adenocarcinomas. Recent recommendations specifically advise preserving a maximal amount of tissue for potential molecular testing and consciously limiting the number of immunohistochemical preparations needed to subclassify a lesion [76, 77].

Detection of an activating EGFR mutation or ALK rearrangement changes the treatment plan for an individual patient. EGFR mutations are present in 10–15 % of NSCLCs in the United States. Tyrosine kinase inhibitors, such as gefitinib and erlotinib, which target the intracellular tyrosine kinase domain of EGFR, have shown dramatic efficacy in advanced-stage NSCLC, with the greatest treatment benefit concentrated in patients harboring a "sensitizing" EGFR mutation [76]. A rearrangement in the ALK gene (most commonly resulting in an *EML4-ALK* fusion gene) is present in approximately 5 % of NSCLCs. Identification of patients with this rearrangement is of key importance because of the availability of crizotinib, a newly approved targeted therapy with activity against the kinases of the products of the *ALK*, *ROS1*, and *MET* genes [76].

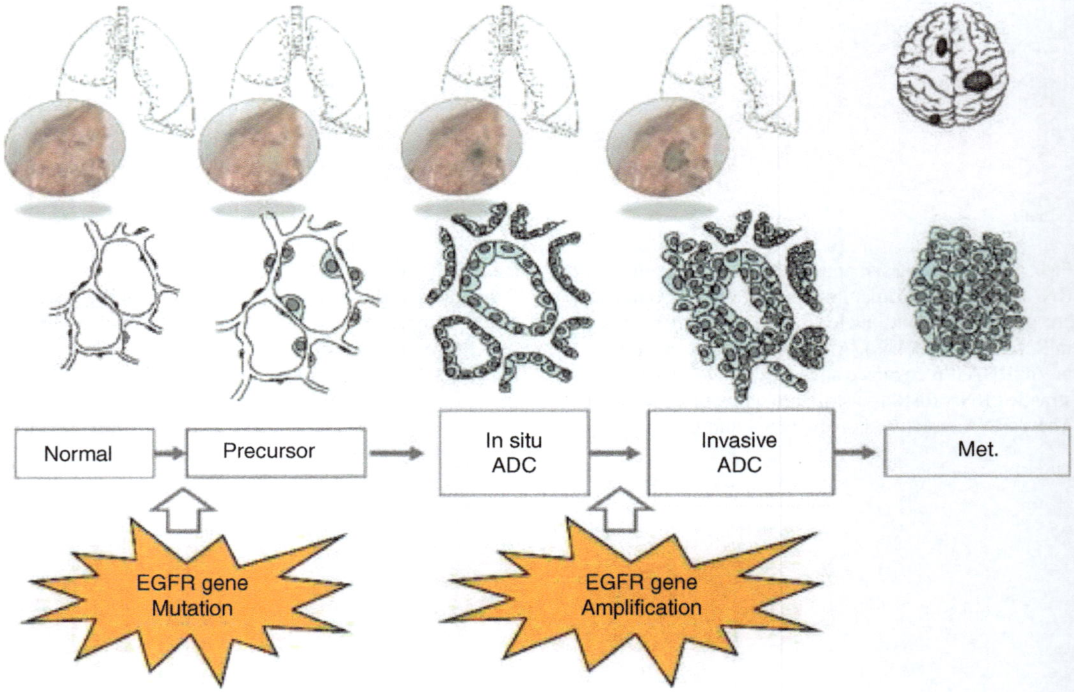

Fig. 1.74 Proposed schema of the progression of lung adenocarcinoma (*ADC*). The development of lung adenocarcinoma is thought to follow a stepwise progression, similar to that of colorectal cancer. A preinvasive lesion, termed *atypical adenomatous hyperplasia*, progresses to an adenocarcinoma in situ, namely a bronchioloalveolar carcinoma, followed by an invasive adenocarcinoma. Thereafter, the adenocarcinoma has the potential to metastasize to other organs. In this schema, epidermal growth factor receptor (*EGFR*) mutation and amplification contribute transformation to the precursor lesion and transition from in situ to invasive adenocarcinoma, respectively. *Met* metastasis (From Yatabe [78])

1.7.3 The Primacy of FNA Cytology in the Management of Pancreatic Cancers

In the not too distant past cytology was the stepchild of histopathology. With the advent of immunocytochemistry, the utility of cytology has increased, and it will increase further as molecular diagnostic methods become widely available. There are three principal reasons for this: (1) Treatment decisions for lung cancer and especially pancreatic cancer are overwhelmingly based on cytology specimens because these tumors have often have already metastasized at the time of diagnosis. Surgical specimens are, therefore, not available. (2) The DNA and RNA content of the typical FNA specimen are quite adequate for most purposes. (3) FNA cytology can be performed repeatedly, and this may become important because therapy strategies will be tailored to the changing genomic signature of metastatic and treated tumors. (4) The process of obtaining FNA cytology may actually enrich tumor cells over stromal cells. The latter two points deserve some expansion.

1.7.3.1 The Clonal Nature of Tumors in Space and Time and the Need for Directed and Repeat Biopsies

Most cancers are ecosystems of evolving clones and have the following features: the existence of clonal genotypes (i.e., not all mutations occur in the same cells); the expansion and decline of clonal populations over time; the existence of internal spatial variation in tumor composition; partial tumor responses to therapy and the emergence of drug-resistant malignant cells; the seeding of metastatic cells from subclones, which may be rare or common in the originating population; the absence of an observable clonal structure based on genome aberrations in some cancers; and the existence of neutral clonal relationships (e.g., arising from random genetic drift) without discernible phenotypic consequences [79].

The variability in responses to therapy that can be seen between metastases and even within a single tumor mass can be explained on the basis of clonal evolution. In the past molecular profiling of tumors was performed in "bulk," ignoring tumor heterogeneity, and the results reflect only mutations that are present in the majority of cancer cells. Whether the heterogeneity of tumors, which is sometimes visible with EUS or other imaging modalities, especially functional imaging, reflects clonal subpopulations of tumors and whether multiple directed biopsies (such as prostate quadrant biopsies), naturally by FNA, can lead to diagnostic material that adequately maps these tumors will need to be evaluated. There is emerging interest in performing molecular imaging in vivo, for example, using confocal fluorescence laser microscopy, and it is possible to advance the confocal fluorescence laser probe through a EUS-type 19-gauge fine needle [80], but this type of work is in the early stages.

A different but related problem is clonal heterogeneity in time. There is evidence of discordance of mutations between primary and corresponding metastatic disease, including pancreatic cancer, in response to the selective pressure of therapy [79]. Personalized tumor therapy will require elucidation of the mutations in metastatic disease, and this will require repeat biopsies for optimal tumor management.

1.7.4 Stroma and Tumor Cells: The Need for Specimen Enrichment and How FNA Can Do It

Pancreatic neoplasms tend to have abundant stroma, and the overall number of tumor nuclei in a tumor mass tends to be fairly low, a fact well known to endosonographers. In practice, this property predicts that genomic DNA (or RNA) isolated directly from a surgical specimen will consist of a mixture representing both tumor and stromal cells. This presents problems for sequencing because the DNA from stromal cells drowns out the signature of the tumor cells unless the sequencing coverage is greatly increased, which increases cost and time requirements. Coverage means the number of times a sequence is read by next-generation sequencers. A different solution consists of producing an immortalized cell line in culture, providing a pure tumor cell population. Although this solution seems ideal in principle, it is presently unknown in practice what additional modifications occur in the genomes of tumor cells as a result of the immortalization process [81]. Alternatively, tumors can be xenografted whereby a portion of the tumor is grown in an immunocompromised mouse, such that human stromal cells are eliminated. Unfortunately, the mouse also makes a stromal component, which partially defeats the purpose of this exercise [81]. Finally, microdissection can be employed. Manual microdissection is performed under a dissecting or light microscope, often with the use of a needle tip, scalpel point, or hollow-bore pipette, to preferentially isolate tumor cells from counterstained slides. Laser-capture microdissection, which is not widely available, uses computer-aided imaging to select specific cells for capture [82]. Interestingly, the process of FNA is itself an enrichment method. Cell enrichment by aspiration is based on the general characteristic of epithelial tumor cells to have decreased adhesion, therefore allowing easy separation from the surrounding stroma, and many authors have obtained satisfactory specimens for molecular analysis using FNA alone [83, 84].

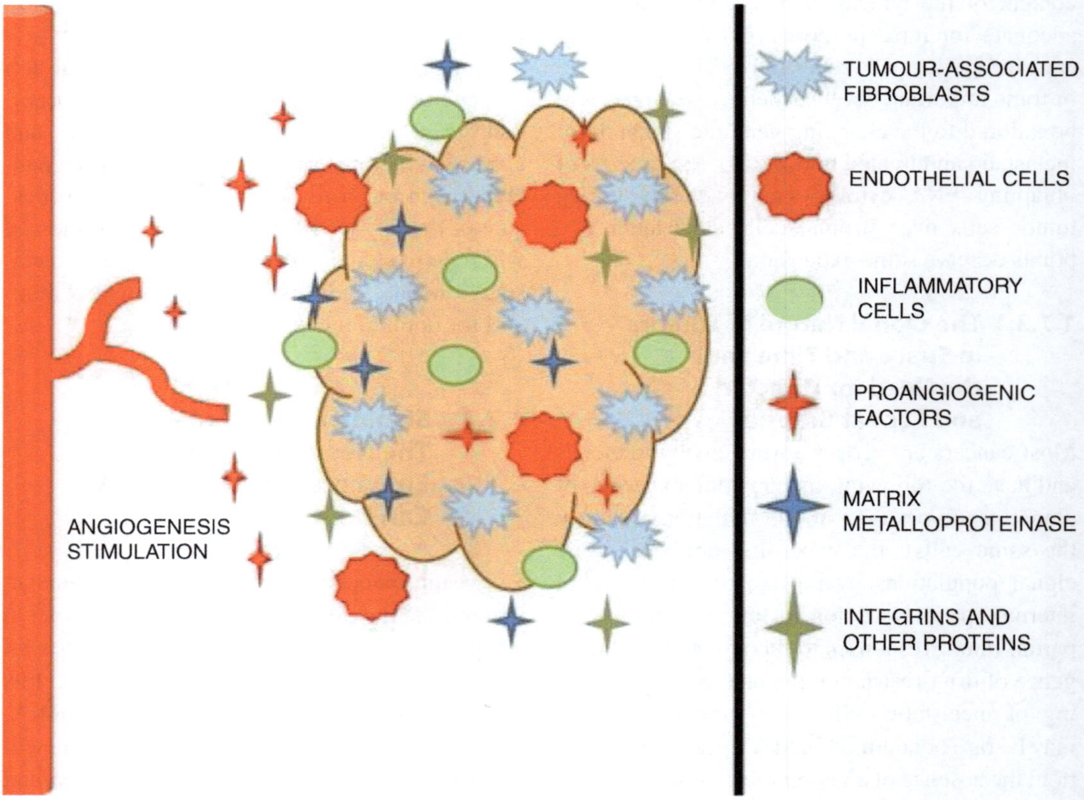

Fig. 1.75 Tumor mass with stroma showing the major supporting noncancer stromal cells and pivotal protein families. Individual cancer cells are not shown (From Nyga et al. [85])

1.7.5 Specimen Handling: Know What Needs to Happen with Your Specimen

Conventional processing of FNA cytology varies from institution to institution, but the protocol described in the box is typical.

> Cytologic preparations are made by using the stylet to expel the sample from the needle onto a slide. If this yields minimal to no sample, air is used to push out the sample. Another slide is placed gently over the first to make a smear. One slide is air dried if rapid on-site evaluation (ROSE) is used for DiffQuik staining. If ROSE is not used, then both slides are sprayed with an alcohol-based fixative for later processing. A needle rinse is then obtained by expelling any remaining sample into Cytolyt (a methanol-based buffered preservative) for cell block preparation. For histologic examination, the stylet is used to expel the sample into formalin. Sterile saline solution is then used to wash any remaining tissue or cells into the formalin. The "core" biopsies then are embedded in paraffin and stained with hematoxylin and eosin [86].

Currently most established molecular testing is done on FFPE slides (cell block in cytology), despite the fact that formalin fixation does not preserve nucleic acids well. This results in RNA that is often significantly degraded; formalin also causes cross-linkage between nucleic acids and proteins [87]. FFPE specimens are, however, so ubiquitous that methodologies were developed to extract and amplify RNA from FFPE tissue. However, these techniques have limitations and for certain applications immediate freezing of the specimen is required.

The determination of the adequacy of the cytology specimen through ROSE is helpful for beginning endosonographers, but many experienced practitioners seem to be able to do just as well without it and dedicate most of their aspirate to the cell block. The advantage is that material does not need to be "wasted" for quick staining and adequate interpretation. FFPE material (paraffin cell block) can be sectioned and subjected to ancillary studies such as immunohistochemistry and molecular testing, and in general, more is better, unless the specimen becomes too bloody.

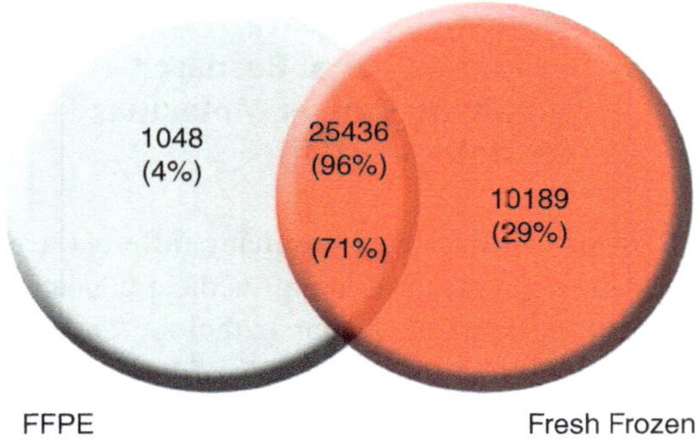

Fig. 1.76 A Venn diagram showing retention of probe sets consistently called present between frozen and formalin-fixed paraffin-embedded (FFPE) samples on the Almac Diagnostics Lung Cancer DSA™ research tool. Sensitivity was 71 %, indicating that 71 % of the genes from the fresh frozen sample was detected in FFPE. Specificity was extremely high, with 96 % of the FFPE genes detected also detected in the fresh frozen sample (From Farragher et al. [87])

It is crucial that there is good communication between the physician who ordered the FNA (or made the referral to the endosonographer), the endosonographer, and the pathology laboratory. For example, if a patient is undergoing additional biopsies for the express purpose of acquiring material for molecular testing, much frustration arises when a specimen submitted is inadvertently exhausted and no material is left for the intended purpose because numerous immunohistochemical stains were performed to classify the tumor (which has already been done). Therefore, it is necessary to clearly communicate the priorities for a specimen. We mentioned earlier that cyst aspiration and analysis for miRNA shows promise and multicenter studies examining their possible value will emerge quickly. Co-investigators in such studies will have to adhere to the protocol for sample collection and preservation. MiRNA tends to be more stable than messenger RNA. Even so, specimens from the pancreas are easily exposed to nucleases and precautions such as the use of special transport media and deep freezing may need to be taken [84].

1.7.6 How to Participate in Translational Research Involving Cancer Molecular Pathology

We recognize that there are many different avenues for pursuing continuing medical education in genomics and molecular pathology and that these depend on personal levels of interest, participation in research programs, and the environment of practice. One of the best approaches could consist of creating an ad hoc local special interest group of oncologists, subspecialty clinicians, and practitioners who have direct access to the diagnostic material, such as endosonographers and interventional radiologists. Oncologists often do not know what endosonographers can do, and endosonographers frequently do not understand what research agendas are of interest to oncologists. A better dialogue could streamline translational research and benefit all. Currently it seems that the Association for Molecular Pathology, which was founded in 1995, will assume, in conjunction with the American College of Pathologists, a leadership role in shaping the field of clinical molecular diagnostics and issue guidelines that will have wide effect. If your institution has a molecular pathology group they will naturally need to be part of your special interest group.

In May 2013 a search of clinicaltrials.gov using the search term *eus fna* (which searches similar and related terms) showed 67 registered prospective clinical studies, of which only a few directly addressed a molecular pathology methodology. The field is wide open with plentiful opportunities.

1.8 Solution to Challenge Case

Hidden Figure Test – A Dalmatian is sniffing the ground.

References

1. Kolb DA. Experiential learning: experience as the source of learning and development. Englewood Cliffs: Prentice-Hall; 1984.
2. Croskerry P. The importance of cognitive errors in diagnosis and strategies to minimize them. Acad Med. 2003;78(8):775–80.
3. Gunderman RB. Biases in radiologic reasoning. AJR Am J Roentgenol. 2009;192(3):561–4. doi:10.2214/AJR.08.1220.
4. Noone TC, Hosey J, Firat Z, Semelka RC. Imaging and localization of islet-cell tumours of the pancreas on CT and MRI. Best Pract Res Clin Endocrinol Metab. 2005;19(2):195–211. doi:10.1016/j.beem.2004.11.013.
5. Krupinski EA. The importance of perception research in medical imaging. Radiat Med. 2000;18(6):329–34.
6. Kundel HL, Nodine CF, Carmody D. Visual scanning, pattern recognition and decision-making in pulmonary nodule detection. Invest Radiol. 1978;13(3):175–81.
7. Shergill HK. Experimental psychology. New Delhi: PHI Learning Pvt. Ltd.; 2012.
8. Daffner RH. Visual illusions in the interpretation of the radiographic image. Curr Probl Diagn Radiol. 1989;18(2):62–87.
9. Kremkau FW, Taylor KJ. Artifacts in ultrasound imaging. J Ultrasound Med. 1986;5(4):227–37.
10. Tole NM. Image Characteristics in Clinical Ultrasound. In: Ostensen H, editor. Basic physics of ultrasonographic imaging. Geneva: World Health Organization; 2005.
11. Barrett JF, Keat N. Artifacts in CT: recognition and avoidance1. Radiographics. 2004;24(6):1679–91. doi:10.1148/rg.246045065.
12. Sawhney MS, Nelson DB, Debol S. The ever-expanding spectrum of GI endoscopy: EUS-guided FNA of thyroid cancer. Gastrointest Endosc. 2007;65(2):319–20. doi:10.1016/j.gie.2006.06.046.
13. Kim DW, Eun CK, In HS, Kim MH, Jung SJ, Bae SK. Sonographic differentiation of asymptomatic diffuse thyroid disease from normal thyroid: a prospective study. AJNR Am J Neuroradiol. 2010;31(10):1956–60. doi:10.3174/ajnr.A2164.
14. Yuen HY, Tong CS-L, Ahuja AT. Sonography of the normal thyroid. In: Ultrasound of the thyroid and parathyroid glands. New York: Springer; 2012. p. 41–60.
15. Dieleman EMT, Senan S, Vincent A, Lagerwaard FJ, Slotman BJ, van Sörnsen de Koste JR. Four-dimensional computed tomographic analysis of esophageal mobility during normal respiration. Int J Radiat Oncol Biol Phys. 2007;67(3):775–80. doi:10.1016/j.ijrobp.2006.09.054.
16. Larsen E, Reddy H, Drewes AM, Arendt-Nielsen L, Gregersen H. Ultrasonographic study of mechanosensory properties in human esophagus during mechanical distension. World J Gastroenterol. 2006;12(28):4517–23.
17. Dumont AE, Rifkind KM. Evolutionary significance of the thoracic duct. Nature. 1968;219(5159):1182–3. doi:10.1038/2191182a0.
18. Parasher VK, Meroni E, Malesci A, et al. Observation of thoracic duct morphology in portal hypertension by endoscopic ultrasound. Gastrointest Endosc. 1998;48(6):588–92. doi:10.1016/S0016-5107(98)70040-9.

19. Casaccia G, et al. Pleural effusion requiring drainage in congenital diaphragmatic hernia: incidence, aetiology and treatment. Pediatr Surg Int. 2006;22(7): 585–8.
20. Faigel DO, Rosen HR, Sasaki A, Flora K, Benner K. EUS in cirrhotic patients with and without prior variceal hemorrhage in comparison with noncirrhotic control subjects. Gastrointest Endosc. 2000;52(4): 455–62. doi:10.1067/mge.2000.107297.
21. Staller K, Braden Kuo MD. Development, anatomy, and physiology of the esophagus. In: Principles of deglutition. New York: Springer; 2013. p. 269–86.
22. Rusch VW, Asamura H, Watanabe H, Giroux DJ, Rami-Porta R, Goldstraw P. The IASLC lung cancer staging project. J Thorac Oncol. 2009;4(5):568–77. doi:10.1097/JTO.0b013e3181a0d82e.
23. Kelloff GJ, Choyke P, Coffey DS. Challenges in clinical prostate cancer: role of imaging. AJR Am J Roentgenol. 2009;192(6):1455–70. doi:10.2214/AJR. 09.2579.
24. Halpern EJ, Cochlin DL, Goldberg BB. Imaging of the prostate. London/New York/Florence: Martin Dunitz; Distributed in the USA by Taylor & Francis; 2002.
25. Kamoi K, Babaian RJ. Contemporary TRUS-guided prostate biopsy for screening and staging. In: Contemporary interventional ultrasonography in urology. London: Springer; 2009. p. 49–62.
26. Kim B, Kawashima A, Ryu J-A, Takahashi N, Hartman RP, King BF. Imaging of the seminal vesicle and vas deferens1. Radiographics. 2009;29(4):1105–21. doi:10.1148/rg.294085235.
27. Wennemuth G, Krause W. The normal genitalia–structure and physiology. In: Sexually transmitted infections and sexually transmitted diseases. Berlin/Heidelberg: Springer; 2011. p. 43–8.
28. Merz E, Miric-Tesanic D, Bahlmann F, Weber G, Wellek S. Sonographic size of uterus and ovaries in pre- and postmenopausal women. Ultrasound Obstet Gynecol. 1996;7(1):38–42. doi:10.1046/j.1469-0705.1996.07010038.x.
29. Gottlieb K. Doppler-endosonography with the GF-UE 160 electronic radial echoendoscope – current use and future potential. J Gastrointestin Liver Dis. 2007; 16(4):455–61.
30. Hansen EF, Bendtsen F, Brinc K. Endoscopic Doppler ultrasound for measurement of azygos blood flow: validation against thermodilution and assessment of pharmacological effects of terlipressin in portal hypertension. Scand J Gastroenterol. 2001;36(3):318–25. doi:10.1080/00365520120159.
31. Nishida H, Giostra E, Spahr L, Mentha G, Mitamura K, Hadengue A. Validation of color Doppler EUS for azygos blood flow measurement in patients with cirrhosis: application to the acute hemodynamic effects of somatostatin, octreotide, or placebo. Gastrointest Endosc. 2001;54(1):24–30.
32. Sato T, Yamazaki K, Toyota J, et al. Usefulness of electronic radial endoscopic color Doppler ultrasonography in esophageal varices: comparison with convex type. J Gastroenterol. 2006;41(1):28–33. doi:10.1007/s00535-005-1719-4.
33. Fujii L, Clain JE, Morris JM, Levy MJ. Anterior spinal cord infarction with permanent paralysis following endoscopic ultrasound celiac plexus neurolysis. Endoscopy. 2012;44(S02):E265–6.
34. Okuda K, Kage M, Shrestha SM. Proposal of a new nomenclature for Budd-Chiari syndrome: hepatic vein thrombosis versus thrombosis of the inferior vena cava at its hepatic portion. Hepatology. 1998;28(5):1191–8. doi:10.1002/hep.510280505.
35. Bargalló X, Gilabert R, Nicolau C, García-Pagán JC, Ayuso JR, Brú C. Sonography of Budd-Chiari syndrome. AJR Am J Roentgenol. 2006;187(1):W33–41. doi:10.2214/AJR.04.0918.
36. Lim AK, Patel N, Eckersley RJ, et al. Can Doppler sonography grade the severity of hepatitis C-related liver disease? AJR Am J Roentgenol. 2005;184(6): 1848–53.
37. Bonekamp S, Kamel I, Solga S, Clark J. Can imaging modalities diagnose and stage hepatic fibrosis and cirrhosis accurately? J Hepatol. 2009;50(1):17–35. doi:10.1016/j.jhep.2008.10.016.
38. Görg C, Riera-Knorrenschild J, Dietrich J. Colour Doppler ultrasound flow patterns in the portal venous system. Br J Radiol. 2002;75(899):919–29.
39. McNaughton DA, Abu-Yousef MM. Doppler US of the liver made simple. Radiographics. 2011;31(1):161–88. doi:10.1148/rg.311105093.
40. Sharma M, Babu CSR, Garg S, Rai P. Portal venous system and its tributaries: a radial endosonographic assessment. Endosc Ultrasound. 2012;1(2):96–107. doi:10.7178/eus.02.008.
41. Sgouros SN, Bergele C, Avgerinos A. Endoscopic ultrasonography in the diagnosis and management of portal hypertension. Where are we next? Dig Liver Dis. 2006;38(5):289–95. doi:10.1016/j.dld.2005.11.012.
42. Lai L, Brugge WR. Endoscopic ultrasound is a sensitive and specific test to diagnose portal venous system thrombosis (PVST). Am J Gastroenterol. 2003;99(1):40–4. doi:10.1046/j.1572-0241.2003.04020.x.
43. Bureau C, Pagan JCG, Layrargues GP, et al. Patency of stents covered with polytetrafluoroethylene in patients treated by transjugular intrahepatic portosystemic shunts: long-term results of a randomized multicentre study. Liver Int. 2007;27(6):742–7. doi:10.1111/j.1478-3231.2007.01522.x.
44. Sato T, Yamazaki K. Endoscopic color Doppler ultrasonography for esophagogastric varices. Diagn Ther Endosc. 2012. doi:10.1155/2012/859213.
45. Wiersema MJ, Chak A, Kopecky KK, Wiersema LM. Duplex Doppler endosonography in the diagnosis of splenic vein, portal vein, and portosystemic shunt thrombosis. Gastrointest Endosc. 1995;42(1):19–26. doi:10.1016/S0016-5107(95)70237-7.
46. Köklü S, Çoban Ş, Yüksel O, Arhan M. Left-sided portal hypertension. Dig Dis Sci. 2007;52(5):1141–9. doi:10.1007/s10620-006-9307-x.

47. Kutlu R, Karaman I, Akbulut A, et al. Quantitative Doppler evaluation of the splenoportal venous system in various stages of cirrhosis: differences between right and left portal veins. J Clin Ultrasound. 2002;30(9):537–43. doi:10.1002/jcu.10114.
48. Madoff DC, Denys A, Wallace MJ, et al. Splenic arterial interventions: anatomy, indications, technical considerations, and potential complications. Radiographics. 2005;25(Suppl_1):S191–211. doi:10.1148/rg.25si055504.
49. Varadarajulu S, Eloubeidi MA. Diagnosis of an aneurysm masquerading as a pancreatic-cyst lesion at EUS. Gastrointest Endosc. 2007;65(4):721–5. doi:10.1016/j.gie.2006.08.037.
50. Robinson M, Richards D, Carr N. Treatment of a splenic artery pseudoaneurysm by endoscopic ultrasound-guided thrombin injection. Cardiovasc Intervent Radiol. 2007;30(3):515–7. doi:10.1007/s00270-006-0081-0.
51. Robb PM, Yeaton P, Bishop T, Wessinger J. Endoscopic ultrasound guided embolization of a pancreatic pseudoaneurysm. Gastroenterol Res. 2013;5(6):239–41.
52. Mitchell EL, Moneta GL. Mesenteric duplex scanning. Perspect Vasc Surg Endovasc Ther. 2006;18(2):175–83. doi:10.1177/1531003506291885.
53. Gielecki J, Zurada A, Sonpal N, Jabłońska B. The clinical relevance of coeliac trunk variations. Folia Morphol (Warsz). 2005;64(3):123–9.
54. Song S-Y, Chung JW, Yin YH, et al. Celiac axis and common hepatic artery variations in 5002 patients: systematic analysis with spiral CT and DSA1. Radiology. 2010;255(1):278–88. doi:10.1148/radiol.09090389.
55. Nelson TM, Pollak R, Jonasson O, Abcarian H. Anatomic variants of the celiac, superior mesenteric, and inferior mesenteric arteries and their clinical relevance. Clin Anat. 1988;1(2):75–91. doi:10.1002/ca.980010202.
56. Yi SQ. A rare case of inferior mesenteric artery arising from the superior mesenteric artery, with a review of the review of the literature. Surg Radiol Anat. 2008;30(2):159. doi:10.1007/s00276-007-0298-x.
57. Higashi N, Hirai K. A case of the three branches of the celiac trunk arising directly from the abdominal aorta. Kaibogaku Zasshi. 1995;70(4):349–52.
58. Losanoff JE. Hepato-spleno-mesenteric trunk. J Am Coll Surg. 2007;204(3):511. doi:10.1016/j.jamcollsurg.2006.07.045.
59. Levy M, Rajan E, Keeney G, Fletcher JG, Topazian M. Neural ganglia visualized by endoscopic ultrasound. Am J Gastroenterol. 2006;101(8):1787–91. doi:10.1111/j.1572-0241.2006.00685.x.
60. Sato T, Yamazaki K, Toyota J, Karino Y, Ohmura T, Akaike J. Diagnosis of rectal varices via color Doppler ultrasonography. Am J Gastroenterol. 2007;102(10):2253–8. doi:10.1111/j.1572-0241.2007.01340.x.
61. Ghosh P, Antani S, Long LR, Thoma GR. Review of medical image retrieval systems and future directions. In: 2011 24th international symposium on Computer-Based Medical Systems (CBMS), Bristol. 2011. p. 1–6. doi:10.1109/CBMS.2011.5999142.
62. Hearst MA, Divoli A, Guturu H, et al. BioText Search Engine: beyond abstract search. Bioinformatics. 2007;23(16):2196–7. doi:10.1093/bioinformatics/btm301.
63. Xu S, McCusker J, Krauthammer M. Yale Image Finder (YIF): a new search engine for retrieving biomedical images. Bioinformatics. 2008;24(17):1968–70. doi:10.1093/bioinformatics/btn340.
64. Gress FG, Savides TJ. Endoscopic ultrasonography. Chichester: Wiley-Blackwell; 2009.
65. Shami VM, Michel K. Endoscopic ultrasound. New York: Humana Press; 2010.
66. Dietrich CF, Allgayer H. Endoscopic ultrasound: an introductory manual and atlas. Stuttgart: Thieme; 2011.
67. Hawes RH, Fockens P, Varadarajulu S. Endosonography. Philadelphia: Elsevier/Saunders; 2011.
68. Akahoshi K, Bapaye A. Practical handbook of endoscopic ultrasonography. Tokyo: Springer; 2012.
69. Brugge WR, Lewandrowski K, Lee-Lewandrowski E, et al. Diagnosis of pancreatic cystic neoplasms: a report of the cooperative pancreatic cyst study. Gastroenterology. 2004;126(5):1330–6. doi:10.1053/j.gastro.2004.02.013.
70. Schmidt CM. Pancreatic cyst cytology: optimization of cancer risk profiling. Cancer Cytopathol. 2013;121(1):2–3. doi:10.1002/cncy.21267.
71. Thomas RM, Fleming JB. MicroRNA dissects out dangerous pancreatic cysts from all the rest. Clin Cancer Res. 2012;18(17):4482–4. doi:10.1158/1078-0432.CCR-12-2089.
72. Duttagupta R, Jones KW. The curious case of miRNAs in circulation: potential diagnostic biomarkers? Wiley Interdiscip Rev RNA. 2013;4(1):129–38. doi:10.1002/wrna.1149.
73. Matthaei H, Wylie D, Lloyd MB, et al. miRNA biomarkers in cyst fluid augment the diagnosis and management of pancreatic cysts. Clin Cancer Res. 2012;18(17):4713–24. doi:10.1158/1078-0432.CCR-12-0035.
74. Lubezky N, Loewenstein S, Ben-Haim M, et al. MicroRNA expression signatures in intraductal papillary mucinous neoplasm of the pancreas. Surgery. 2013. doi:10.1016/j.surg.2012.11.016.
75. Sørensen KD, et al. The application of microRNAs in cancer diagnostics. In: RNA interference from biology to therapeutics. New York: Springer; 2013. p. 259–98
76. Aisner DL, Marshall CB. Molecular pathology of non-small cell lung cancer a practical guide. Am J Clin Pathol. 2012;138(3):332–46. doi:10.1309/AJCPFR12WJKCEEZZ.
77. Travis W, Rekhtman N. Pathological diagnosis and classification of lung cancer in small biopsies and cytology: strategic management of tissue for

molecular testing. Semin Respir Crit Care Med. 2011;32(01):022–31. doi:10.1055/s-0031-1272866.

78. Yatabe Y. EGFR mutations and the terminal respiratory unit. Cancer Metastasis Rev. 2010;29(1):23–36.
79. Aparicio S, Caldas C. The implications of clonal genome evolution for cancer medicine. N Eng J Med. 2013;368(9):842–51. doi:10.1056/NEJMra1204892.
80. Eser S, Messer M, Eser P, et al. In vivo diagnosis of murine pancreatic intraepithelial neoplasia and early-stage pancreatic cancer by molecular imaging. Proc Natl Acad Sci USA. 2011;108(24):9945–50. doi:10.1073/pnas.1100890108.
81. Mardis ER. Applying next-generation sequencing to pancreatic cancer treatment. Nat Rev Gastroenterol Hepatol. 2012;9(8):477–86. doi:10.1038/nrgastro.2012.126.
82. Aisner DL, Sams SB. The role of cytology specimens in molecular testing of solid tumors: techniques, limitations, and opportunities. Diagn Cytopathol. 2012; 40(6):511–24. doi:10.1002/dc.22820.
83. Crnogorac-Jurcevic T, et al. Gene expression profiles of pancreatic cancer and stromal desmoplasia. Oncogene. 2001;20(50):7437. doi:10.1038/sj.onc.1204935.
84. Bournet B, Pointreau A, Delpu Y, et al. Molecular endoscopic ultrasound for diagnosis of pancreatic cancer. Cancers. 2011;3(4):872–82. doi:10.3390/cancers3010872.
85. Nyga A, Cheema U, Loizidou M. 3D tumour models: novel in vitro approaches to cancer studies. J Cell Commun Signal. 2011;5(3):239–48.
86. Toth JW, Zubelevitskiy K, Strow JA, Kaifi JT, Kunselman AR, Reed MF. Specimen processing techniques for endobronchial ultrasound-guided transbronchial needle aspiration. Ann Thorac Surg. 2013;95(3):976–81. doi:10.1016/j.athoracsur.2012.11.058.
87. Farragher SM, Tanney A, Kennedy RD, Harkin DP. RNA expression analysis from formalin fixed paraffin embedded tissues. Histochem Cell Biol. 2008;130(3): 435–45. doi:10.1007/s00418-008-0479-7.

Esophagus and Mediastinum

2

Contents

2.1 **General Principles** 71
2.1.1 The Esophagus: A Window into the Mediastinum 71
2.1.2 The Esophagus Is Not a Pipe 72
2.1.3 Endobronchial Ultrasound 72
2.1.4 Lymph Node Maps for the Mediastinum 73
2.1.5 Mediastinal Biopsies 73
2.1.6 Examination of the Esophagus 73

2.2 **Cases and Discussions** 74
2.2.1 Mediastinum 74
2.2.1.1 Aortic Aneurysms 74
2.2.1.2 Aortic Dissection 76
2.2.1.3 New Pulmonary Emboli, Aortic Dissection, and Right Heart Strain 78
2.2.1.4 Subcarinal Lymph Node Biopsy 83
2.2.1.5 Biopsies of Upper Paratracheal Lymph Nodes: Melanoma or Lymphoma? 85
2.2.1.6 Recurrent Hodgkin's Lymphoma 87
2.2.1.7 Bronchial Carcinoid 90
2.2.1.8 Bronchogenic Cysts 94
2.2.1.9 Mediastinal Pseudocyst 97
2.2.1.10 Mediastinal Plasmacytoma 99
2.2.1.11 Posterior Mediastinal Paravertebral Mass 101
2.2.1.12 Pleural and Pericardial Effusion 103
2.2.1.13 Consolidated Lung 105
2.2.1.14 Dysphagia Caused by Carcinoma of the Lung 107
2.2.1.15 Centrally Located Primary Lung Lesions 109
2.2.1.16 Restaging of Lung Cancer Following Mediastinoscopy and Treatment by EUS 113
2.2.1.17 False-Positive PET Scan 117
2.2.1.18 Triple Cytology for Lung Cancer Diagnosis 119
2.2.1.19 Malignant Invasion of the Pulmonary Artery 122
2.2.2 Esophagus 125
2.2.2.1 Carcinosarcoma of the Esophagus 125
2.2.2.2 T1N1 Esophageal Cancer 129
2.2.2.3 Esophageal Leiomyoma Arising from the Muscularis Mucosae 130
2.2.2.4 Granular Cell Tumor of the Esophagus 132
2.2.2.5 Esophageal Intramucosal Cyst 134
2.2.2.6 Esophageal Duplication Cyst 135
2.2.2.7 Esophageal Leiomyoma 137
2.2.2.8 Intramural Metastasis of Esophageal Cancer 140
2.2.2.9 Recurrent Esophageal Cancer 142
2.2.2.10 Challenge Question 144
References 145

2.1 General Principles

2.1.1 The Esophagus: A Window into the Mediastinum

The esophagus is, from an endosonographer's perspective, the window into the mediastinum, and it makes sense to consider both anatomic regions together. A good understanding of mediastinal anatomy is a prerequisite for competent image interpretation. After a basic review of cross-sectional and traditional anatomy, the endosonographer should approach mediastinal anatomy from the perspective of the ultrasound transducer in the esophagus. Numerous resources on the Internet allow familiarization of 3-dimensional anatomy of the mediastinum from every possible angle and vantage point, allowing structures and layers to be peeled away and added as desired (see Box 2.1). The number of possible cross sections that can be achieved with linear

K. Gottlieb, G. Marino, *Diagnostic Endosonography*,
DOI 10.1007/978-3-642-39118-7_2, © Springer-Verlag Berlin Heidelberg 2014

and radial endosonography probes vastly exceed those that can be reasonably expected to be represented in image collections even if they are dedicated to the topic (e.g., in an endoscopic ultrasound [EUS] anatomy atlas), although these collections are certainly helpful. Therefore, the endosonographer should make a point of identifying mediastinal structures every time an upper EUS exam is being conducted until such time when the mediastinum becomes a "second home."

Box 2.1: Open Access Resources for the Esophagus and Mediastinum

- Websites
  - Anatronica: 3D Interactive Anatomy www.anatronica.com
- Articles
  - Direct Nodal Sampling by Echo-endoscopy in Lung Cancer: The Clinician's Expectations. *Insights Imaging* 2011 http://www.ncbi.nlm.nih.gov/pmc/articles/PMC3259317/
  - Lung Cancer Staging by Endoscopic and Endobronchial Ultrasound-Guided Fine-Needle Aspiration http://is.gd/dm58CC
  - Mediastinoscopy vs. Endosonography for Mediastinal Nodal Staging of Lung Cancer: A Randomized Trial. *JAMA* 2010 http://is.gd/vLtRLm
  - Cancer Staging Poster and Stage Grouping of Lung Cancer, Seventh Edition http://is.gd/X6BAwy
- Videos
  - EBUS Lymph node map: http://is.gd/R6Jaxk
  - Band Ligation Endoscopic Mucosal Resection of a Distal Esophageal Granular Cell Tumor http://is.gd/cwmBdF
  - Esophagus – Esophageal cancer EUS example 3 http://is.gd/YFe0ZQ
  - Esophagus – Adenocarcinoma Arising in Barrett's Staged with EUS FNA http://is.gd/un1xMr
  - Mediastinum – EUS of Pericardial Cyst http://is.gd/7Joota
  - ASGE Learning Video Sample – EUS-Guided Tissue Sampling Techniques: Cytology and Biopsy http://is.gd/6UCGmY

2.1.2 The Esophagus Is Not a Pipe

Chest radiologists have exquisite knowledge of mediastinal anatomy, and frequent consultation with them is essential for two reasons: (1) to learn and (2) to teach. Almost always it is the radiologist who, as consultant to the original requestor of the chest computed tomography (CT) or positron emission tomography (PET) scan, makes further recommendations for how a lesion could best be biopsied or further investigated. However, even chest radiologists often have an incomplete understanding of what locations can be successfully biopsied by EUS-guided fine-needle aspiration (FNA). Part of this is related to semantics, for example, mediastinal lymph nodes often are referred to by their relation to the trachea even if they are just as close to the esophagus, and this may already predicate the advice of performing an endobronchial ultrasound or mediastinoscopy instead of a transesophageal ultrasound. Furthermore, radiologists are accustomed to static images. How much the esophagus can be displaced in one direction or another by the gentle push from the tip of the echoendoscope is most often not appreciated. Lesions that appear on cross-sectional imaging as if they could not be "seen" or biopsied from a probe in the esophagus are, in fact, often within reach, and some of the cases that follow make this clear.

2.1.3 Endobronchial Ultrasound

There are clearly situations when endobronchial ultrasound (EBUS) is the imaging modality of choice in the mediastinum and others where transesophageal EUS is the best modality. In general, EUS is most appropriate for evaluation of the posterior inferior mediastinum, whereas mediastinoscopy or EBUS are best for evaluating the anterior superior mediastinum. In many cases there will be overlap from a purely anatomic point of view. From a clinical standpoint many patients who require biopsies of lesions in the mediastinum will have coexisting pulmonary disease, and biopsies through the esophagus may be preferable to a procedure with a bronchoscope in the trachea or bronchus. The quality of biopsies (false negatives) is also correlated with how much time is available to localize the lesion and find the best biopsy trajectory and the number of biopsy passes that can be made uninterrupted by coughing and other signs of patient distress. Perspectives on the relative merits of EBUS versus EUS from the point of view of gastroenterologists and pulmonologist are listed in Box 2.1.

2.1.4 Lymph Node Maps for the Mediastinum

North American clinicians have traditionally used the Mountain-Dressler thoracic lymph node map. To reconcile differences from the Japanese Naruke system, the International Association for the Study of Lung Cancer proposed a new lymph node map in 2009 (Box 2.1). The relevant stations for the endosonographer remain the same: upper paratracheal 2L and 2R, lower paratracheal 4L and 4R, aortopulmonary window 5, subcarinal 7, and paraesophageal 8.

2.1.5 Mediastinal Biopsies

Mediastinal lymph node biopsies are relatively easy to perform compared with biopsies of, for example, the pancreas. The American Society for Gastrointestinal Endoscopy has an excellent video describing FNA biopsies of various anatomic locations (see Box 2.1).

2.1.6 Examination of the Esophagus

The examination of small esophageal lesions and high-quality demonstrations of the esophageal wall layers is actually one of the more difficult techniques to master. An overinflated balloon that pushes hard on the esophageal wall will distort the anatomy and may lead to incorrect staging. In contrast to the stomach and rectum, it is not possible to use copious amounts of water to improve acoustic coupling. With patience and practice it is possible to combine moderate balloon inflation and small amounts of water instillation to temporarily view excellent demonstrations of small lesions. If this approach is used, regurgitation and possibly coughing and aspiration are risks. It is, therefore, preferable to elevate the head of the endoscopy table by 30 degrees.

One of the most frequent indications for EUS is the staging of esophageal carcinomas. We assume that most of our readers are familiar with the TNM (tumor, node, metastasis) system and the principles of esophageal tumor staging. There are excellent introductory textbooks that deal with this subject matter, and we will not present many esophageal tumor cases here. The problem with correct TNM staging of esophageal tumors is related to not only technical factors or operator experience but also the basic technology. Even with optimal technique there are inherent limitations, and other imaging modalities have caught up so that the contribution of EUS in the preoperative staging of esophageal cancer for surgical resection has been questioned [1]. Leading institutions discourage the restaging of esophageal cancer after combination chemotherapy and radiation [2]. A related but somewhat different problem is the evaluation of small esophageal lesions that are potentially amenable to endoscopic mucosal resection (EMR). It was previously thought that this would be an indication where EUS evaluation before the procedure would have the biggest effect. Diagnostic EMR as a first step is increasingly being promoted over EUS evaluation before EMR because the depth of submucosal invasion is difficult to accurately determine using EUS [3]. When submucosal involvement is found the patient is referred for surgical resection because of the high risk of early lymph node metastasis, which would be undetectable by imaging. We still believe that EUS is reasonable before EMR to obtain accurate measurements of the tumor, especially for those practioners who are more comfortable resecting smaller lesions and would refer larger lesions to surgeons with more experience. Furthermore, it seems that EUS will continue to contribute to the optimal management of esophageal cancers. Esophageal tumor length recently has been found to be a strong, independent predictor of long-term survival even when controlled for pTNM criteria in patients with early-stage disease who have not received neoadjuvant chemotherapy [4].

It seems that endoscopy better determines esophageal tumor length than other imaging modalities, and perhaps disease length and tumor volume defined by endoluminal ultrasound could add further value [5].

2.2 Cases and Discussions

2.2.1 Mediastinum

2.2.1.1 Aortic Aneurysms

The aorta is typically ignored by endosonographers. However, even transaortic EUS-guided biopsies have been done successfully [6]. Here we demonstrate an aorta with calcified plaques and an aneurysm with clot. Segmental arteries are shown in Chap. 1 (posterior intercostal arteries). The practical point is that transaortic biopsies should probably not be done through a clot/aneurysm or heavily calcified plaque to avoid a showering of cholesterol emboli.

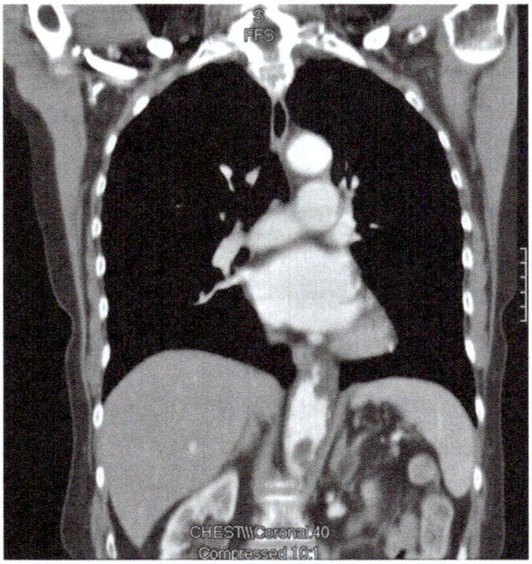

Fig. 2.1 This coronal computed tomography reconstruction shows plaque and clot

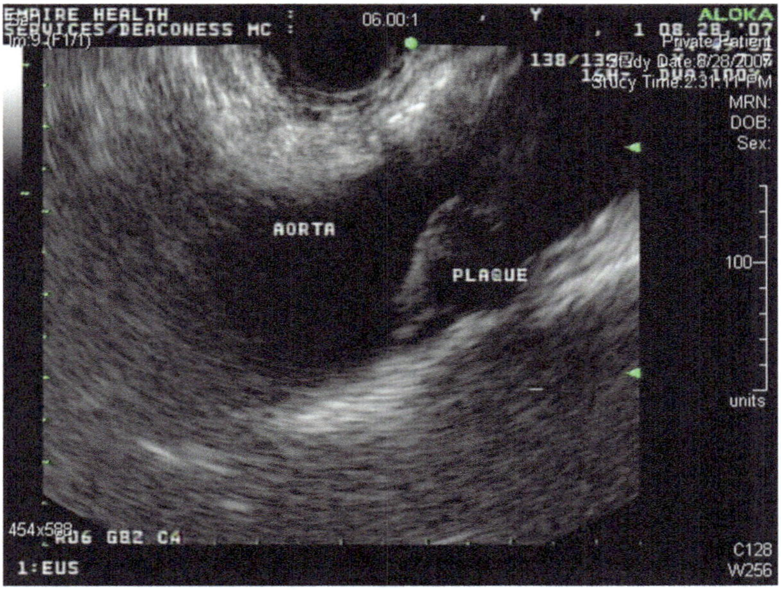

Fig. 2.2 This calcified plaque seems to correspond to the lesion seen more distally in the abdominal aorta on the reconstructed computed tomography scan

2.2.1.2 Aortic Dissection

Aortic dissections are infrequently observed during EUS. This is a 74-year-old patient with a type A chronic aortic dissection who was referred for esophageal cancer staging. The DeBakey classification scheme (I, II, or III) is based on the location of the intimal tear and the extension of the false lumen, whereas in the Stanford classification type A indicates involvement of the ascending aorta and type B indicates no involvement of the ascending aorta.

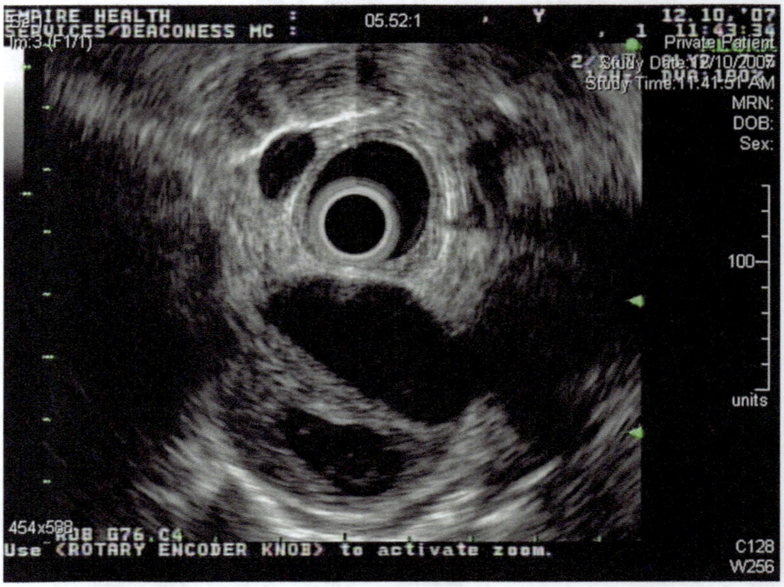

Fig. 2.3 This radial endoscopic ultrasound image shows the thoracic aorta in cross section with two lumina, one of which is false

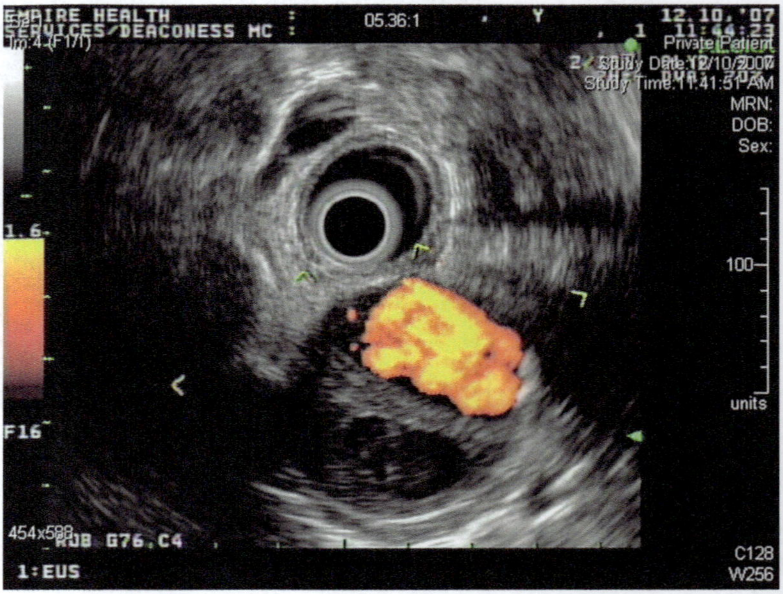

Fig. 2.4 Power Doppler clarifies the location of the true and false lumen in this type A (Stanford classification) aortic dissection

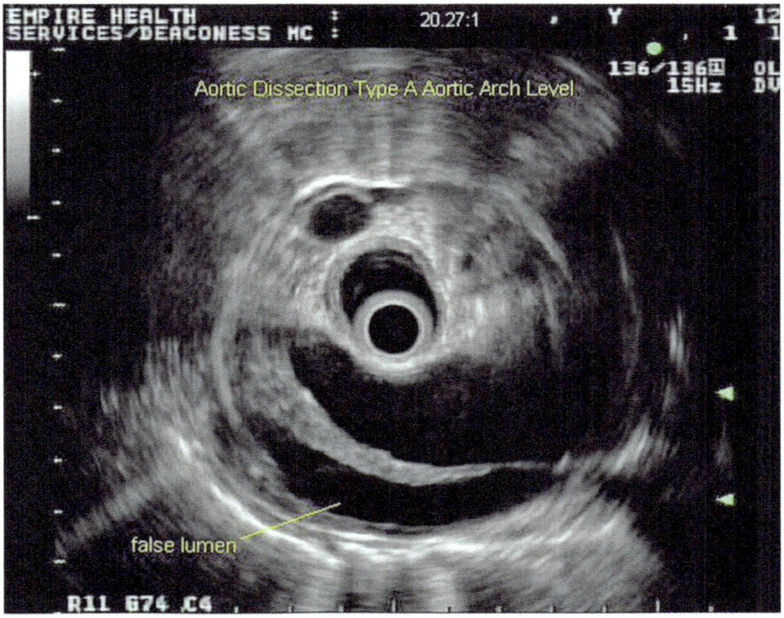

Fig. 2.5 This is the same aorta as in Fig. 2.4 at the level of the aortic arch. The true lumen is next to the esophagus

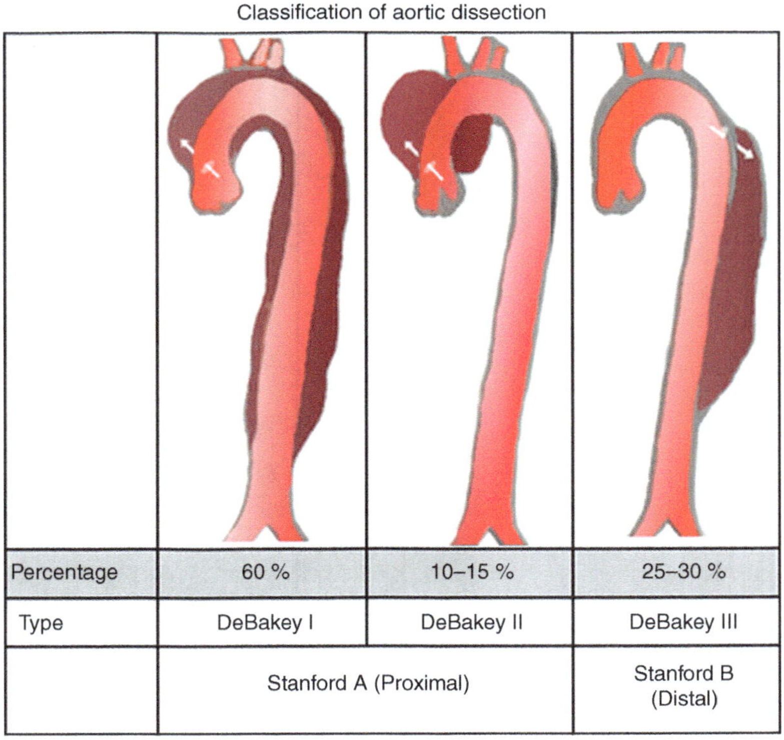

Percentage	60 %	10–15 %	25–30 %
Type	DeBakey I	DeBakey II	DeBakey III
	Stanford A (Proximal)		Stanford B (Distal)

Fig. 2.6 Stanford type A means involvement of the ascending aorta, whereas type B indicates no involvement of the ascending aorta (From Wikimedia Commons)

2.2.1.3 New Pulmonary Emboli, Aortic Dissection, and Right Heart Strain

This sequence of images describes pulsatile bidirectional flow in the azygos vein as a sign of right heart strain in the same 74-year-old patient discussed above, who was referred for EUS evaluation of esophageal cancer. Four months earlier she had almost died when she presented with a type A aortic dissection, which was emergently repaired. Doppler EUS shows true and false aortic lumina together with flow in the false channel. To complete staging of her esophageal cancer, a CT scan was done immediately following the EUS exam. CT of the chest revealed new bilateral pulmonary emboli, which were thought to be the likely cause of her disturbed regurgitant azygos flow seen on Doppler endosonography. For didactic purposes the CT scans are shown first, followed by the EUS images. Azygos vein diameters have been correlated with outcomes in cases of pulmonary embolus [7]. Another important and more frequently seen cause of enlarged azygos veins and increased flow rates is, of course, portal hypertension [8].

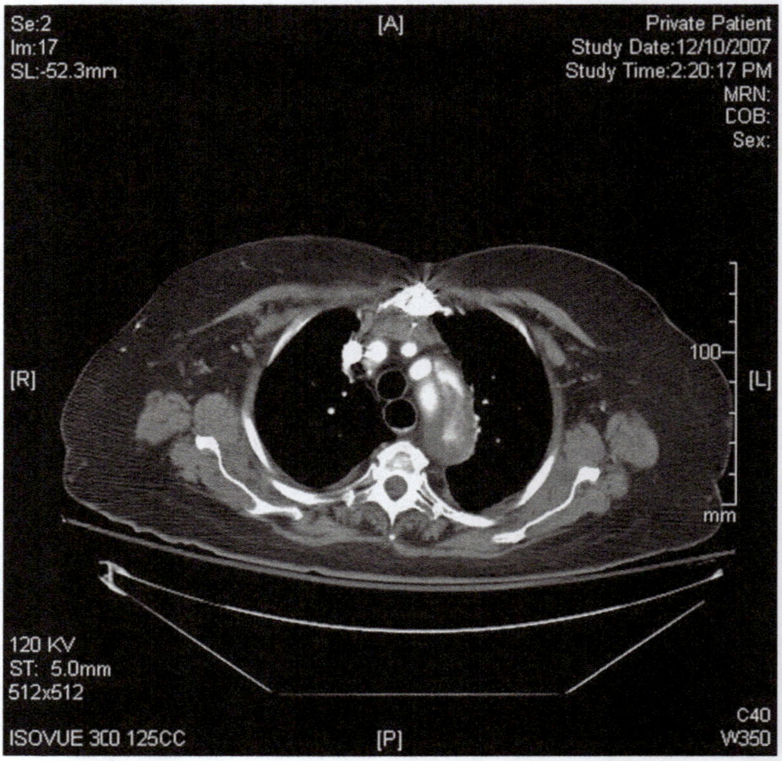

Fig. 2.7 This computed tomography scan shows flow in the true and false lumen in this chronic type A aortic dissection

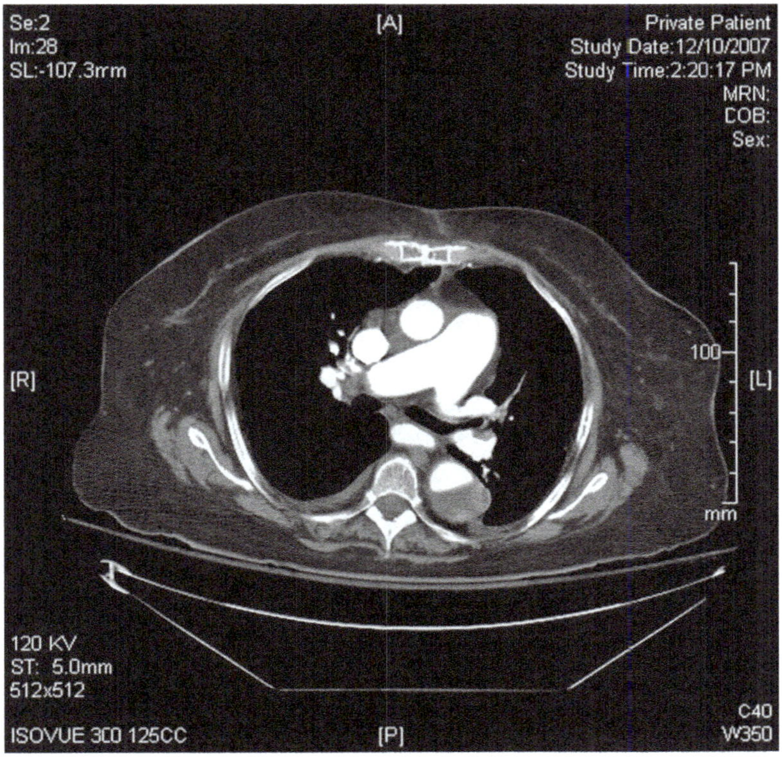

Fig. 2.8 The computed tomography scan performed for esophageal cancer staging shows new bilateral pulmonary artery emboli (only right side shown)

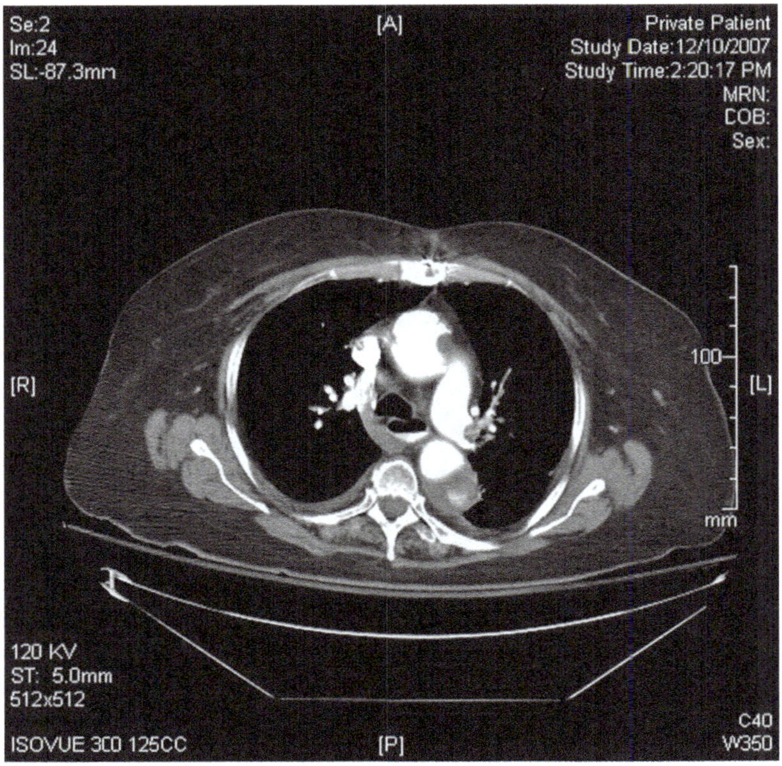

Fig. 2.9 Azygos vein reflux from the superior vena cava is seen on this slice. It commonly represents right heart strain but can sometimes be seen in healthy individuals

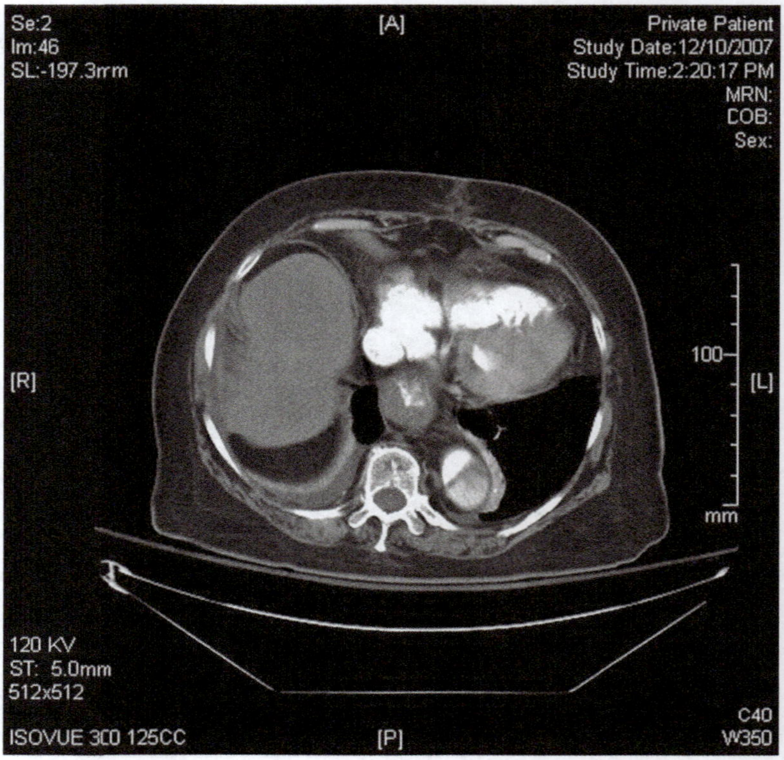

Fig. 2.10 This slice shows thickening of the distal esophageal wall. Note the continuation of the aortic dissection into the abdominal aorta

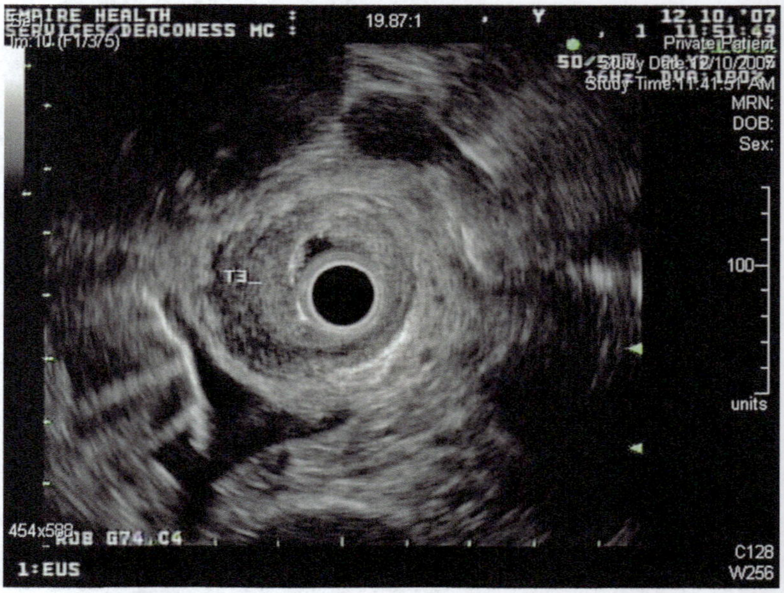

Fig. 2.11 Endoscopic ultrasound shows a T3 adenocarcinoma of the distal esophagus but no apparent lymphadenopathy. A pleural effusion is also present

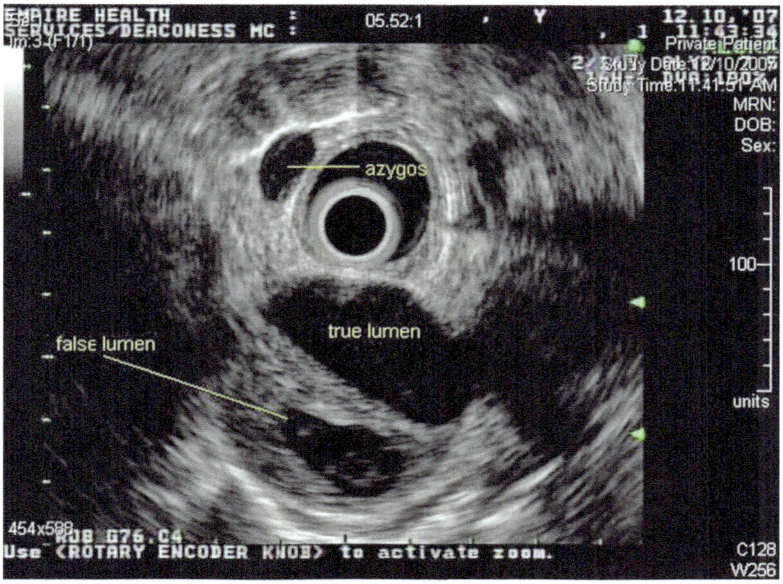

Fig. 2.12 This image with the GF-UE160 electronic radial echogastroscope shows true and false lumen of the descending aorta and a prominent azygos vein

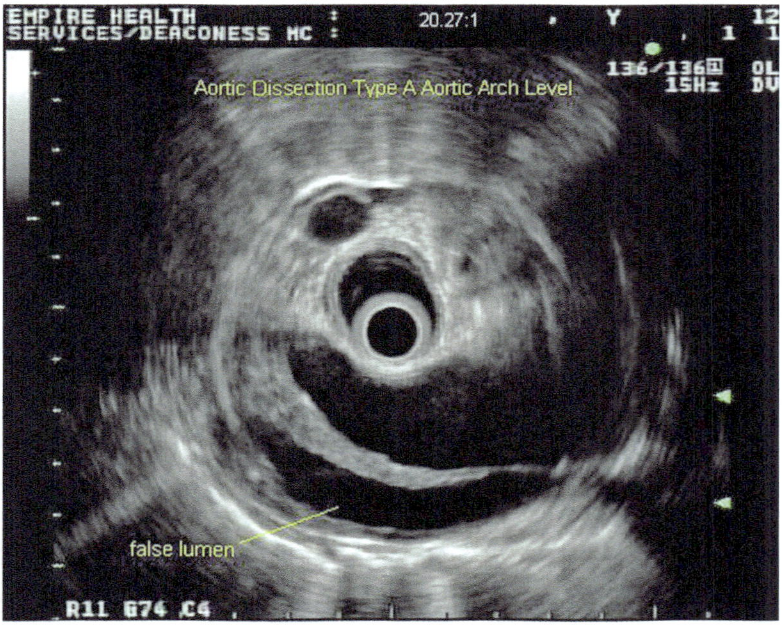

Fig. 2.13 This endoscopic ultrasound image shows the dissection at the level of the aortic arch

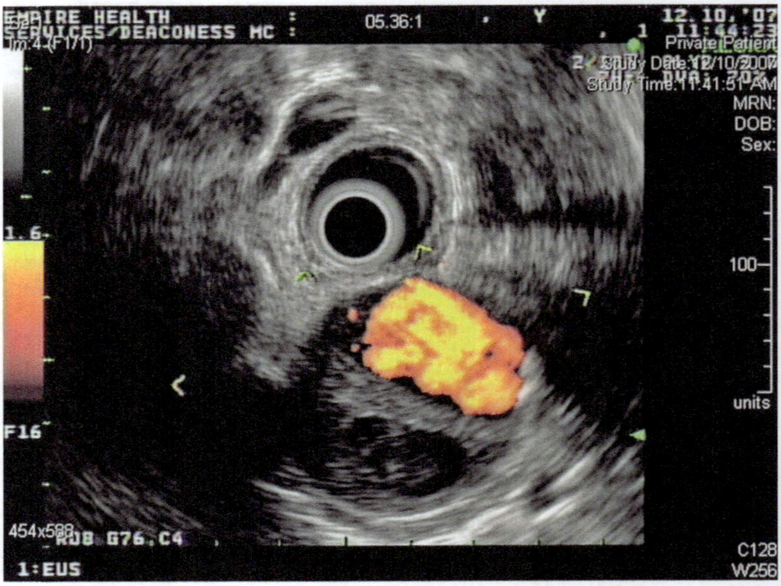

Fig. 2.14 The aortic dissection investigated with power Doppler. The Doppler gate is not positioned to show flow in the false channel

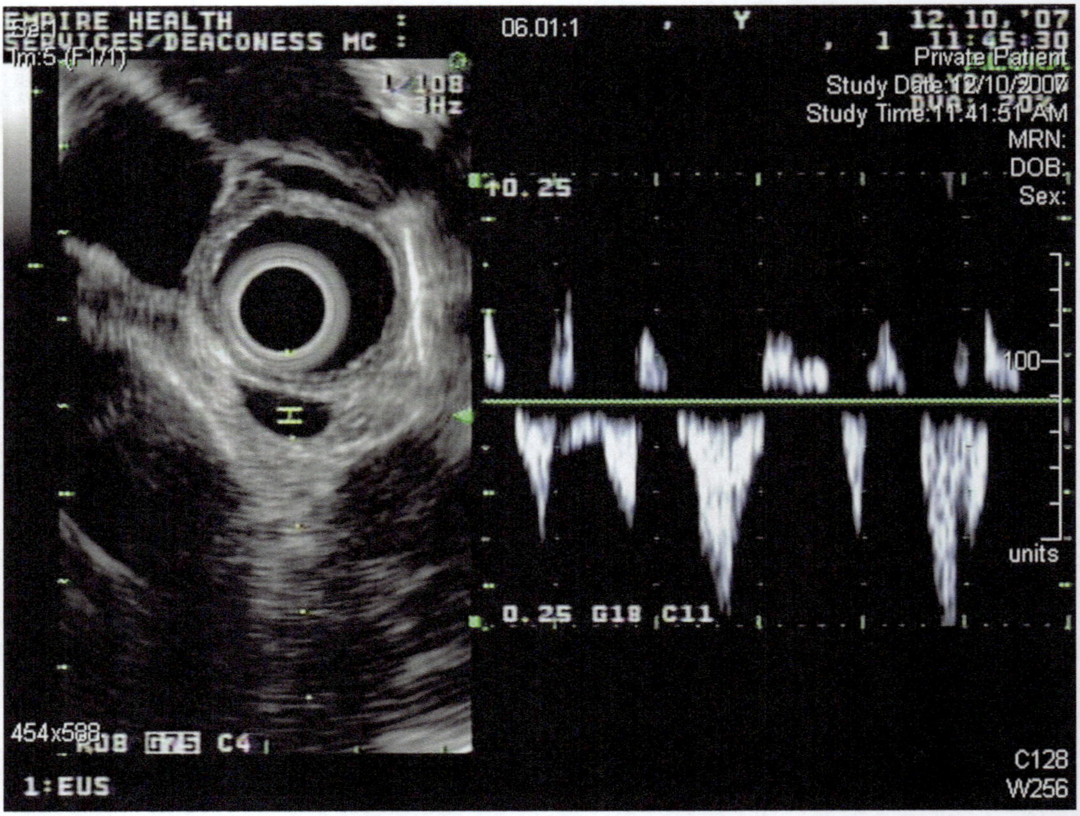

Fig. 2.15 This image shows pulsatile complete reversal of flow in the azygos vein (azygos reflux, bidirectional flow), reflecting right heart strain from the pulmonary embolism

2.2.1.4 Subcarinal Lymph Node Biopsy

EUS-guided FNA has high sensitivity, specificity, and diagnostic accuracy that is comparable to mediastinoscopy and transbronchial FNA, and it allows sampling of nodes that cannot be easily accessed by other methods. This is a 65-year-old patient who presented 10 months earlier with atelectasis of his left lower lobe of the lung. Noninvasive staging revealed that the cancer was resectable. During surgery it was found to be a T2N1 lesion. Unfortunately, 10 months after the surgery a CT scan of the chest showed a subcarinal lymph node suspicious for recurrent disease. Bronchoscopic evaluation was negative or nondiagnostic. EUS-guided FNA was performed, and cytology confirmed recurrent adenocarcinoma EUS-guided FNA of American Thoracic Society area 7 (subcarinal) and area 5 (aortopulmonary window) lymph nodes is easy but is unfortunately underused.

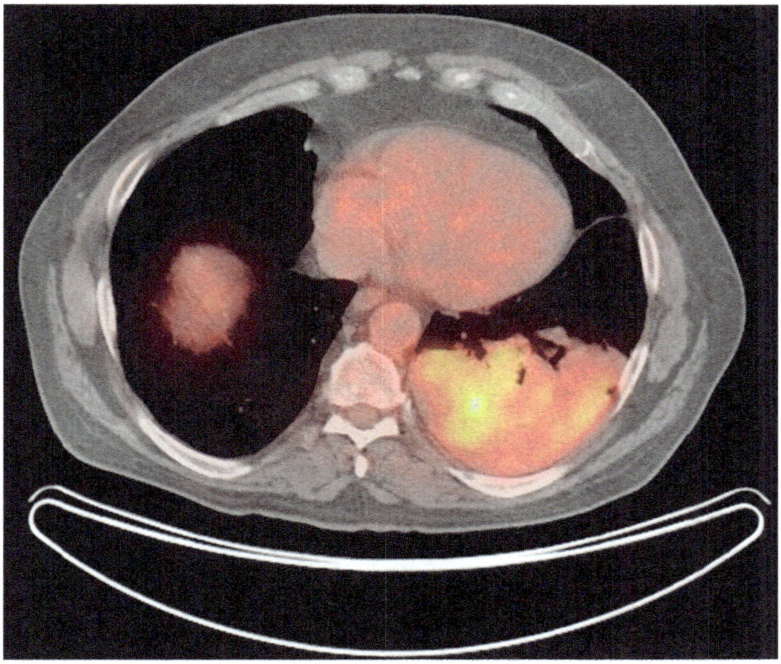

Fig. 2.16 Positron emission tomography scan shows the original cancer in the left lower lobe of the lung

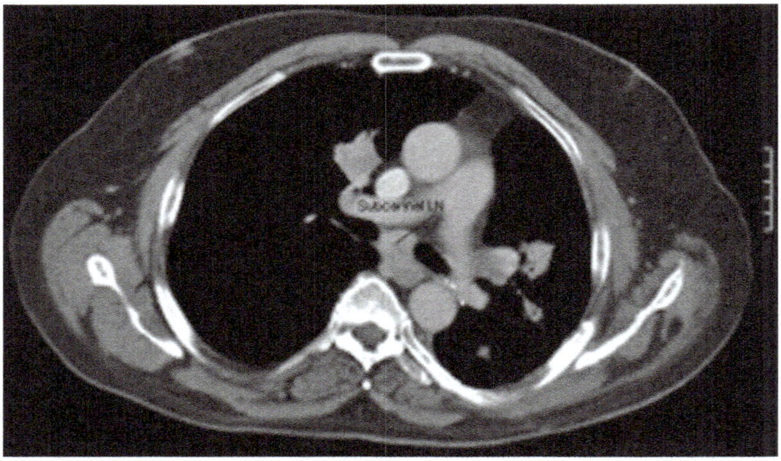

Fig. 2.17 Ten months later, subcarinal lymphadenopathy (*LN*) is seen

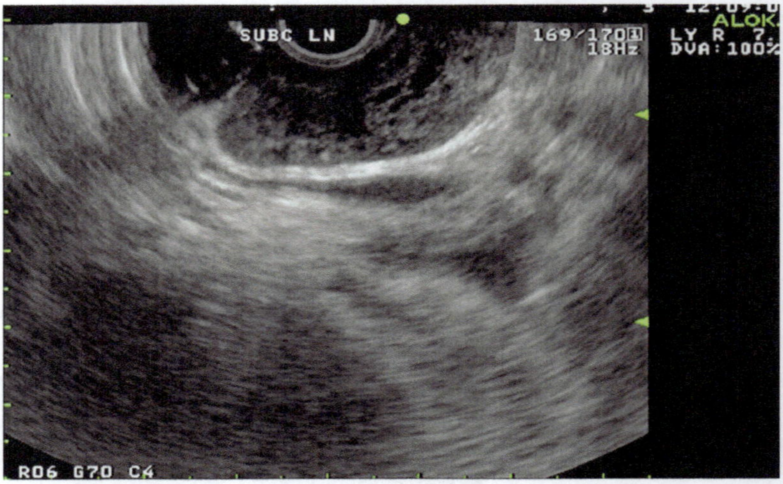

Fig. 2.18 Endoscopic ultrasound shows a large partially necrotic lymph node

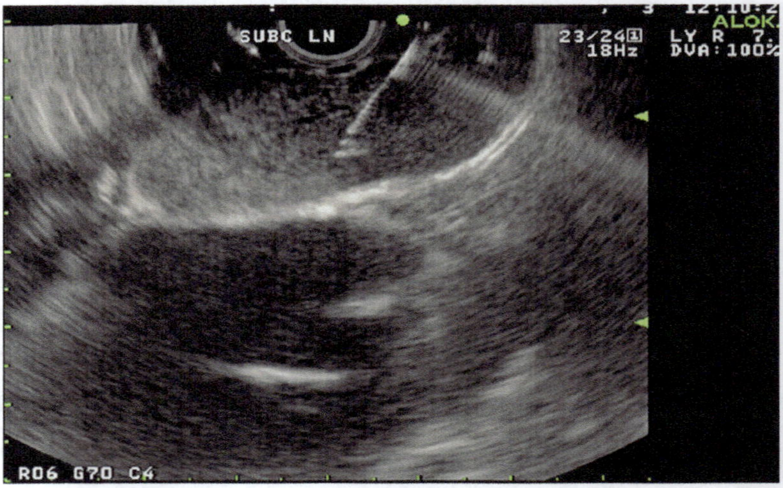

Fig. 2.19 Fine-needle aspiration

2.2.1.5 Biopsies of Upper Paratracheal Lymph Nodes: Melanoma or Lymphoma?

This is a 74-year-old patient who generally feels well but developed a lump in his neck, which he noticed while shaving. Initial percutaneous FNA biopsy was suspicious for neoplasm but essentially nondiagnostic. A modified radical neck dissection was performed, which revealed the simultaneous presence of mantle cell lymphoma and amelanotic melanoma in the same lymph nodes, confirmed by outside consultation. EUS was performed to biopsy a large right-sided upper paratracheal lymph node to determine whether this station was affected by melanoma or lymphoma. Only lymphoma cells were seen.

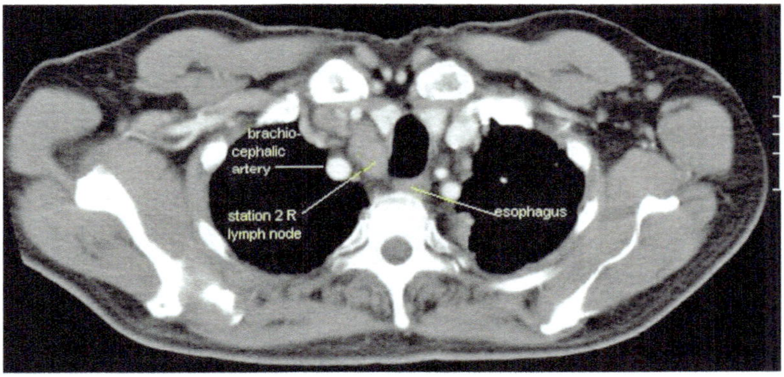

Fig. 2.20 This patient with coexisting mantle cell lymphoma and metastatic melanoma found in lymph nodes of the neck also had enlarged upper paratracheal lymph nodes

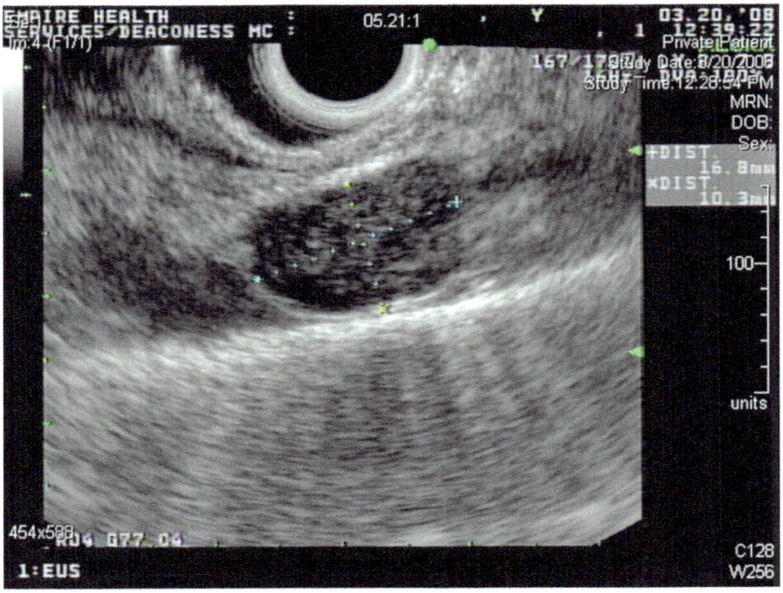

Fig. 2.21 This is the endoscopic ultrasound view of the 2R lymph node

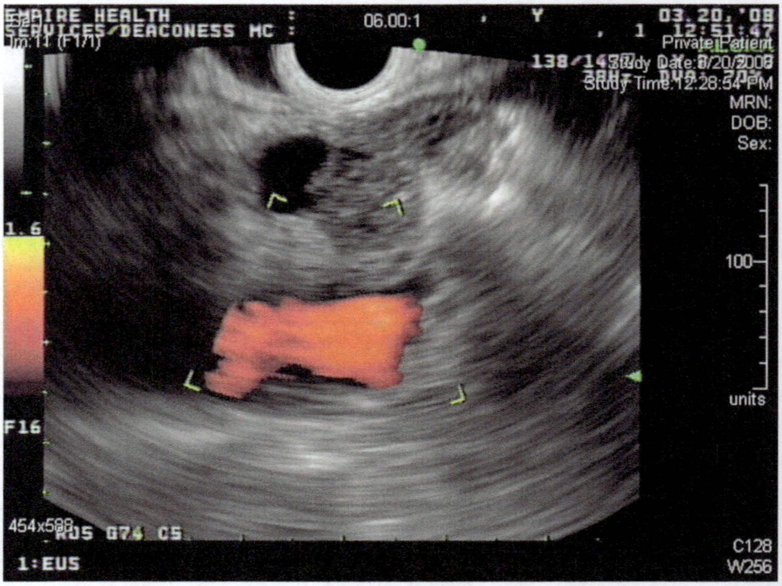

Fig. 2.22 This initially appeared to be a necrotic cervical lymph 3 cm proximal to the 2R lymph node. The carotid is shown

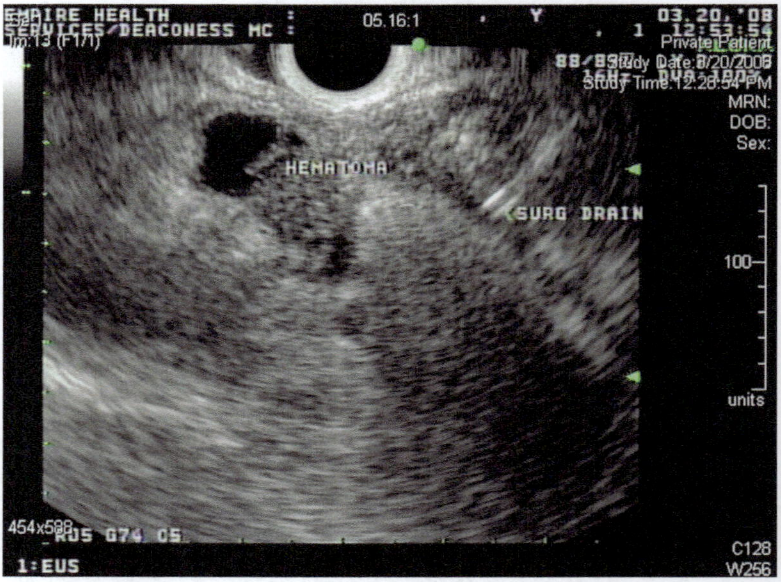

Fig. 2.23 A closer look at this "lymph node" reveals its irregular features and a surgical drain close by. Given the fact that a neck dissection had jut been performed the day before this EUS, a small hematoma is the most likely explanation

2.2.1.6 Recurrent Hodgkin's Lymphoma

This 14-year-old boy was diagnosed with a nodular sclerosing type Hodgkin's lymphoma 2 years earlier. He had cervical lymphadenopathy. He finished treatment 6 months later and had a comprehensive follow-up examination 2 years after the first diagnosis. He was feeling well but had several mediastinal hot spots on a positron emission tomography scan. The pediatric oncologist referred him for EUS-guided FNA as the least invasive modality to make a diagnosis. If positive for recurrent disease the patient would need to undergo high-dose chemotherapy and a bone marrow transplant. The EUS-guided FNA was positive for two different lymph node groups: subcarinal and aortopulmonary window.

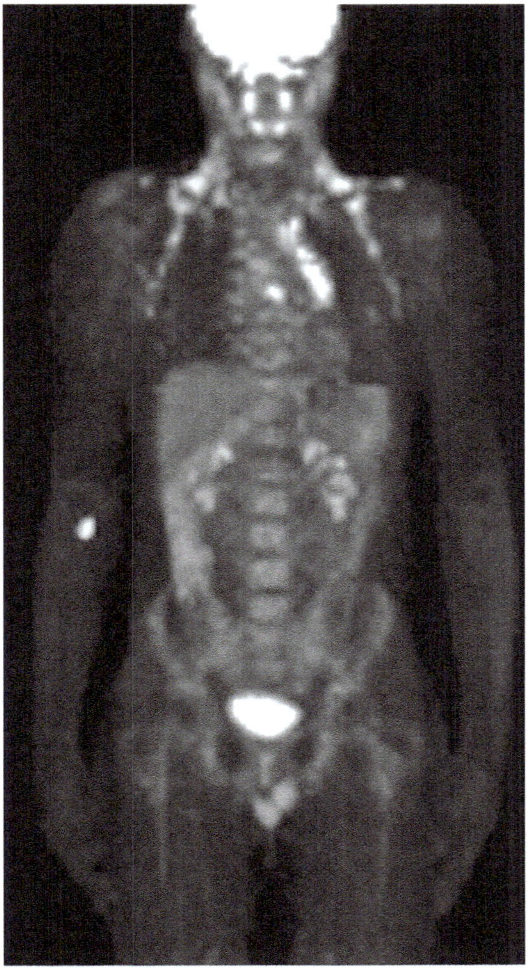

Fig. 2.24 Several hot spots in the mediastinum are suspicious for recurrent Hodgkin's disease

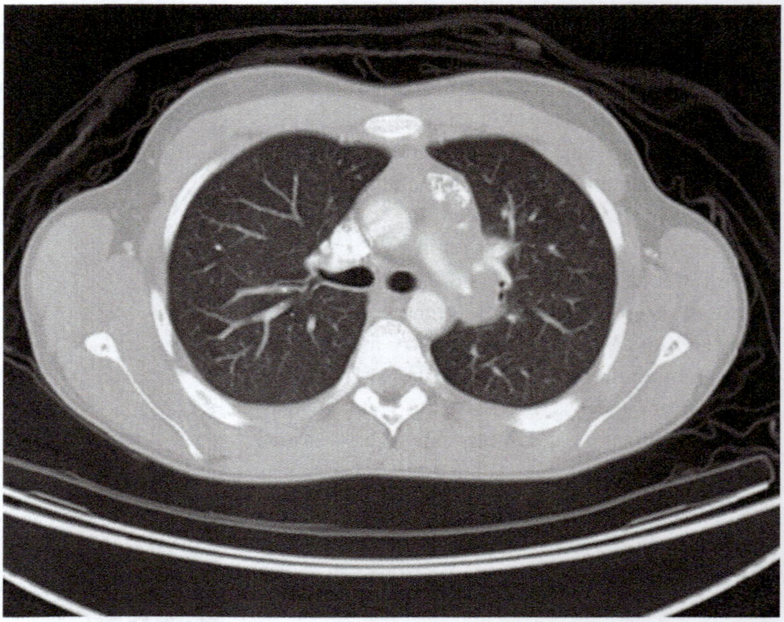

Fig. 2.25 A computed tomography scan shows a white-out between the subcarina and the spine. Individual structures are difficult to determine

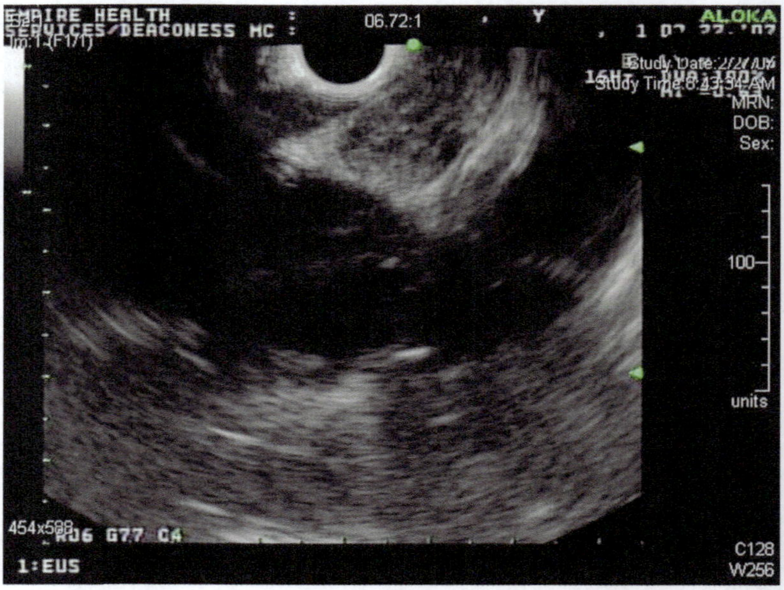

Fig. 2.26 Linear endoscopic ultrasound shows a rather unimpressive subcarinal lymph node with a short-axis dimension of barely 10 mm

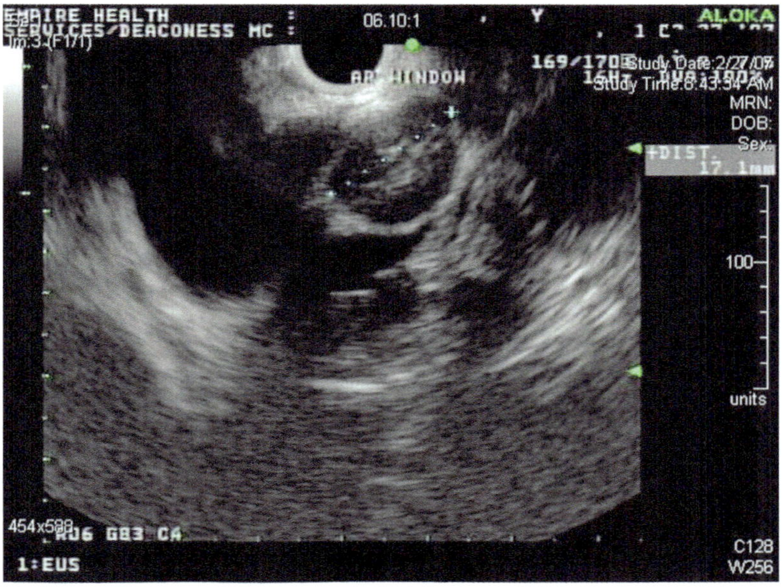

Fig. 2.27 This is an enlarged aortopulmonary (*AP*) window lymph node. Biopsies were difficult and the aspirate repeatedly "dry"

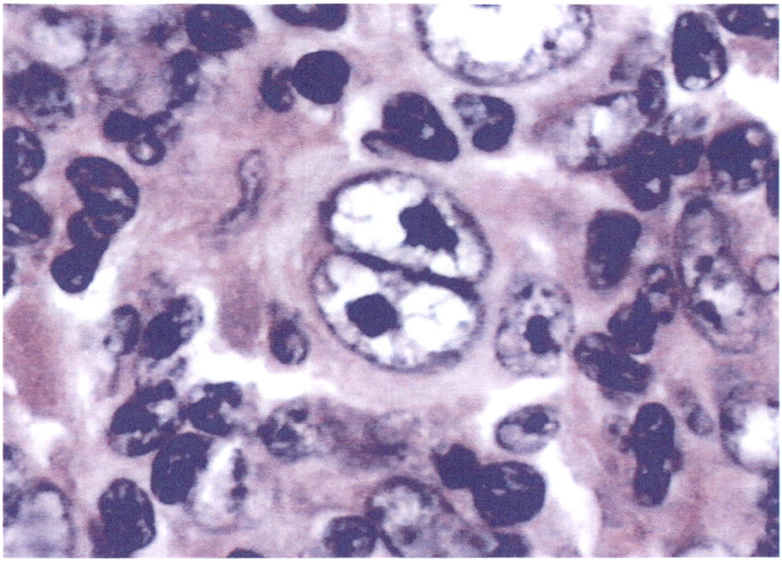

Fig. 2.28 The cytology was positive both for the subcarinal and aortopulmonary window lymph nodes, showing Reed-Sternberg cells and a compatible immunohistochemistry

2.2.1.7 Bronchial Carcinoid

This case illustrates the principle that lesions that are distant to the esophagus on static cross-sectional imaging may still be amenable to biopsy through a flexible esophagus. This is a 74-year-old woman with cirrhosis of the liver who was incidentally found to have a centrally located lung tumor on an abdominal CT scan. She was referred for EUS-guided FNA, which revealed cytology characteristic of a bronchial carcinoid. Bronchial carcinoids are tumors that, depending on the subtype, may have relatively low-grade malignant potential associated with slow growth and a corresponding favorable prognosis [9]. In view of the patient's comorbidities, no further treatment was planned.

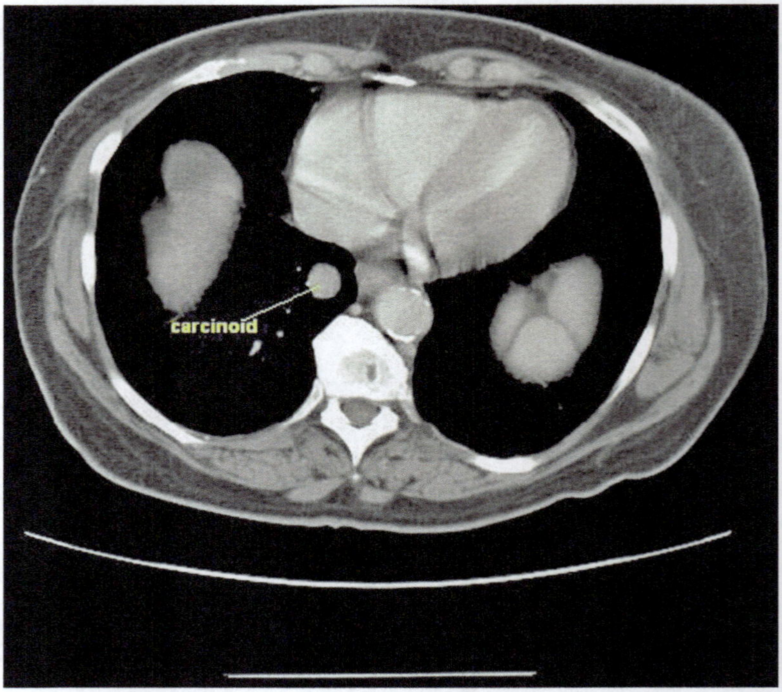

Fig. 2.29 This chest computed tomography shows a small mass in the right lower lobe. Note the intervening normal lung between the lesion and the esophagus

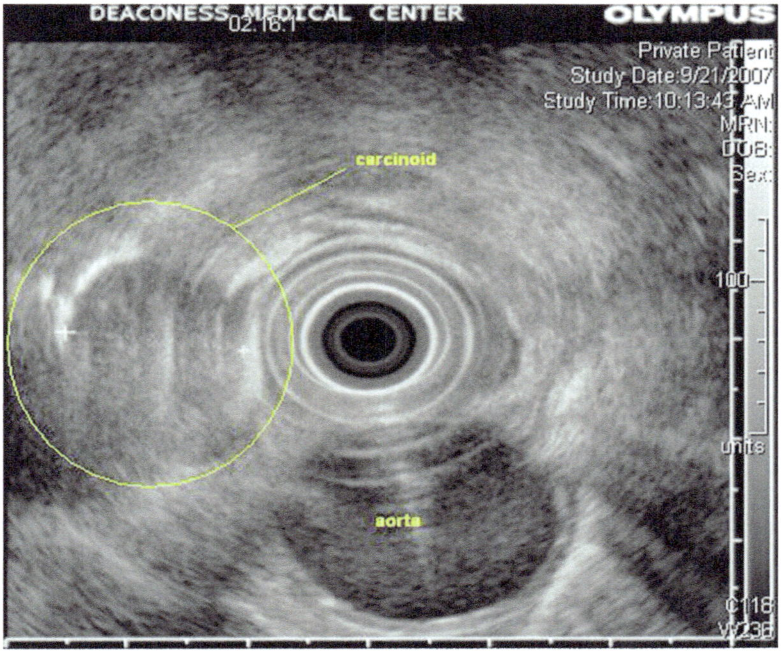

Fig. 2.30 The tumor can be seen on the radial endoscopic ultrasound image despite the intervening normal lung

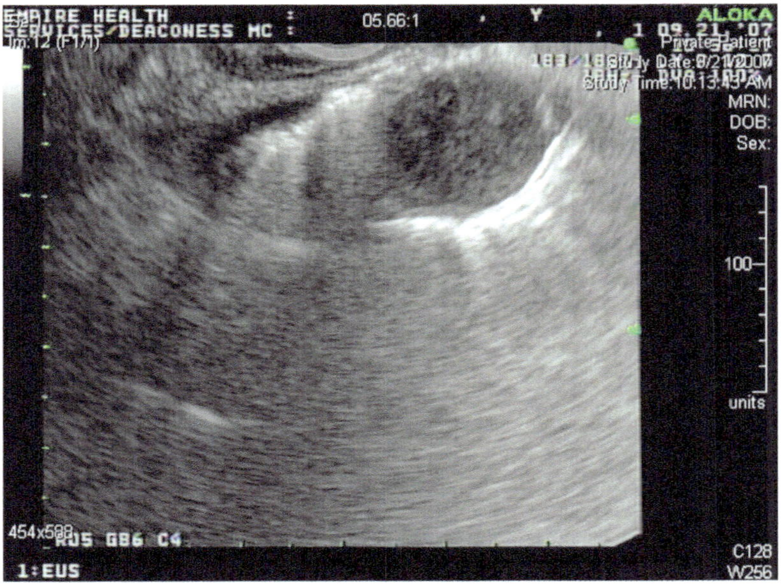

Fig. 2.31 Visualization of the lesion was better with the electronic curved-linear array echoendoscope. Note the echo pattern of normal lung

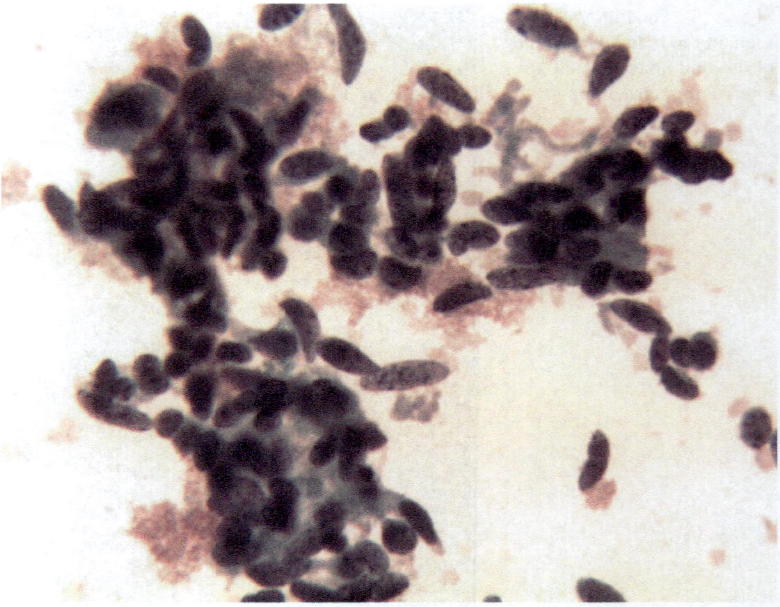

Fig. 2.32 A concentrated smear (magnification ×40) using a Pap stain shows spindle cells, friable cytoplasm, and elongated oval nuclei in clusters and as single cells (image courtesy of Vann Schaffner, MD)

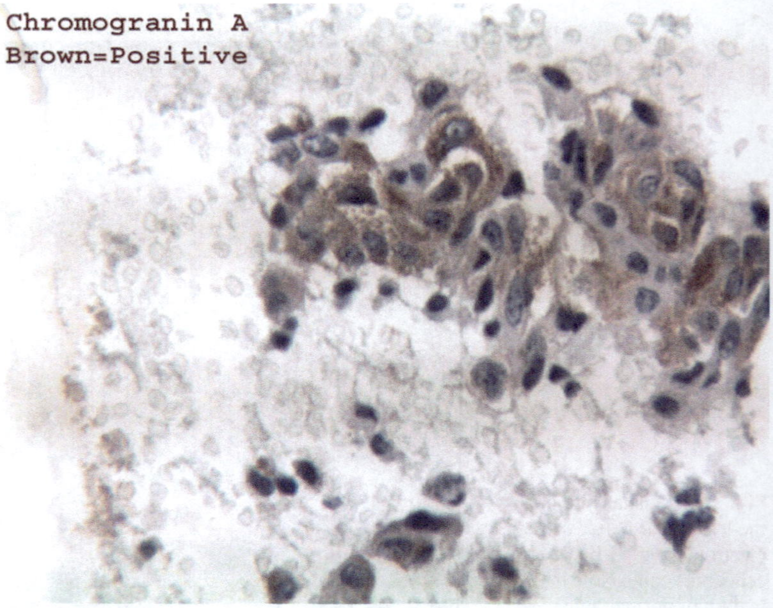

Fig. 2.33 A cytokeratin 7 immunostain demonstrates cytoplasmic positivity and proves epithelial differentiation. Chromogranin A and synaptophysin also are focally positive, showing neuroendocrine differentiation (image courtesy of Vann Schaffner, MD)

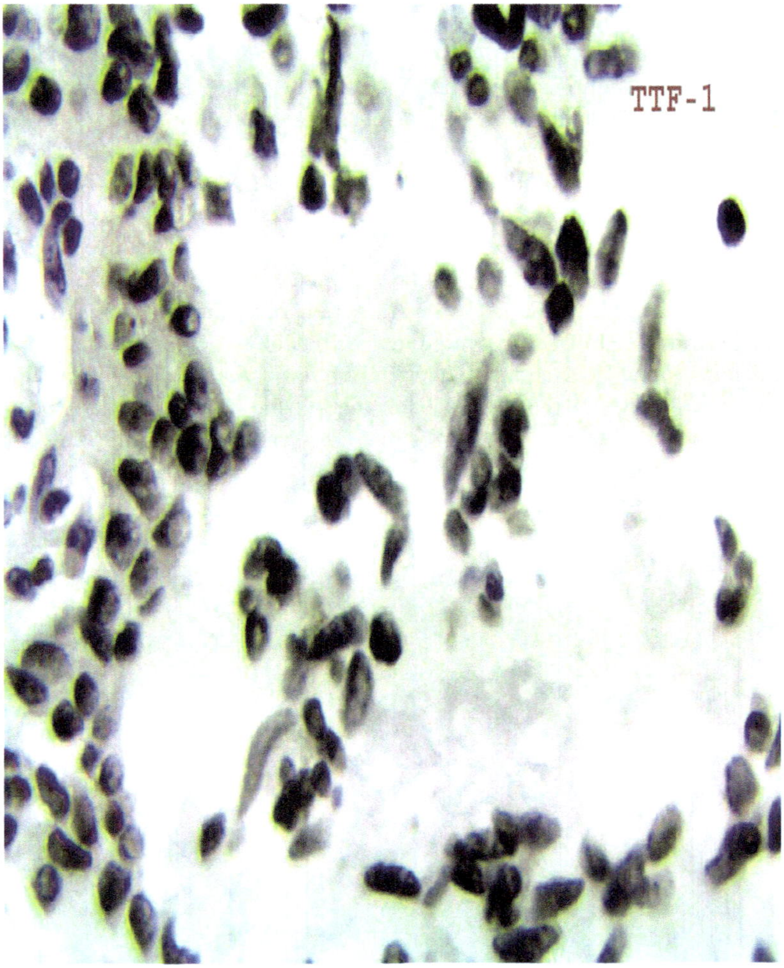

Fig. 2.34 The thyroid transcription faction (TTF)-1 immunostain shows nuclear positivity, strongly supporting lung origin. CDX2 was negative, arguing against a metastatic intestinal carcinoid (image courtesy of Vann Schaffner, MD)

2.2.1.8 Bronchogenic Cysts

Bronchogenic cysts are uncommon and represent a cystic reduplication of the bronchial tree. They are most frequent in the mediastinum; if present in the lung parenchyma they may represent a form of pulmonary sequestration. If asymptomatic, as they mostly are, they are best left alone [10].

This is a 60-year-old patient who was incidentally found to have a large cystic structure in her mediastinum. She had no symptoms attributable to the lesion. EUS and possible FNA biopsies were requested. In this case we felt that all the imaging was consistent with that diagnosis and we did not pursue FNA biopsies because of the risk of infection [10].

In contrast to the above case, this 36-year-old otherwise healthy patient was symptomatic, with a 2-year history of dyspepsia and chest pain. Endoscopy was unremarkable. A CT scan of the chest was eventually obtained (see Fig. 2.38) and showed a mediastinal mass. EUS revealed classic features of a bronchogenic cyst. The material inside the cyst appeared pasty with bright echogenic "floaters." Again, the imaging features were characteristic of bronchogenic cysts, no biopsies were performed, and the patient was referred to a thoracic surgeon.

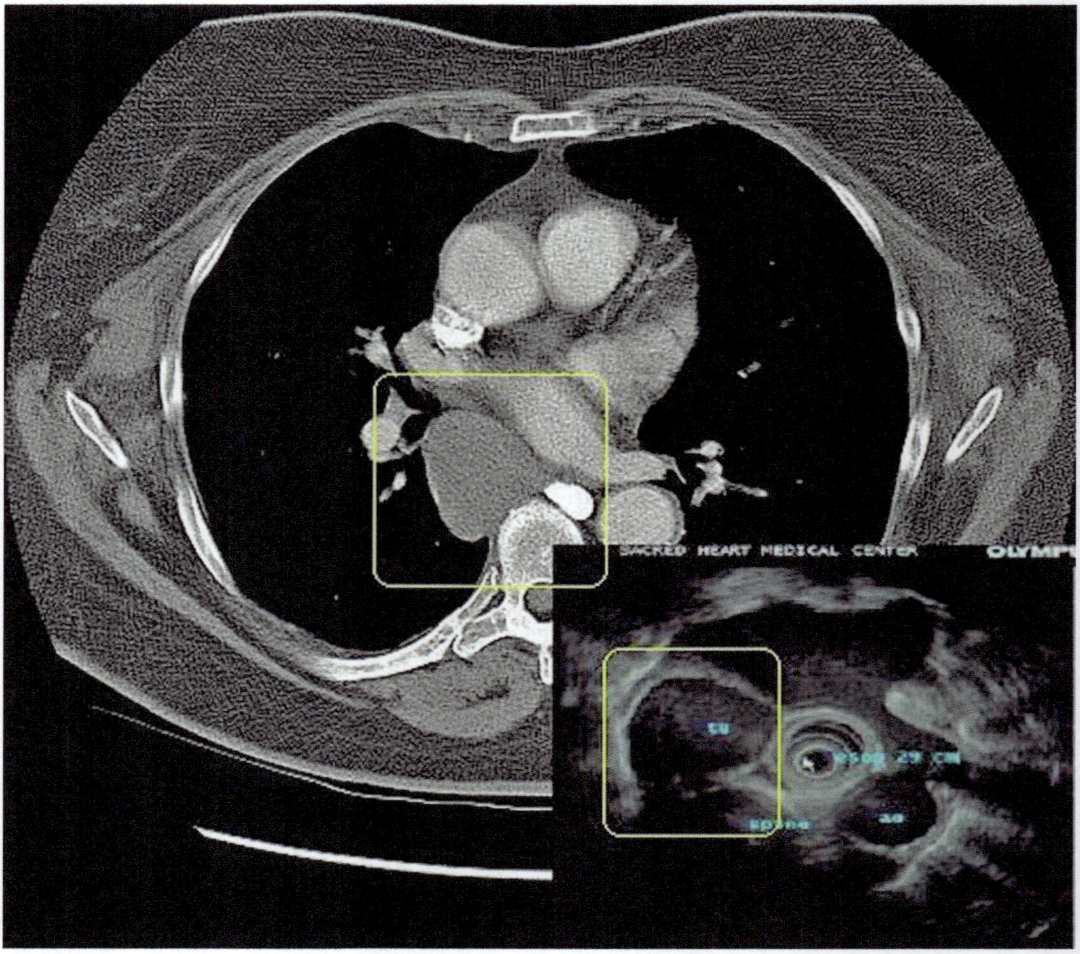

Fig. 2.35 This is a patient with a 4-cm-diameter mediastinal cyst adjacent to the esophagus. A computed tomography scan is shown with an endoscopic ultrasound image inset

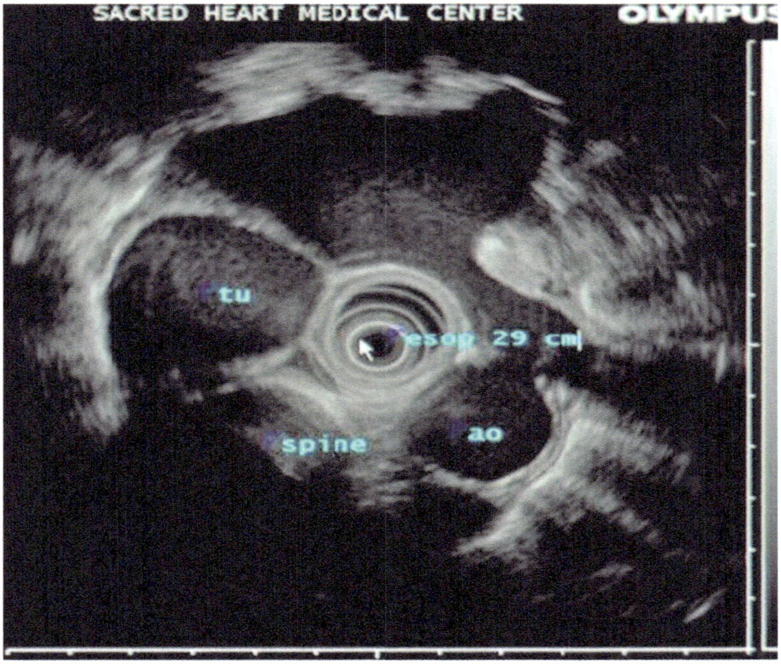

Fig. 2.36 This endoscopic ultrasound image is a larger version of the one shown in Fig. 2.35. The cyst is somewhat misleadingly labeled *tu*. *AO esoph* esophagus

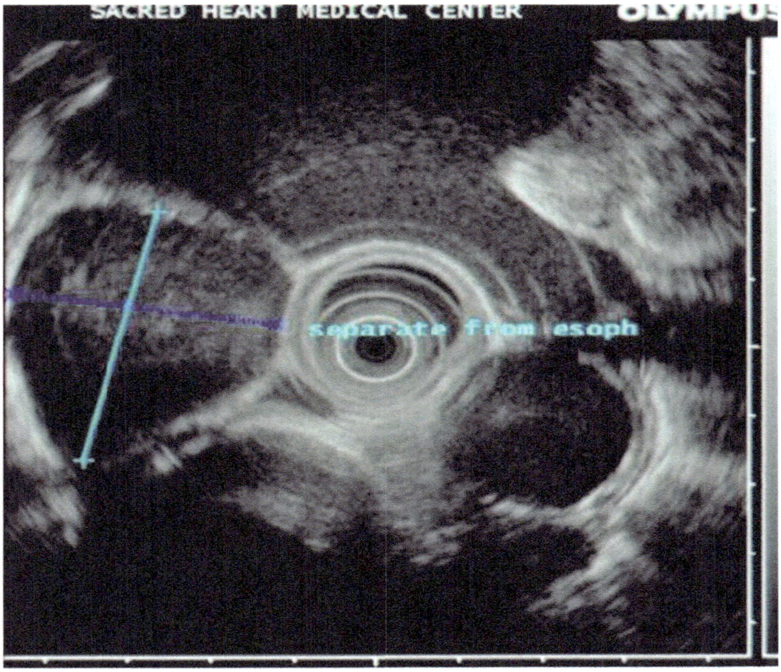

Fig. 2.37 As can be seen on this endoscopic ultrasound image, the 4-cm-diameter structure is not an esophageal duplication cyst but has the classic appearance of a bronchogenic cyst. *esoph* esophagus

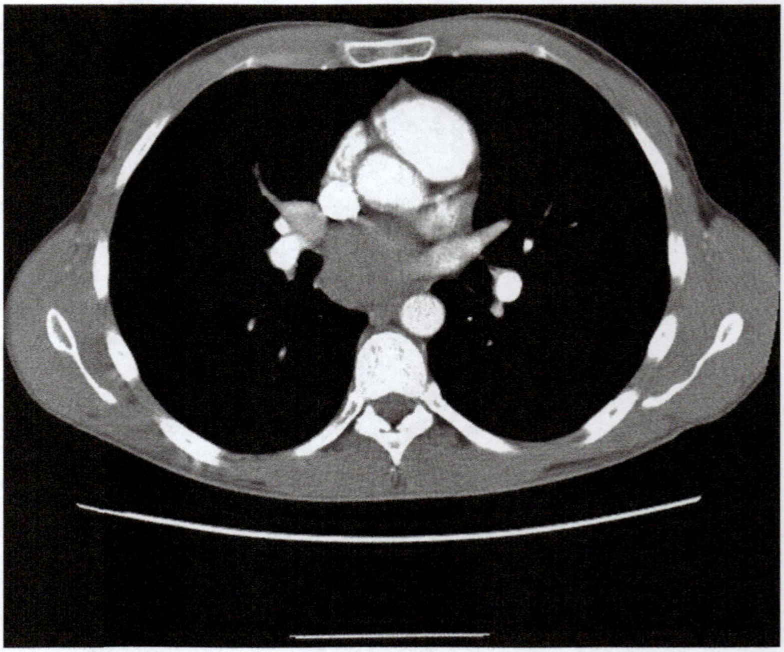

Fig. 2.38 A mediastinal mass with low Hounsfield units on computed tomography

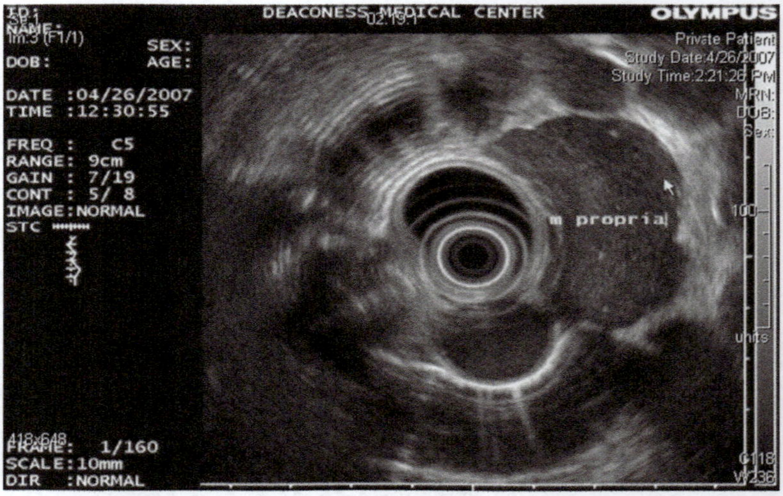

Fig. 2.39 The same mediastinal mass as seen on endoscopic ultrasound is not arising from the esophagus. It has the typical appearance of a bronchogenic cyst

2.2.1.9 Mediastinal Pseudocyst

Mediastinal pseudocysts are rare; only approximately 50 cases are described in the world literature. Obviously, there are no standardized treatment approaches. It is thought that mediastinal pseudocysts develop after rupture of the pancreatic duct posteriorly into the retroperitoneal space. In most cases the pancreatic fluid enters the mediastinum through the esophageal or aortic hiatus. Therapeutic options include surgery with internal or external drainage of the pseudocysts (cystogastrostomy and cystoenterostomy); percutaneous, transpapillary, transgastric and transesophageal endoscopic drainage; and conservative management [11]. This is a 36-year-old patient with a history of alcohol abuse and recurrent pancreatitis who complained of chest pain. Conservative treatment was thought to be the best initial option.

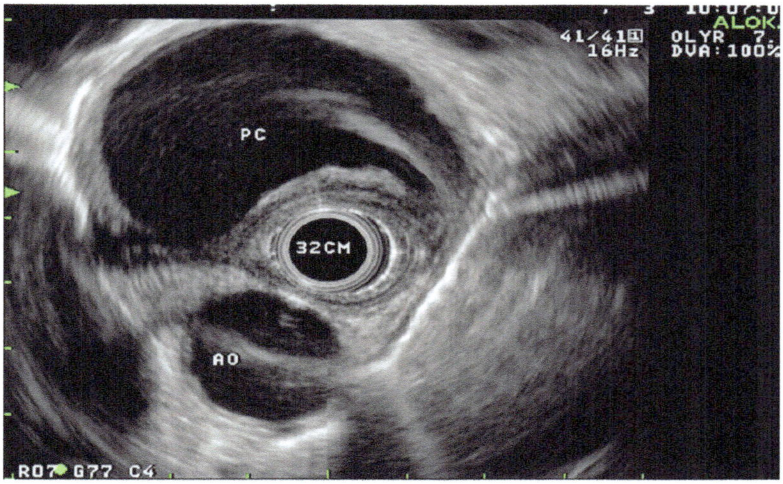

Fig. 2.40 This endoscopic ultrasound image shows the mediastinal pseudocyst (*PC*) anterior to the esophagus, with the aorta (*AO*) in the 7 o'clock position 32 cm from the incisors

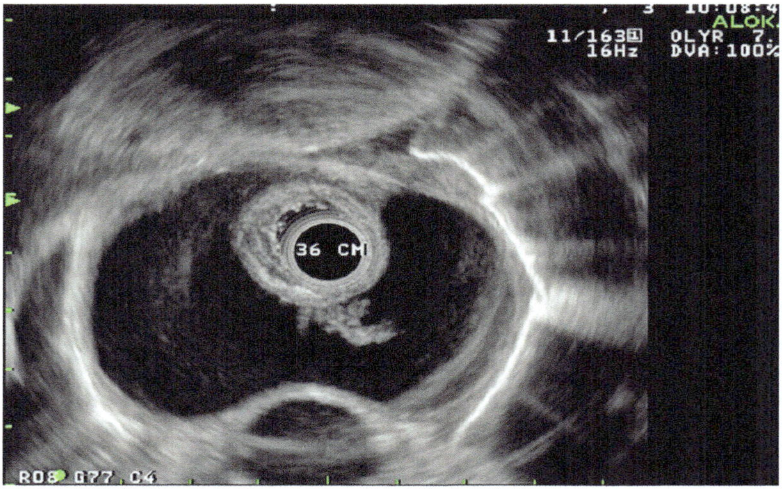

Fig. 2.41 The pseudocyst wraps around the esophagus more distally (at 36 cm from the incisors) and is mostly posterior, abutting the aorta

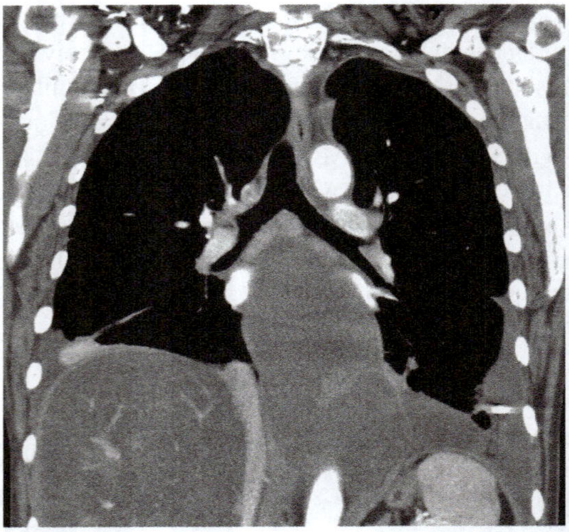

Fig. 2.42 This coronally reformatted computed tomography scan shows the extent of the pseudocyst

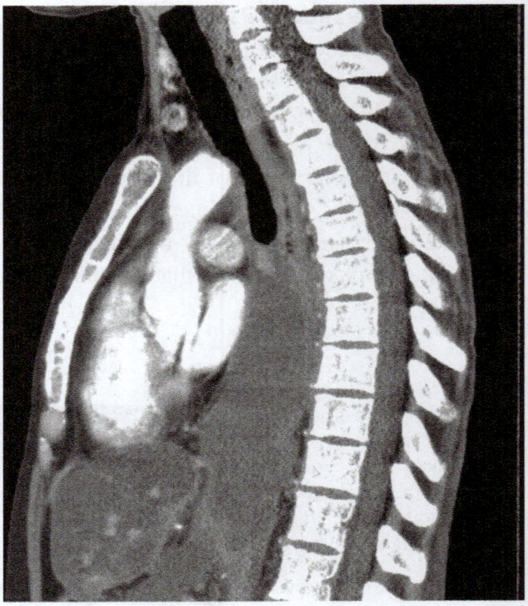

Fig. 2.43 A sagittal computed tomography scan of the same mediastinal pseudocyst

2.2.1.10 Mediastinal Plasmacytoma

Plasmacytomas (or plasmocytomas) are a localized proliferation of plasma cells in the bone marrow. They are less frequently seen in extraosseous organs or tissues. Extramedullary plasmacytoma is a rare malignant neoplasm and is especially rare when it arises in the mediastinum. This is a 65-year-old patient with coronary artery disease who developed chest pain that was atypical for ischemia. An echocardiogram was unremarkable except for a mediastinal mass. A CT scan of the chest was obtained. EUS evaluation showed the lower mediastinal tumor shown in Figs. 2.44, 2.45, and 2.46. In contrast to the two preceding cases, the etiology of this mass was unclear, but malignancy was suspected. FNA biopsies were consistent with plasmacytoma. Flow cytometry studies showed plasma cells with kappa light-chain restriction [12]. Treatment with radiation is effective, but 17 to 33 % of cases progress to multiple myeloma [13].

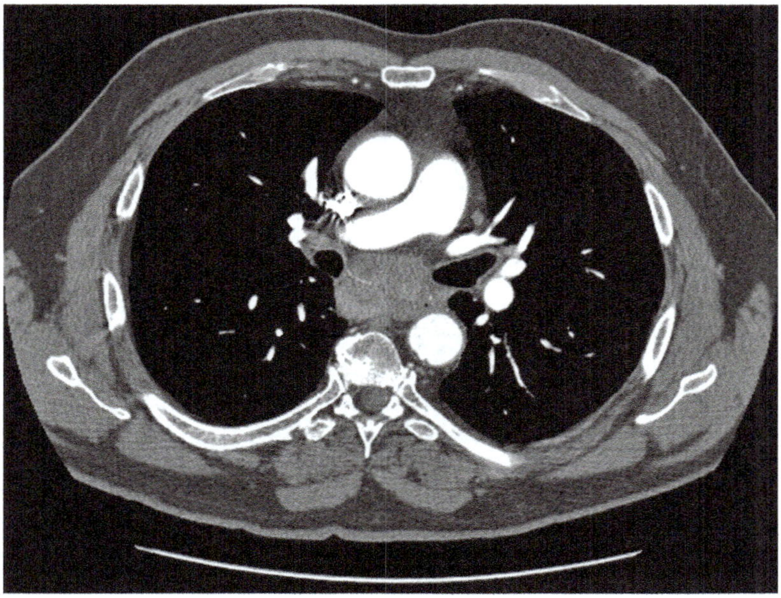

Fig. 2.44 This is a large tumor in the lower mediastinum that turned out to be a plasmacytoma

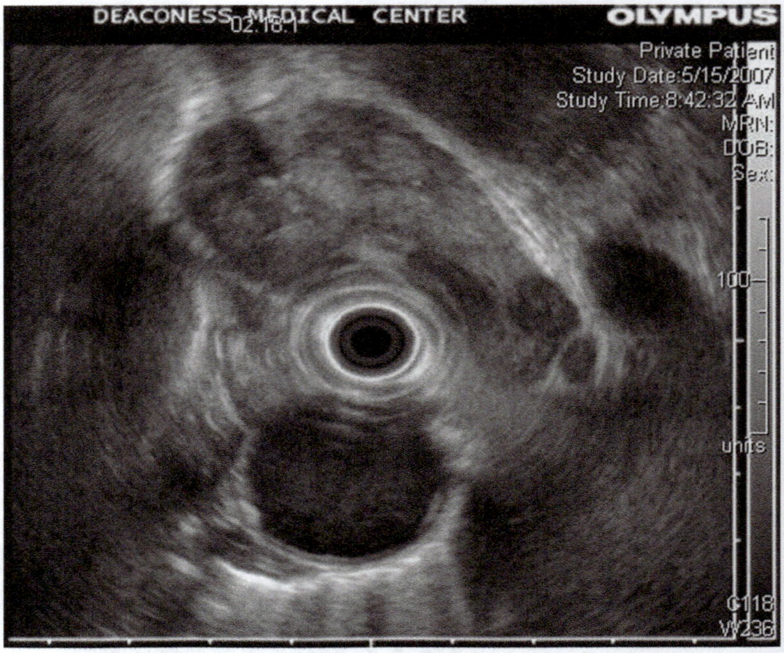

Fig. 2.45 This is the mediastinal plasmacytoma as seen by radial endoscopic ultrasound

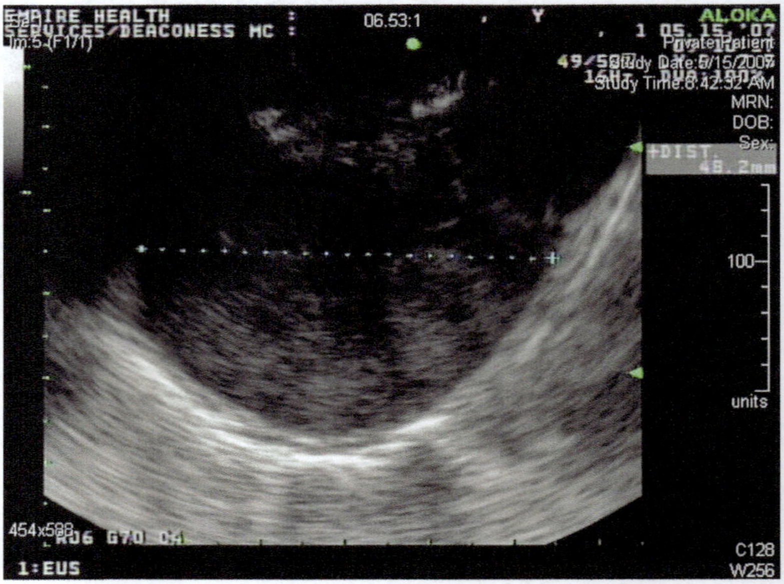

Fig. 2.46 The same mediastinal plasmacytoma seen with linear endoscopic ultrasound before fine-needle aspiration biopsy

2.2.1.11 Posterior Mediastinal Paravertebral Mass

This is a 75-year-old patient with a history of prostate cancer and rising prostate-specific antigen levels who was previously diagnosed with polymyalgia rheumatica. He took steroids for 3 years. He developed chest pain, and after cardiac causes were eliminated, magnetic resonance imaging of the thoracic spine was obtained, which showed a paravertebral mass measuring 6 cm in length and extending from T3 to T6. EUS evaluation and guided biopsies were requested. FNA cytology shows carcinoma cells most consistent with a prostate origin.

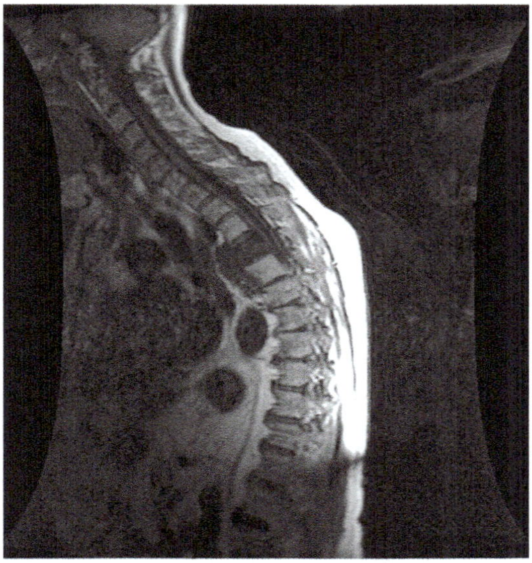

Fig. 2.47 The paraspinal/prevertebral tumor appears to originate from the vertebral body on this magnetic resonance image

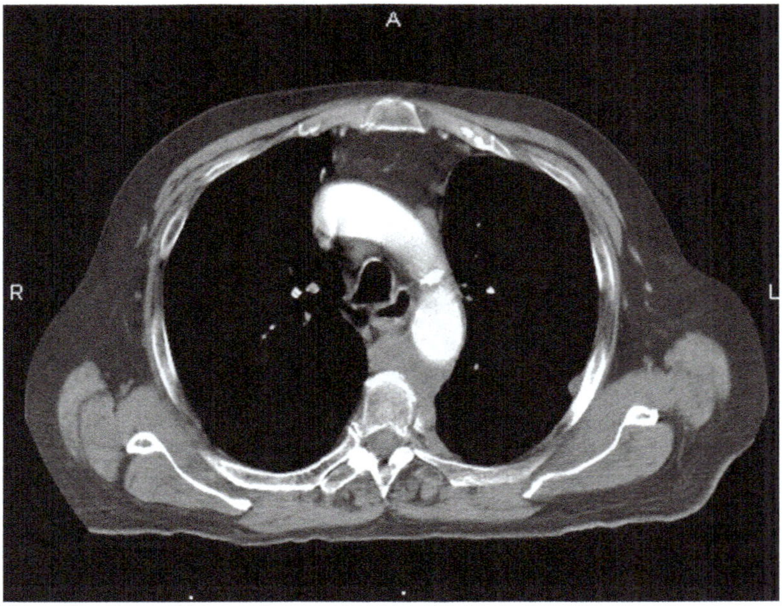

Fig. 2.48 The same mass as in Fig. 2.47 seen on computed tomography

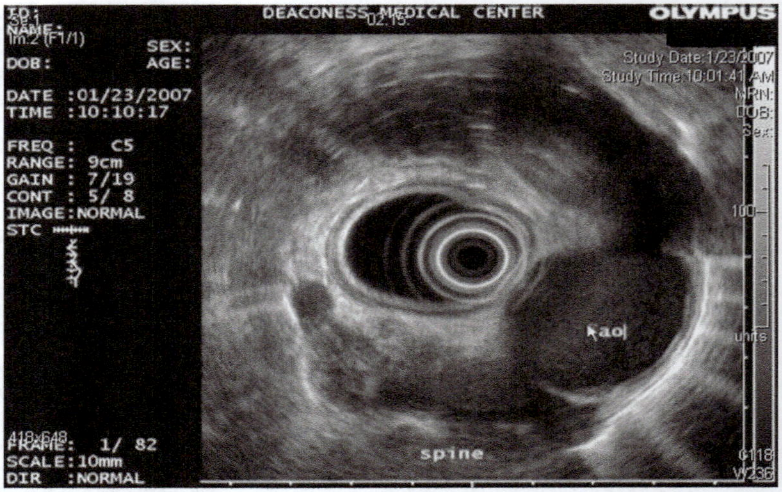

Fig. 2.49 An ill-defined prevertebral hypoechoic mass on radial endoscopic ultrasound

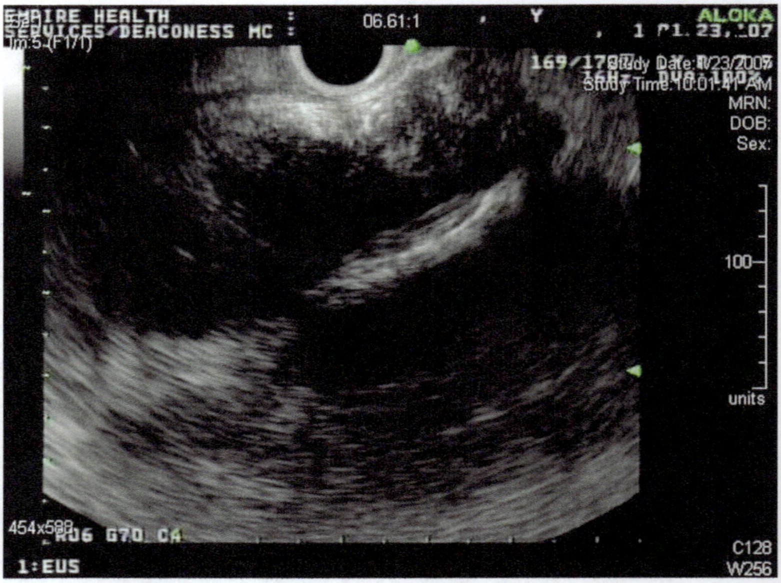

Fig. 2.50 The same mass as in Fig. 2.49 seen with a linear endoscopic ultrasound instrument before fine-needle aspiration biopsy

2.2.1.12 Pleural and Pericardial Effusion

This is a 91-year-old patient who was referred for EUS evaluation of an abnormal barium esophagogram. She was scheduled to undergo aortic valve replacement for critical aortic stenosis. The esophagus was intact, but a large pleural effusion and a small pericardial effusion were incidentally noted. The CT scan (Fig. 2.51) shows approximately the same level as the EUS images. According to the internal echogenicity, effusions can be subclassified as anechoic, complex nonseptated, complex septated, and homogenously echogenic. The effusion is defined as anechoic if totally echo-free spaces are present between the visceral and parietal pleura, complex nonseptated if echogenic materials are inside the anechoic effusions, complex septated if floating fibrin strands or septa are inside the effusions, and homogenously echogenic if homogenously echogenic spaces are present between the visceral and parietal pleura [14].

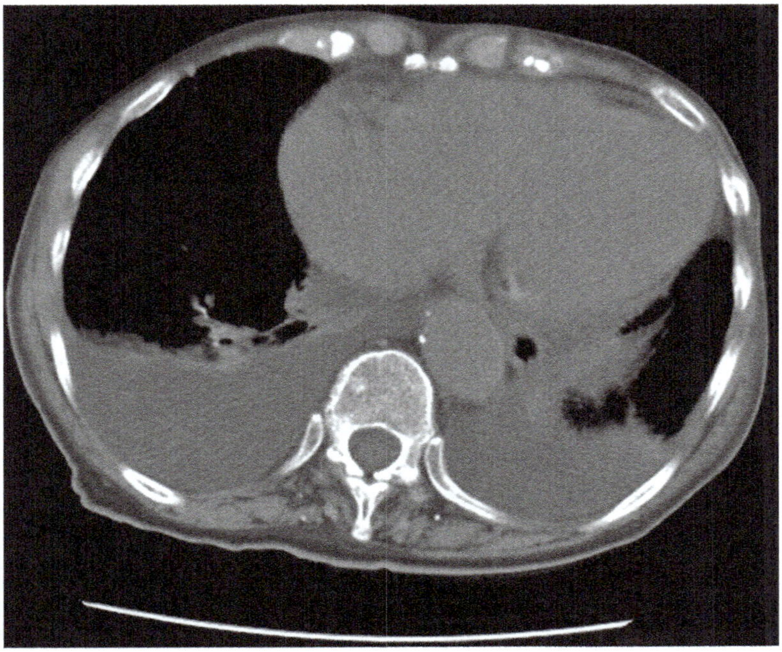

Fig. 2.51 Computed tomography with pleural effusion

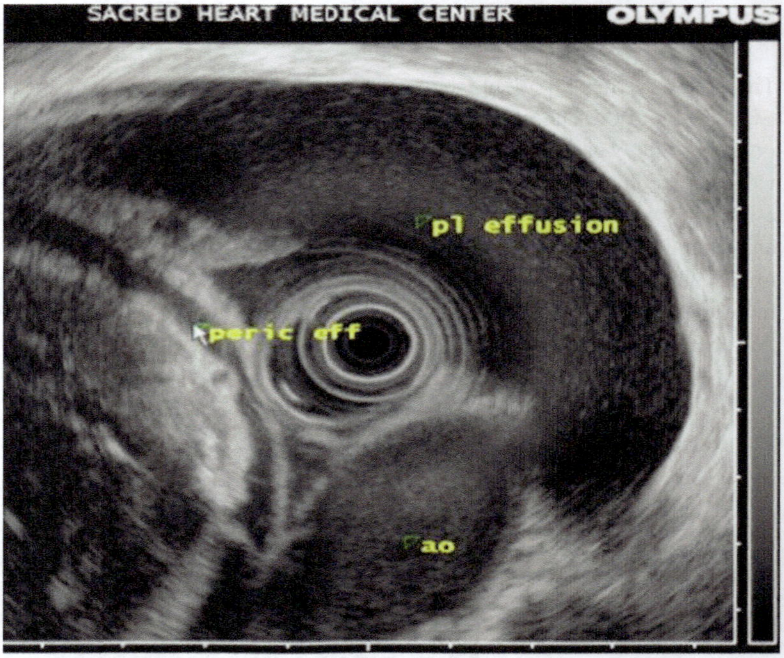

Fig. 2.52 Endoscopic ultrasound shows a pericardial effusion as well. *ao* aorta, *pl* plural

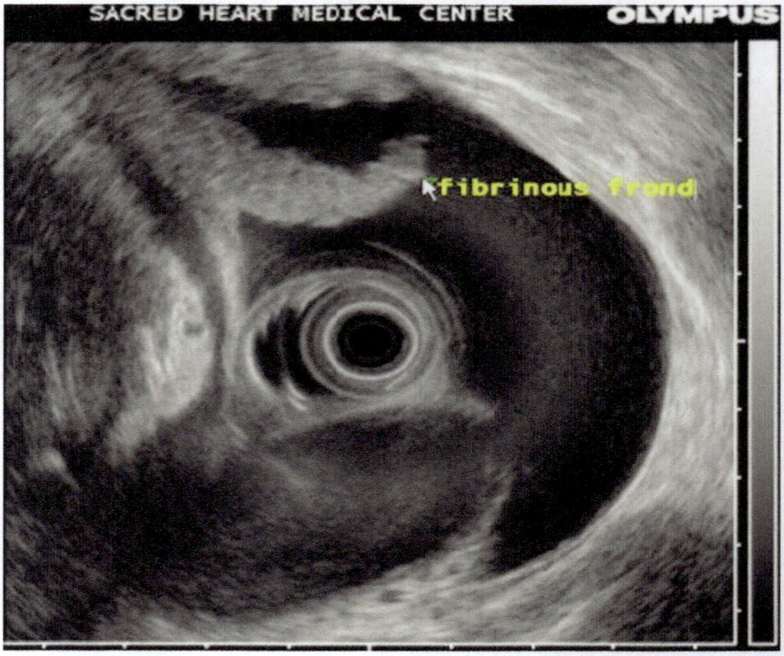

Fig. 2.53 Fibrin strands in the effusion

2.2.1.13 Consolidated Lung

This is a 83-year-old patient referred for the evaluation of a small pancreatic hypodense area. No pancreatic abnormalities were seen. The case is being presented to demonstrate consolidated lung tissue surrounded by pleural fluid, which may be encountered occasionally during an EUS exam for other reasons.

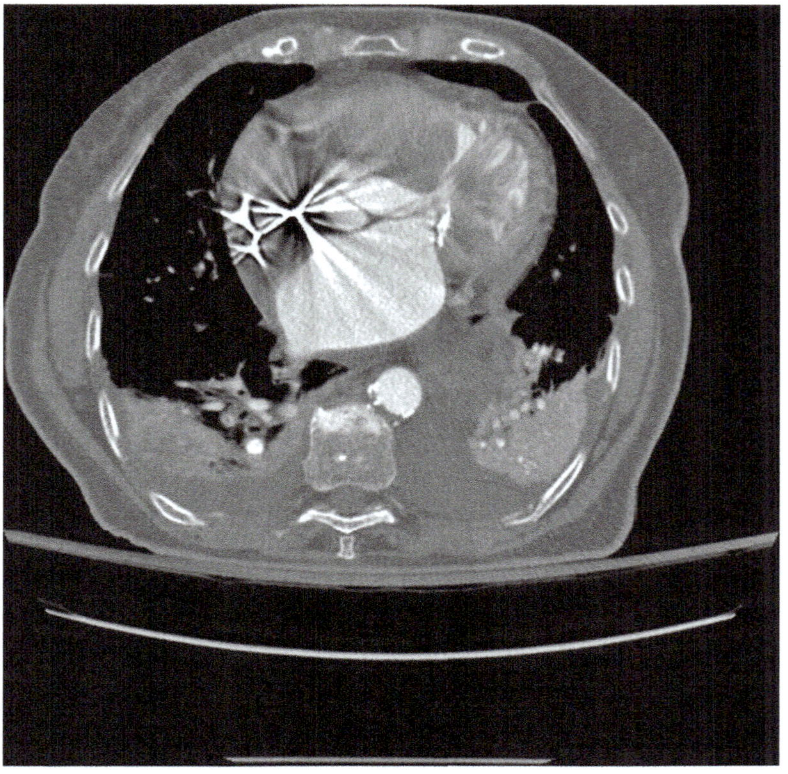

Fig. 2.54 This computed tomography image shows a pleural effusion surrounding consolidated lung (sometimes called hepatization)

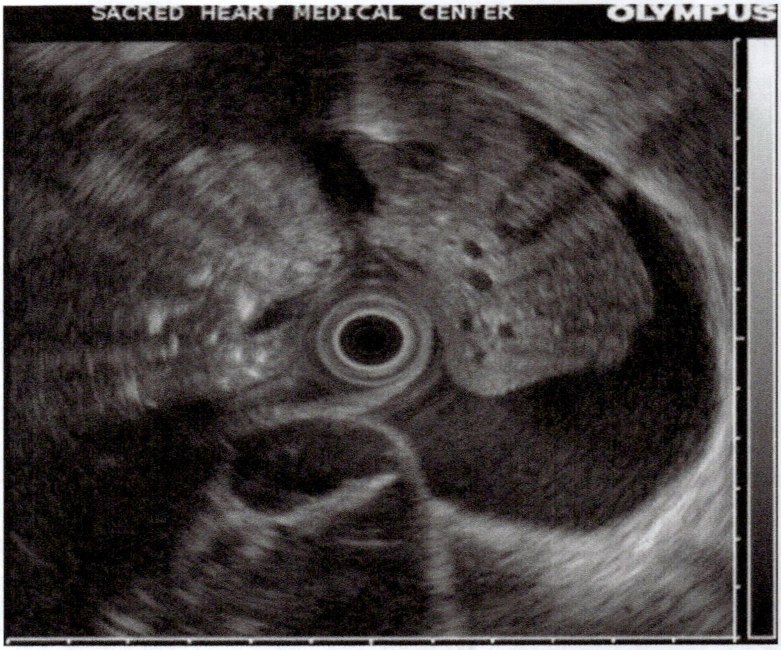

Fig. 2.55 The same consolidated left lower lobe seen by endoscopic ultrasound

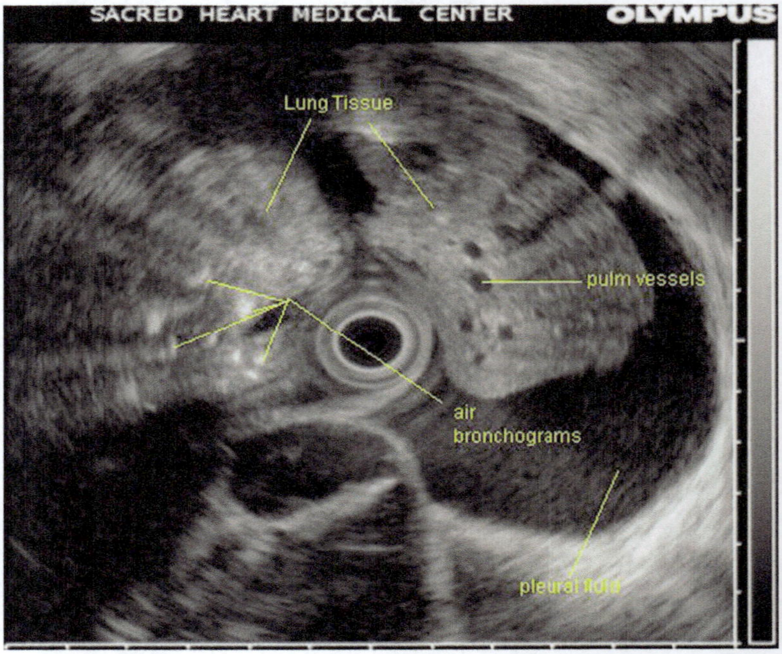

Fig. 2.56 This image shows the different stages of pulmonary consolidation. Air bronchograms (indicated by *white echo foci* with reverberation artifact) are still seen on one side but not the other

2.2.1.14 Dysphagia Caused by Carcinoma of the Lung

The most commonly reported cause of dysphagia associated with lung cancer is mediastinal disease, especially that caused by enlarging lymph nodes in the subcarina. The lateral growth of these is limited by the rigid bronchi and they tend to expand posteriorly into the esophagus. This is a 74-year-old patient who presented with fever and a cough as well as dysphagia. He smokes several packs of cigarettes a day. A CT scan of the chest was interpreted at an outside institution as showing pneumonia (it was not available for review). Endoscopy revealed extrinsic-appearing compression of the mid-esophagus with a friable esophageal wall; biopsies revealed squamous cell carcinoma. EUS evaluation was requested. It appears that the patient actually has a primary lung cancer with postobstructive pneumonia with massive subcarinal lymphadenopathy and direct invasion of the (metastatic) tumor into the esophagus.

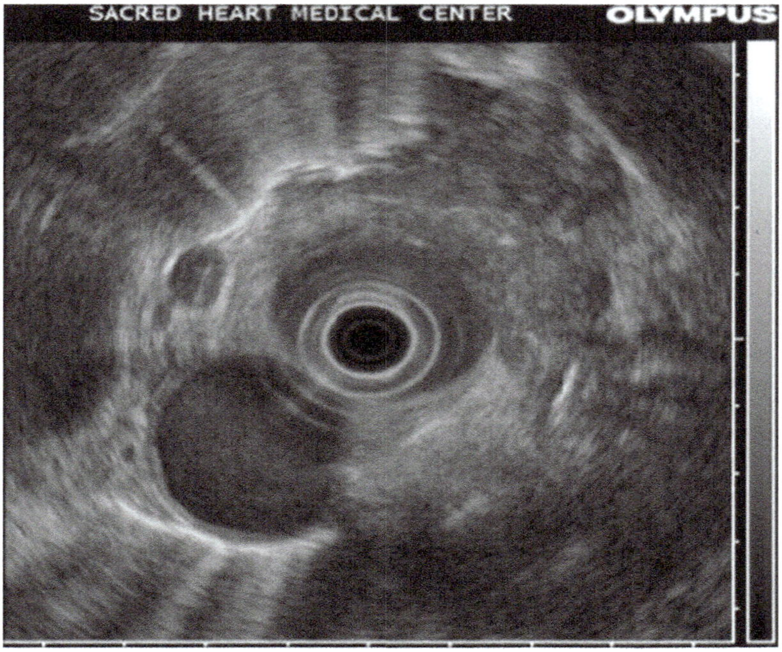

Fig. 2.57 This radial endoscopic ultrasound image shows a large confluent mass of subcarinal lymph nodes

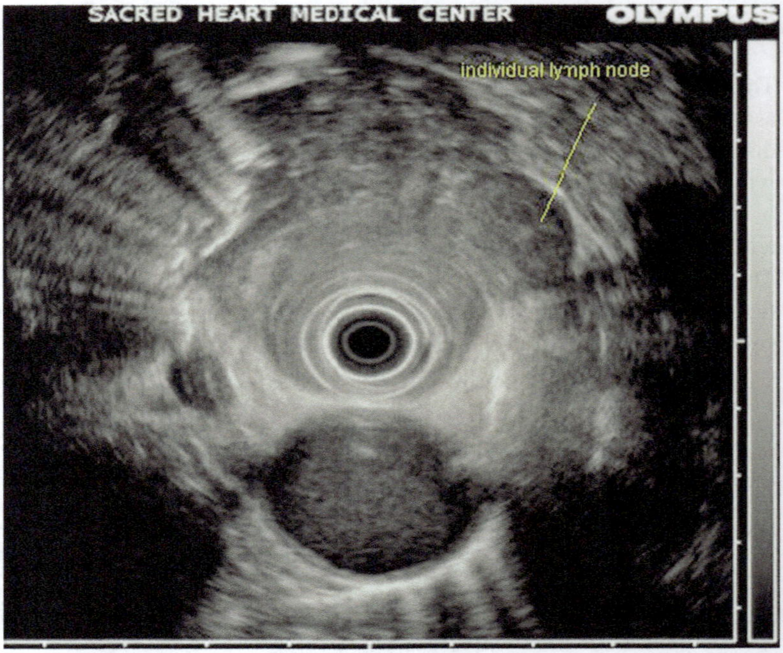

Fig. 2.58 In this image of the same subcarinal lymph node conglomerate, at least one individual lymph node can be identified

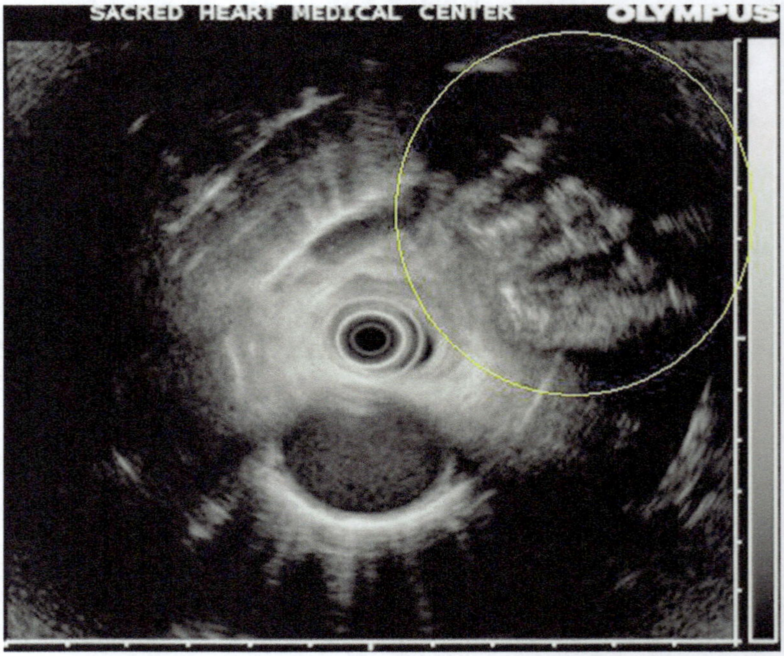

Fig. 2.59 This radial endoscopic ultrasound image shows a hypoechoic lesion (several centimeters in size) in the left lung (scanned from the upper third of the esophagus), probably representing a primary lung cancer with or without obstructive pneumonia

2.2.1.15 Centrally Located Primary Lung Lesions

EUS and EBUS are increasingly being used to diagnose centrally located primary lung lesions (as opposed to metastatic mediastinal lymph nodes) [15, 16]. The first patient (Figs. 2.60 and 2.61) had a nondiagnostic bronchoscopy and was referred for EUS. This was a bulky tumor that wrapped around the aortic arch but could also be directly accessed through the esophagus. This again illustrates our experience that the esophagus allows a degree of flexibility in positioning the transducer that allows biopsies that appear to be difficult or impossible to access on CT scan. The cytology showed squamous cell carcinoma. Although not necessary in this case, transaortic FNA would have been an option.

EUS-guided FNA can or should be the initial diagnostic modality for centrally located primary lung cancers. Unfortunately, when first seen on CT, often little or no thought is given to referring the patient for EUS. This 72 year old woman (Figs. 2.62–2.65), a life-long non-smoker with a centrally located lung mass, was, however, directly referred for EUS. Transesophageal biopsies of this mass were accomplished in less than 20 min and revealed non–small cell carcinoma (adenocarcinoma). Special stains were performed because she also has a remote history of early stage breast cancer. Immunohistochemistry was most consistent with a lung primary tumor.

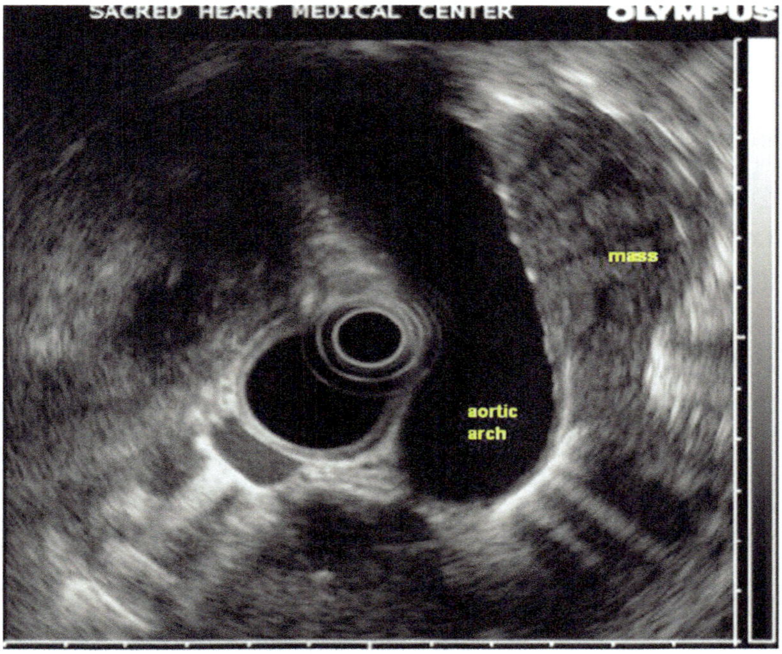

Fig. 2.60 This radial endoscopic ultrasound image shows a left upper lobe lung mass that is largely behind the aortic arch

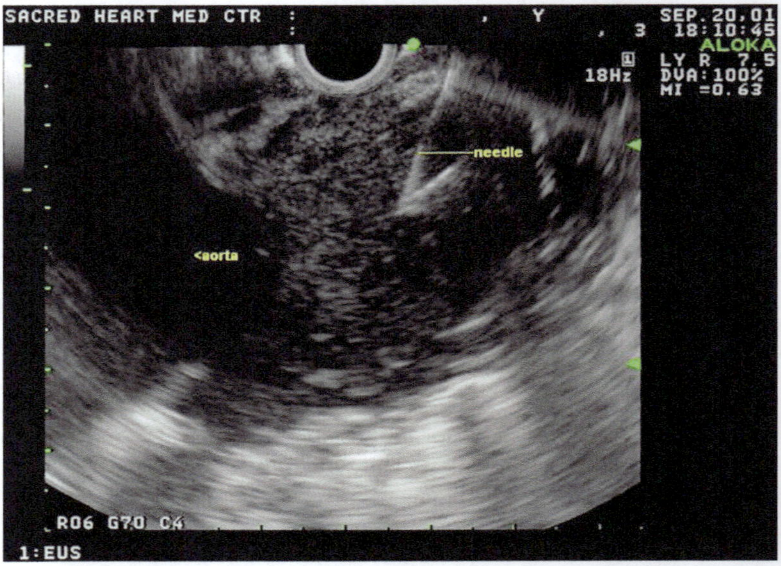

Fig. 2.61 Nevertheless, a biopsy window was fairly easily found with the curved-linear array echoinstrument. EUS-guided FNA revealed non–small cell carcinoma consistent with squamous cell carcinoma

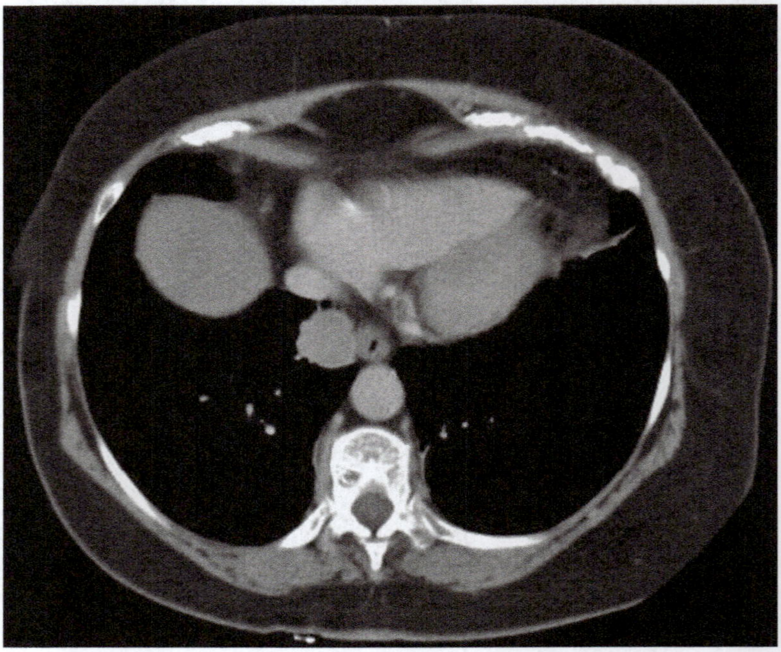

Fig. 2.62 This is a centrally located spiculated lung mass suspicious for a primary lung cancer. Mediastinal adenopathy was not encountered

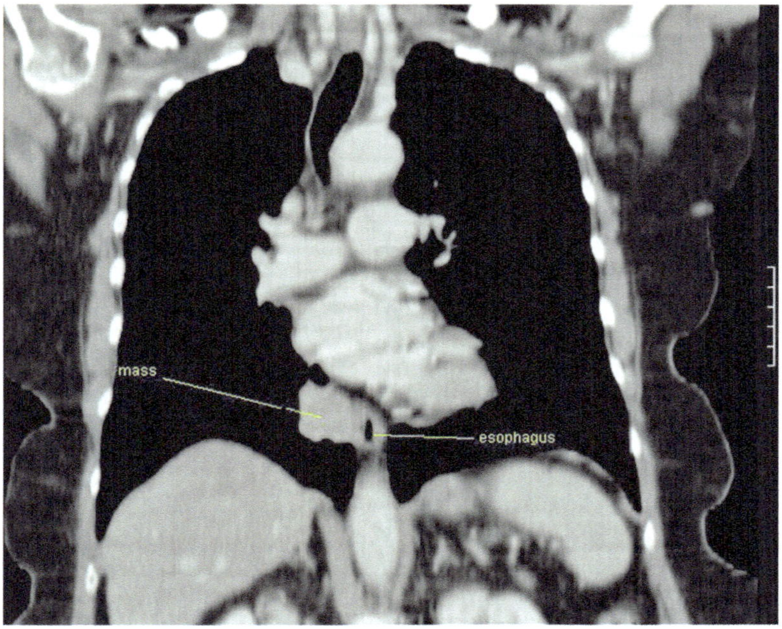

Fig. 2.63 A coronal reconstruction of the same lung mass seen on computed tomography

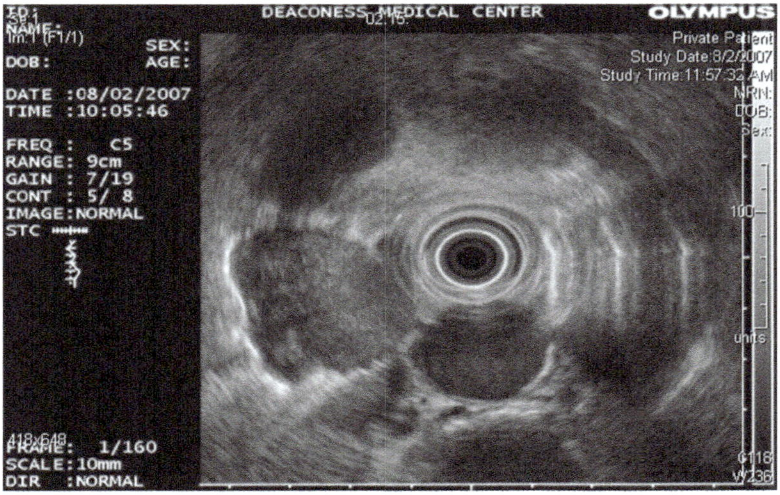

Fig. 2.64 The lung mass as observed with radial endoscopic ultrasound

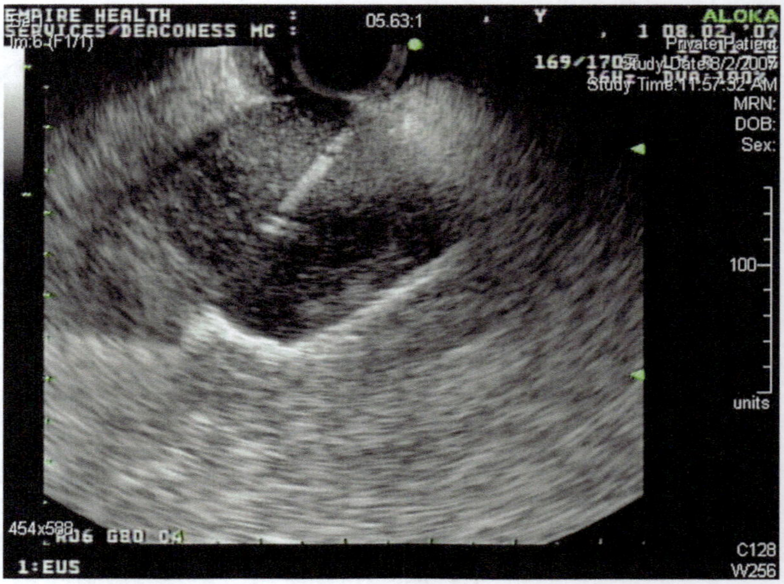

Fig. 2.65 Fine-needle aspiration biopsy of the lung mass under direct endoscopic ultrasound control

2.2.1.16 Restaging of Lung Cancer Following Mediastinoscopy and Treatment by EUS

According to the American College of Chest Physicians lung cancer staging guidelines [17], in patients with discrete node enlargement, staging by CT or PET is not sufficiently accurate, and staging by sampling is recommended. This is a 39-year-old otherwise healthy woman who developed sharp chest pain that was worse during inspiration. She was diagnosed with a right posterior upper lobe lung mass (seen on CT scan) without mediastinal lymph node enlargement. A subsequent PET scan, however, did reveal abnormal glucose uptake in a subcarinal and right pretracheal lymph node. Mediastinoscopy confirmed adenocarcinoma involving stations 4R, 4R (tracheobronchial angle), and 7 (subcarina). Area 5 lymph nodes (the aortopulmonary window) were not sampled. The patient underwent induction chemotherapy and radiation and PET for restaging showed decreased intensity of the right upper lung nodule (standardized uptake values decreased from 7.1 to 3.1) and resolution of the previously noted mediastinal lymphadenopathy. Before planned surgery the patient was referred by the thoracic surgeon for a restaging EUS. During EUS small subcarinal lymph nodes were seen but attention was focused on two small, round, hypoechoic, 4- to 6-mm-diameter lymph nodes in the aortopulmonary window. These were biopsied under EUS guidance and were positive for non–small cell carcinoma, falsifying the PET scan results and resulting in a pathologic stage of IIIB after induction, making it unlikely that the patient would benefit from surgery. This case makes the following points:

- PET results need to be confirmed because of the high rates of false positives and false negatives
- Mediastinoscopy is a gold standard modality that is losing its luster because it is invasive and cannot evaluate the area 5 (aortopulmonary window)
- Thoracic surgeons dislike restaging mediastinoscopies because of the subsequent scarring; EUS may be the easiest invasive restaging modality

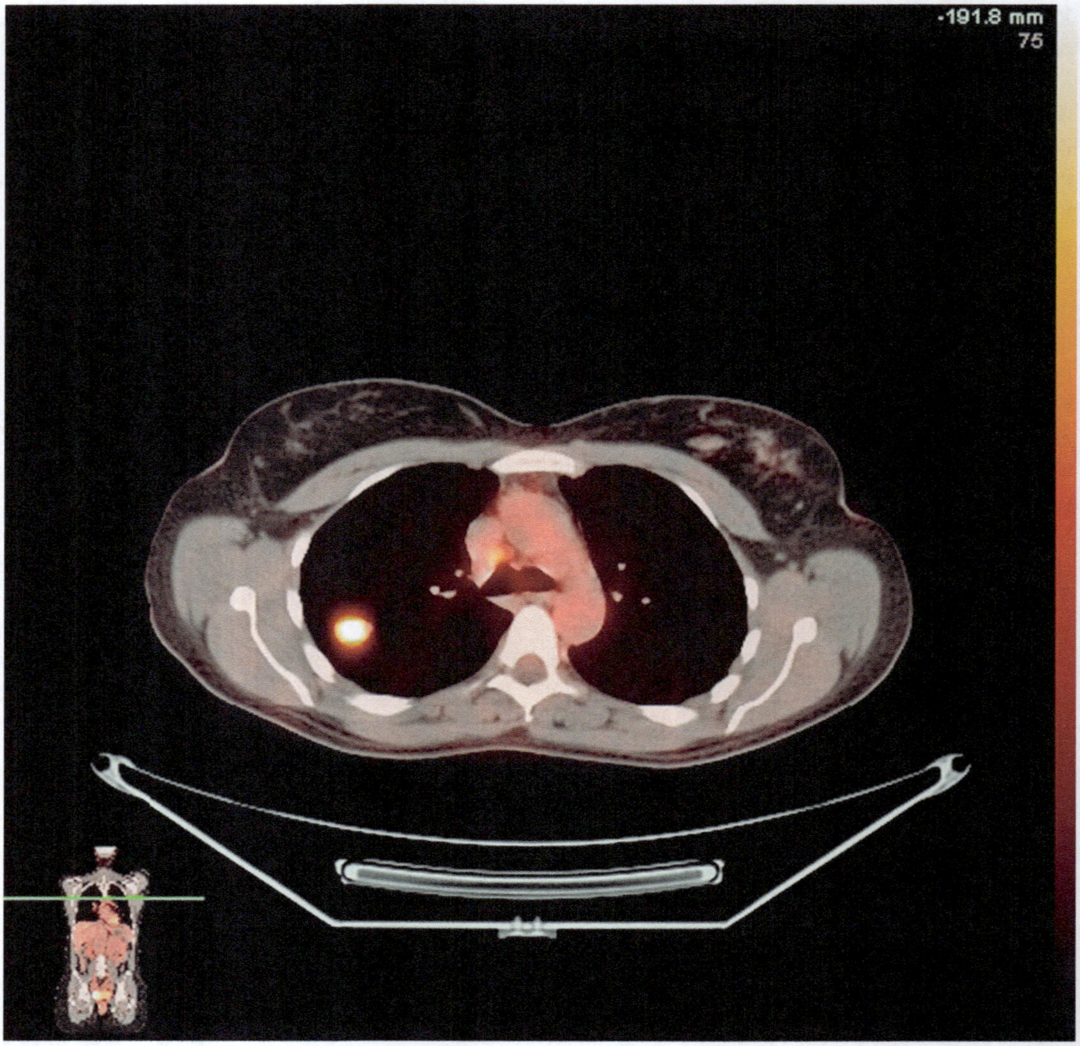

Fig. 2.66 This is the original staging positron emission tomography scan showing a hot spot in the right upper lobe (standardized uptake value, 7.1)

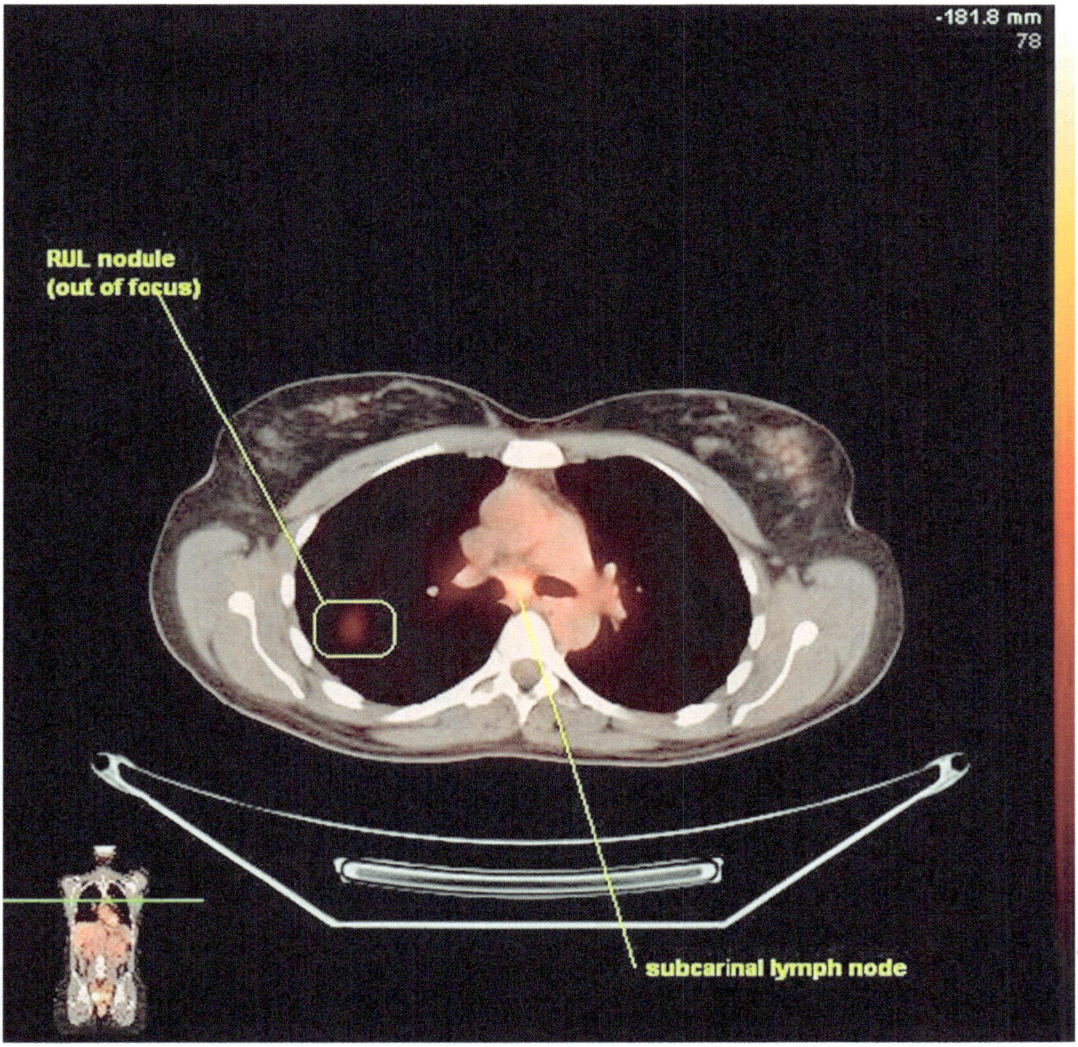

Fig. 2.67 This slice of the initial staging positron emission tomography scan shows a high degree of glucose avidity in the subcarinal region, consistent with lymph node metastasis. *RUL* right upper lobe

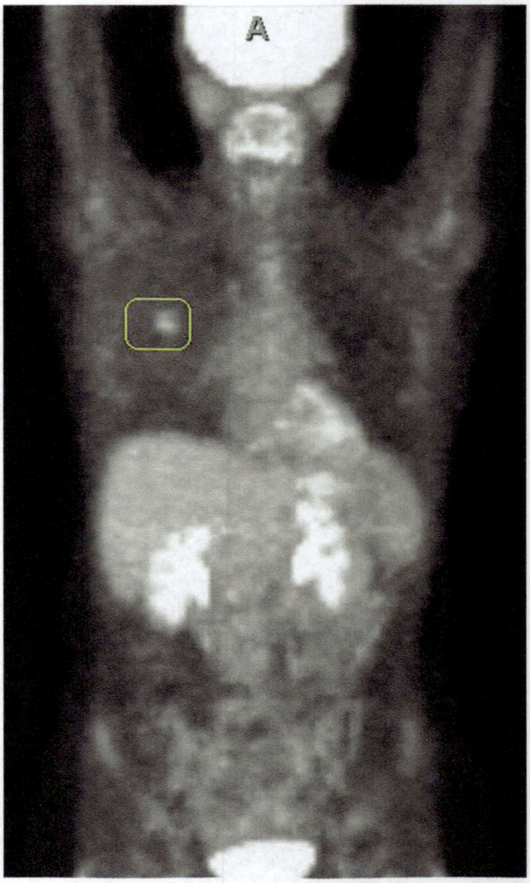

Fig. 2.68 This restaging positron emission tomography scan after induction chemotherapy and radiation shows a reduction in the intensity of the right upper lobe mass and no activity in the mediastinum, consistent with a good treatment response

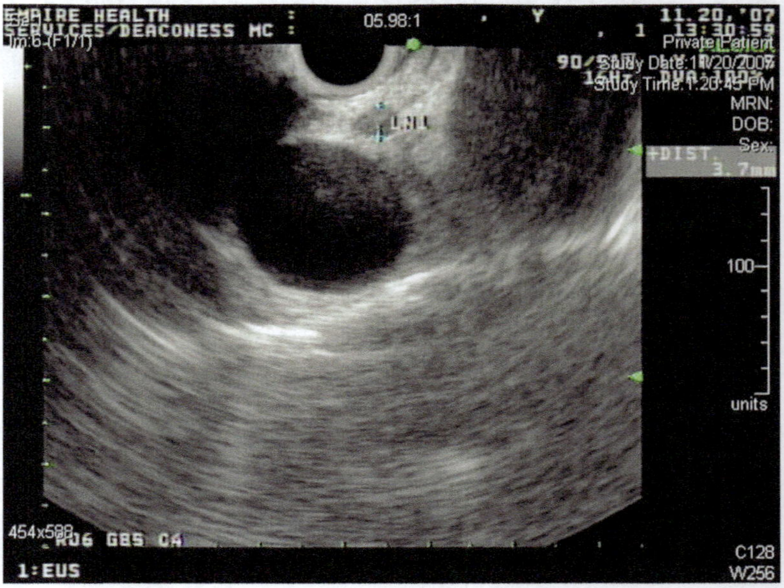

Fig. 2.69 There were two small lymph nodes (*LN*; 3.7 mm) in the aortopulmonary window visible on endoscopic ultrasound. Nevertheless, the biopsies showed non–small cell lung carcinoma

2.2.1.17 False-Positive PET Scan

If distant metastases have been ruled out, the status of the mediastinum becomes crucial in the staging of lung cancer. The pooled sensitivity and specificity of CT for identifying mediastinal lymph node metastasis are 51 and 85 %, respectively; for PET scanning the respective values are 74 % (95 % confidence interval, 69–79 %) and 85 % (95 % confidence interval, 82–88 %) [18]. Therefore, in many clinical situations confirmation of the status of the mediastinal nodes by sampling will be necessary; sampling is recommended in the 2007 guidelines of the American College of Chest Physicians. This is a 76-year-old patient with a small right upper lobe lung nodule. PET scan suggested N3 mediastinal disease, but the EUS-guided FNA of the most active lymph nodes in the subcarina showed only anthracotic lymph node material. Therefore the patient was offered surgery. Intraoperative mediastinoscopy with frozen section was negative, and the patient had a successful wedge resection with a final tumor stage of T1N0.

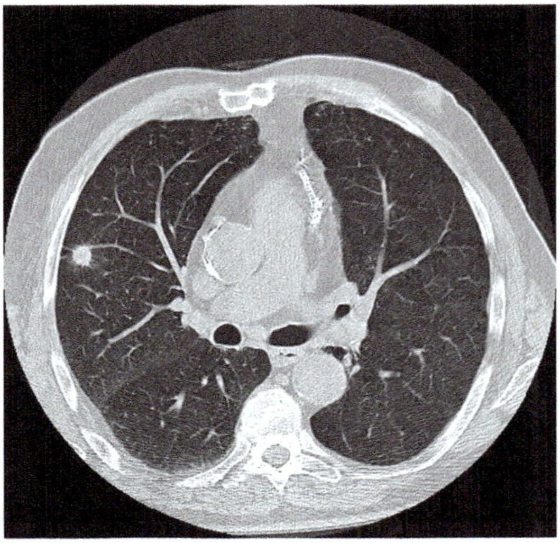

Fig. 2.70 This chest computed tomography scan shows a small right upper lobe nodule, which was resected and found to be an adenocarcinoma

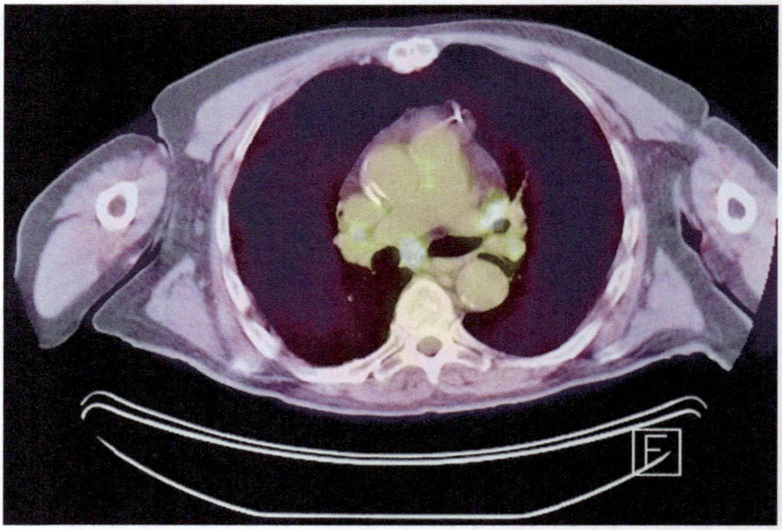

Fig. 2.71 A positron emission tomography scan showing several glucose-avid mediastinal lymph nodes, consistent with metastasis

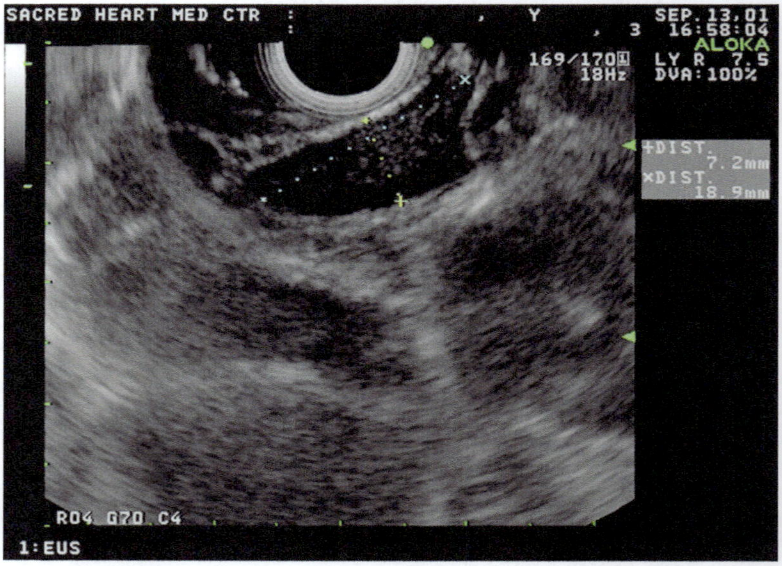

Fig. 2.72 This endoscopic ultrasound image shows subcarinal lymph nodes, which were extensively sampled by fine-needle aspiration. The cytology was negative. This was confirmed by a subsequent mediastinoscopy. A wedge resection of the right upper lobe tumor was then performed (final stage, T1N0)

2.2.1.18 Triple Cytology for Lung Cancer Diagnosis

This is a 83-year-old patient who 3 years before this presentation was diagnosed with stage IIIB lung cancer and had radiation and chemotherapy. He was in apparent remission until recently, when CT showed multiple abnormalities. PET-CT indicated several areas of mildly increased activity, with one hot spot located close to the right hilum. The patient was referred directly for EUS evaluation. The EUS showed a pleural effusion and two relatively small but still suspicious subcarinal lymph nodes. Pleural fluid and the lymph nodes were aspirated with EUS guidance for cytology. During portions of the procedure the patient repeatedly coughed and produced sputum, which was submitted as a third sample. All three samples (pleural fluid, lymph nodes, and sputum) were negative for malignancy. Sputum samples for cytology to diagnose lung cancer have largely fallen out of favor but their value is not trivial. The sensitivity of sputum cytology depends heavily on the circumstances (central vs. peripheral tumors, sputum quality, number of samples), but in this case the situation is not unlike that of older studies where sputum samples were obtained before bronchoscopy. In these circumstances a sensitivity of 0.10–0.74 (mean, 0.22) was obtained [17].

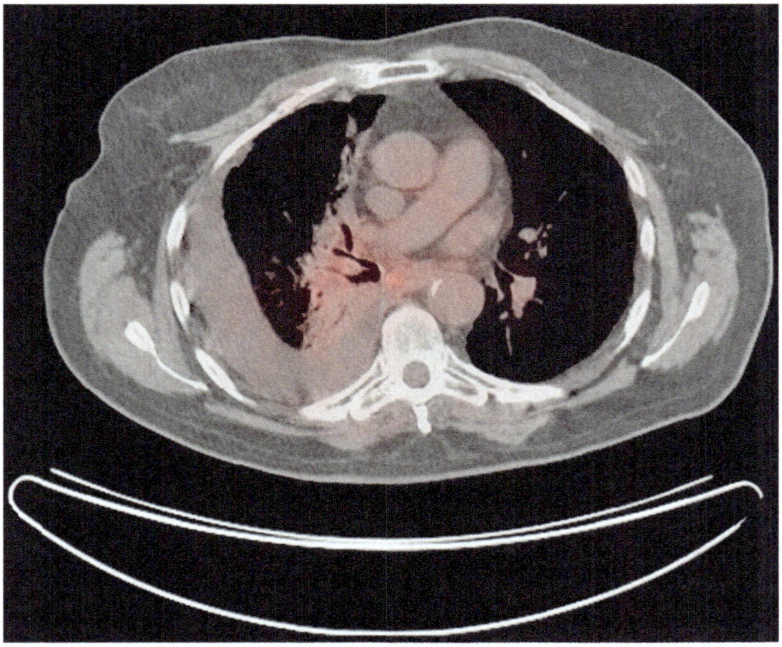

Fig. 2.73 This fusion positron emission tomography–computed tomography scan shows airspace disease and a pleural effusion. Recurrent non–small cell carcinoma of the lung is suspected

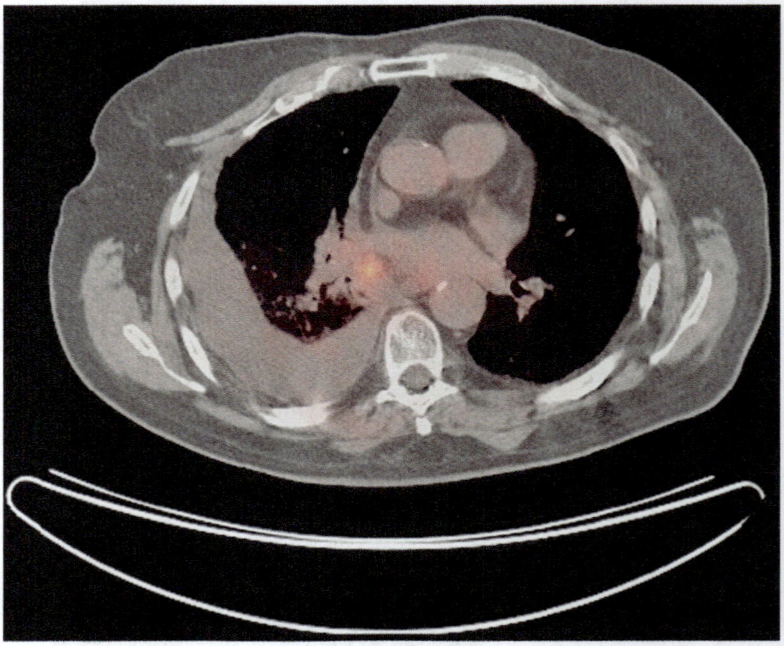

Fig. 2.74 This positron emission tomography–computed tomography fusion study shows a hot spot close to the right hilum

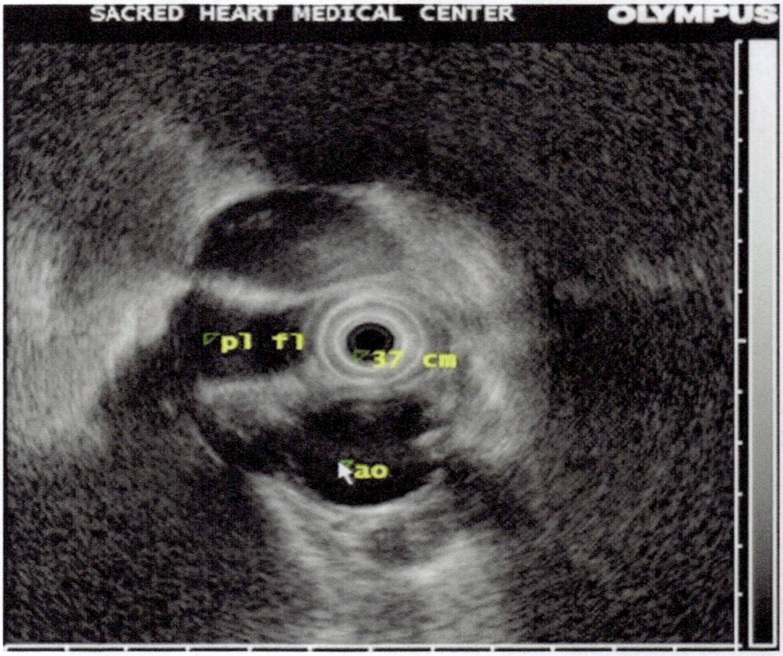

Fig. 2.75 The corresponding endoscopic ultrasound study shows a pleural effusion but no large masses or lymph nodes. *ao* aorta, *pl fl* pleural fluid

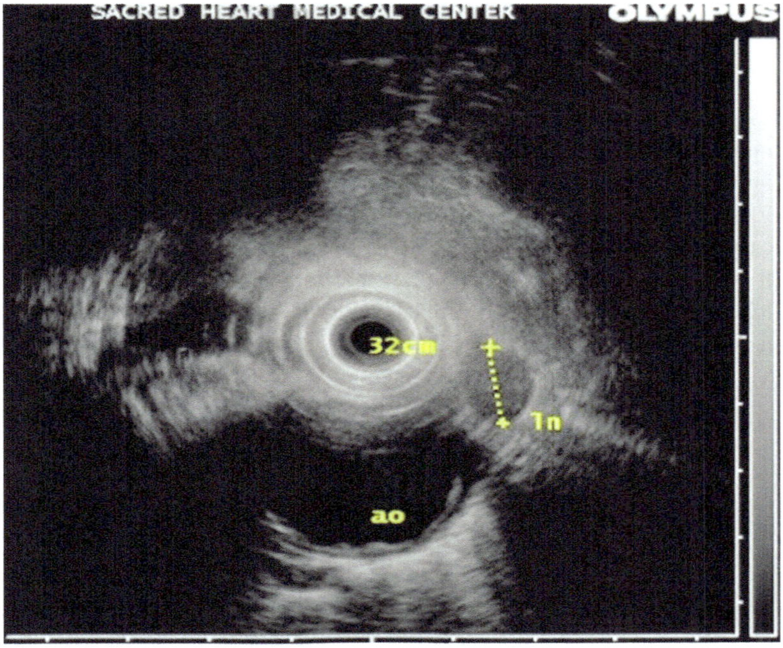

Fig. 2.76 Endoscopic ultrasound reveals two relatively small, subcarinal, round, hypoechoic lymph nodes (*ln*). *ao* aorta

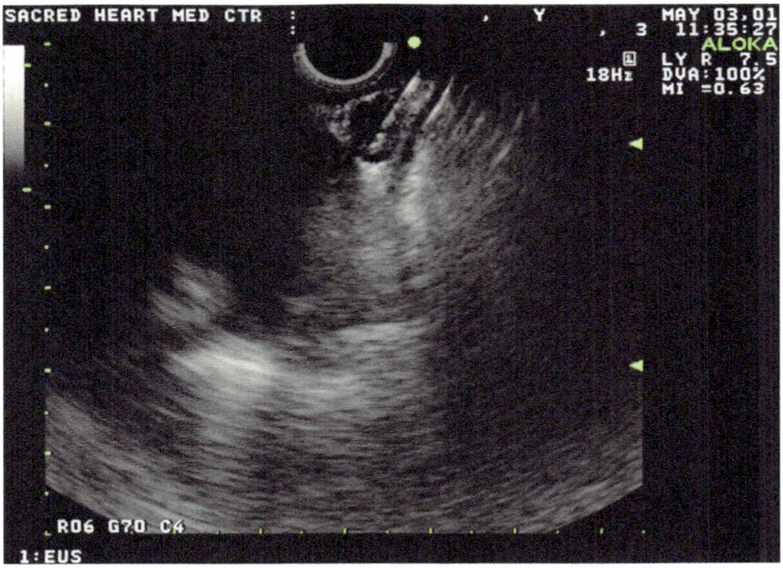

Fig. 2.77 This image shows that even small (in this case, 11-mm diameter) lymph nodes can easily biopsied using real-time guidance with endoscopic ultrasound

2.2.1.19 Malignant Invasion of the Pulmonary Artery

This is a 79-year-old woman with a non–small cell carcinoma of the right lower lobe of the lung who underwent preoperative bronchoscopy (nondiagnostic), CT-guided transthoracic FNA (positive), PET, and staging mediastinoscopy of the precarinal and paratracheal lymph nodes (negative), followed by a right lower lobe and right middle lobe lobectomy that was complicated by an air leak. The final surgical pathology was T2N1M0. Six weeks after surgery she was readmitted with complaints of fever and weakness, and treatment for pneumonia was started. Suspecting metastatic cancer, EUS was performed, revealing a malignant-appearing subcarinal lymph node and evidence of a tumor thrombus in the pulmonary artery. FNA of the lymph node was positive for metastatic non–small-cell lung carcinoma. Magnetic resonance imaging of the brain showed multiple metastatic foci. There is an increasing body of literature showing that EUS in addition to mediastinoscopy (instead of mediastinoscopy alone) can help avoid futile thoracotomies [19].

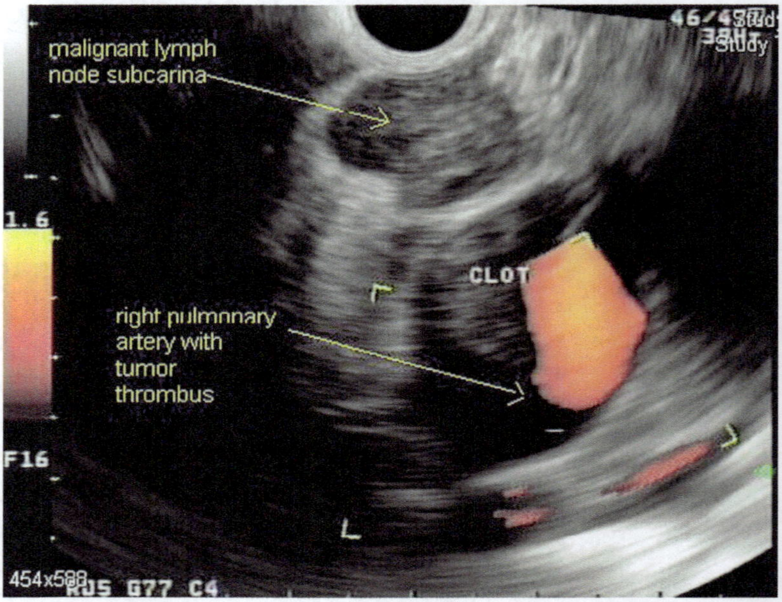

Fig. 2.78 This linear endoscopic ultrasound with power Doppler reveals a thrombus in the pulmonary artery and a hypoechoic subcarinal lymph node

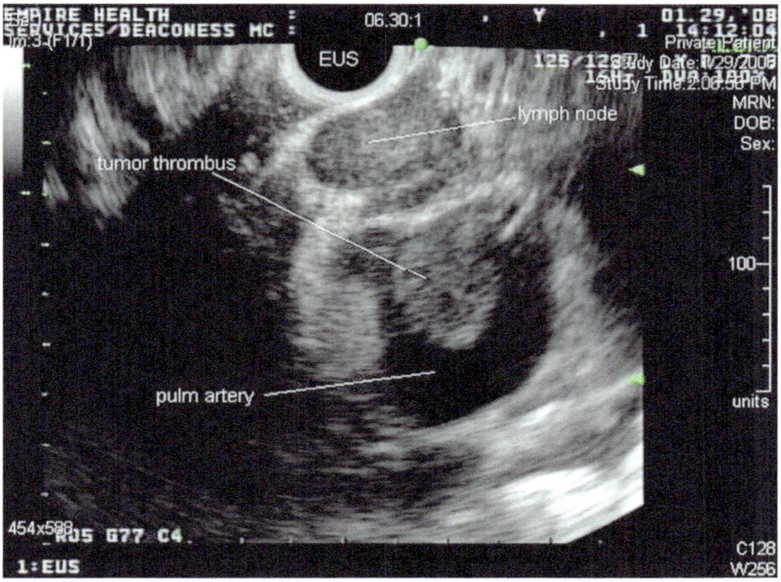

Fig. 2.79 Using the Doppler deteriorates the grayscale imaging. This is a crisp image of the thrombus, which, based on the findings on computed tomography, in all likelihood represents an invading tumor

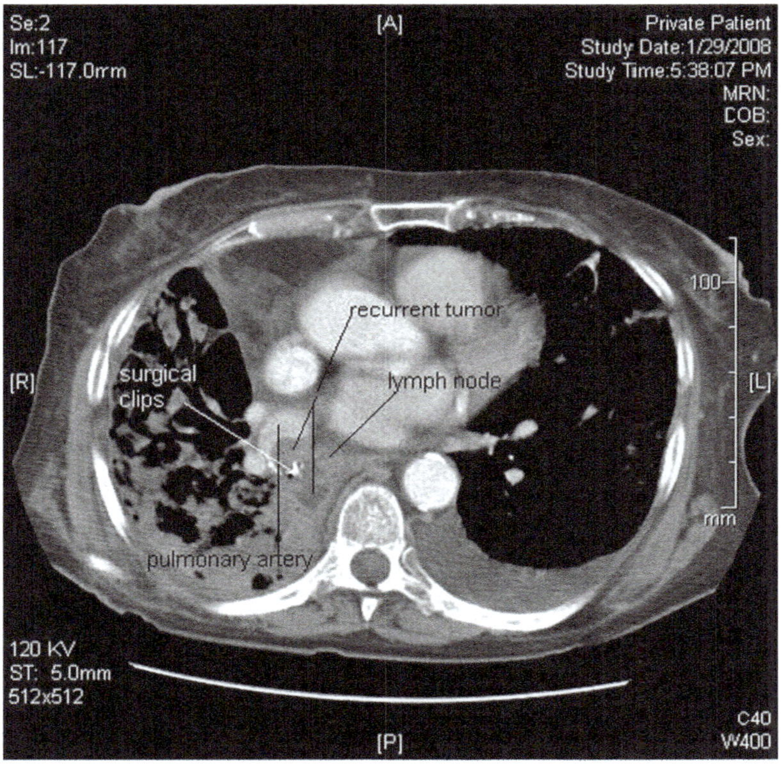

Fig. 2.80 The labels on this computed tomography scan reflect the structural relationships of the tumor and surrounding anatomy

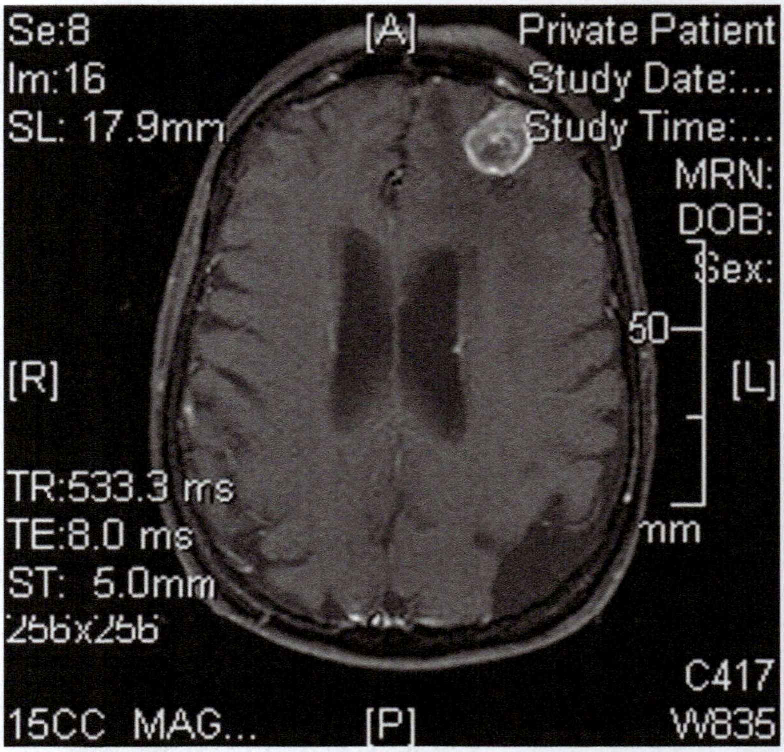

Fig. 2.81 This section of a T1-weighted magnetic resonance image shows one of several metastatic lesions

2.2.2 Esophagus

2.2.2.1 Carcinosarcoma of the Esophagus

This is a 66-year-old patient with a 4-month or longer history of progressive dysphagia. He was initially evaluated with a barium swallow, which showed a peculiar polypoid tumor of the esophagus. He was reluctant to seek further care, and an upper endoscopy was performed only when swallowing became next to impossible (4 months later). CT showed a sausage-shaped tumor of the esophagus. EUS revealed a tumor that focally (probably at the site of its attachment) had T3 features. No lymphadenopathy was seen. Surgical removal confirmed the stage that was determined using ultrasound.

Carcinosarcoma of the esophagus is a rare tumor, accounting for less than 2 % of esophageal neoplasms. Histologically, sarcomatoid carcinomas of the esophagus are biphasic; the epithelial component is usually limited to a few areas, and the bulk of the tumor has a pleomorphic sarcomatoid appearance [20]. The tumor appears to grow rapidly, assuming a polypoid shape; this fast growth may lead to earlier symptoms and an earlier stage at first diagnosis. Light microscopy typically reveals tumors with variable amounts of carcinomatous and sarcomatous tissue. Immunohistochemistry reveals carcinomatous cells with features of mesenchymal cells and vice versa.

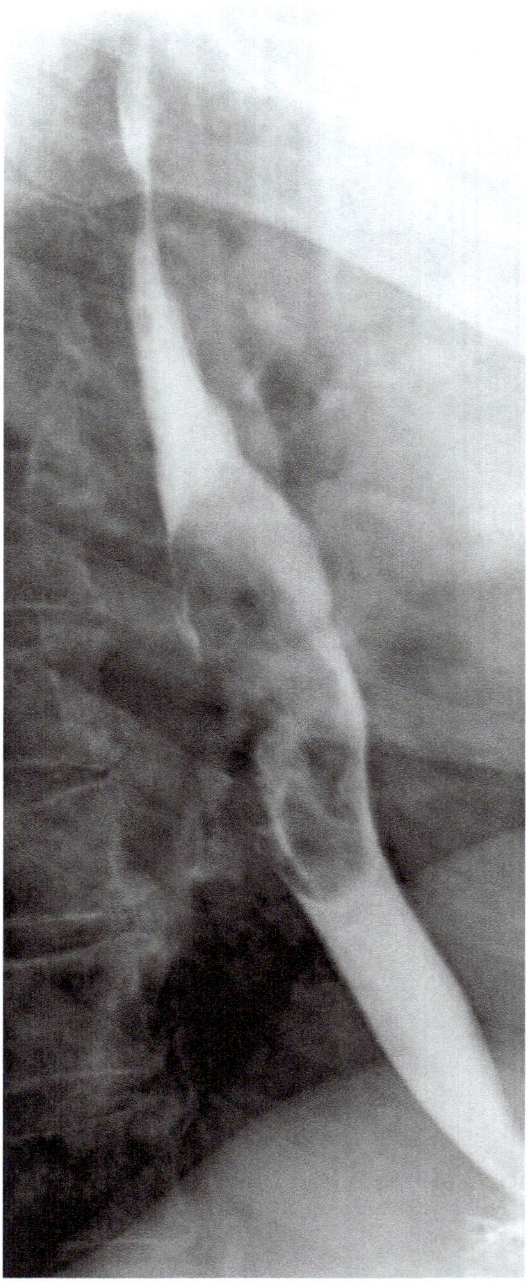

Fig. 2.82 This barium esophagogram shows the tumor 4 months before the current presentation. Note the narrow base where the carcinosarcoma attaches to the posterior wall of the mid-esophagus

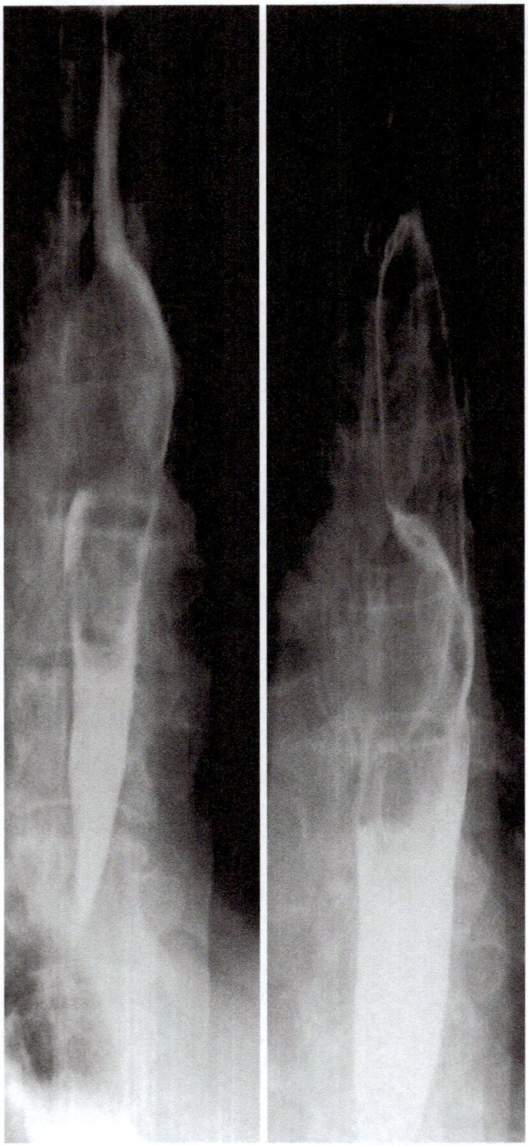

Fig. 2.83 This is another view of the same esophagogram, emphasizing the polypoid nature of the carcinosarcoma

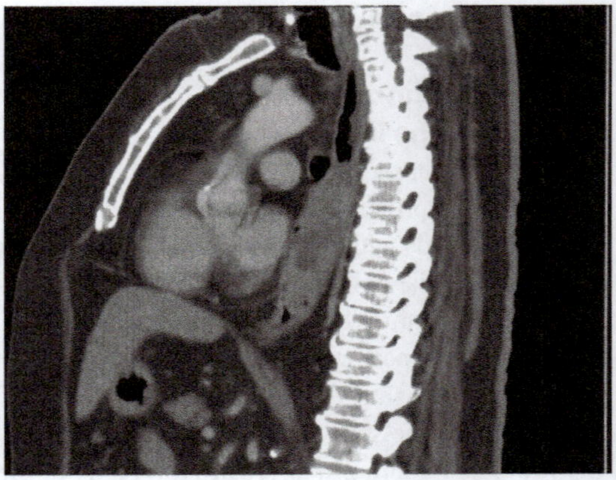

Fig. 2.84 This sagittal reconstruction of a chest computed tomography scan shows a sausage-shaped tumor in the esophagus, which enhances nonhomogenously

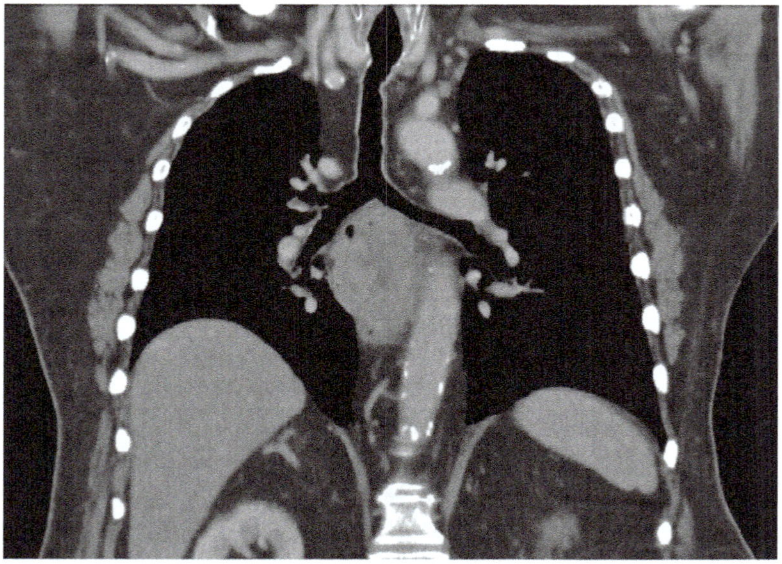

Fig. 2.85 This is a coronal reconstruction of the computed tomography of the chest showing a peculiar mass in the esophagus

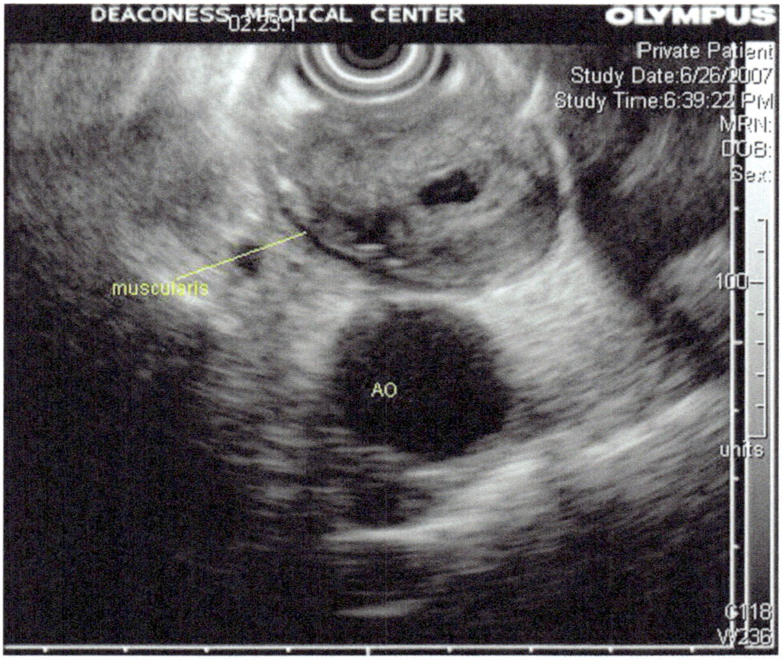

Fig. 2.86 This radial endoscopic ultrasound image of the tumor shows areas of cystic degeneration. The muscularis appears intact. *AO* aorta

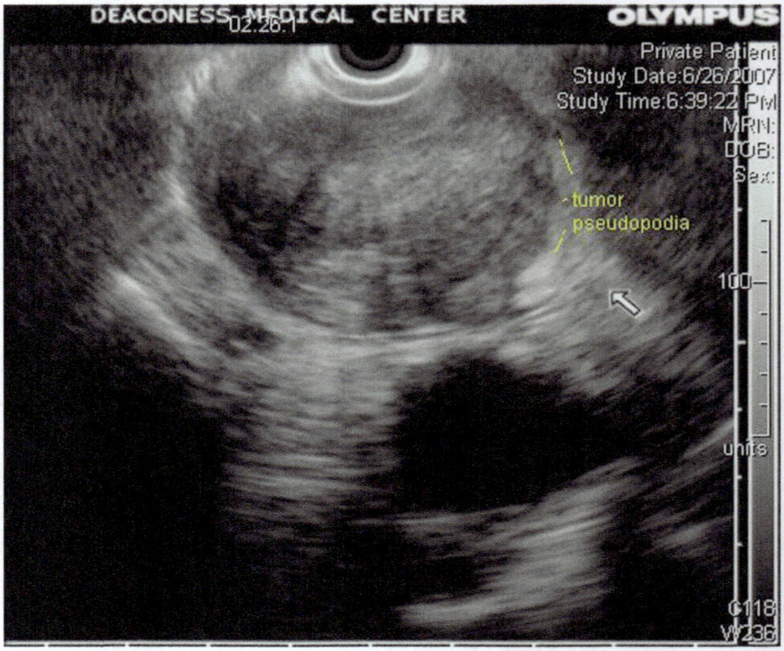

Fig. 2.87 In the mid-esophagus the tumor assumes T3 features with tumor pseudopodia

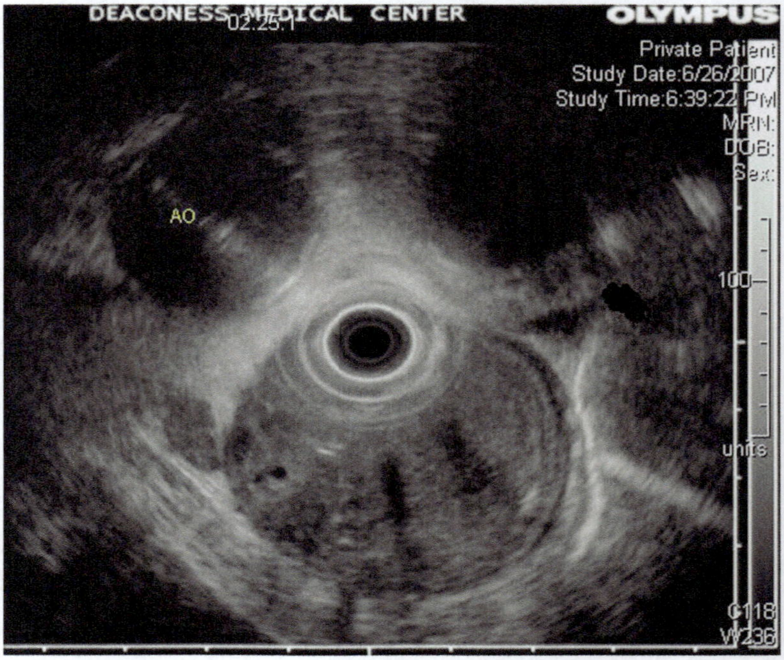

Fig. 2.88 This endoscopic ultrasound image shows the exophytic nature of the tumor. It fills approximately 90 % of the lumen of the esophagus but apparently attaches only to one portion of the wall

2.2.2.2 T1N1 Esophageal Cancer

When symptomatic, esophageal cancers present in the majority of patients with transmural involvement and malignant lymphadenopathy. This is a 83-year-old patient with an adenocarcinoma at the gastroesophageal junction (grouped with esophageal cancers) who turned out to have lymphadenopathy with a T1 tumor.

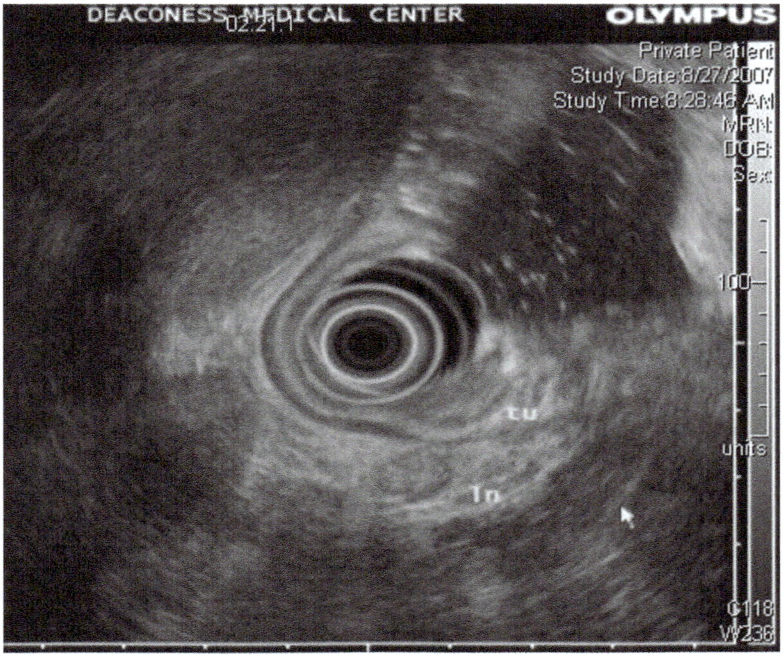

Fig. 2.89 This adenocarcinoma of the gastroesophageal junction (*tu*) is confined to the mucosa and submucosa but, unfortunately, a 1-cm-diameter, malignant-appearing lymph node (*ln*) is close by

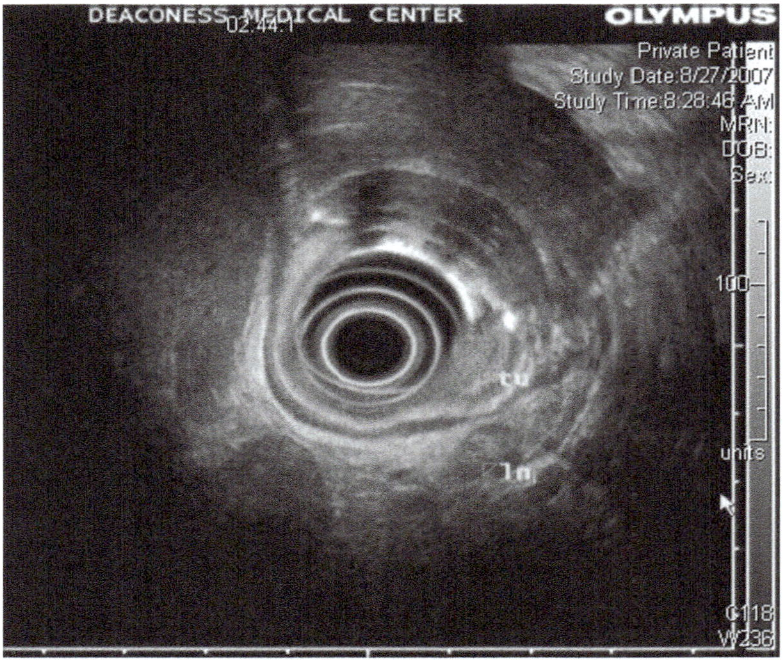

Fig. 2.90 The same situation seen in Fig. 2.89 is shown here at 12 MHz. *ln* lymph node, *tu* tumor

2.2.2.3 Esophageal Leiomyoma Arising from the Muscularis Mucosae

More than 95 % of esophageal leiomyomas arise from the muscularis propria and have an intramural growth pattern. The rare leiomyomas that arise from the muscularis mucosae may become polypoid and pedunculated. This is a 49-year-old patient referred for EUS evaluation of a submucosal lesion in the mid-esophagus that was found during upper endoscopy for abdominal pain.

The lesion resembles a leiomyoma in all respects except that it clearly does not originate from the muscularis propria on EUS. Therefore, biopsies were obtained. In theory, FNA biopsies could have been done, but we were confident that tunneling biopsies with a large-capacity biopsy forceps would be easier and provide a larger sample. Histology confirmed leiomyoma, special stains were negative for the CD117 antigen, and the layer of origin was immediately subepithelial.

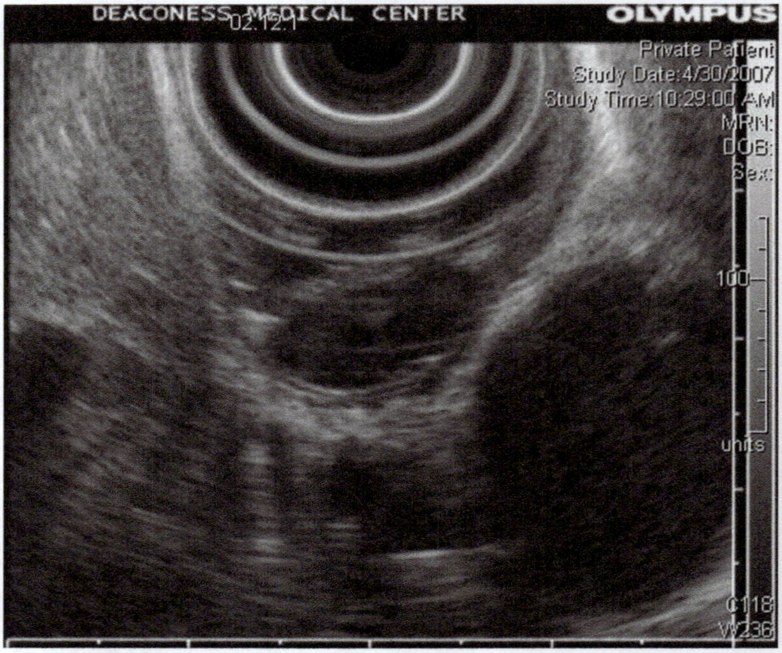

Fig. 2.91 This is a biopsy-proven esophageal leiomyoma arising from the muscularis mucosa (subepithelial)

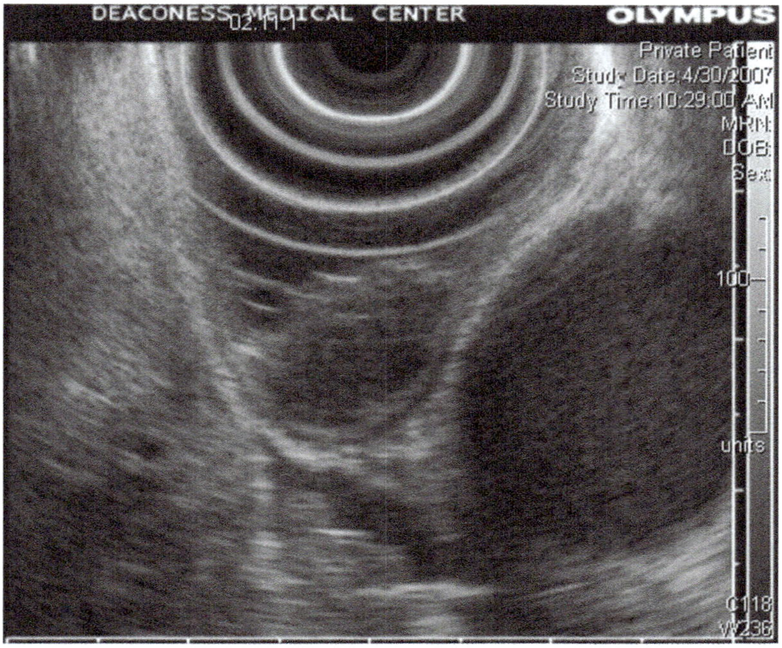

Fig. 2.92 A different view seen on radial endoscopic ultrasound of the same leiomyoma presented in Fig. 2.91. The scale is 5 mm

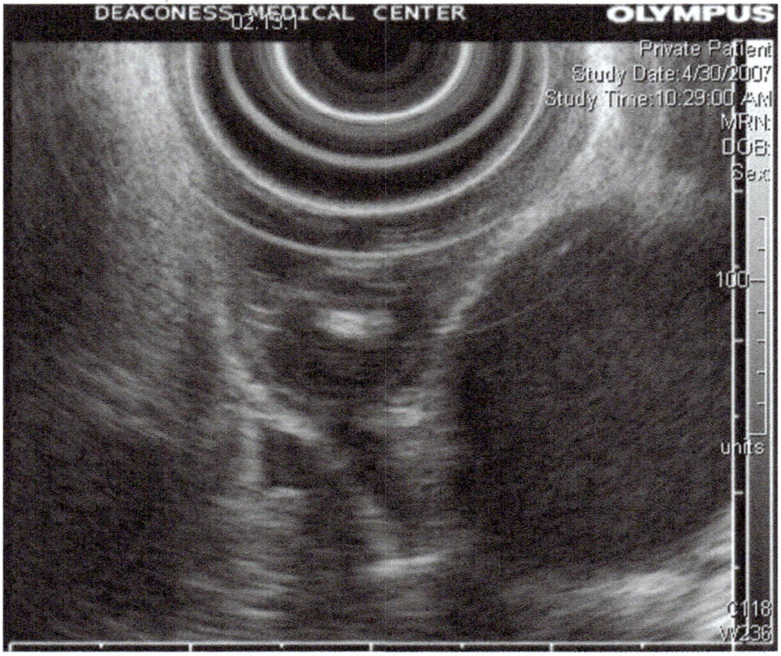

Fig. 2.93 The leiomyoma has a central bright or echogenic focus that is probably not calcium since there is no posterior shadowing

2.2.2.4 Granular Cell Tumor of the Esophagus

Granular cell tumors are typically found in the skin or soft tissues; in the gastrointestinal tract they are rare. They may be derived from Schwann cells since they stain positive for the S-100 protein on immunohistochemistry. In the United States, granular cell tumors of the esophageal tract are more common in African American women than in other ethnic groups [21]. They can be solitary or multiple and present as yellow submucosal tumors on surface endoscopy. The majority (>95 %) are benign. There are no standardized management guidelines, but many experts believe that they do not need to be removed unless they are larger than 1 cm in diameter or have atypical features (infiltrative pattern) on EUS. This is a 44-year-old African-American woman with noncardiac chest pain. Surface endoscopy showed two submucosal yellow nodules. Biopsies confirmed the clinical impression. EUS revealed that the larger of the two nodules was 3–4 mm in size and both were confined to the submucosa.

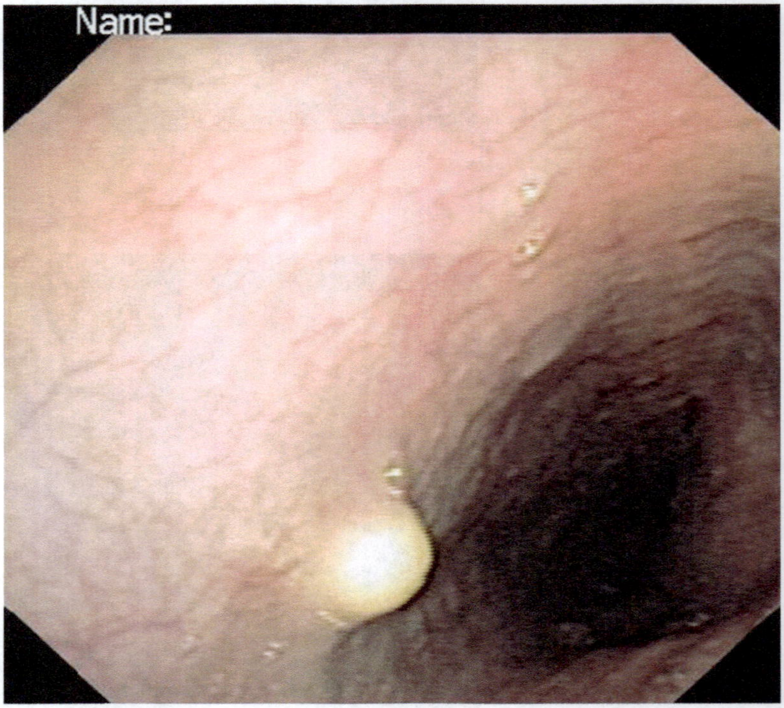

Fig. 2.94 Granular cell tumors of the esophagus are submucosal and appear yellow on esophagogastroduodenoscopy

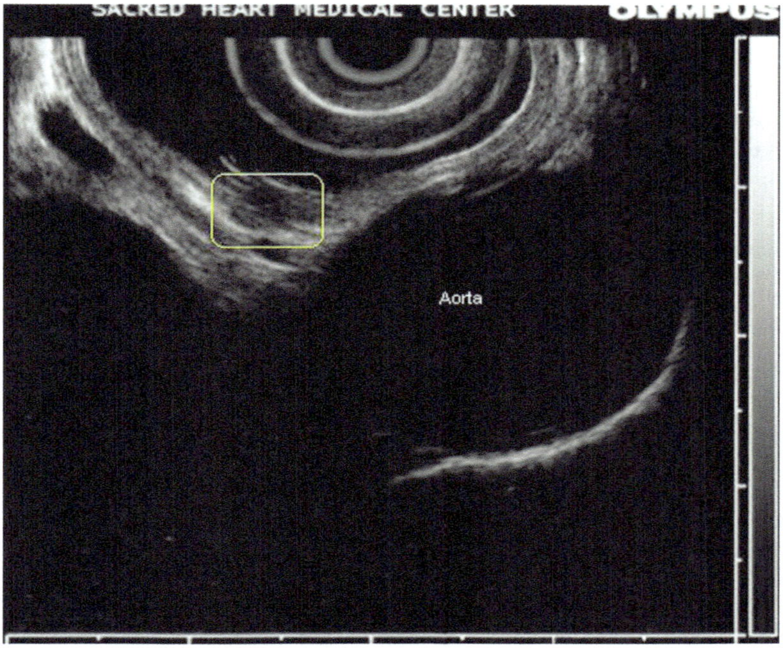

Fig. 2.95 The esophageal granular cell tumor seen on this endoscopic ultrasound image measured only 3–4 mm in size and was confined to the submucosa

2.2.2.5 Esophageal Intramucosal Cyst

This is a 79-year-old woman who was found to have a small apparently submucosal lesion in the cervical esophagus on upper endoscopy. EUS evaluation was requested. The lesion consists of a 12-mm-diameter anechoic space in the mucosa of the esophageal wall. Esophageal cysts are typically classified according to their embryological site of origin as inclusion cysts (lined by squamous or columnar epithelium, sometimes ciliated); retention cysts, also called mucoceles (arising from cystic dilatation of submucosal glands); and developmental or duplication cysts (of esophageal, bronchial, or gastric origin). It is obvious that EUS cannot duplicate histology; however, in this case, a retention cyst is suspected.

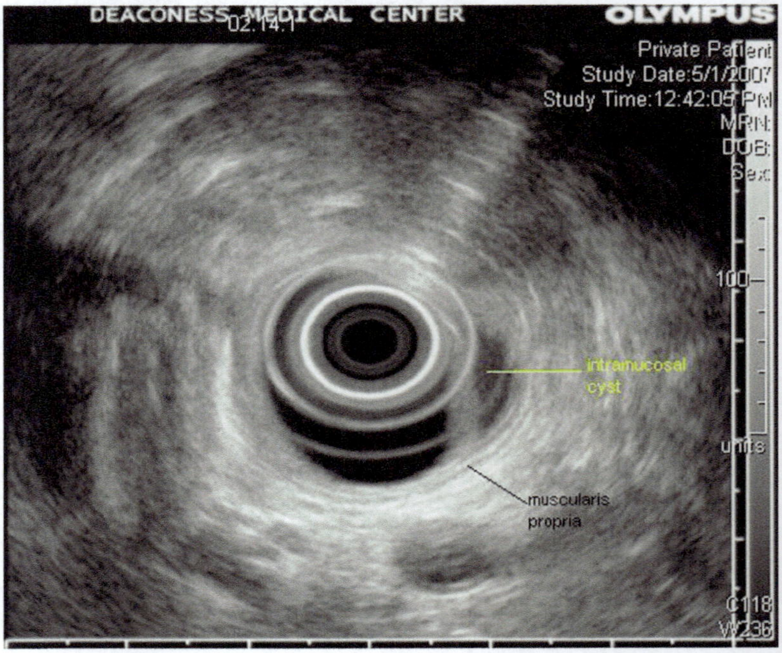

Fig. 2.96 Intramucosal cyst of the esophagus

2.2.2.6 Esophageal Duplication Cyst

Duplication cysts of the gastrointestinal tract are rare benign anomalies that can be recognized by a "duplication" of the wall of the gastrointestinal tract in the cyst lining. This is a 70-year-old patient who presented with dysphagia. The esophageal mucosa was unremarkable on endoscopy, which showed a large submucosal mass. EUS demonstrated a cystic structure with a complex interior consisting of swirls of debris. The cyst clearly originates from the esophagus. The muscularis propria could be followed around the cyst. In addition, a second hypoechoic layer could be identified in the cyst wall, which is characteristic of a duplication cyst.

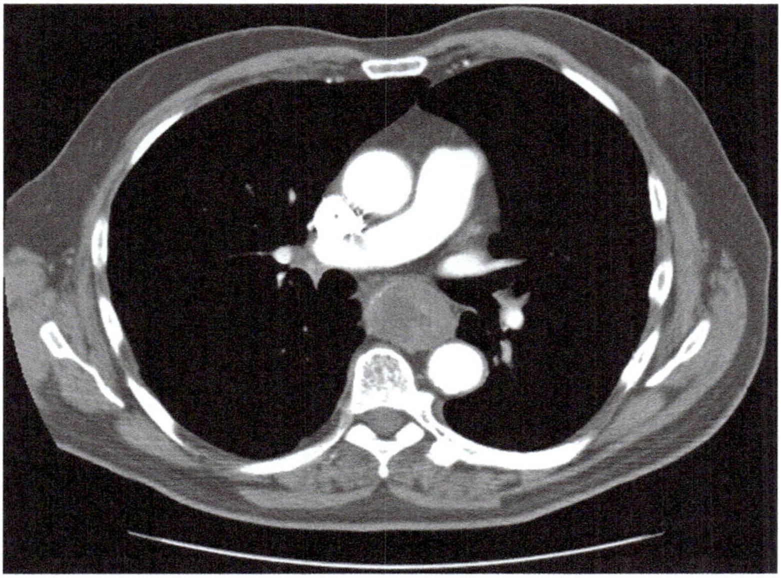

Fig. 2.97 This computed tomography scan shows a large mediastinal mass with a broad differential diagnosis

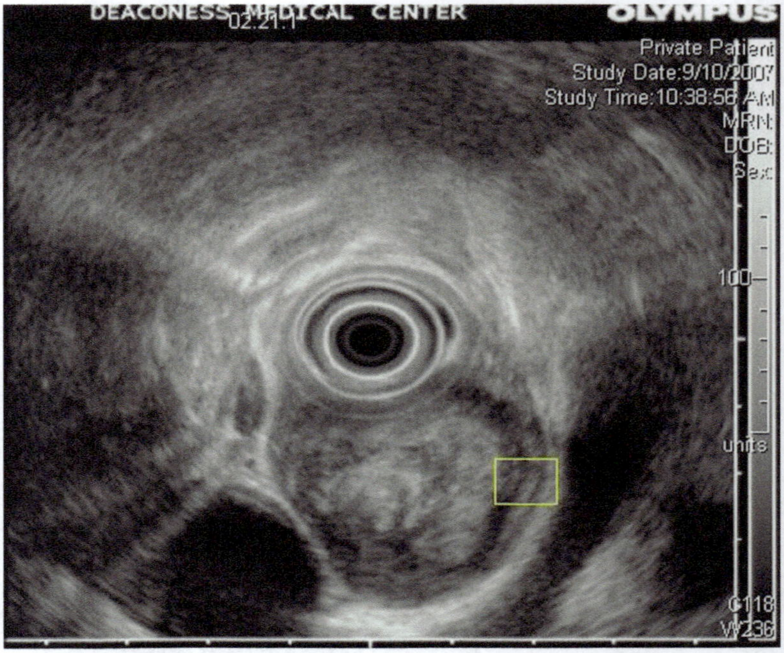

Fig. 2.98 The cyst wall seems to contain several layers of the gastrointestinal tract wall. This is characteristic of an esophageal duplication cyst

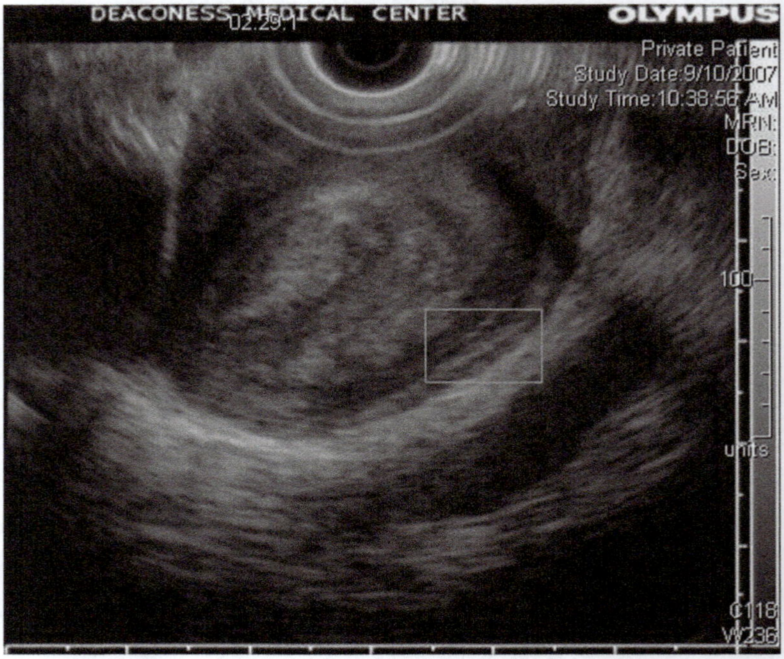

Fig. 2.99 Note the sebaceous appearance of the contents of this duplication cyst, representing cellular debris

2.2.2.7 Esophageal Leiomyoma

This is a 63-year-old patient who underwent a CT scan of the chest for pain under the right rib cage. A small esophageal lesion of unclear etiology was found incidentally. This case also shows nice coronal and sagittal reconstructions of the original CT scan. EUS clearly reveals the layer of origin of the tumor, the muscularis propria, making it virtually certain that this is a benign esophageal leiomyoma. Esophageal tumors arising from the muscularis propria in the esophagus are overwhelmingly leiomyomas, whereas those in the rest of the gastrointestinal tract, especially the stomach, are predominantly gastrointestinal stromal tumors.

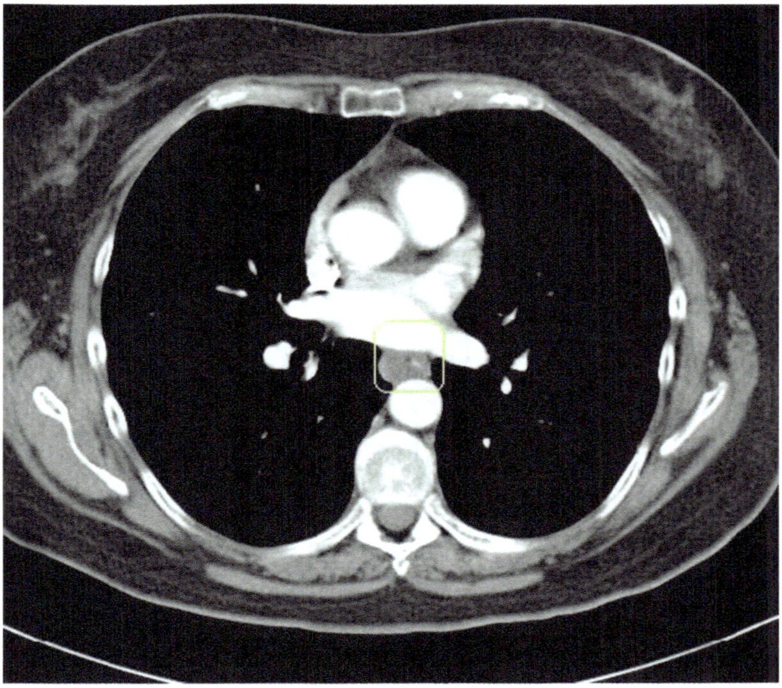

Fig. 2.100 Esophageal leiomyoma seen on computed tomography (horizontal sections)

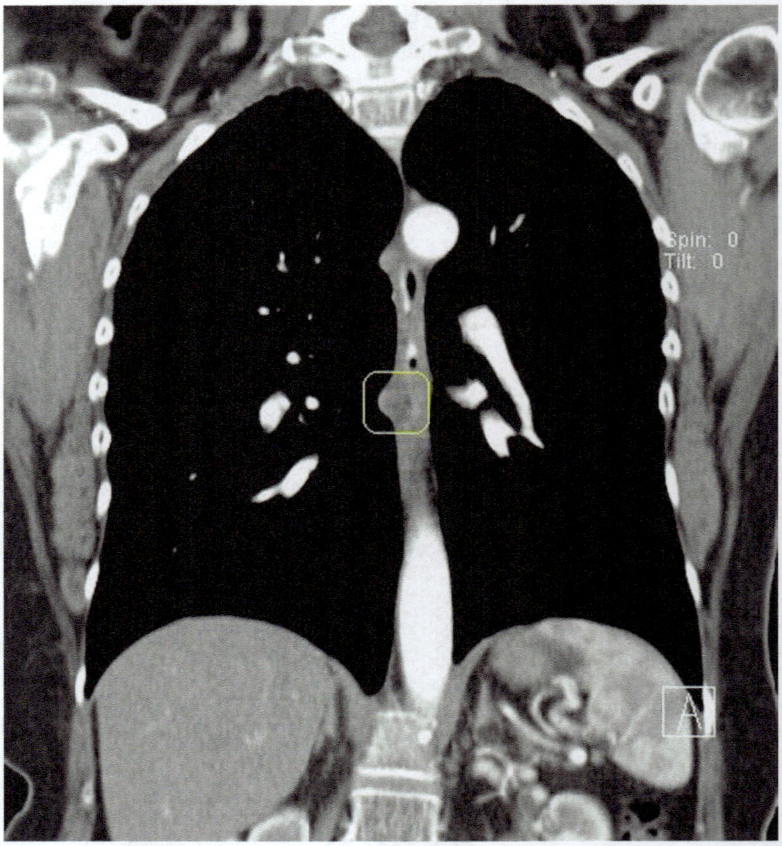

Fig. 2.101 The same esophageal leiomyoma seen on coronal reconstructions of computed tomography

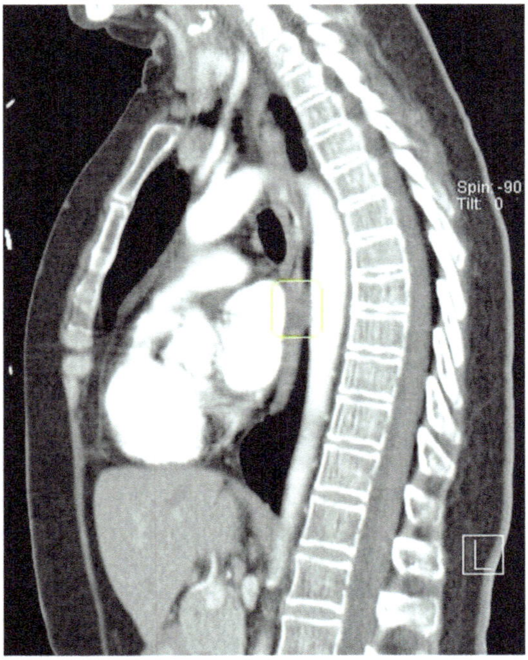

Fig. 2.102 Sagittal computed tomography reconstruction

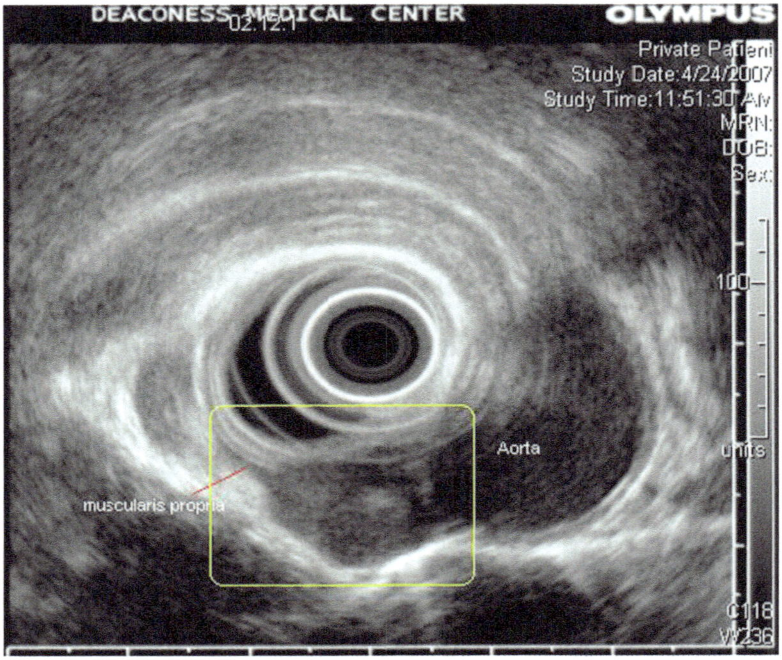

Fig. 2.103 Radial endoscopic ultrasound nicely demonstrates the layer of origin of this esophageal leiomyoma (dimensions, 1.2 × 1.0 cm)

2.2.2.8 Intramural Metastasis of Esophageal Cancer

This is a 62-year-old patient who 8 years earlier had an orthotopic liver transplantation and has done well in this regard. Unfortunately, 18 months before this presentation he was diagnosed with a locally advanced distal esophageal adenocarcinoma. He responded well to radiation and chemotherapy but during a recent follow-up endoscopy a submucosal recurrence was found in the cervical esophagus. Given the rich lymph supply of the esophageal wall, it is interesting that intramural metastases are not seen more often. When found at initial presentation they predict a poor prognosis. In this rare case, indicating recurrent disease, the prognosis is unclear. The patient underwent endoluminal brachytherapy.

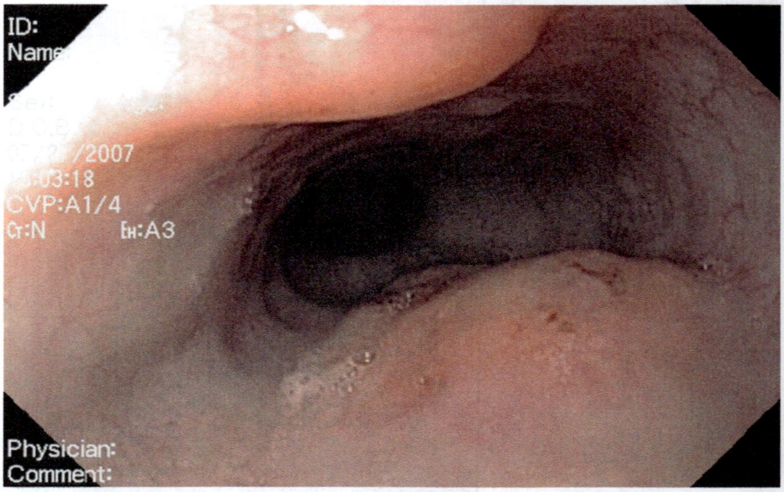

Fig. 2.104 This upper endoscopy image shows a bulge in the cervical esophagus with the mucosa largely intact. Nevertheless, surface biopsies showed underlying adenocarcinoma

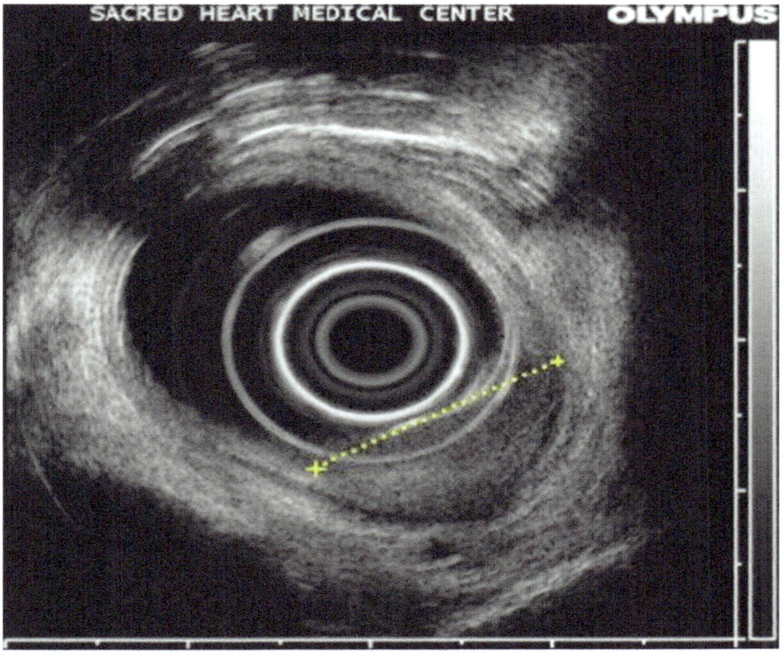

Fig. 2.105 Radial endoscopic ultrasound reveals a 1.5-cm-diameter intramural mass

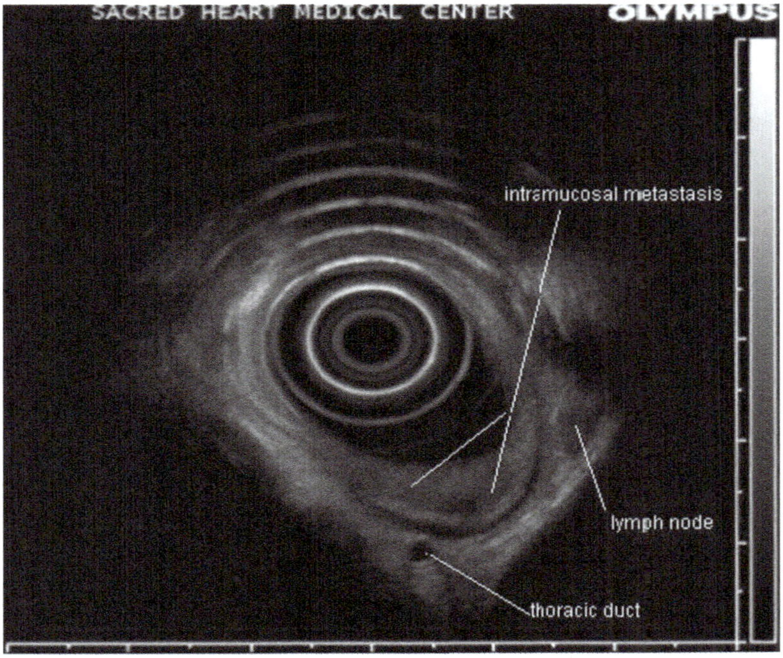

Fig. 2.106 This endoscopic ultrasound image shows the adjacent lymph node

2.2.2.9 Recurrent Esophageal Cancer

Esophageal squamous cell carcinoma has a high postoperative recurrence rate. This 63-year-old man had a chronic esophageal stricture secondary to lye ingestion some 40 years earlier. He was accustomed to frequent small meals of soft food. His symptoms started to worsen and an esophageal dilation was performed elsewhere. This was complicated by perforation, and the patient had an Ivor-Lewis esophagectomy. The final pathology showed an unexpected T3N0 squamous cell carcinoma of the esophagus. He did not receive postoperative radiation and chemotherapy (he apparently refused this treatment). His symptoms worsened again and 5 months after the esophagectomy a PET scan showed three suspicious hot spots in the mediastinum. Surface endoscopy revealed a tight anastomotic stricture but no evidence of recurrent tumor in the lumen. EUS, however, showed an apparent tumor mass adjacent to the esophagus, which FNA determined was positive for squamous cell carcinoma. While PET can suggest the diagnosis of recurrence, radiation and medical oncologists are reluctant to base their treatment decisions on PET findings alone because of the substantial false-positive rate seen postoperatively.

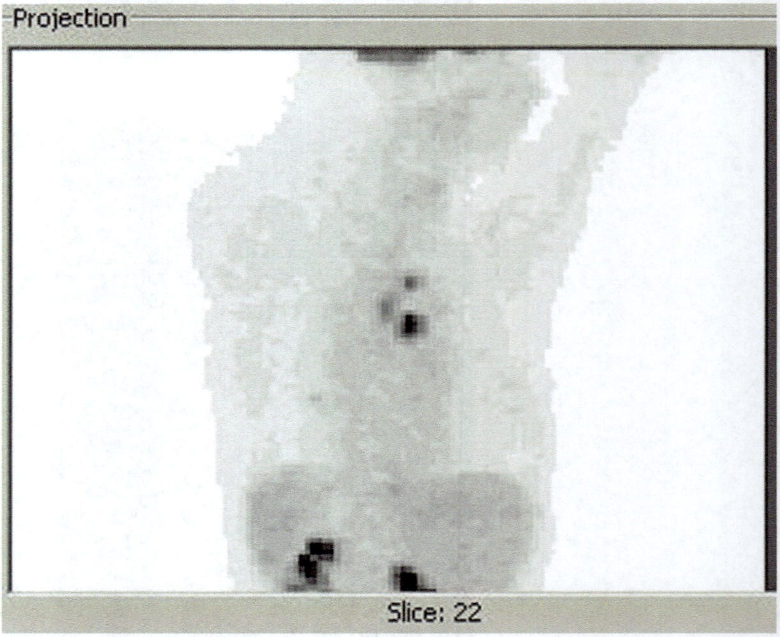

Fig. 2.107 This positron emission tomography scan shows several glucose-avid areas in the mediastinum suspicious for recurrent esophageal squamous cell carcinoma

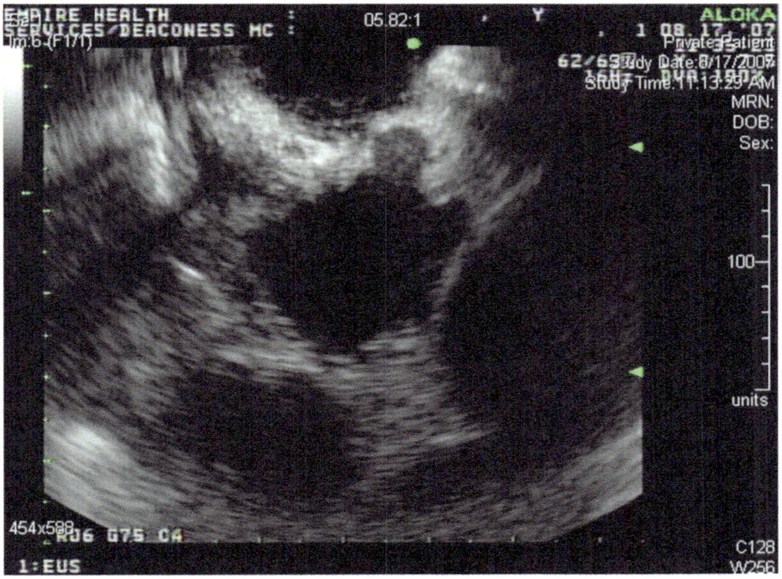

Fig. 2.108 This endoscopic ultrasound image shows a hypoechoic tumor mass outside the lumen of the esophagus. Biopsies were positive for a poorly differentiated squamous cell carcinoma

2.2.2.10 Challenge Question

1. A 60-year-old man was referred for EUS evaluation of recurrent pancreatitis of unknown etiology. EUS revealed no evident cause of pancreatitis, including a normal gallbladder without stones or sludge, a normal pancreatic duct, and no evidence of focal lesions in the pancreas or periampullary area. The endoscope was withdrawn carefully, revealing an oval mass measuring 23 × 18 mm at the level of the left atrium that appeared to arise from the interatrial septum but did not involve the mitral valve. What is the differential diagnosis of this lesion? What is the most likely diagnosis?

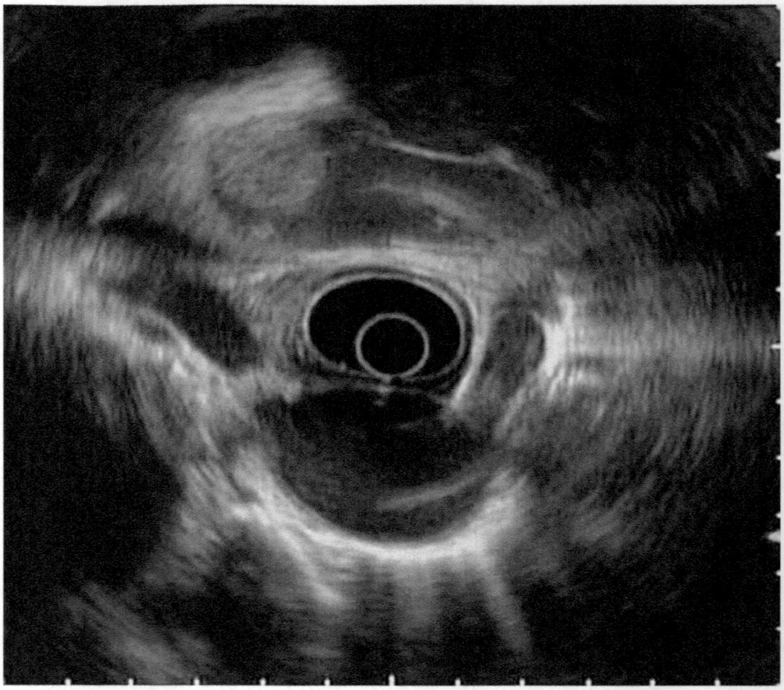

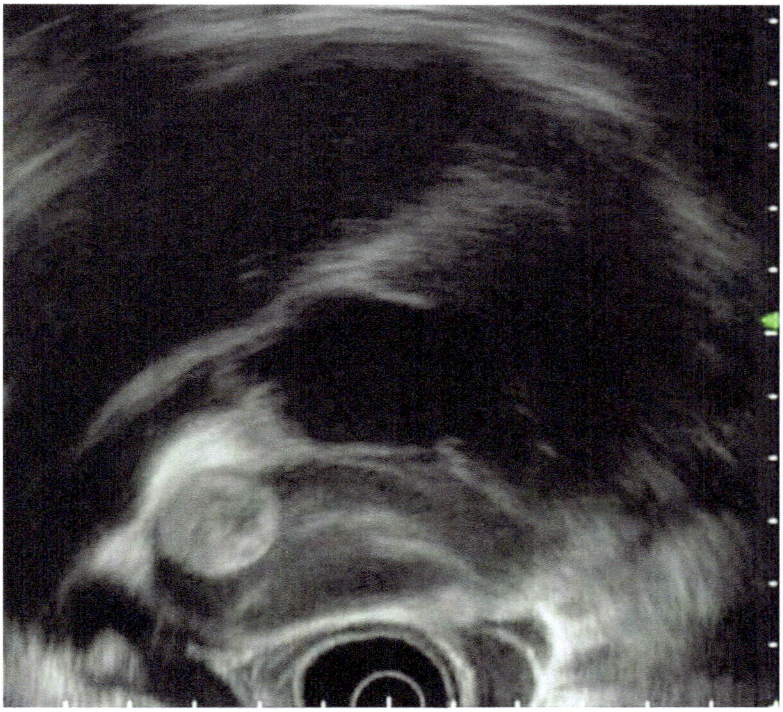

References

1. van Zoonen M, van Oijen M, van Leeuwen M, et al. Low impact of staging EUS for determining surgical resectability in esophageal cancer. Surg Endosc. 2012;26(10):2828–34.
2. Griffin JM, Reed CE, Denlinger CE. Utility of restaging endoscopic ultrasound after neoadjuvant therapy for esophageal cancer. Ann Thorac Surg. 2012;93(6):1855–60.
3. Pouw RE, Heldoorn N, Herrero LA, et al. Do we still need EUS in the workup of patients with early esophageal neoplasia? A retrospective analysis of 131 cases. Gastrointest Endosc. 2011;73(4):662–8.
4. Davies L, Mason J, Roberts S, et al. Prognostic significance of total disease length in esophageal cancer. Surg Endosc. 2012;26(10):2810–6.
5. Twine CP, Roberts SA, Lewis WG, Dave BV, Rawlinson CE, Chan D, Robinson M, Crosby TD. Prognostic significance of endoluminal ultrasound-defined disease length and tumor volume (EDTV) for patients with the diagnosis of esophageal cancer. Surg Endosc. 2010;24(4):870–8.
6. Wallace MB, Woodward TA, Raimondo M, Al-Haddad M, Odell JA. Transaortic fine-needle aspiration of centrally located lung cancer under endoscopic ultrasound guidance: the final frontier. Ann Thorac Surg. 2007;84(3):1019–21.
7. Zhao D-J, Ma D-Q, He W, et al. Cardiovascular parameters to assess the severity of acute pulmonary embolism with computed tomography. Acta Radiol. 2010;51(4):413–9.
8. El-Saadany M, Jalil S, Irisawa A, et al. EUS for portal hypertension: a comprehensive and critical appraisal of clinical and experimental indications. Endoscopy. 2008;40(8):690–6.
9. Bertino EM, Confer PD, Colonna JE, Ross P, Otterson GA. Pulmonary neuroendocrine/carcinoid tumors. Cancer. 2009;115(19):4434–41.
10. Diehl DL, Cheruvattath R, Facktor MA, Go BD. Infection after endoscopic ultrasound-guided aspiration of mediastinal cysts. Interact Cardiovasc Thorac Surg. 2010;10(2):338–40.
11. Drescher R, Köster O, Lukas C. Mediastinal pancreatic pseudocyst with isolated thoracic symptoms: a case report. J Med Case Reports. 2008;2:180.
12. Mallo R, Gottlieb K, Waggoner D, Wittenkeller J. Mediastinal plasmacytoma detected by echocardiography and biopsied with EUS-FNA. Echocardiography. 2008;25(9):997–8.
13. Dores GM, Landgren O, McGlynn KA, et al. Plasmacytoma of bone, extramedullary plasmacytoma, and multiple myeloma: incidence and survival in the United States, 1992–2004. Br J Haematol. 2009;144(1):86–94.
14. Anon. Ultrasound in the diagnosis and management of pleural disease. Curr Opin Pulm Med. Available at

http://journals.lww.com/co-pulmonarymedicine/Fulltext/2003/07000/Ultrasound_in_the_diagnosis_and_management_of.7.aspx. Accessed 20 July 2012.
15. Annema JT, Veseliç M, Rabe KF. EUS-guided FNA of centrally located lung tumours following a non-diagnostic bronchoscopy. Lung Cancer. 2005;48(3):357–61.
16. Tournoy KG, Rintoul RC, van Meerbeeck JP, et al. EBUS-TBNA for the diagnosis of central parenchymal lung lesions not visible at routine bronchoscopy. Lung Cancer. 2009;63(1):45–9.
17. Schreiber G, McCrory DC. Performance characteristics of different modalities for diagnosis of suspected lung cancer summary of published evidence. Chest. 2003;123(1_suppl):115S–28.
18. Silvestri GA, Gould MK, Margolis ML, Tanoue LT, McCrory D, Toloza E, Detterbeck F. Noninvasive staging of non-small cell lung cancer: ACCP evidenced-based clinical practice guidelines. Chest. 2007;132(3 Suppl):178S–201.
19. Talebian M, von Bartheld MB, Braun J, et al. EUS-FNA in the preoperative staging of non-small cell lung cancer. Lung Cancer. 2010;69(1):60–5.
20. Raza MA, Mazzara PF. Sarcomatoid carcinoma of esophagus. Arch Pathol Lab Med. 2011;135(7):945–8.
21. Lack EE, Worsham RGF, Callihan MD, et al. Granular cell tumor: a clinicopathologic study of 110 patients. J Surg Oncol. 1980;13(4):301–16.

Stomach

3

Contents

3.1 **General Principles** 147
3.1.1 Anatomy 147
3.1.2 EUS Probes 148
3.1.3 Technique 148
3.1.4 Preparation 149

3.2 **Cases and Discussions** 150
3.2.1 Gastric Cancer 150
3.2.2 Linitis Plastica of the Stomach 154
3.2.3 Linitis Plastica with Bone Metastases 156
3.2.4 Stage 1 Mucosa-Associated Lymphoid Tissue Lymphoma 159
3.2.5 MALT Lymphoma with Local and Distant Lymph Node Involvement 162
3.2.6 Subepithelial Gastric Tumors 166
3.2.7 Gastrointestinal Stromal Tumor with Central Ulceration 167
3.2.8 Metastatic Gastrointestinal Stromal Tumor 170
3.2.9 Gastrointestinal Stromal Tumors and Interstitial Cells of Cajal 172
3.2.10 An Unusual Gastrointestinal Stromal Tumor in a Patient with Situs Inversus 174
3.2.11 Gastrointestinal Stromal Tumors: Principles of Biopsy 177
3.2.12 Gastric Carcinoid 179
3.2.13 Gastric Lipoma 182
3.2.14 Thickened Gastric Folds, Gastric Varix, or Subepithelial Lesion? 184
3.2.15 Pancreatic Rest 188
3.2.16 Submucosal Gastric Pseudotumor 191
3.2.17 Perigastric Abscess 193

References 195

3.1 General Principles

Endoscopic ultrasound (EUS) is a well-established method used in the evaluation of gastric lesions. This procedure provides information that is key for the diagnosis and management of patients with gastric lymphomas, adenocarcinoma, gastrointestinal stromal tumors (GISTs), and subepithelial lesions, among others.

EUS as a staging modality for gastric malignancies has been extensively evaluated, and it is an excellent modality to obtain a histologic/cytologic diagnosis in cases that are otherwise difficult to diagnose for diagnostic or staging purposes. A clear knowledge of technique, indications, appropriate interpretation of findings, and limitations is fundamental for EUS practice.

3.1.1 Anatomy

EUS can assess the layers of the gastric wall, determining the layer of origin of many lesions as well as the deepest level of local involvement. A pattern of five layers of the gastric wall is easy to recognize with standard EUS endoscopes:

Layer	EUS appearance	Anatomic correlation
First	Hyperechoic (echorich)	Interface between the lumen and mucosa (superficial mucosa)
Second	Hypoechoic (echopoor)	Deep mucosa
Third	Hyperechoic (echorich)	Submucosa
Fourth	Hypoechoic (echopoor)	Muscularis propria
Fifth	Hyperechoic (echorich)	Serosa

K. Gottlieb, G. Marino, *Diagnostic Endosonography*,
DOI 10.1007/978-3-642-39118-7_3, © Springer-Verlag Berlin Heidelberg 2014

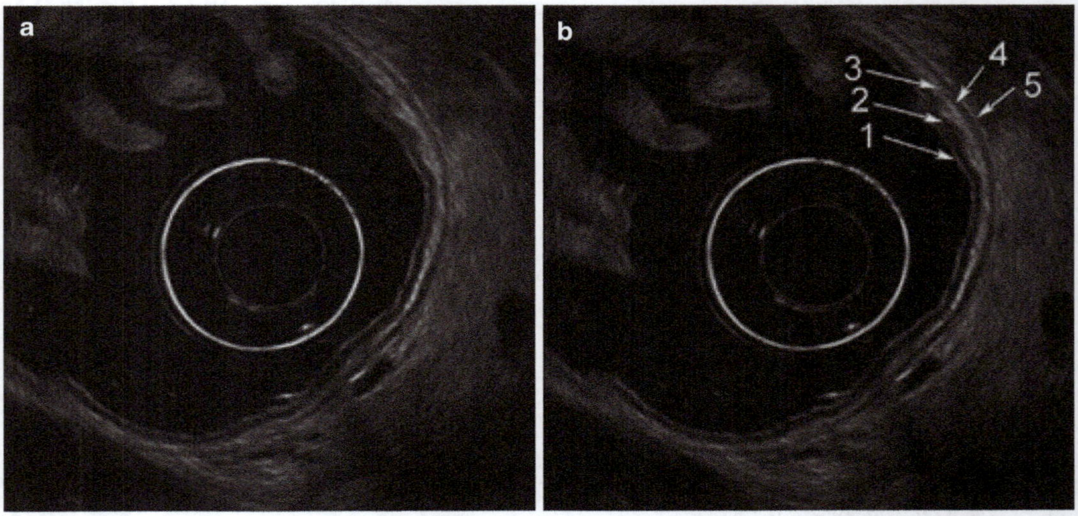

Fig. 3.1 Endoscopic ultrasound images of a normal gastric wall with a five-layered structure using an SU-8000 system (**a**, **b**). *1* first hyperechoic layer, *2* second hypoechoic layer (mucosa), *3* third hyperechoic layer (submucosa), *4* fourth hypoechoic layer (muscularis propria), *5* fifth hyperechoic layer (subserosa and serosa) (From Akahoshi [1])

3.1.2 EUS Probes

EUS examination of the stomach is usually performed with flexible radial scanning echoendoscopes, which provide optimal staging information for gastric malignancies. Miniprobes are also available in some centers and are ideal for the evaluation of small superficial or subepithelial lesions since they have a higher frequency (12–20 MHz) and provide greater resolution. Their disadvantage is that they have limited depth of evaluation and therefore are not recommended for larger lesions.

Linear EUS endoscopes have recently become the echoendoscope of choice for some endoscopists, although many endosonographers still prefer the radial scanning probes for the initial exam. Linear EUS endoscopes allow fine-needle aspiration (FNA) if necessary.

3.1.3 Technique

It is ideal to cover areas of interest with water to enhance acoustic coupling. To better evaluate these areas, air has to be aspirated completely. Air bubbles in the water covering the lesion may also interfere with EUS imaging; suction and repeat filling with water may be necessary to remove these air bubbles. However, some areas, including the cardia, fundus, anterior wall, and lesser curve of the antrum, may be difficult to evaluate. Position changes including supine, right lateral decubitus, or Trendelenburg (flat on the back with the feet higher than the head) may be helpful to cover these areas with water, although these changes may increase the risk of aspiration and patients may need airway protection. Use of an EUS balloon is therefore necessary in some cases to facilitate the examination and minimize the risk of aspiration.

Endoscopic visualization of lesions in the wall of the stomach with oblique view endoscopes allows the endoscopist to position the EUS probe to obtain appropriate sonographic evaluation. This endoscopic visualization should be done with the least amount of air distension possible, preferably under water, to enable optimal acoustic coupling. Recent EUS scopes and electronic consoles allow electronic control of the focal distance; this feature is not available with EUS miniprobes or older models, and in these cases it is important to place the probe at an optimal distance from the wall to obtain a detailed examination of the gastric layers.

To obtain appropriate measurement of wall or lesion thickness, ultrasound waves should approach the wall perpendicularly. Excessive compression should also be avoided; this can impair visualization of subtle lesions or distort the interface between wall layers.

3.1.4 Preparation

EUS evaluation is done with standard preparation for upper endoscopy. Patients are placed in the left lateral decubitus position. Position changes with water filling of the stomach should be done carefully, and appropriate airway protection should be provided to avoid aspiration.

Box 3.1: Resources

- National Comprehensive Cancer Network (NCCN) Clinical Practice Guidelines in Oncology: Soft Tissue Sarcoma http://www.globalgist.org/docs/NCCN_guidelines.pdf
- American Cancer Society: Cancer facts and statistics http://www.cancer.org/Research/CancerFactsFigures/index
- Paris staging system for primary gastrointestinal lymphomas (*Gut* 2003) http://www.ncbi.nlm.nih.gov/pmc/articles/PMC1773680/pdf/gut05200912.pdf
- Small gastric lymphoma diagnosed by EUS images (YouTube) https://www.youtube.com/watch?v=OWC7-1ar5W0

3.2 Cases and Discussions

3.2.1 Gastric Cancer

This is an 87-year-old Japanese woman who was referred for the evaluation of a gastric abnormality. Eighteen months before this presentation a gastric polyp was biopsied and showed only adenoma. The patient returned to her physician again 3 months before her referral to us and again the biopsies showed adenoma. The referring physician felt uneasy with this situation and the patient was referred for EUS. The lesion turned out to be rather large (3.2 cm). Repeat biopsies were performed with the Radial Jaw® 4 Jumbo Biopsy Forceps (Boston-Scientific), and invasive adenocarcinoma was found.

In the United States, gastric cancer ranks 14th in incidence among the major types of malignancies, with approximately 21,320 new cases per year and 10,540 deaths estimated in 2012 [2]. The site of origin within the stomach has changed in frequency in the United States over recent decades. The incidence of tumors of the distal half of the stomach have been decreasing in the Western world since the 1930s, with the incidence of cancer of the cardia and gastroesophageal junction increasing over the past two decades. This elderly patient from Japan, however, illustrates the exception. For reasons not entirely clear but probably related to diet, the incidence of distal gastric cancers remains high in Japan, Chile, and Iceland.

Staging of this disease is critical; unfortunately, in the United States most patients have advanced disease at presentation and therefore their prognosis is poor. However, if detected at an early stage, the management of gastric cancer can be successful. Patients with early gastric cancer (T1 mucosal disease) can be resected endoscopically and patients with T1–T3 locoregional disease without distant metastases are candidates for surgical resection [3].

EUS is considered the most accurate preoperative test for T staging; however, its actual accuracy for T staging varies between 57 and 92 % [3]. EUS is more accurate with advanced disease. Accuracy of N staging using EUS has been reported between 50 and 87 %, with results similar to computed tomography (CT) and magnetic resonance.

Ulcerated lesions may cause fibrosis and inflammatory changes that cannot be differentiated from actual tumoral invasion by EUS [4, 5]. Inflammatory changes indistinguishable from cancer on EUS can also be found after chemotherapy, and therefore this technique is not recommended to assess response after neoadjuvant therapy [6].

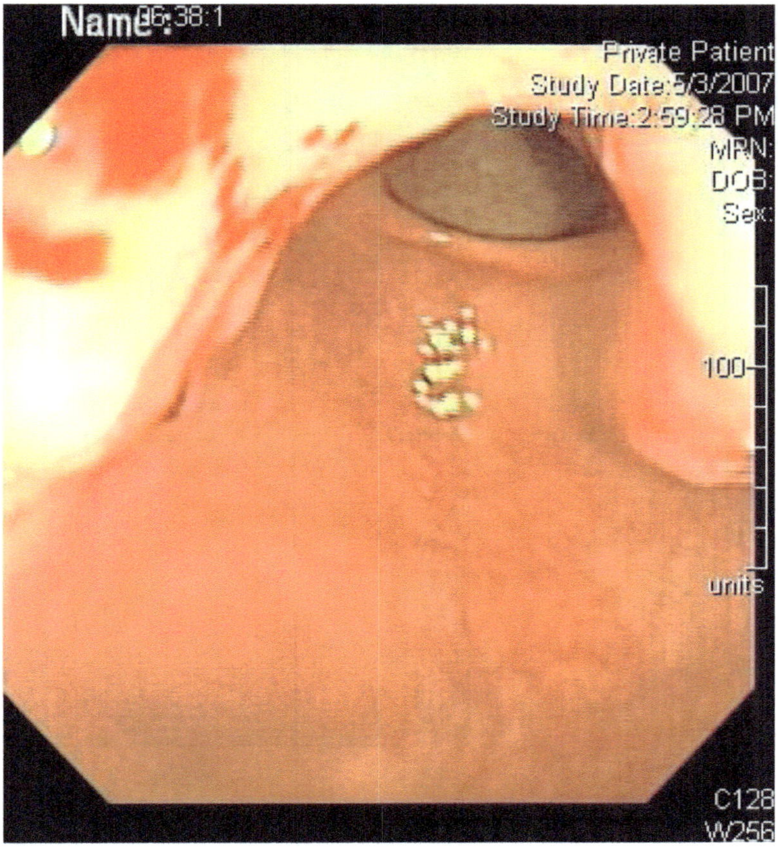

Fig. 3.2 This is how the adenocarcinoma appeared on esophagogastroduodenoscopy

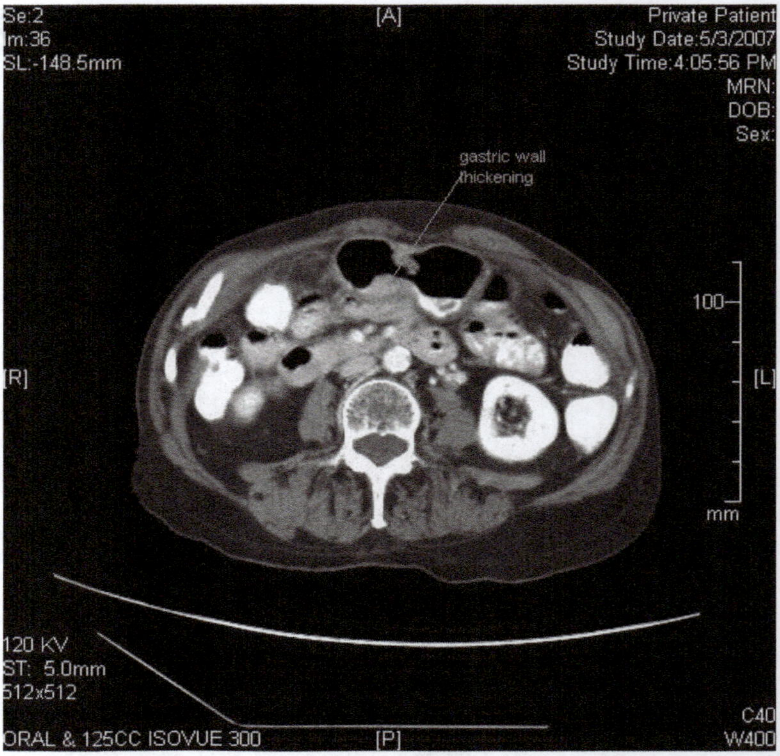

Fig. 3.3 Nonspecific thickening of the gastric wall is seen on this computed tomography scan, which was obtained after the endoscopic ultrasound to rule out distant metastasis

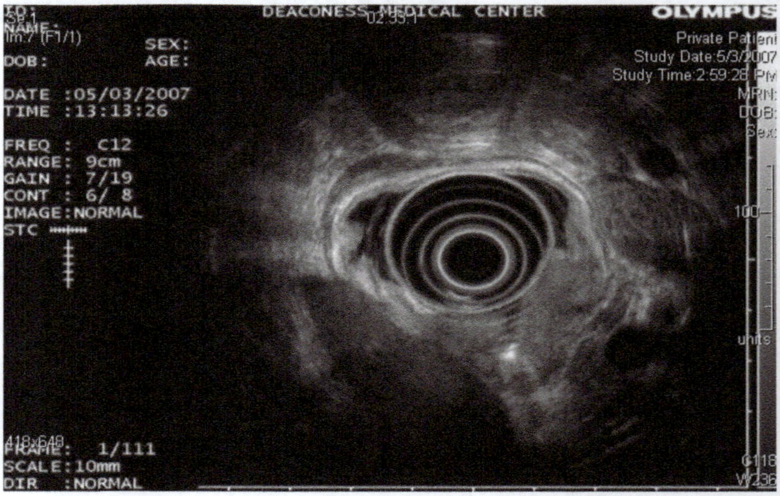

Fig. 3.4 The endoscopic ultrasound shows a gastric cancer obliterating the muscularis propria (T3)

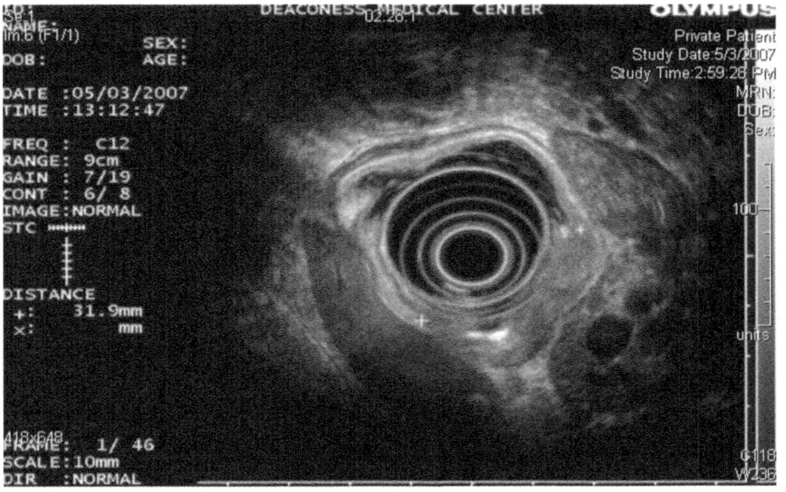

Fig. 3.5 A different endoscopic ultrasound image of the same gastric cancer. No lymphadenopathy was seen

3.2.2 Linitis Plastica of the Stomach

This 58-year-old man presented with nausea and weight loss. Initial endoscopy showed thickened gastric folds suspicious for the condition but biopsies (performed on two separate occasions) were nondiagnostic. On the basis of the CT and EUS appearance, linitis plastic was strongly suspected and the patient referred for laparotomy, at which time the diagnosis was confirmed with a full-thickness biopsy.

Linitis plastica is a diffuse infiltration of the wall of a hollow viscus with severe desmoplastic response, fixing the superficial layers to the muscularis propria and producing a rigid, thickened appearance of the organ. In the stomach this has been called "leather bottle" and is found in up to 10 % of adenocarcinomas, although it can also be secondary to metastatic disease such as infiltrating lobular breast carcinoma [7]. The prognosis is generally poor.

Endoscopically the stomach appears rigid and nondistensible. It affects the antrum and pyloric regions more commonly than the fundus. EUS findings include increased wall thickness (>6 mm) and loss of architecture of the gastric layers.

The superficial gastric mucosa is frequently spared and the malignant cells can be scarcely distributed in the fibrous stroma, making the endoscopic diagnosis challenging [8]; endoscopic biopsies are negative for malignancy in up to a third of cases of linitis plastica adenocarcinomas [9, 10]. Additional endoscopic techniques to obtain a better yield include "tunnel" biopsy, in which biopsies are taken at the same site to obtain deeper samples, and large particle biopsy, in which a fragment of a thickened fold is resected with a diathermic snare or EUS-guided FNA [10].

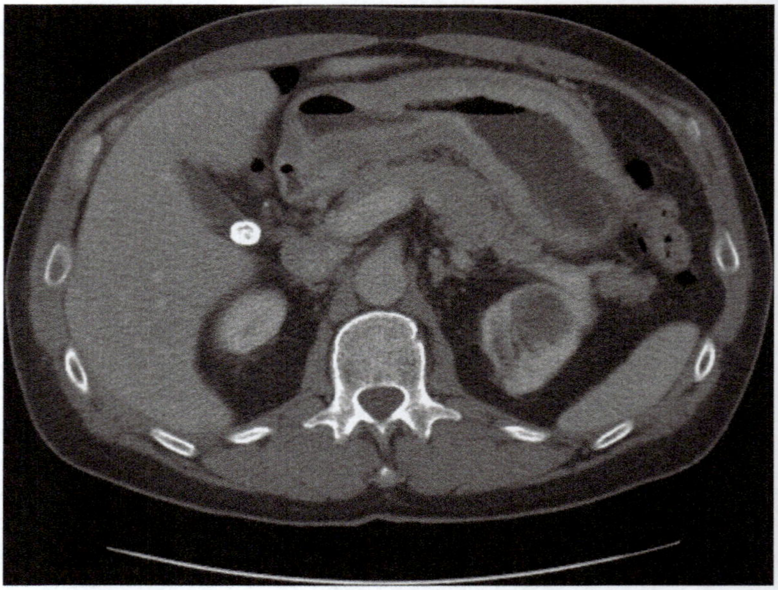

Fig. 3.6 A markedly thickened gastric wall on computed tomography

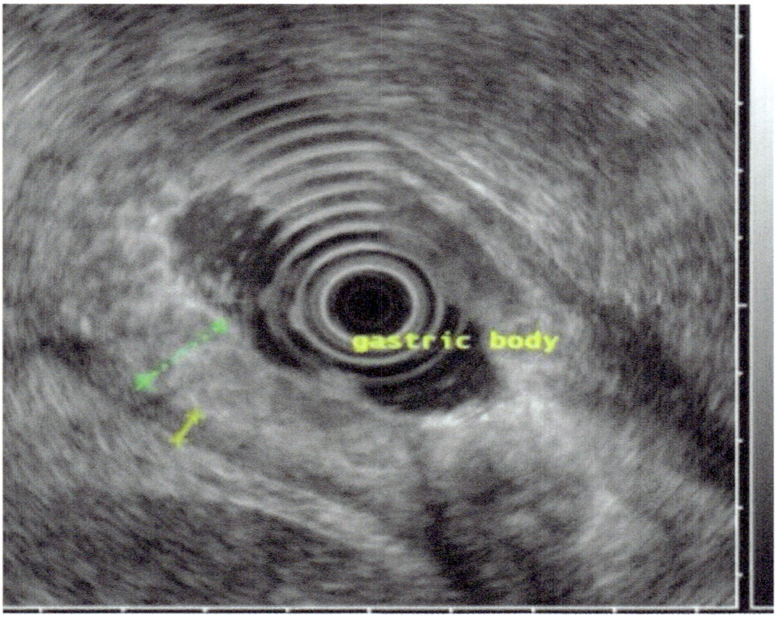

Fig. 3.7 Linitis plastica. The mucosa measures 11 mm, the muscularis 4 mm, *green line* mucosa and submucosa; *yellow line* muscularis propria

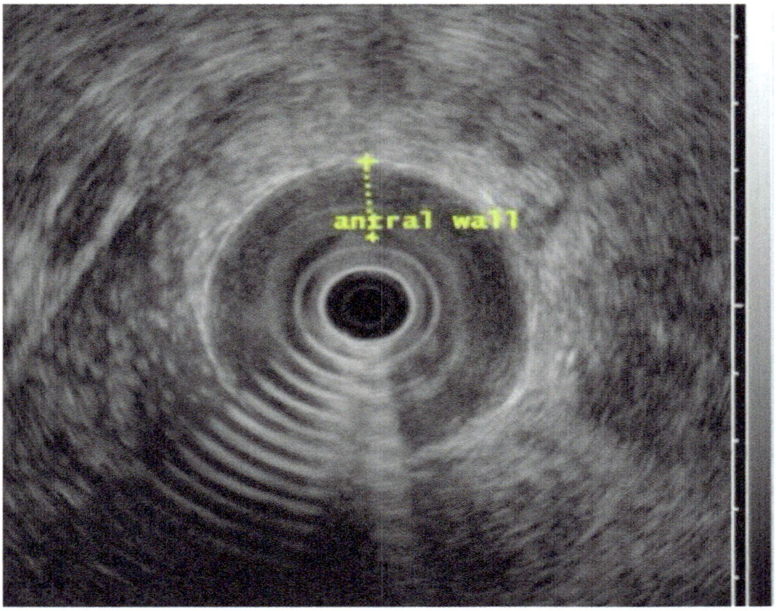

Fig. 3.8 The antral wall is thickened to 12 mm and uniformly hypoechoic

3.2.3 Linitis Plastica with Bone Metastases

This is a 48-year-old woman who was found to have a single bone lesion, which biopsy found to be metastatic adenocarcinoma. Subcarinal lymph node enlargement was found on a chest CT scan. EUS-guided FNA was requested. The lymph nodes seen during the examination with the linear EUS instrument were rather unimpressive. Instead, a markedly abnormal-appearing gastric mucosa was encountered both by surface endoscopy and ultrasound. The CT scan also showed impressive thickening of the gastric wall. The stomach was biopsied twice, once with a regular biopsy forceps and subsequently as a large particle biopsy performed with a polypectomy snare. Both samples were nondiagnostic.

Linitis plastica is a proliferative condition of the connective tissue. It is triggered by the presence of malignant signet-ring cells, which spread diffusely through the layers of the gastric wall. Malignant cells are usually absent from otherwise grossly abnormal-appearing gastric mucosa. The mucosal layer can be so expanded that even very aggressive biopsies do not get to the layer that contains the malignant cells. Ordinary cancers that originate from the mucosa and spread partially through the muscularis propria without eliciting a connective tissue response of this sort should not be called linitis plastica.

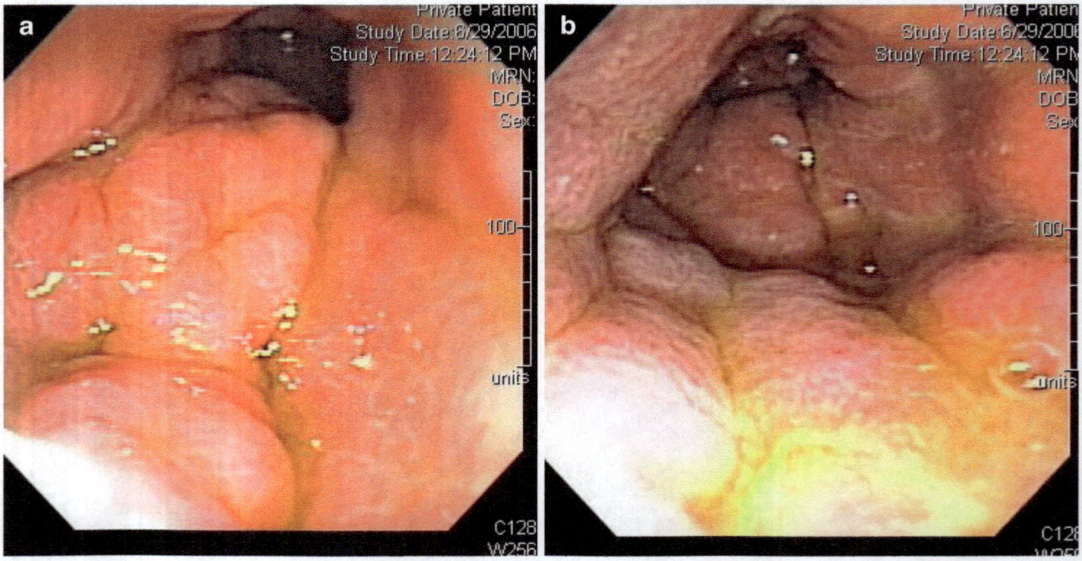

Fig. 3.9 Linitis plastica: Appearance of the gastric mucosa on esophagogastroduodenoscopy

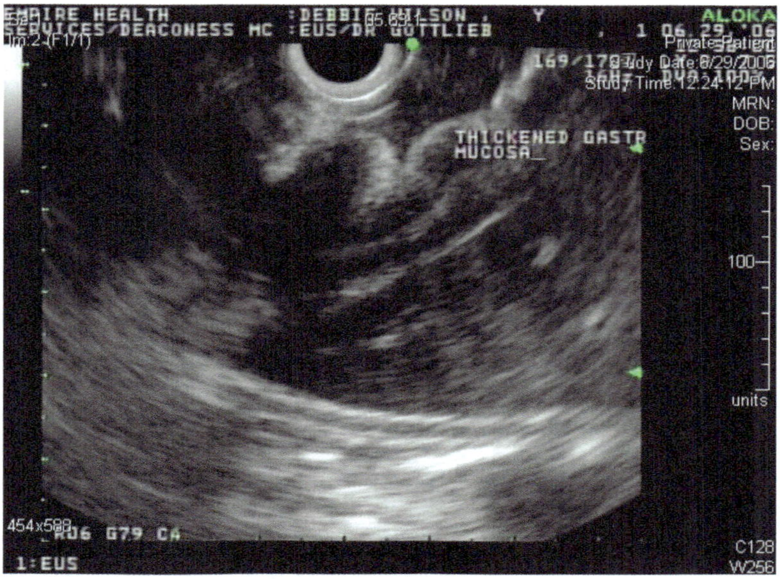

Fig. 3.10 The marked thickening of the gastric wall is apparent on this linear endoscopic ultrasound image

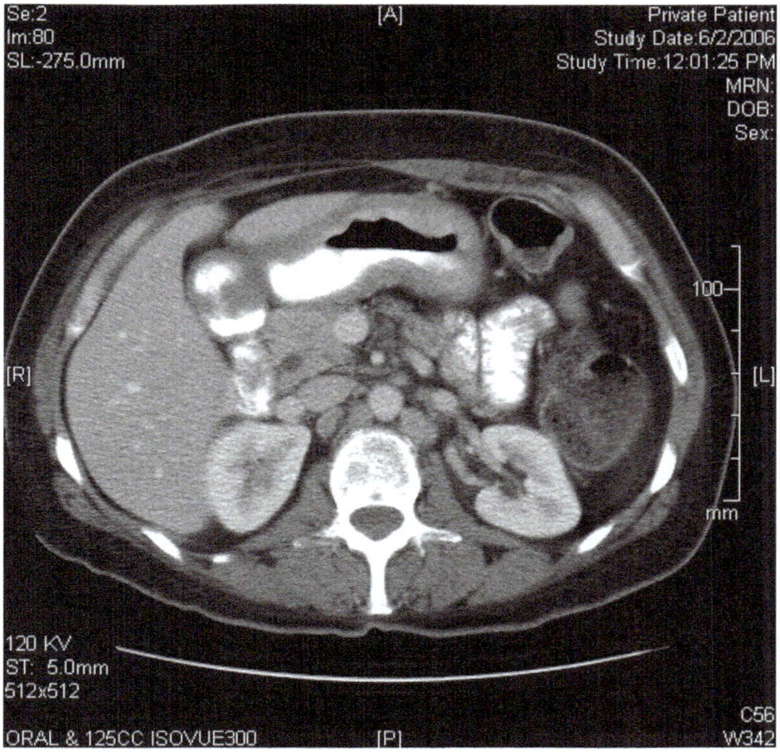

Fig. 3.11 Marked thickening of the wall of the stomach on a computed tomography scan

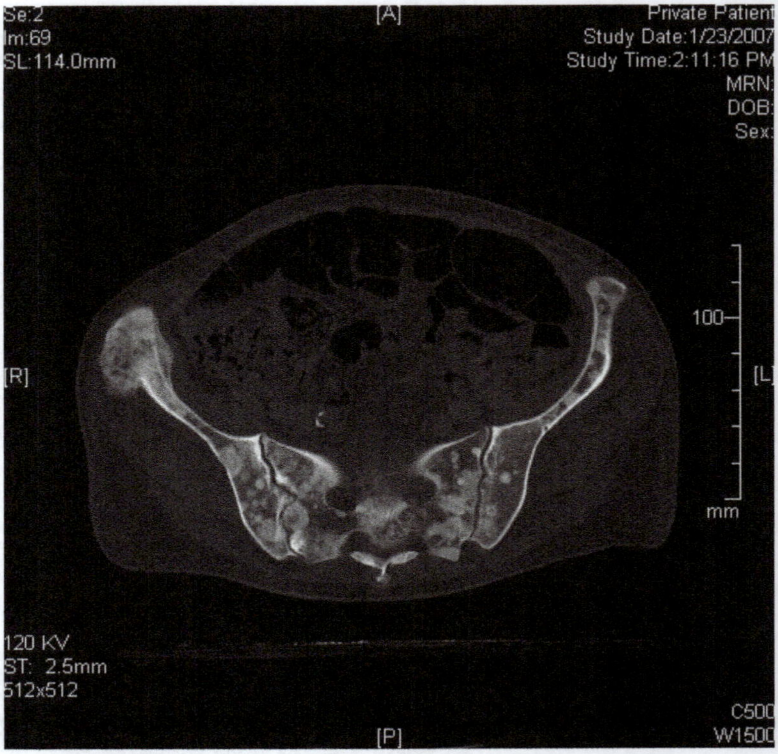

Fig. 3.12 Several months later multiple bone metastases are apparent on this pelvic computed tomography scan

3.2.4 Stage 1 Mucosa-Associated Lymphoid Tissue Lymphoma

This is a 59-year-old patient with a history of a peptic ulcer that had healed when viewed on follow-up endoscopy. However, the endoscopist noted severe hemorrhagic-appearing gastritis along the greater curvature. Biopsies showed an "increased amount of intraepithelial lymphocytes," and a process such as a mucosa-associated lymphoid tissue (MALT) lymphoma could not be ruled out. The patient was referred for EUS evaluation and repeat biopsies, which were performed with the Radial Jaw® 4 Jumbo Biopsy Forceps (Boston-Scientific), and a battery of immunostains confirmed the presence of a low-grade MALT lymphoma.

In the new World Health Organization classification of lymphoid tumors, MALT lymphomas are more correctly called "extranodal marginal zone B-cell lymphomas." This is because there is now strong evidence to suggest that the type of cell from which the lymphoma develops is a specific B-cell that is found in a compartment of the lymphoid tissue called the marginal zone.

Lymphomas represent approximately 5 % of all gastric malignancies, and the most common of them are extranodal marginal zone B-cell lymphomas. Ninety percent of these gastric MALT lymphomas are associated with the presence of *Helicobacter pylori*. These patients will have a monoclonal B-cell infiltration as opposed to the polyclonal response seen in chronic gastritis; additional immunohistochemistry is necessary to differentiate it from other gastric B-cell lymphomas such as mantle cell, lymphocytic gastric, and follicular gastric lymphomas [11]. EUS-guided FNA can be helpful in establishing the diagnosis of non-Hodgkin's lymphoma in up to 89 % of suspicious cases with inconclusive endoscopic biopsies, as shown by Wiersema et al. [12].

There is no generally agreed-upon staging protocol or classification scheme for gastric MALT lymphomas. Adapted versions of the Ann Arbor staging system, such as the Lugano modification of the Blackledge staging scheme [13] and the adapted version of Musshoff's modified Ann Arbor staging system [14], have been used for this purpose; more recently the Paris staging system [15] was developed for gastrointestinal lymphomas (the Paris classification is available at: http://www.ncbi.nlm.nih.gov/pmc/articles/PMC1773680/pdf/gut05200912.pdf). The latter allows stratifying patients using a TNM (tumor, node, metastasis) scheme. T staging in this classification is based on the deepest layer involved, which can be estimated by EUS. Regardless, EUS is considered the most accurate locoregional method of staging [3].

The spectrum of MALT lymphomas ranges from involvement of the mucosa layer alone to all layers of the gastric wall and spread to the lymph nodes and spleen. Increasing depth of invasion through the stomach wall is closely correlated with decreasing responsiveness to treatment to eradicate *H. pylori*. Other EUS-based studies have shown that involvement of the regional lymph nodes is associated with considerably reduced response rates to either antibiotics to eradicate *H. pylori* or conventional lymphoma treatment; response in T1N0 disease is approximately 75 %, decreasing to 50 % in T1N1 and 25 % in T2N0 disease.

The role of EUS in the evaluation of response to therapy or as a surveillance method to detect relapsing MALT lymphoma is controversial; some authors have documented a long time lag between histological and endosonographic remission and sonographic normalization despite histologically ongoing disease [16].

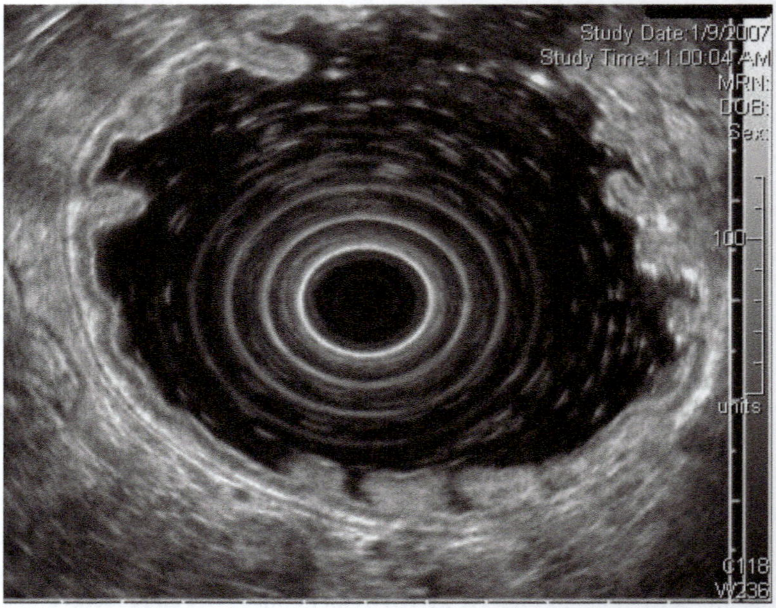

Fig. 3.13 In this mucosa-associated lymphoid tissue case the mucosal layer is subtly expanded

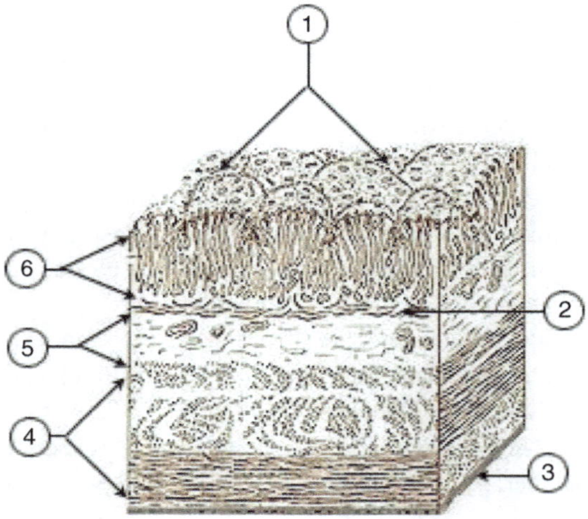

Fig. 3.14 Typically the mucosa occupies one third of the gastric wall thickness (Wikimedia Commons)

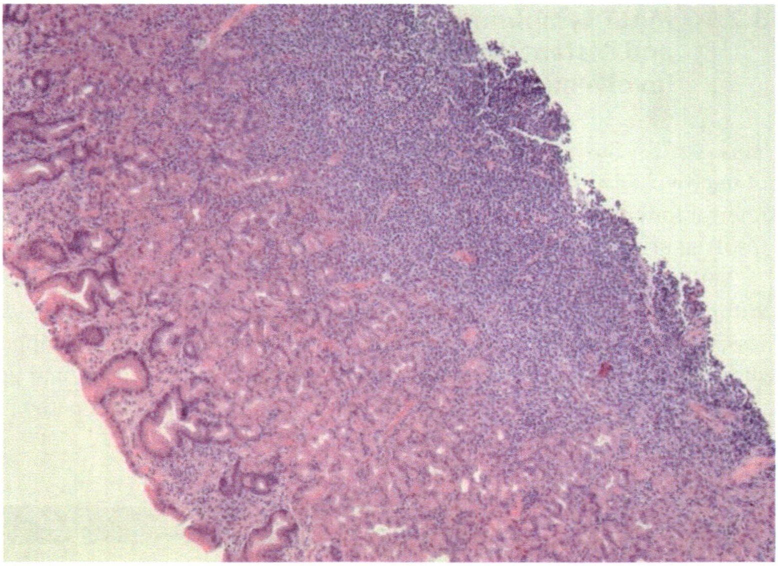

Fig. 3.15 Hematoxylin and eosin stain of the gastric mucosa-associated lymphoid tissue lymphoma shows the dense infiltrate of small lymphocytes

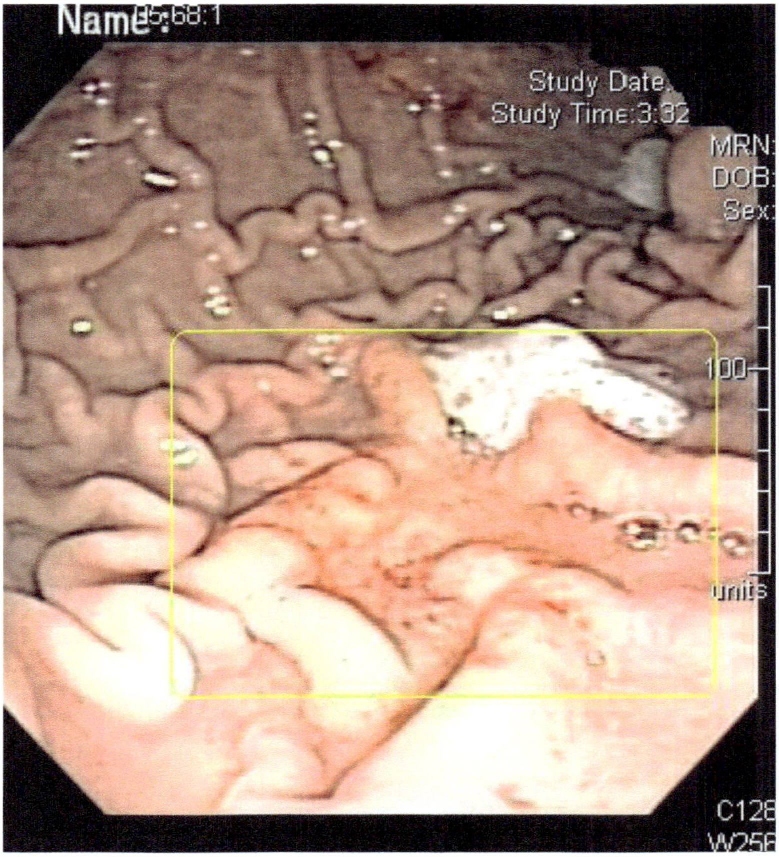

Fig. 3.16 Eight weeks after eradication of the *Helicobacter pylori* organism the area involved by "gastritis" had receded to approximately. 5 cm in diameter, as shown here

3.2.5 MALT Lymphoma with Local and Distant Lymph Node Involvement

This is a 78-year-old patient who had complained of unprovoked vomiting several weeks before her referral for endoscopy. All of her symptoms have resolved and she now feels well.

Endoscopy showed a deep ulcer associated with abnormal surrounding tissue along the lesser curvature of the stomach. Biopsies showed MALT lymphoma confirmed by immunohistochemistry. A CT scan showed what initially was interpreted as a mass in the cecum, but colonoscopy was normal. In fact, what was seen were distant lymph node metastases. There were also enlarged regional perigastric lymph nodes, which were well demonstrated on EUS. Per the World Health Organization classification, this MALT lymphoma is more appropriately called extranodal marginal zone B-cell lymphoma. In this case with regional and distant nodal metastasis. Less than 10 % of patients with MALT lymphoma have distant lymph node involvement, and up to 30 % may have regional lymphadenopathy.

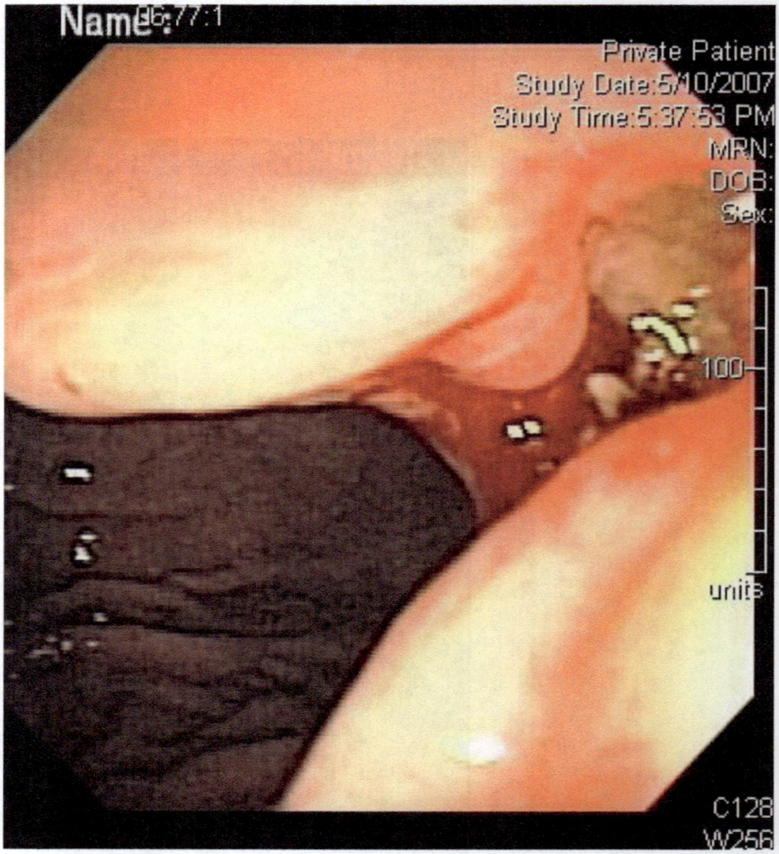

Fig. 3.17 This deep gastric ulcer seen on upper endoscopy with surrounding thickened mucosa turned out to be secondary to a mucosa-associated lymphoid tissue lymphoma

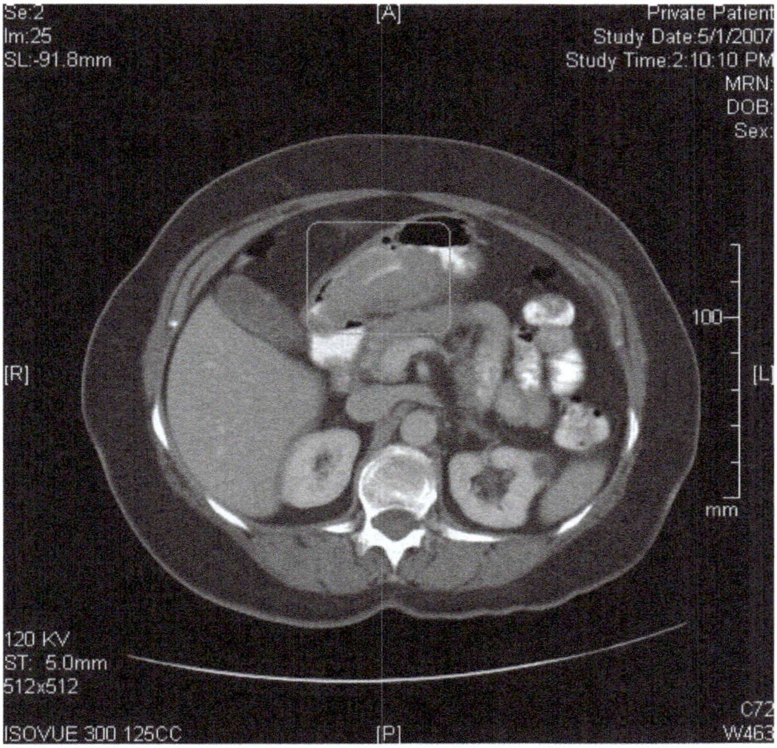

Fig. 3.18 On this computed tomography scan a large gastric mass is seen; in fact, it appears much larger than appreciated on endoscopy

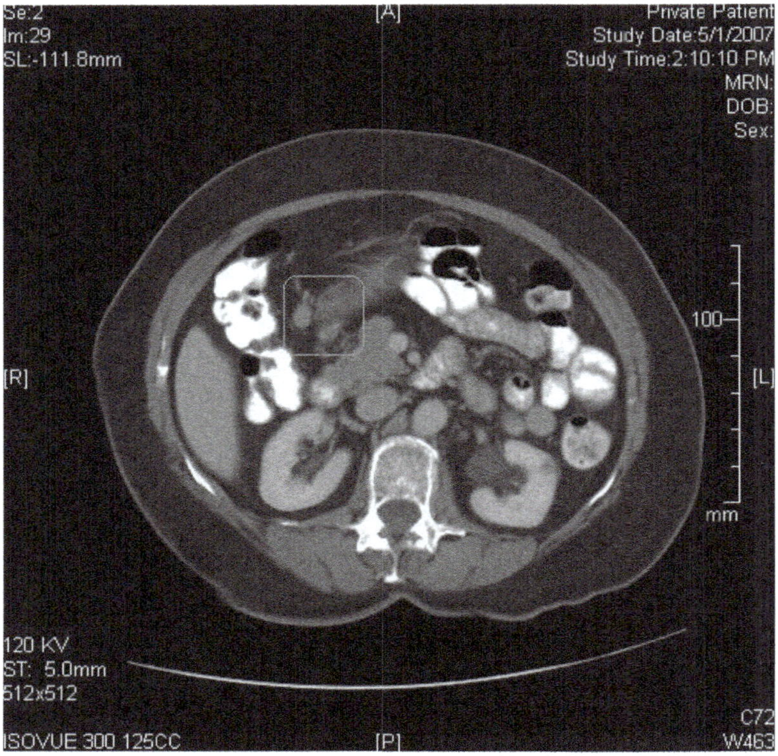

Fig. 3.19 This computed tomography scan shows perigastric lymph node enlargement

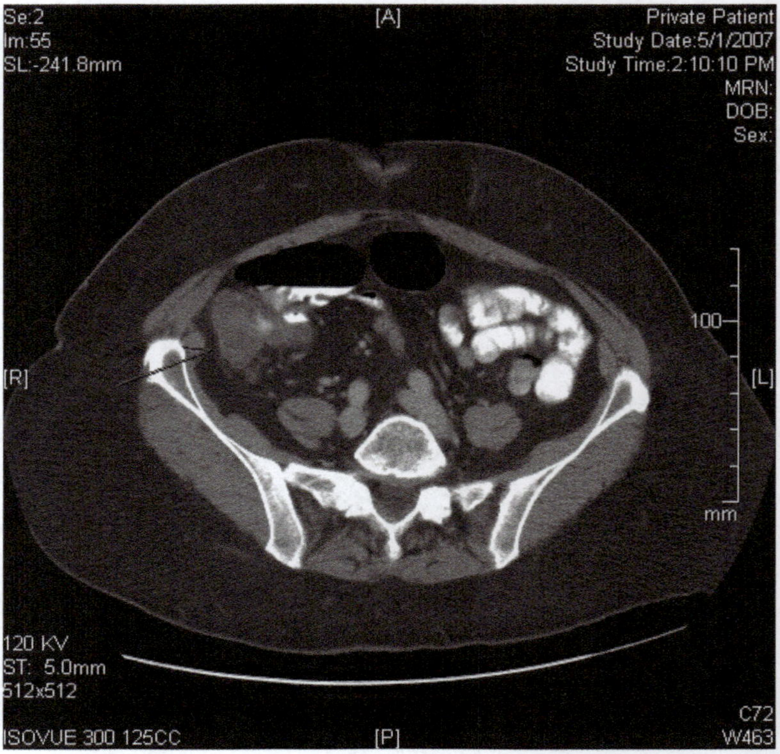

Fig. 3.20 A right lower quadrant lymph node conglomerate is also present. This was initially interpreted as a cecal mass

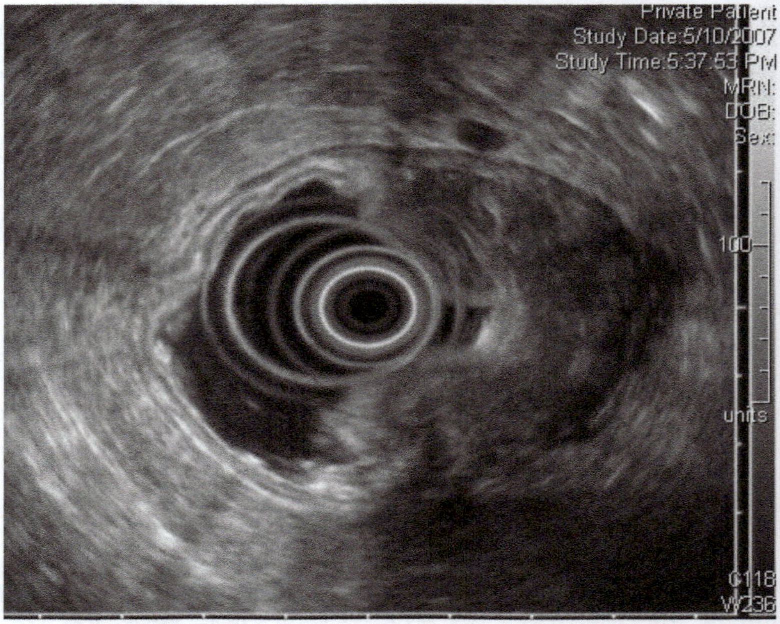

Fig. 3.21 The endoscopic ultrasound image demonstrates transmural involvement of the gastric wall by the lymphoma

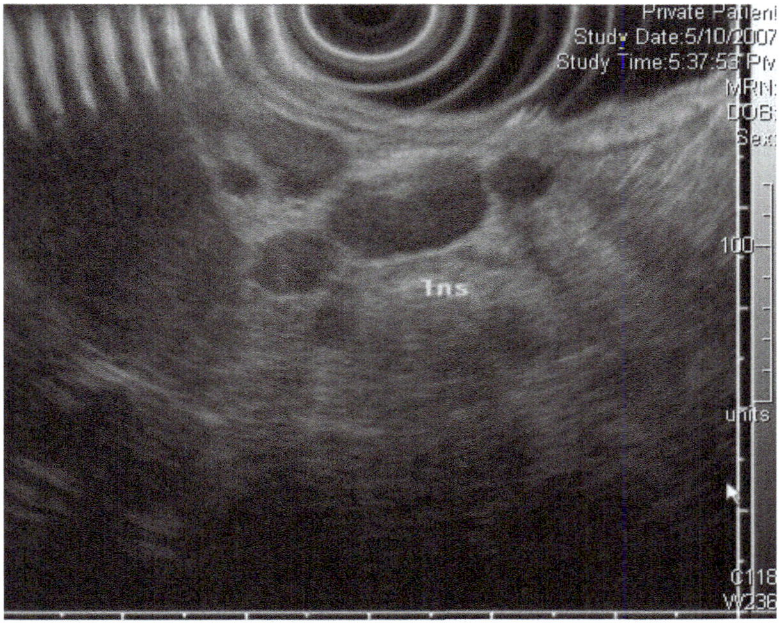

Fig. 3.22 Perigastric lymphadenopathy as seen by endoscopic ultrasound

3.2.6 Subepithelial Gastric Tumors

Subepithelial gastric tumors include lesions that arise from the gastric wall but are covered by normal mucosa; therefore they can originate from deep mucosa to serosa. Subepithelial lesions are commonly found on endoscopy, although most of them are asymptomatic. Unfortunately, it is difficult to establish their malignant potential by endoscopy alone, and EUS has become the study of choice to narrow the differential diagnosis. EUS can exclude extrinsic compression and vascular lesions; determine their nature (solid vs. cystic), and allow tissue sampling.

Differential diagnosis of subepithelial gastric lesions
Gastrointestinal stromal tumors
Leiomyoma
Leiomyosarcoma
Schwannoma
Granular cell tumors
Carcinoid
Lipoma
Glomus tumor
Metastases
Neurofibroma
Kaposi's sarcoma
Duplication cyst
Submucosal cyst
Gastric varices
Lymphangioma
Pancreatic rest
Hemangiomas

In the following cases we illustrate some of most common presentations of subepithelial gastric lesions.

3.2.7 Gastrointestinal Stromal Tumor with Central Ulceration

This is a patient with a history of bleeding in the upper gastrointestinal tract. Surface endoscopy shows a submucosal lesion with overlying central ulceration in the body of the stomach. EUS shows a hypoechoic well-circumscribed tumor that connects to the muscularis propria. This tumor was surgically removed and the final pathology confirmed GIST.

GISTs have an incidence between 5,000 and 10,000 cases per year in the United States [17]. They can develop in any segment of the gastrointestinal tract, but their most common primary location (approximately 50 % of GISTs) is the stomach [18].

Bleeding, as found in this case, is the most common clinical manifestation. Patients can also present with signs or symptoms related to mass effect, including early satiety, bloating, or a palpable mass. In about 20 % of patients these tumors are found incidentally [17].

GISTs in the upper gastrointestinal tract appear as subepithelial bulging lesions; they are occasionally ulcerated. Endoscopic biopsies are usually not able to provide adequate tissue for histologic diagnosis [19]. EUS is considered the procedure of choice to obtain histologic confirmation of GISTs, but its main role is to establish a differential diagnosis with other subepithelial or vascular lesions. Most GISTs arise from the fourth hypoechoic layer (muscularis propria) Fig. 3.25, although occasional cases can arise from the muscularis mucosa, as demonstrated in one of the following cases Fig. 3.34. These tumors have a hypoechoic appearance. Large GIST tumors may have a heterogeneous sonographic pattern due to necrosis, hemorrhage, and cystic or hyaline degeneration. Some authors have reported that the accuracy of EUS without FNA in establishing the diagnosis of subepithelial tumors is suboptimal [20, 21], emphasizing the importance of histologic diagnosis. However, if the lesion has a classic endoscopic appearance, as demonstrated in this case, and the lesion appears resectable without neoadjuvant therapy, then preoperative biopsy or FNA are not necessary [22].

A clear management algorithm recommended by the NCCN is available at: http://www.global-gist.org/docs/NCCN_guidelines.pdf.

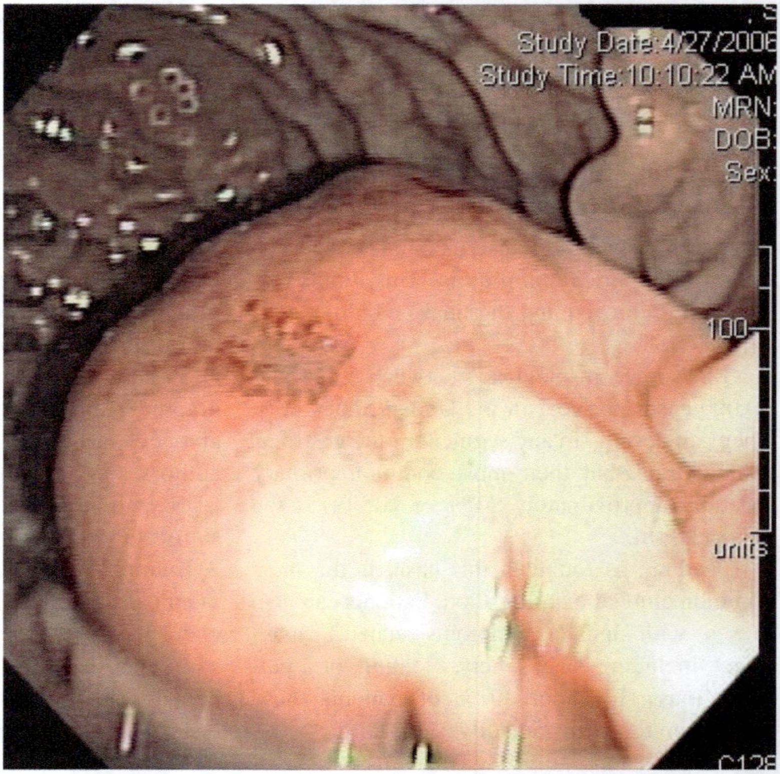

Fig. 3.23 A gastrointestinal stromal tumor on surface endoscopy with central ulceration

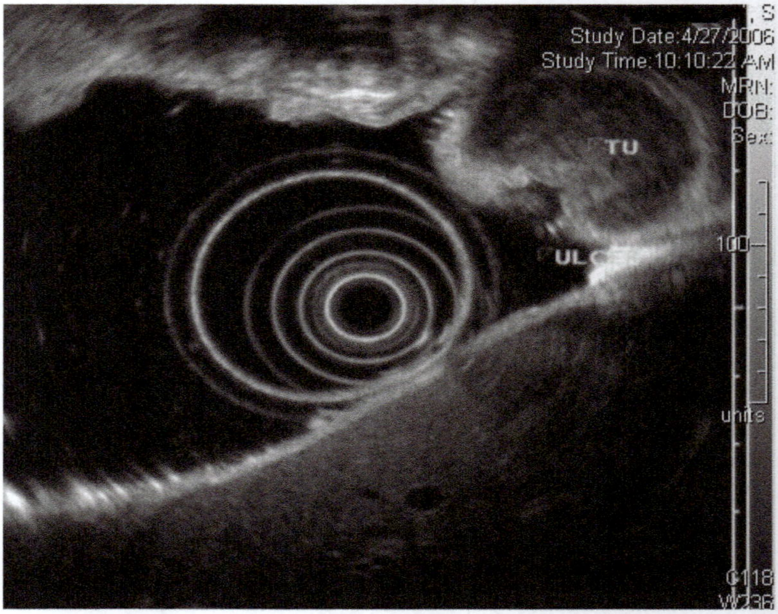

Fig. 3.24 This endoscopic ultrasound image clearly shows the central ulceration

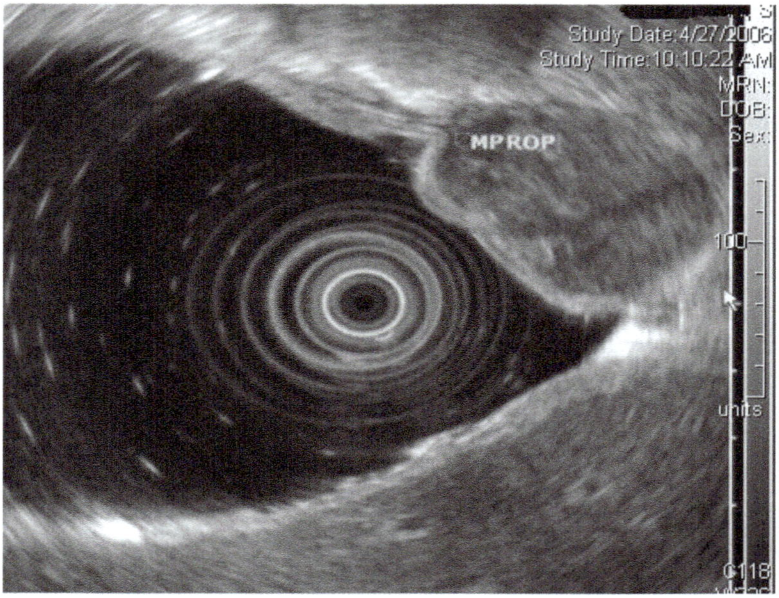

Fig. 3.25 This EUS image clearly shows the layer of origin of the gastrointestinal stromal tumor

3.2.8 Metastatic Gastrointestinal Stromal Tumor

Most GISTs are small and benign. This tumor is rather large (8 cm in diameter). It has a deceptively innocuous appearance on surface endoscopy. Despite the size of the tumor the layer of origin (muscularis propria) is clearly visible. There are internal cystic spaces consistent with tumor necrosis. This and the large size are suspicious for malignant behavior. Indeed, a small liver metastasis was seen with EUS that was not appreciated on CT. The tumor was biopsied to confirm its nature (immunohistochemistry with CD 117 staining) to determine whether the patient is a candidate for tyrosine kinase inhibitors.

Up to 47 % of patients with GISTs have been found to have metastasis at initial presentation, and nearly two thirds of those with metastasis have hepatic involvement. Lymph node metastases are relatively uncommon [23].

CT is recommended to evaluate for metastases. Contrast CT will reveal homogeneous enhancement of the tumor, although large masses can have patchy enhancement due to areas of tumor necrosis. MRI can also be used, demonstrating enhancement with gadolinium, low signal intensity on T1-weighted images, and high signal intensity on T2-weighted images [17].

According to the American Joint Cancer Committee [24] T staging of GISTs is based on the largest diameter of the tumor, allowing EUS to provide this information preoperatively. This classification is available online at http://goo.gl/xys4L.

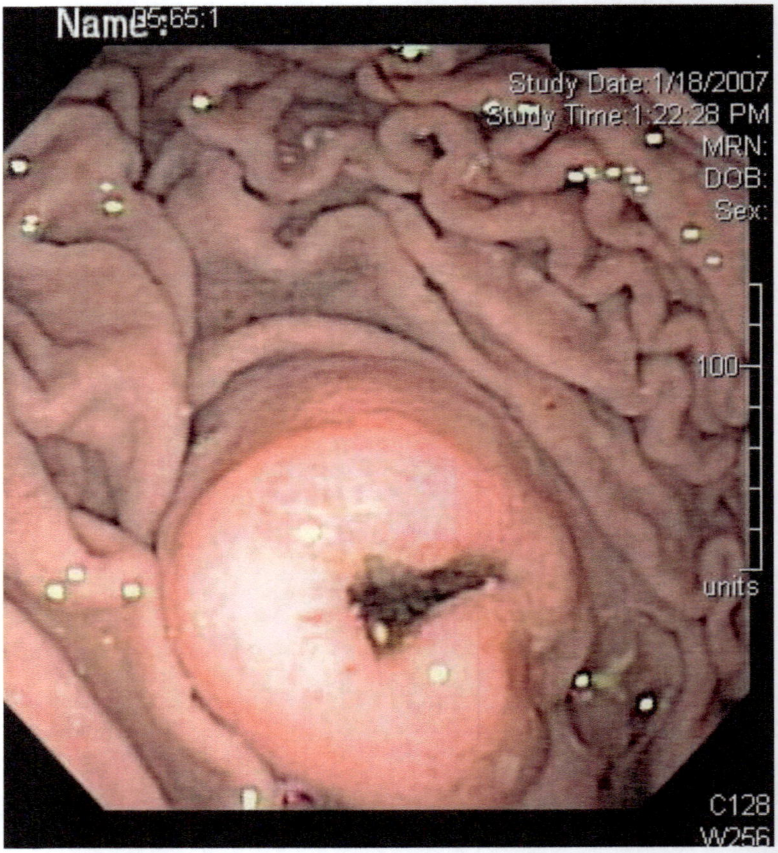

Fig. 3.26 Endoscopic appearance of the gastrointestinal stromal tumor

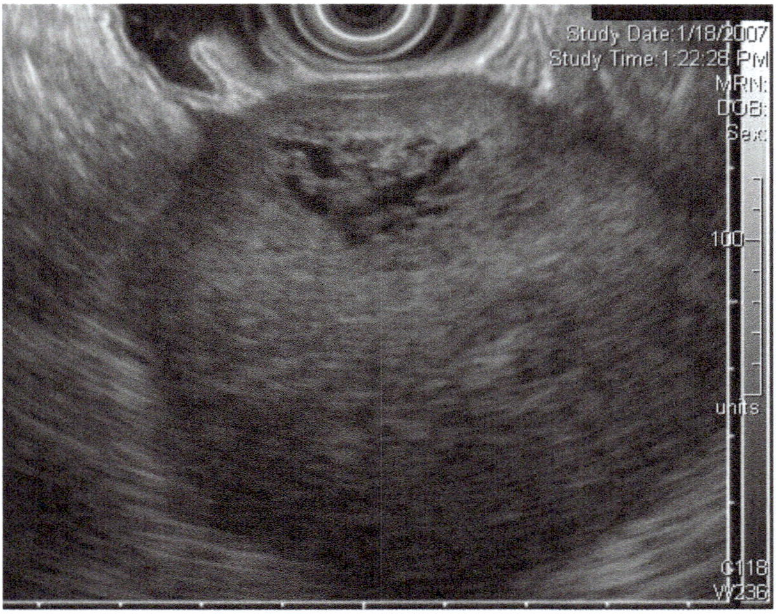

Fig. 3.27 A large (8-cm-diameter) gastrointestinal stromal tumor arising from the gastric wall

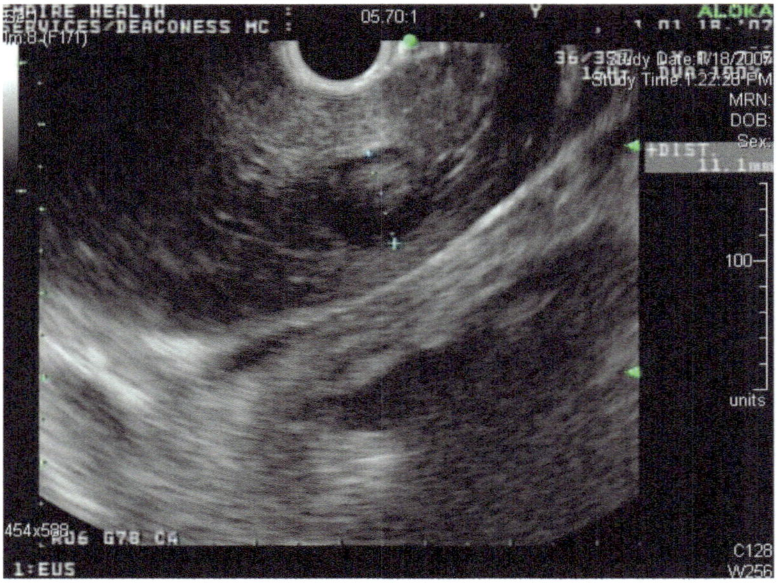

Fig. 3.28 Metastasis in the tip of the left lobe of the liver

3.2.9 Gastrointestinal Stromal Tumors and Interstitial Cells of Cajal

GISTs are believed to be neoplastic proliferations of the interstitial cells of Cajal (ICCs) or their progenitors. Five types of ICCs can be distinguished:

1. ICC-MY: At the level of the myenteric plexus of Auerbach. These are the pacemaker cells of the stomach and small intestine.
2. ICC-IM: These are intramuscular ICCs in the wall of the stomach, which seem to act as mediators of neurotransmission.
3. ICC-DMP or ICC-SEP: These are located in the deep muscular plexus of the small intestine and may be similar to the ICC-IM in function.
4. ICC-SM: These are distributed along the submucosal surface of the circular layer of the gastric antrum and colon. In the colon they are believed to be pacemaker cells.
5. ICC-S: These are located in the subserosal layer of the colon.

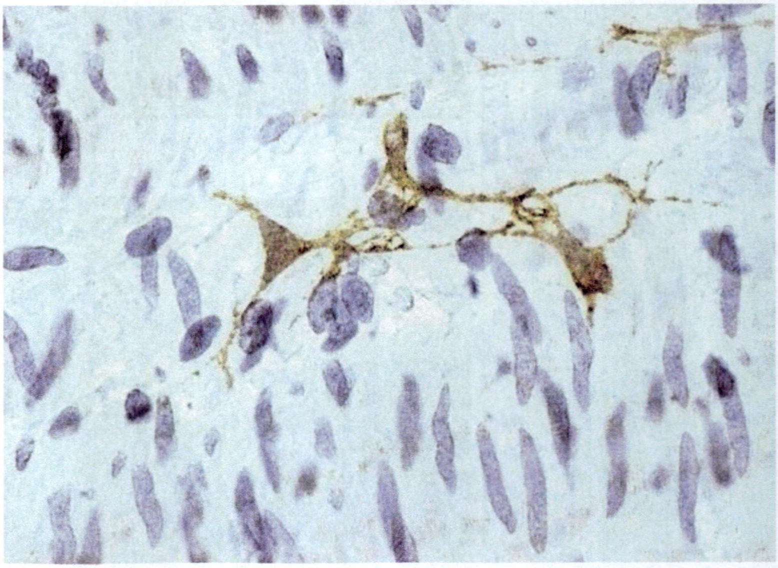

Fig. 3.29 Interstitial cells of Cajal (*brown stain*) in the circular muscle layer of an aganglionic colon segment (c-Kit immunohistochemistry, ×400) (From Newman et al. [25])

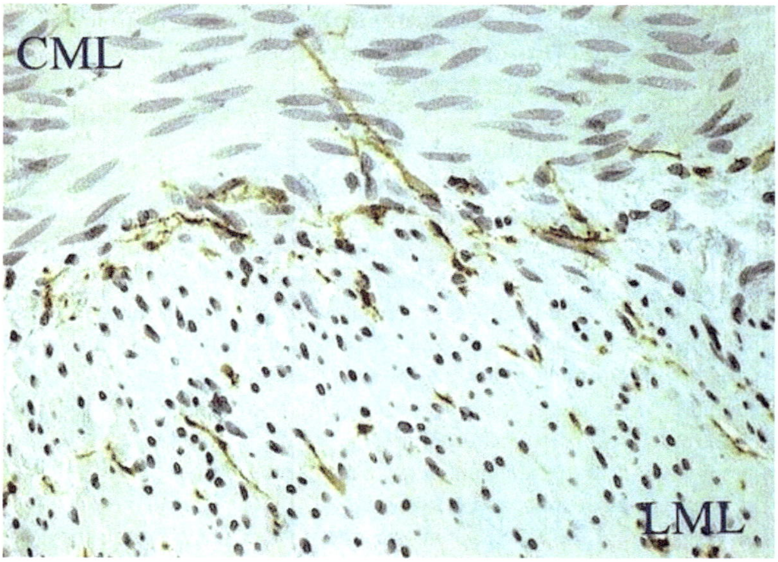

Fig. 3.30 Interstitial cells of Cajal (*brown stain*) in an aganglionic colon segment (c-Kit immunohistochemistry, ×200). *CML* circular muscle layer, *LML* longitudinal muscle layer (From Newman et al. [25])

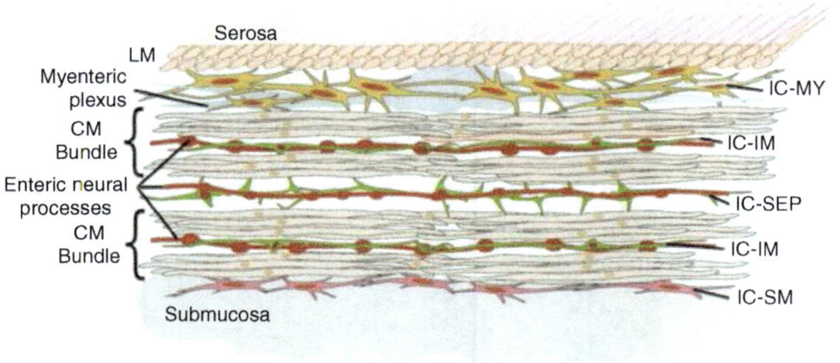

Fig. 3.31 Schematic diagram showing the basic organization of interstitial cells of Cajal (ICCs) in the canine antrum and their relationships with enteric motor nerves. ICCs are found in the region of the myenteric plexus (*IC-MY*), within muscle bundles (*IC-IM*), between muscle bundles (*IC-SEP*), and along the submucosal surface of the circular muscle layer (*IC-SM*). IC-IM and IC-SEP are closely associated with varicose processes of enteric motor neurons (colored *red*). *CM* circular muscle, *LM* longitudinal muscle (From Horiguchi et al. [26])

3.2.10 An Unusual Gastrointestinal Stromal Tumor in a Patient with Situs Inversus

This is a 56-year-old patient who was referred to us for mediastinal lymph node biopsies after bronchoscopy and transthoracic lung biopsies had been nondiagnostic. EUS-guided FNA of an American Thoracic Society area 2 lymph node established the diagnosis of non-small-cell carcinoma of the lung (mediastinal lymph node map demonstrated online at http://is.gd/AmQiJh). A CT scan showed complete situs inversus. A positron emission tomography scan demonstrated an area of high glucose avidity in the stomach. Surface endoscopy revealed an intact mucosa throughout. The EUS showed two subsurface lesions: one was in the gastric antrum with features characteristic of a small GIST (well circumscribed hypoechoic arising from the muscularis propria); the other one, which was much larger (2.8 cm in diameter) and corresponded to the lesion seen on the CT scan, was hypoechoic granular and arose from the submucosa. Nevertheless, EUS-guided FNA cytology with immunohistochemistry showed classic indications of a GIST.

Multiple synchronous GISTs have been found in 2 % of patients with this type of tumor in a large consecutive series of cases [27].

GISTs arising from layers other than the fourth layer of the gastric wall (muscularis propria) are rare. There are no clear statistics in the literature but we estimate that they constitute less than 2 % of all GISTs. This case is also interesting because it shows that GISTs must be a certain size before they show up on a positron emission tomography scan: 2.8 cm seems to be sufficient, whereas 1 cm (an antral lesion) is not.

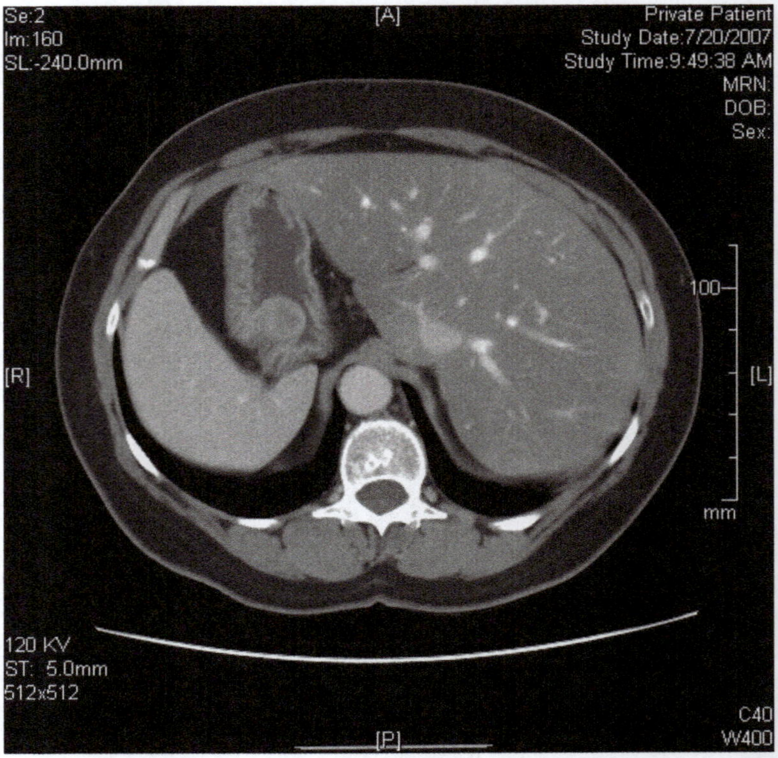

Fig. 3.32 This abdominal computed tomography scan shows situs inversus and a mass originating from the wall of the stomach

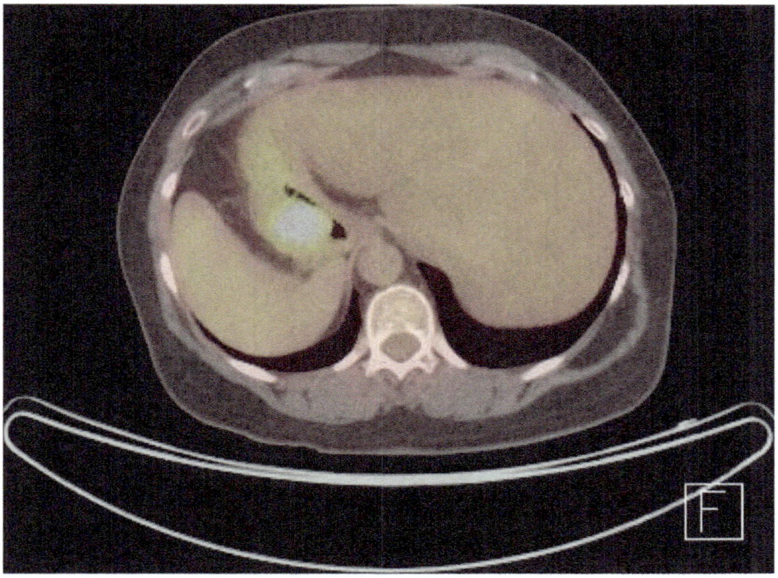

Fig. 3.33 The positron emission tomography–computed tomography scan shows that the tumor in the stomach is very glucose avid

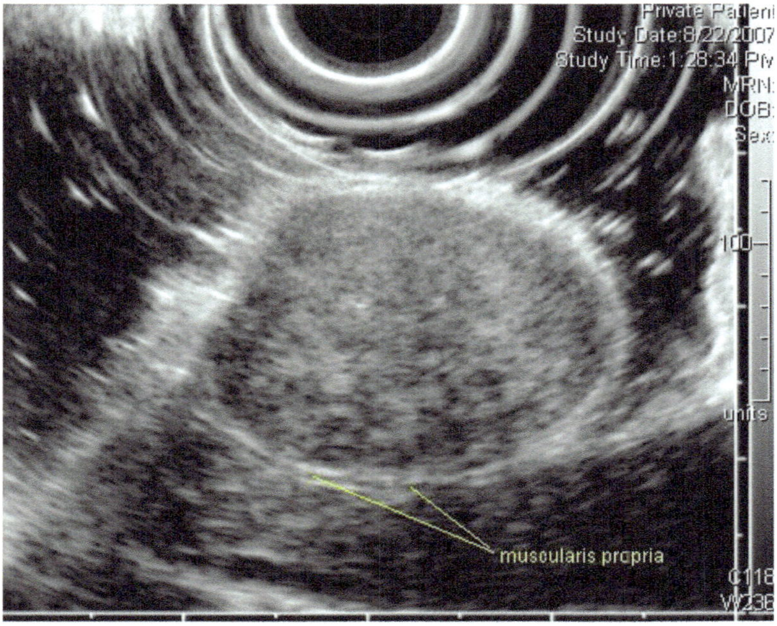

Fig. 3.34 This is a submucosal gastrointestinal stromal tumor confirmed by biopsy that originates from the submucosa rather than the muscularis propria of the gastric wall

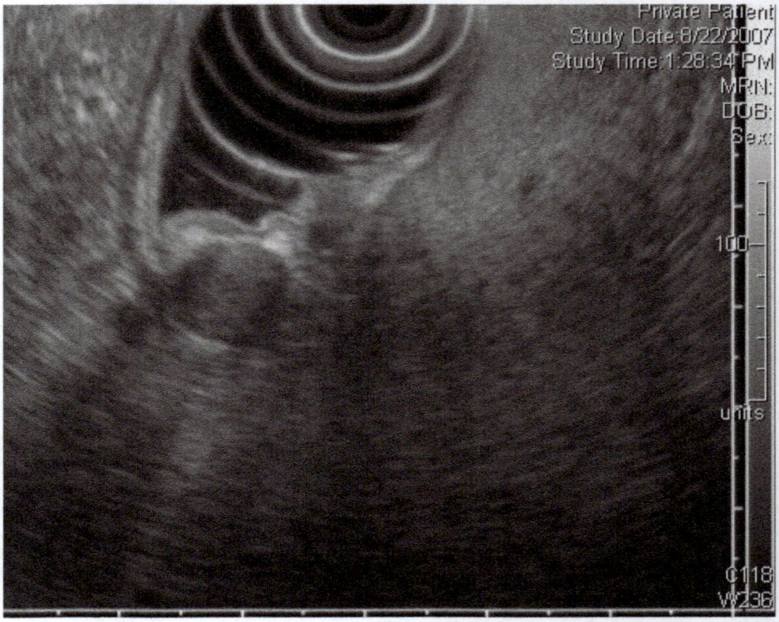

Fig. 3.35 The same patient harbored a more conventional-appearing gastrointestinal stromal tumor in the antrum. Note that the layer of origin is properly the muscularis propria

3.2.11 Gastrointestinal Stromal Tumors: Principles of Biopsy

GISTs should preferentially be biopsied by EUS; percutaneous biopsy has a theoretical risk of peritoneal spread of disease and is usually avoided except in selected cases with unresectable disease. The relevant passage of the Sarcoma/GIST guideline from the NCCN is available online at http://www.globalgist.org/docs/NCCN_guidelines.pdf.

This 78-year-old patient had undergone a percutaneous biopsy instead of EUS because the diagnosis of GIST had not been suspected. Indeed, on abdominal CT scan the tumor appeared cystic and not connected to the gastric wall. A referral for EUS was made later as part of the surgical planning, and the origin from the muscularis propria can be shown clearly.

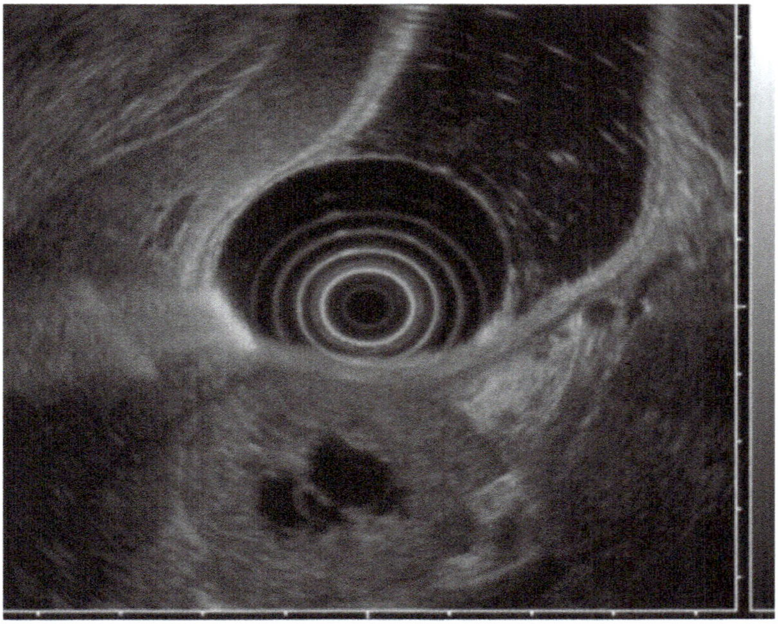

Fig. 3.36 This necrotic retrogastric gastrointestinal stromal tumor was not initially recognized as such and was biopsied percutaneously

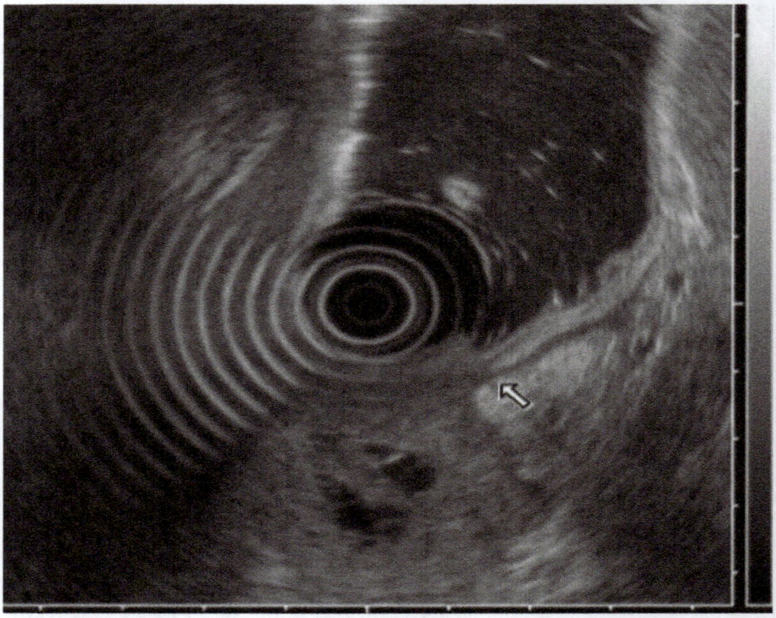

Fig. 3.37 The layer of origin of this gastrointestinal stromal tumor – the muscularis propria – is quite clear on this radial endoscopic ultrasound image

3.2.12 Gastric Carcinoid

This is a 49-year-old morbidly obese patient who was referred for the evaluation of anemia. A colonoscopy had been normal. Upper endoscopy showed the lesion seen in Fig. 3.38. EUS showed a hypoechoic tumor, which measured 15 mm in the largest extension. EUS imaging was difficult secondary to a difficult sedation process, but it appeared that there was early invasion of the muscularis propria from a tumor originating from the submucosa. Biopsies showed a carcinoid tumor but no gastric atrophy. This patient showed no evidence of multiple endocrine neoplasia type 1 or Zollinger-Ellison syndrome.

Gastric carcinoid tumors are rare and originate from gastric enterochromaffin-like cells in the oxyntic mucosa. There are three types of gastric carcinoid tumors:

- Type I, the most common (70–80 % of gastric carcinoids), is associated with autoimmune chronic atrophic gastritis resulting in achlorydria, antral G-cell hyperplasia, and hypergastrinemia. This type has good prognosis and the 5- and 10-year survival is similar to that in the age-matched population [28].
- Type II develops in patients with combined multiple endocrine neoplasia type 1 and the Zollinger-Ellison syndrome and accounts for approximately 5 % of gastric carcinoids. Up to 30 % of these tumors can metastasize [29].
- Type III is sporadic, developing despite normal gastrin levels and accounting for 15–20 % of gastric carcinoids. These tumors have a high malignant potential even when small and their risk of metastasis is >50 % [29]. Therefore, in the case presented above the tumor was a type III.

Clinical evaluation including gastrin level, gastric juice pH, secretin in questionable cases and gastric body biopsies to evaluate for autoimmune atrophic gastritis is necessary to determine tumor type as described above. Somatostatin-receptor scintigraphy in addition to standard contrast enhanced CT or MRI is recommended to evaluate for metastatic disease.

Gastric carcinoid tumor size >10 mm is an important prognostic variable but is insufficient to determine the management of these tumors. A large study of a Japanese tumor registry of almost 2,000 gastrointestinal tract carcinoids revealed that gastric carcinoids between 10.1 and 20 mm in size had a metastatic rate of 23 % [30]. Additional prognosis is determined by histologic features that require complete resection, including angioinvasion, mitotic index, and Ki67 index [31].

The T (tumor) component of the TNM staging system for gastric carcinoids considers the size of the carcinoid and depth of penetration into the wall. This staging system is available online at http://goo.gl/YOzF8.

Endoscopic resection is appropriate for single type I or II gastric carcinoids that are smaller than 2 cm and do not demonstrate involvement of the muscularis propria or distant metastases [32]. However, more aggressive lesions may require surgical intervention; type III lesions are usually treated with partial or total gastrectomy with local lymphadenectomy [33].

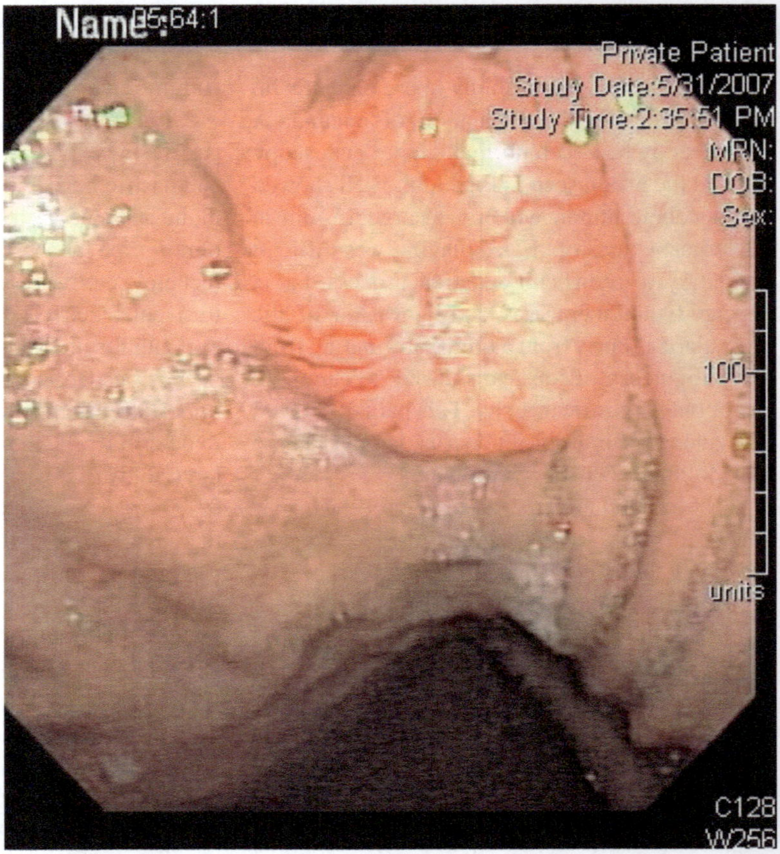

Fig. 3.38 Gastric carcinoid on upper endoscopy

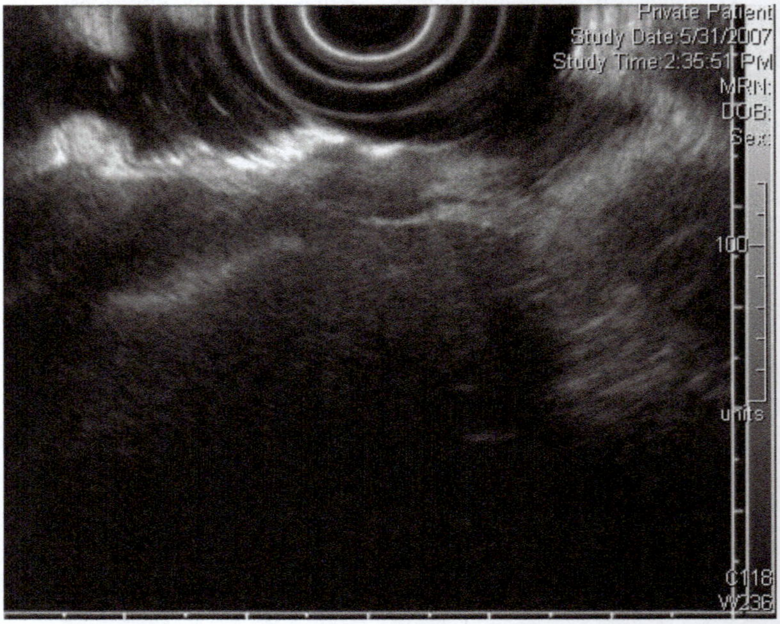

Fig. 3.39 This radial endoscopic ultrasound seems to show invasion of the carcinoid into the muscularis propria

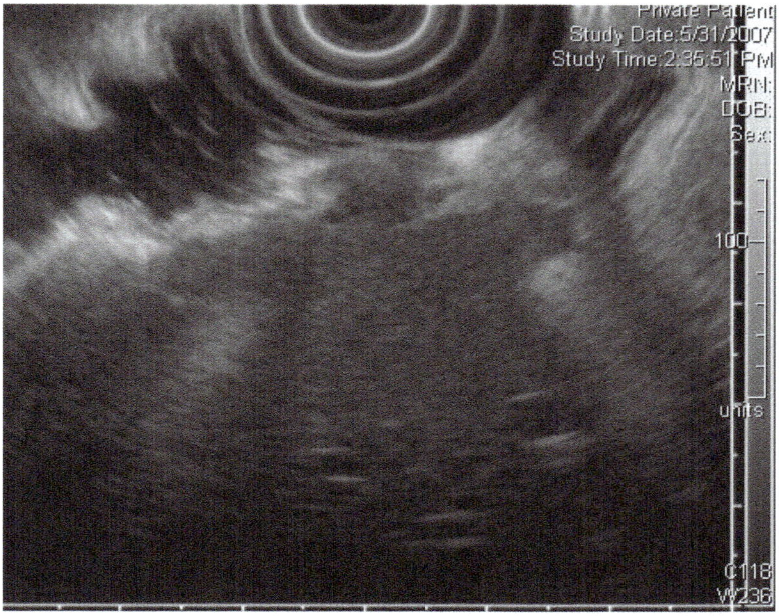

Fig. 3.40 A different view of the same carcinoid tumor with endoscopic ultrasound

3.2.13 Gastric Lipoma

This is a 48-year-old patient who we found to have a gastric lipoma on EUS 8 years before this presentation. He was referred to us again for a follow-up EUS because his primary gastroenterologist thought that the size of the lipoma had increased by approximately 25 %. We found no worrisome features on this EUS but noticed instead that the patient's abdominal girth had also increased by 25 %.

The development of a liposarcoma from a preexisting benign lipoma is rare. Most cases arise de novo. Liposarcomas most frequently arise from the deep stroma rather than the submucosal or subcutaneous fat. Most lipomas in the gastrointestinal tract do not require EUS for diagnosis if they demonstrate the characteristic "pillow sign" when depressed with the tip of a closed biopsy forceps.

Gastrointestinal lipomas are subepithelial lesions formed by mature lipocytes. These lesions can occur in any segment of the gastrointestinal tract; they are most commonly found in the colon but occasionally are seen in the stomach. Large lipomas can cause partial obstruction, abdominal pain, or bleeding but most are asymptomatic and found incidentally during endoscopic procedures. Lipomas appear endoscopically as yellowish bulges with a smooth border and normal-appearing overlying mucosa. Gentle pressure with an endoscopic tool can produce an indentation, called the pillow sign. EUS examination at the level of the bulge reveals a pathognomonic appearance: a hyperechoic lesion with homogeneous pattern and well-defined borders arising from the submucosa (third sonographic layer) is the usual pathognomonic finding.

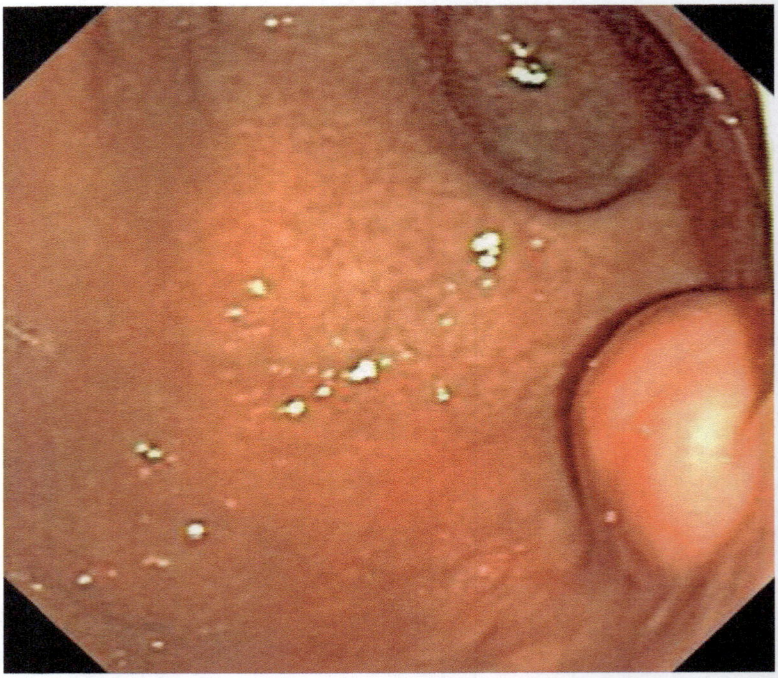

Fig. 3.41 This upper endoscopy view shows a submucosal mass identified on endoscopic ultrasound to be a lipoma

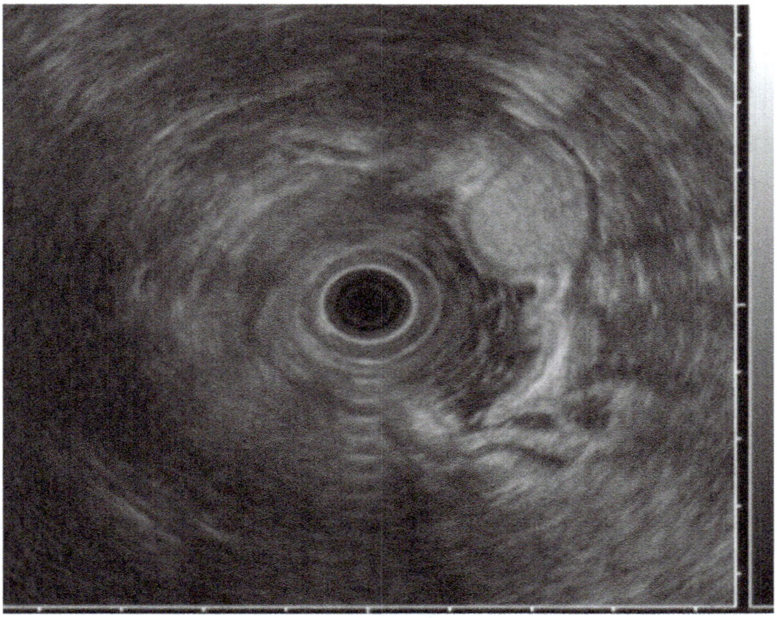

Fig. 3.42 This endoscopic ultrasound image shows the mucosa and muscularis propria surrounding a hyperechoic tumor originating from the submucosa. These findings are characteristic of a gastric lipoma

3.2.14 Thickened Gastric Folds, Gastric Varix, or Subepithelial Lesion?

This is a 79-year-old patient S/P Billroth II surgery for gastric cancer (T3N3) who developed melena several weeks following the surgery. Upper endoscopy revealed a protuberant lesion at the cardia with normal-appearing overlying mucosa. EUS with Doppler revealed the typical serpiginous, tubular structures with venous flow, diagnostic of gastric varices.

Gastric varices classically appear as serpiginous protuberances with a bluish venous hue in the fundus of the stomach. However, the diagnosis of gastric varices can sometimes be difficult based on endoscopic appearance alone. Their differential diagnosis may include submucosal tumors and thickened gastric folds. Diagnosis of gastric varices by EUS is considered very accurate given its capacity to visualize them as intramural curved, serpiginous structures; venous flow can be confirmed by Doppler ultrasound [35]. Perigastric venous collaterals can also be accurately detected by EUS [36].

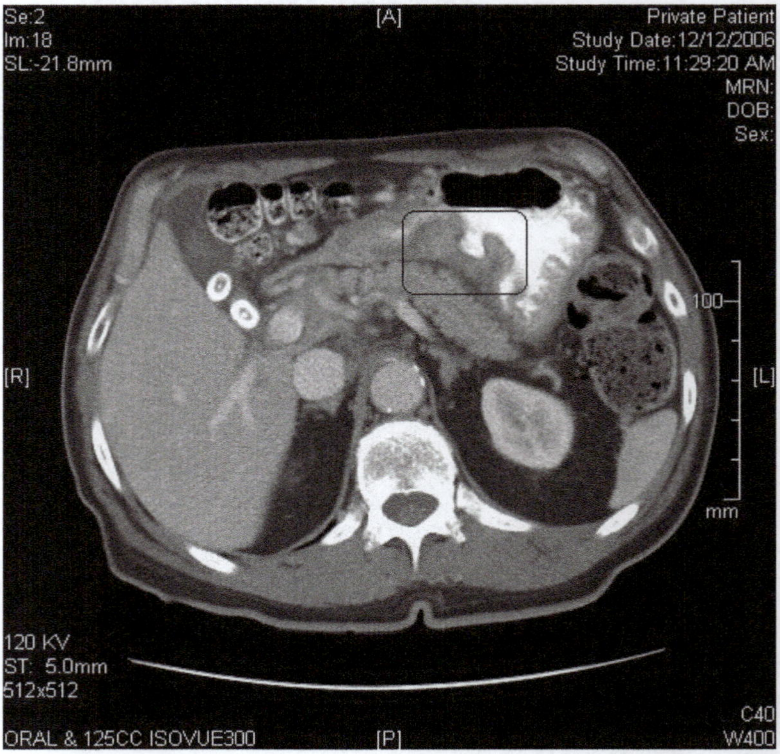

Fig. 3.43 The original gastric cancer on computed tomography

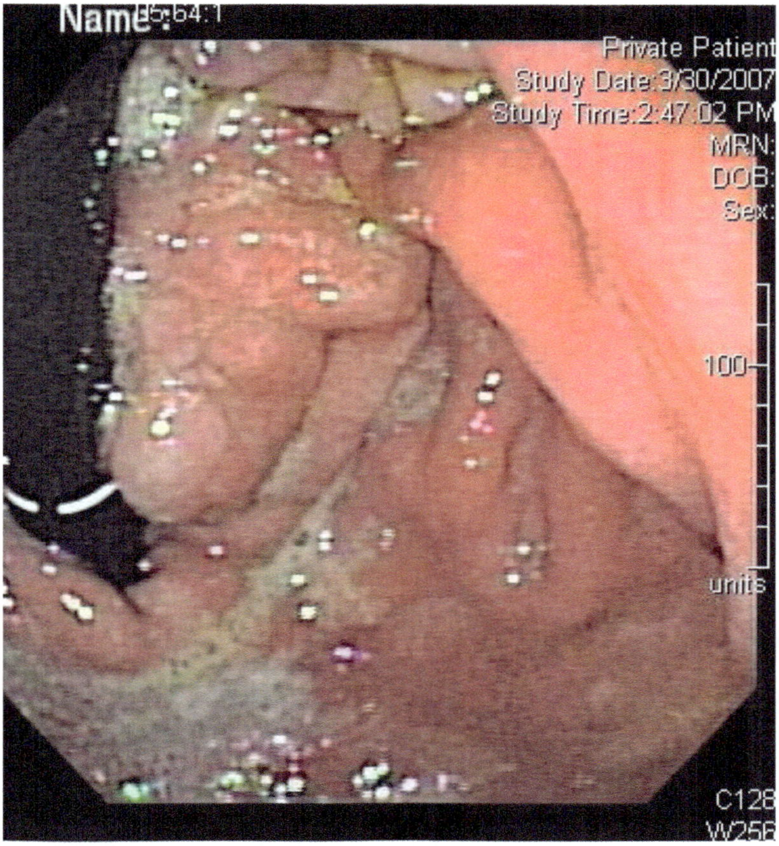

Fig. 3.44 This retroflexed view of the gastric cardia shows an enlarged protuberant lesion suspicious for gastric varices

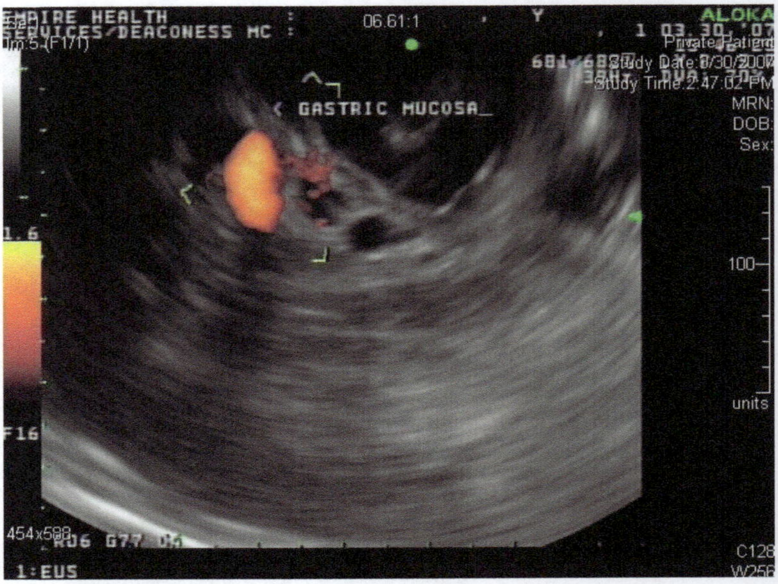

Fig. 3.45 Examination of this structure with the linear array Doppler-capable echoinstrument reveals a large (dilated) vessel in the submucosa

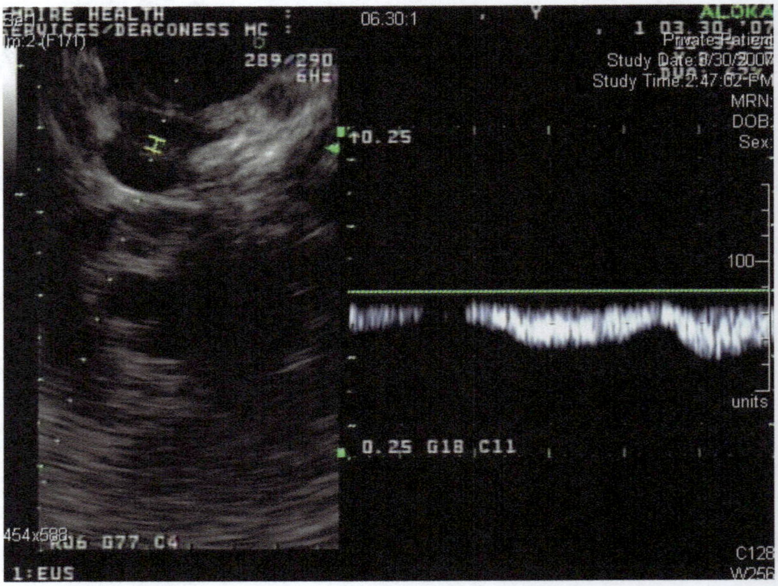

Fig. 3.46 The spectral Doppler signature unmistakably belongs to the portal venous system

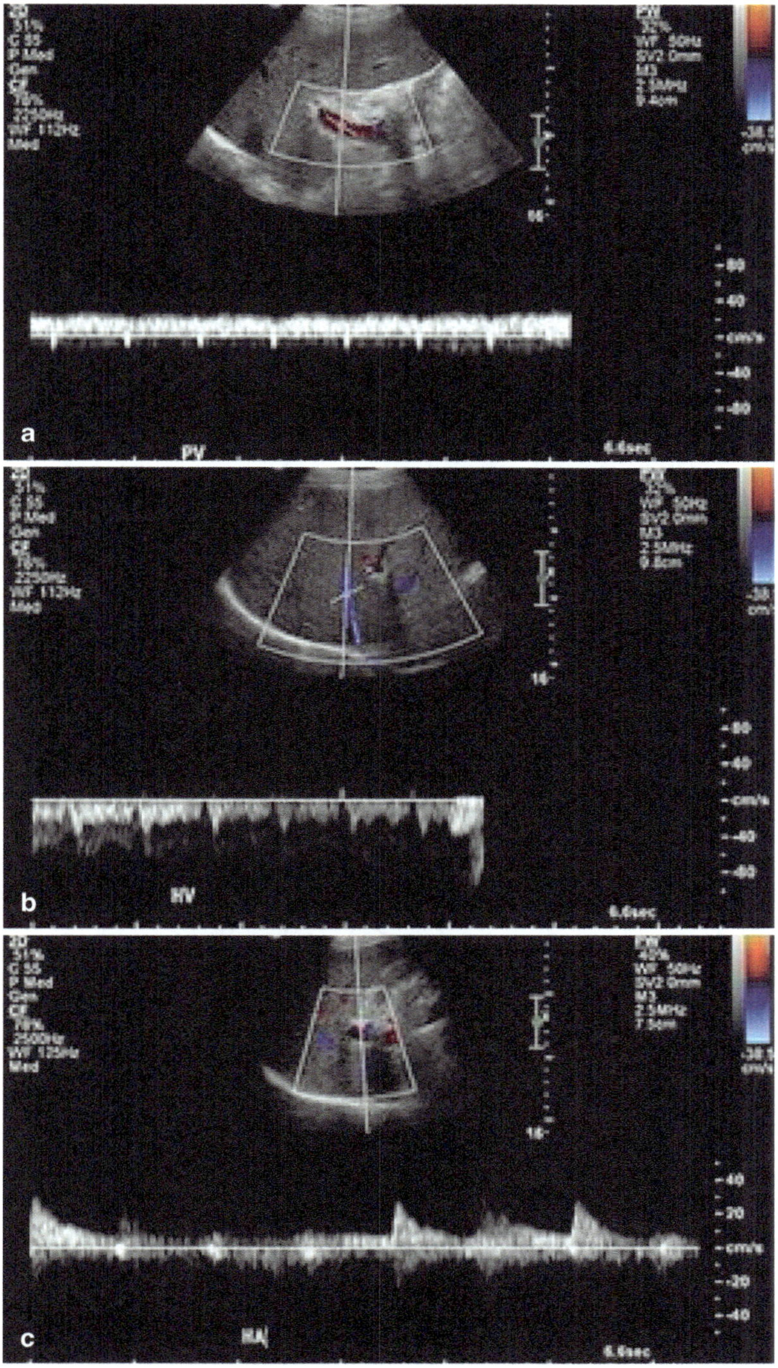

Fig. 3.47 Blood flow patterns seen on Doppler ultrasound: (**a**) portal vein; (**b**) hepatic artery; and (**c**) hepatic vein (From Singal et al. [34])

3.2.15 Pancreatic Rest

This is a 37-year-old woman with abdominal pain who was found to have a submucosal mass in the gastric antrum with central umbilication (see Fig. 3.48) that was suspicious for pancreatic heterotopia. An EUS was requested and showed a well-circumscribed generally hypoechoic lesion with echogenic foci with cystic spaces arising from or connecting to the muscularis propria. The largest cystic space appeared to connect to the surface. A differential diagnosis of a GIST was entertained. EUS-guided FNA did not show spindle cells but "cytologically bland epithelial cells." The patient had surgery because of persistent abdominal pain, which confirmed this tumor as being a pancreatic rest with pancreatic exocrine and endocrine components; chronic active inflammation also was seen. In other words, the echogenic foci seen on EUS were probably a representation of chronic pancreatitis in heterotopic pancreatic tissue.

The presence of pancreatic tissue outside the normal location without anatomic or vascular connection with the pancreas is called pancreatic rest, or heterotopic pancreas. This phenomenon occurs more often in stomach, duodenum, or jejunum, but it is found rarely in other locations of the gastrointestinal tract, abdomen, and chest. Some patients have abdominal pain, although the correlation of pain with this entity is not clear unless they present with pancreatitis or develop obstruction or intussusception with this ectopic tissue as the lead point [37].

The typical endoscopic appearance is a subepithelial lesion in the antrum with central umbilication or indentation, as shown in our case. EUS can assist in the differential diagnosis with subepithelial lesions and metastatic cancers, providing additional information about the involvement of gastric layers and ruling out invasive features. FNA can also be performed. These lesions have a poorly defined margin with a heterogeneous sonographic pattern that is predominantly hypoechoic mixed with small hyperechoic areas and frequently anechoic areas that correspond to ductal dilatation. They are found in the submucosa and muscularis propria [38].

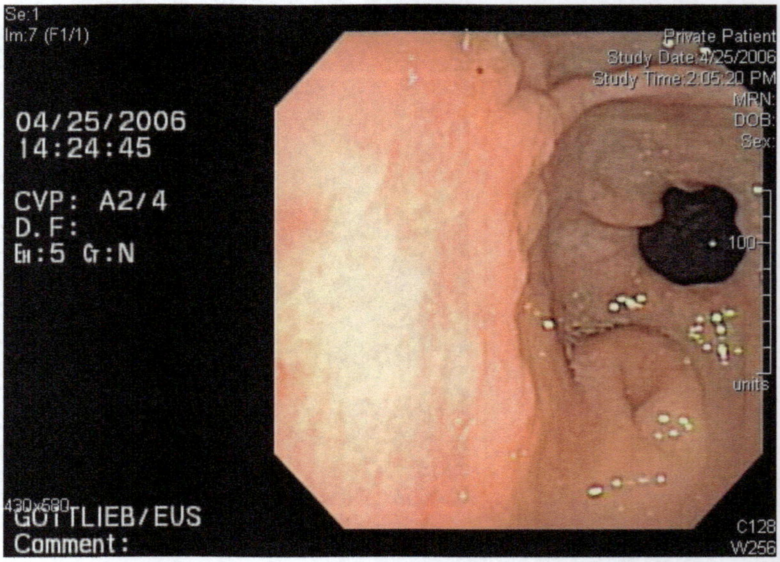

Fig. 3.48 Esophagogastroduodenoscopy shows a submucosal mass with central umbilication in the gastric antrum

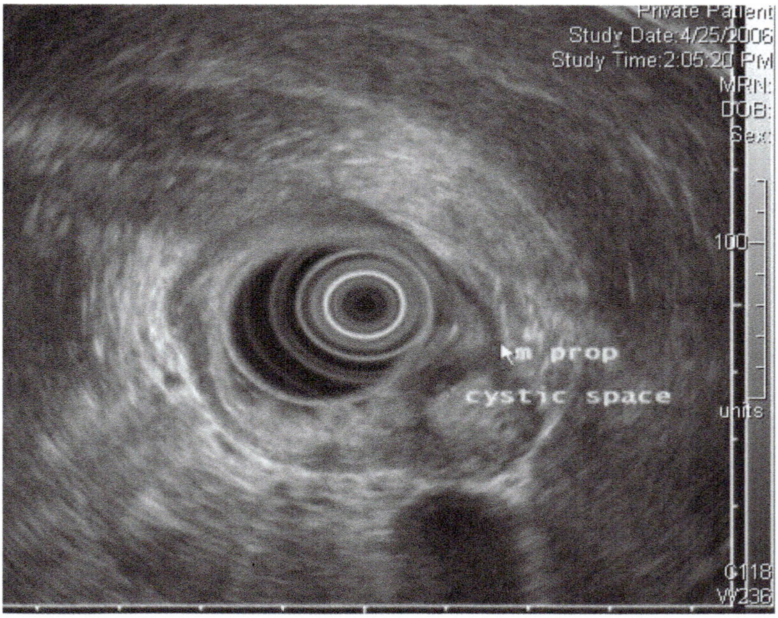

Fig. 3.49 Cystic spaces in the mass suggest a pancreas rest

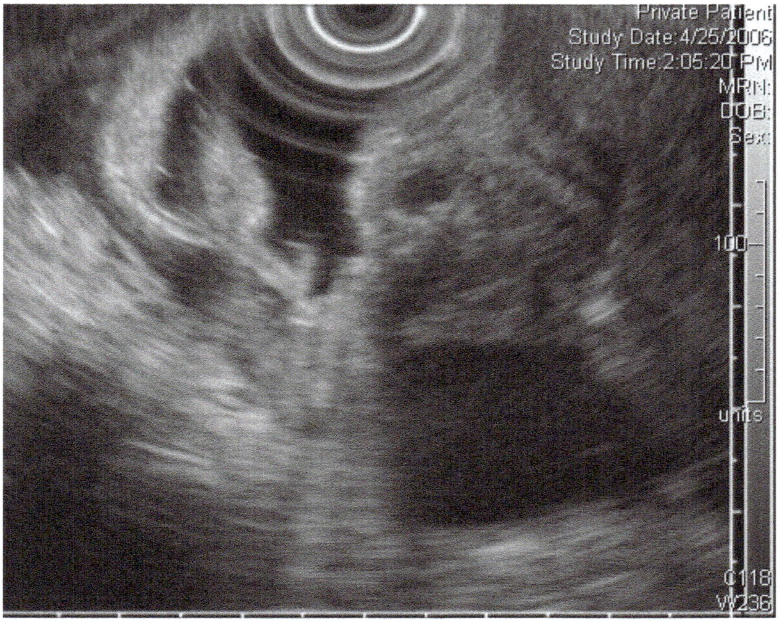

Fig. 3.50 A close-up of the suspected ectopic pancreas

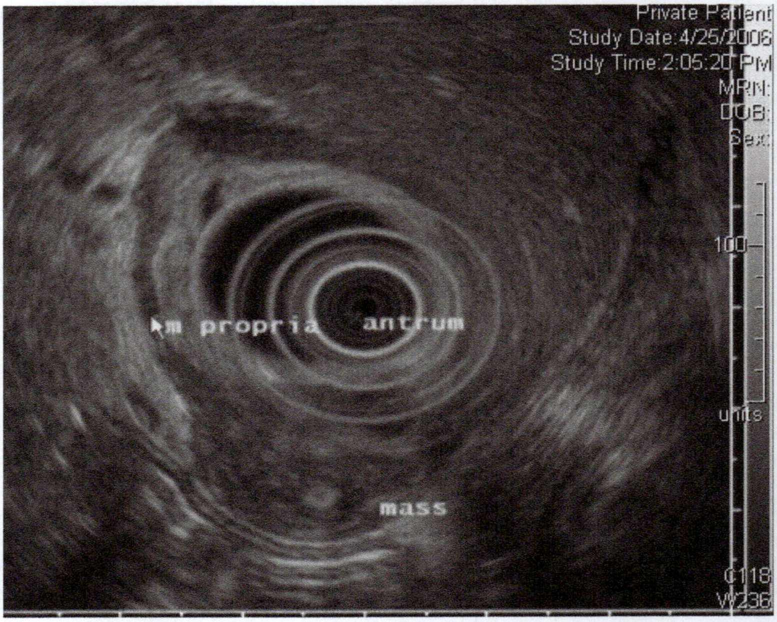

Fig. 3.51 This endoscopic ultrasound image of the ectopic pancreatic tissue shows echogenic foci

3.2.16 Submucosal Gastric Pseudotumor

This is a 50-year-old woman with a long history of functional gastrointestinal complaints who underwent repeated endoscopic investigations. On her most recent upper endoscopy a submucosal tumor in the gastric fundus was suspected. A CT scan was negative. EUS was requested and showed that the only gastric impression in this location was caused by a normal structure, the splenic hilum, or, specifically, the splenic hilar vessels.

Endoscopy alone has a limited capacity to differentiate subepithelial lesions from extramural lesions compressing the gastric wall. EUS is an excellent tool to establish this difference; Rösch et al. [40] have shown a sensitivity of 92 % and specificity of 100 % in differentiating subepithelial lesions from extramural compression in a prospective series. As shown in Figs. 3.52 and 3.53, the splenic vessels are located adjacent to the posterior wall of the stomach and can occasionally cause an impression at that level between the fundus and body of the stomach [41]. EUS with Doppler can also establish the vascular nature of these cases, ruling out solid tumors or enlarged organs causing a compression effect. A differential diagnosis of extraluminal lesions compressing the stomach at that level includes pancreatic cancer, pancreatic cystic lesions, peripancreatic abscess splenic cyst, vascular aneurysms, metastases, lymphoma, and splenomegaly [42].

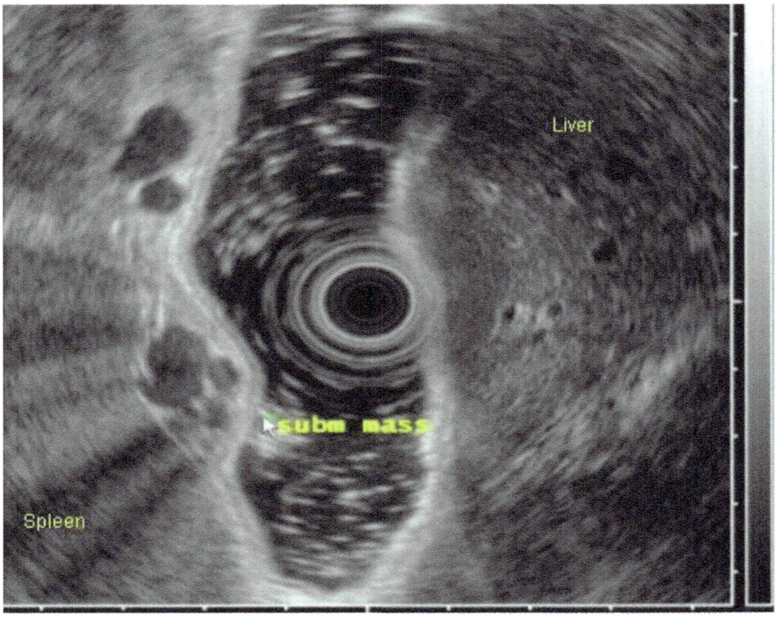

Fig. 3.52 This endoscopic ultrasound shows a gastric impression caused by the splenic hilar vessels. Not always are pulsations visible, which would suggest this as the cause of the suspected submucosal tumor on surface endoscopy

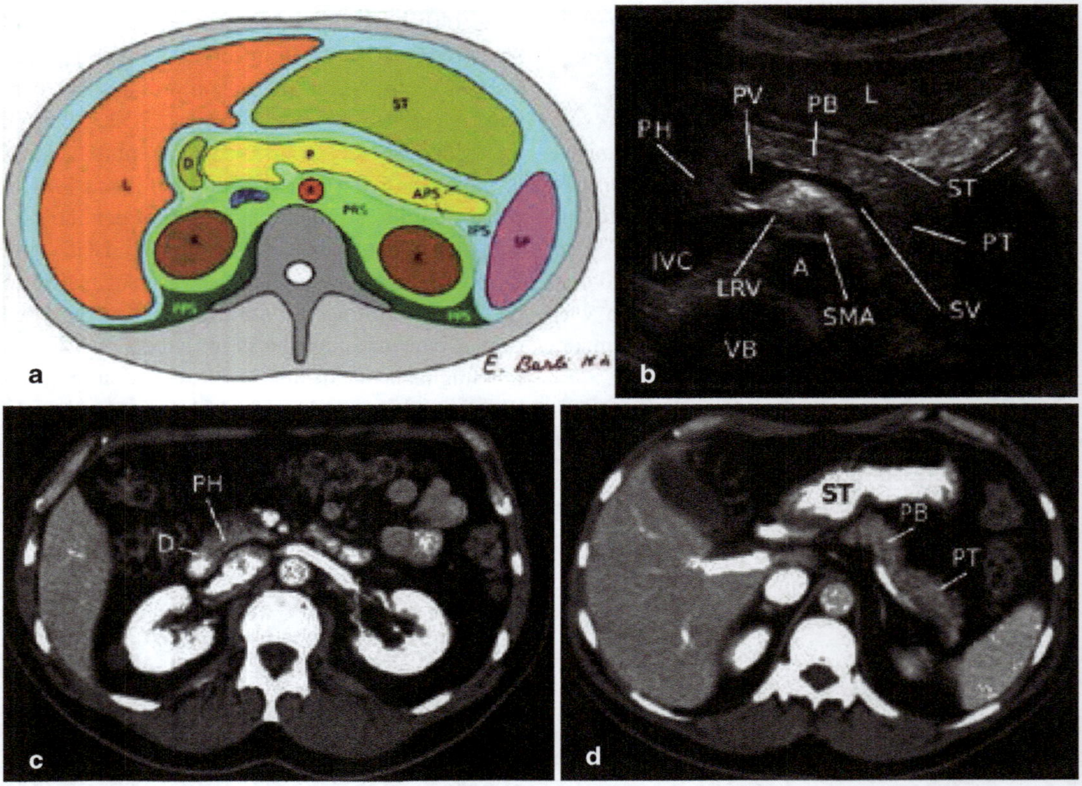

Fig. 3.53 Axial anatomy of the pancreas (*P*). (**a**) Anatomic features of the pancreas and its relations with the surrounding organs. The anterior pararenal space (*APS*, *light green*) in the front; the perirenal space (*PRS*, *medium green*) and the posterior pararenal space (*PPS*, *dark green*) behind; and the intraperitoneal space (*IPS*, *sky blue*) anterior and lateral. (**b**) Ultrasound of the pancreas showing the head (*PH*), body (*PB*), and tail (*PT*). (**c**, **d**) Computed tomography scan of the pancreas passing through the head (*PH*) without visualization of the body or tail (**c**) or passing through the body and tail without visualization of the head (was). *A* aorta, *D* duodenum, *IVC* inferior vena cava, *K* kidney, *L* liver, *LRV* left renal vein, *PV* portal vein, *SMA* superior mesenteric artery, *SP* spleen, *ST* stomach, *SV* splenic vein, *VB* vertebral body (From Barbi et al. [39])

3.2.17 Perigastric Abscess

This is a 75-year-old woman who had a Whipple pancreaticoduodenectomy for cholangiocarcinoma 2 years ago at an outside institution. She came back complaining of early satiety, vomiting, and diffuse abdominal pain. CT showed multiple abnormalities including a dilated biliary tree and a central hypodense liver mass, which proved to be recurrent adenocarcinoma. The obstruction of bile drainage was thought to be related to obstruction of the afferent limb and improved after percutaneous transhepatic drainage. Upper endoscopy confirmed progressive narrowing of the afferent limb, which connected to a fistula. The CT scan was reviewed and it was thought that there was a retrogastric abscess cavity, probably through the fistula, filled with barium. An EUS was performed immediately after the regular gastroscopy and indeed showed a large abscess cavity in the expected location. The abscess was subsequently drained and was growing *Klebsiella oxytoca* and *Enterococcus* spp.

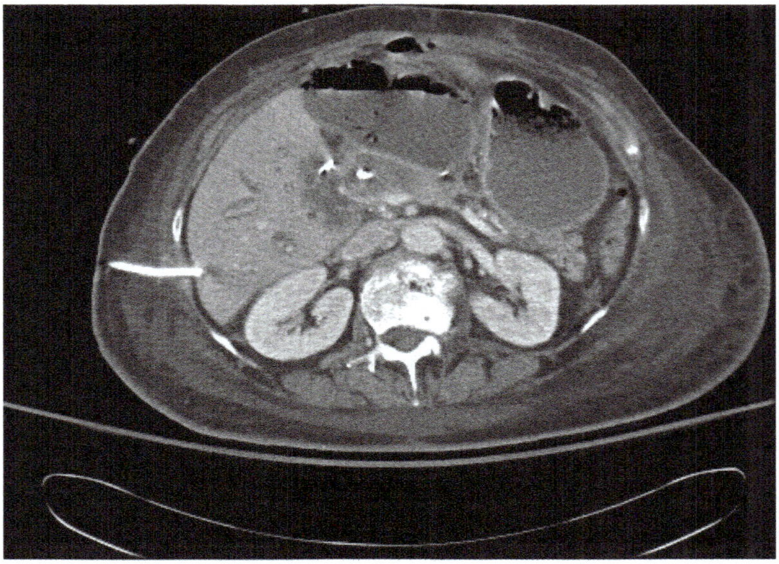

Fig. 3.54 This computed tomography scan shows recurrent cholangiocarcinoma following a Whipple pancreaticoduodenectomy. Note the presence of a percutaneous transhepatic drainage tube

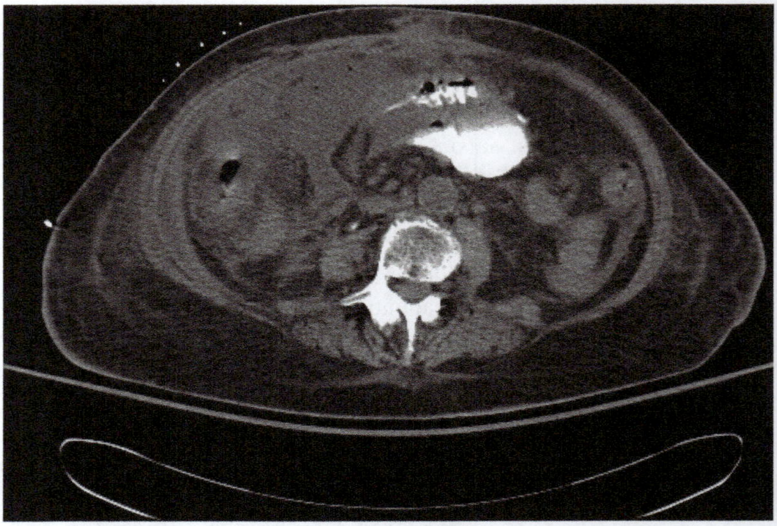

Fig. 3.55 The same computed tomography scan shows barium in what initially was interpreted as the stomach

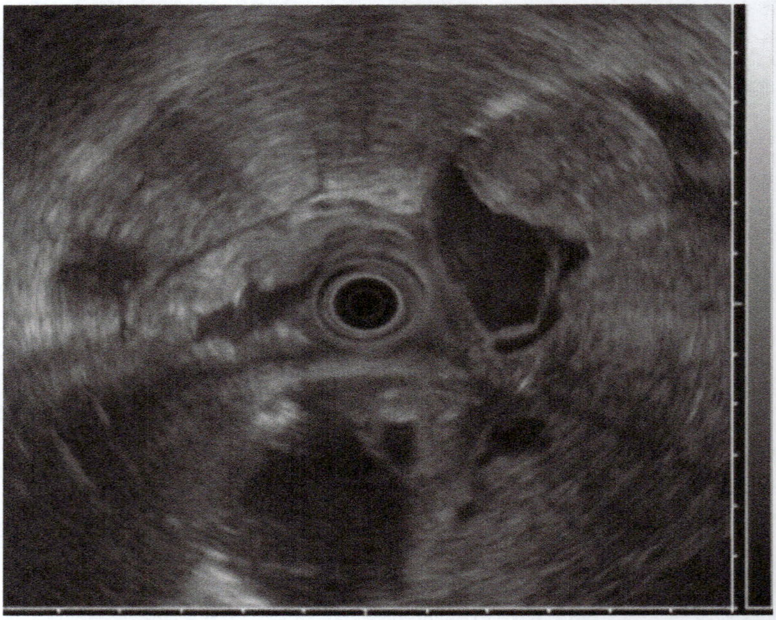

Fig. 3.56 A radial endoscopic ultrasound shows the presence of a large complex abscess cavity immediately adjacent to the stomach. A fistulous tract was shown endoscopically to connect to the afferent limb of the stomach

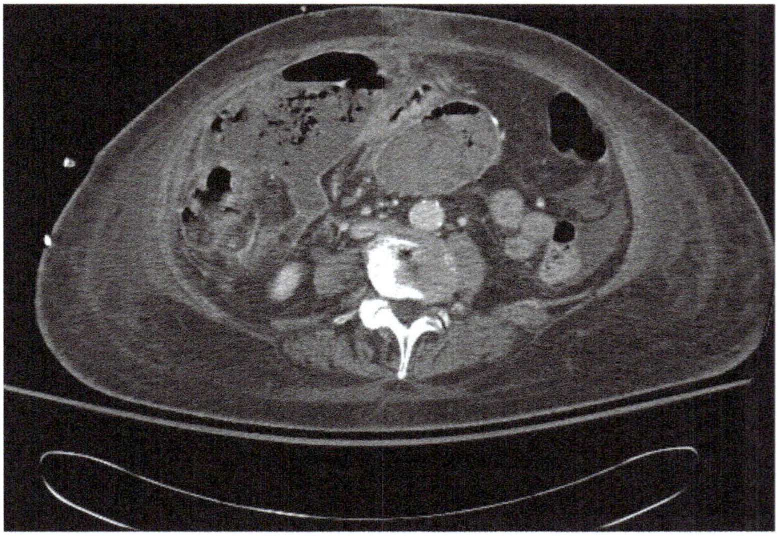

Fig. 3.57 This computed tomography scan obtained after the barium had a chance to drain shows the relationship of the abscess cavity to the stomach

References

1. Akahoshi K. Radial EUS of the stomach. In: Practical handbook of endoscopic ultrasonography. Tokyo: Springer; 2012. p. 49–63.
2. American Cancer Society. What are the key statistics about stomach cancer? [Internet]. http://www.cancer.org/Cancer/StomachCancer/DetailedGuide/stomach-cancer-key-statistics. 2013.
3. Nagler AK, Aslanian HR, Siddiqui UD. Endoscopic ultrasound and gastric lesions. J Clin Gastroenterol. 2011;45(3):215–21.
4. Bentrem D, Gerdes H, Tang L, Brennan M, Coit D. Clinical correlation of endoscopic ultrasonography with pathologic stage and outcome in patients undergoing curative resection for gastric cancer. Ann Surg Oncol. 2007;14(6):1853–9.
5. Akashi K, Yanai H, Nishikawa J, Satake M, Fukagawa Y, Okamoto T, et al. Ulcerous change decreases the accuracy of endoscopic ultrasonography diagnosis for the invasive depth of early gastric cancer. Int J Gastrointest Cancer. 2006;37(4):133–8.
6. Park SR, Lee JS, Kim CG, Kim HK, Kook M-C, Kim Y-W, et al. Endoscopic ultrasound and computed tomography in restaging and predicting prognosis after neoadjuvant chemotherapy in patients with locally advanced gastric cancer. Cancer. 2008;112(11):2368–76.
7. Lorimier G, Binelli C, Burtin P, Maillart P, Bertrand G, Verriele V, et al. Metastatic gastric cancer arising from breast carcinoma: endoscopic ultrasonographic aspects. Endoscopy. 1998;30(9):800–4.
8. Negreanu L, Assor P, Bumsel F, Metman E-H. An endoscopic view in gastric linitis. A case report. J Gastrointestin Liver Dis. 2007;16(3):321–3.
9. Andriulli A, Recchia S, De Angelis C, Mazzucco D, Berti E, Arrigoni A, et al. Endoscopic ultrasonographic evaluation of patients with biopsy negative gastric linitis plastica. Gastrointest Endosc. 1990;36(6):611–5.
10. Carter JE, Nelson JJ, Eves M, Boudreaux C. Diagnosis of linitis plastica-type gastric adenocarcinoma by endoscopic ultrasound-guided fine needle aspiration: a case report. Acta Cytol. 2008;52(6):725–8.
11. Caletti G, Fusaroli P, Togliani T. EUS in MALT lymphoma. Gastrointest Endosc. 2002;56(4 Suppl):S21–6.
12. Wiersema MJ, Vilmann P, Giovannini M, Chang KJ, Wiersema LM. Endosonography-guided fine-needle aspiration biopsy: diagnostic accuracy and complication assessment. Gastroenterology. 1997;112(4):1087–95.
13. Rohatiner A, d'Amore F, Coiffier B, Crowther D, Gospodarowicz M, Isaacson P, et al. Report on a workshop convened to discuss the pathological and staging classifications of gastrointestinal tract lymphoma. Ann Oncol. 1994;5(5):397–400.
14. Chang A, et al. Oncology [Internet]. New York: Springer; 2006. p. 737. http://www.springer.com/medicine/oncology/book/978-0-387-24291-0. Cited 3 Sep 2012.
15. Ruskoné-Fourmestraux A, Dragosics B, Morgner A, Wotherspoon A, De Jong D. Paris staging system for primary gastrointestinal lymphomas Gut. 2003;52(6):912–3.
16. Püspök A, Raderer M, Chott A, Dragosics B, Gangl A, Schöfl R. Endoscopic ultrasound in the follow up and response assessment of patients with primary gastric lymphoma. Gut. 2002;51(5):691–4.
17. Bennett JJ, Rubino MS. Gastrointestinal stromal tumors of the stomach. Surg Oncol Clin N Am. 2012;21(1):21–33.
18. Tran T, Davila JA, El-Serag HB. The epidemiology of malignant gastrointestinal stromal tumors: an analysis

of 1,458 cases from 1992 to 2000. Am J Gastroenterol. 2005;100(1):162–8.
19. Tio TL, Tytgat GN, den Hartog Jager FC. Endoscopic ultrasonography for the evaluation of smooth muscle tumors in the upper gastrointestinal tract: an experience with 42 cases. Gastrointest Endosc. 1990;36(4): 342–50.
20. Karaca C, Turner BG, Cizginer S, Forcione D, Brugge W. Accuracy of EUS in the evaluation of small gastric subepithelial lesions. Gastrointest Endosc. 2010;71(4):722–7.
21. Hwang JH, Saunders MD, Rulyak SJ, Shaw S, Nietsch H, Kimmey MB. A prospective study comparing endoscopy and EUS in the evaluation of GI subepithelial masses. Gastrointest Endosc. 2005;62(2):202–8.
22. National Comprehensive Cancer Network. NCCN clinical practice guidelines in oncology. Soft tissue sarcoma. V.2.2007 [Internet]. 2007. http://www.globalgist.org/docs/NCCN_guidelines.pdf. Cited 4 Sep 2012.
23. DeMatteo RP, Lewis JJ, Leung D, Mudan SS, Woodruff JM, Brennan MF. Two hundred gastrointestinal stromal tumors: recurrence patterns and prognostic factors for survival. Ann Surg. 2000;231(1): 51–8.
24. Edge S, Byrd D, Compton C. Gastrointestinal stromal tumour (GIST). In: AJCC cancer staging manual. 7th ed. New York: Springer; 2010. p. 175–80.
25. Newman CJ, et al. Interstitial cells of Cajal are normally distributed in both ganglionated and aganglionic bowel in Hirschsprung's disease. Pediatr Surg Int. 2003;19(9–10):662–8.
26. Horiguchi K, Sanders KM, Ward SM. Enteric motor neurons form synaptic-like junctions with interstitial cells of Cajal in the canine gastric antrum. Cell Tissue Res. 2003;311(3):299–313.
27. Xu C, Liu Y-L, Yu H-Y, Hou Y-Y, Lu S-H, Zhao L-J, et al. Synchronous and metachronous multiple gastrointestinal stromal tumors. Histol Histopathol. 2012;27(2):225–34.
28. Borch K, Ahrén B, Ahlman H, Falkmer S, Granérus G, Grimelius L. Gastric carcinoids: biologic behavior and prognosis after differentiated treatment in relation to type. Ann Surg. 2005;242(1):64–73.
29. Burkitt MD, Pritchard DM. Review article: pathogenesis and management of gastric carcinoid tumours. Aliment Pharmacol Ther. 2006;24(9):1305–20.
30. Soga J. Early-stage carcinoids of the gastrointestinal tract: an analysis of 1914 reported cases. Cancer. 2005;103(8):1587–95.
31. Rindi G, Azzoni C, La Rosa S, Klersy C, Paolotti D, Rappel S, et al. ECL cell tumor and poorly differentiated endocrine carcinoma of the stomach: prognostic evaluation by pathological analysis. Gastroenterology. 1999;116(3):532–42.
32. Varas MJ, Gornals JB, Pons C, Espinós JC, Abad R, Lorente FJ, et al. Usefulness of endoscopic ultrasonography (EUS) for selecting carcinoid tumors as candidates to endoscopic resection. Rev Esp Enferm Dig. 2010;102(10):577–82.
33. Delle Fave G, Kwekkeboom DJ, Van Cutsem E, Rindi G, Kos-Kudla B, Knigge U, et al. ENETS Consensus Guidelines for the management of patients with gastroduodenal neoplasms. Neuroendocrinology. 2012; 95(2):74–87.
34. Singal AK, Ahmad M, Soloway RD. Duplex Doppler ultrasound examination of the portal venous system: an emerging novel technique for the estimation of portal vein pressure. Dig Dis Sci. 2010;55(5):1230–40.
35. Caletti GC, Brocchi E, Ferrari A, Fiorino S, Barbara L. Value of endoscopic ultrasonography in the management of portal hypertension. Endoscopy. 1992;24 Suppl 1:342–6.
36. El-Saadany M, Jalil S, Irisawa A, Shibukawa G, Ohira H, Bhutani MS. EUS for portal hypertension: a comprehensive and critical appraisal of clinical and experimental indications. Endoscopy. 2008;40(8):690–6.
37. Ormarsson OT, Gudmundsdottir I, Mårvik R. Diagnosis and treatment of gastric heterotopic pancreas. World J Surg. 2006;30(9):1682–9.
38. Matsushita M, Hajiro K, Okazaki K, Takakuwa H. Gastric aberrant pancreas: EUS analysis in comparison with the histology. Gastrointest Endosc. 1999;49(4 Pt 1):493–7.
39. Barbi E, et al. Pancreatic anatomy, variants and pseudolesions of the pancreas. In: Ultrasonography of the pancreas. Milan: Springer; 2012. p. 63–81
40. Rösch T, Kapfer B, Will U, Baronius W, Strobel M, Lorenz R, et al. Accuracy of endoscopic ultrasonography in upper gastrointestinal submucosal lesions: a prospective multicenter study. Scand J Gastroenterol. 2002;37(7):856–62.
41. Rösch T, Lorenz R, von Wichert A, Classen M. Gastric fundus impression caused by splenic vessels: detection by endoscopic ultrasound. Endoscopy. 1991;23(2):85–7.
42. Chen TK, Wu CH, Lee CL, Lai YC, Yang SS, Tu TC. Endoscopic ultrasonography to study the causes of extragastric compression mimicking gastric submucosal tumor. J Formos Med Assoc. 2001;100(11):758–61.

Duodenum

4

Contents

4.1 **General Principles** 197
4.1.1 Anatomy 197
4.1.2 EUS Probes 197
4.1.3 Technique 197

4.2 **Cases and Discussions** 198
4.2.1 Duodenal Cancer 198
4.2.2 Duodenal Diverticulum 201
4.2.3 Duodenal Perforation by Foreign Body 203
4.2.4 Duodenal Pseudocyst 207
4.2.5 Ampullary Carcinoma 211
4.2.6 Familial Adenomatous Polyposis 213
4.2.7 Periduodenal Collaterals 215
4.2.8 Primary Duodenal Non-Hodgkin's Lymphoma 218
4.2.9 Transduodenal Abscess Drainage 222
4.2.10 Zollinger-Ellison Syndrome: An Imaging Odyssey 230

References 233

4.1 General Principles

4.1.1 Anatomy

Endoscopic ultrasound (EUS) examination of the duodenal wall reveals a five-layer sonographic pattern similar to that of the esophagus, stomach, and rectum, as described in Chaps. 2, 3, and 8, respectively. Wall thickness varies depending on the tension applied. The bile duct and pancreatic duct converge at the major papilla, which usually appears as a small hypoechoic structure.

4.1.2 EUS Probes

High-frequency probes, including miniprobes (catheter EUS probes) advanced through the standard endoscope channel, have the advantage of higher resolution. However, these high-frequency probes provide limited depth of sonographic visualization. Evaluation of deep involvement, adjacent anatomical structures, and lymph nodes is better with dedicated EUS radial and linear scanning endoscopes.

4.1.3 Technique

Endoscopic ultrasound examination of focal small lesions can be targeted after initial endoscopic visualization while a systematic insertion and withdrawal technique allows for the identification of anatomic landmarks such as the major

K. Gottlieb, G. Marino, *Diagnostic Endosonography*,
DOI 10.1007/978-3-642-39118-7_4, © Springer-Verlag Berlin Heidelberg 2014

papilla and larger lesions. An appropriate ultrasound wave conduction interface is necessary; this can be accomplished by suctioning all luminal air and direct contact of the endoscope with or without a water-filled balloon or with water infusion filling the lumen. Focal distance can be adjusted by processors to improve the resolution, according to the depth of the area of interest. Endosonographers have variable preferences but should be able to combine these techniques, depending on the location of the lesion. Compression and tangential scanning of the wall should be minimized to avoid false interpretation of the findings.

Box 4.1: Resources

- American Society for Gastrointestinal Endoscopy guidelines: The role of endoscopy in ampullary and duodenal adenomas http://www.asge.org/assets/0/71542/71544/8f8a3952917f4fe78f3855ff0ec77d07.pdf
- Familial adenomatous polypopsis: APC-Associated Polyposis Conditions (Review) Jasperson KW, Burt RW. APC-Associated Polyposis Conditions. 1998 Dec 18 (Updated 2011 Oct 27). In: Pagon RA, Bird TD, Dolan CR, et al., editors. GeneReviews™ [Internet]. Seattle (WA): University of Washington, Seattle; 1993. Available from: http://www.ncbi.nlm.nih.gov/books/NBK1345/
- Surgical management of neuroendocrine tumors of the gastrointestinal tract Lyen C. Huang, MD, MPH, George A. Poultsides, MD, Jeffrey A. Norton, MD Aug 15, 2011. CancerNetwork.com: http://www.cancernetwork.com/gastrointestinal-cancer/content/article/10165/192182
- DAVE Project – Gastroenterology: Duodenum, carcinoid tumor With EUS FNA http://daveproject.org/duodenum-carcinoid-tumor-with-eus-fna/2009-03-25/
- DAVE Project – Gastroenterology: Duodenum, adenoma treated with argon plasma coagulation in a patient with FAP http://daveproject.org/duodenum-adenoma-treated-with-argon-plasma-coagulation-in-a-patient-with-fap/2006-03-09/
- DAVE Project – Gastroenterology: Duodenum, malignant mass evaluated by EUS http://daveproject.org/duodenum-malignant-mass-evaluated-with-eus/2004-05-07/

4.2 Cases and Discussions

4.2.1 Duodenal Cancer

This is a 66-year-old man who was evaluated for anemia by upper endoscopy and colonoscopy. The colonoscopy was unremarkable but, based on the results of the endoscopic biopsies, the upper endoscopy showed what appeared to be a benign villous adenoma in the third portion of the duodenum. The patient was referred for EUS evaluation, and this study showed a superficial tumor that did not involve the muscularis propria. However, there was one 1.7-cm-diameter lymph-node-like structure immediately adjacent to the involved area. EUS-guided fine-needle aspiration (FNA) of the lymph node revealed adenocarcinoma.

In this case the presence of metastatic lymphadenopathy proven by EUS allowed the diagnosis of adenocarcinoma and indicated the need for surgery. An article from UCLA Medical Center summarizing 40 years of experience with this rare tumor reported that prognosis of duodenal cancers was related more to tumor size, local invasion, and histologic grade than tumor spread to local lymph nodes and that the disease can be potentially curable by surgery even with local lymph node involvement [1]. However, more recent articles have found that metastatic lymph node involvement decreases the rate of survival.

A study from the Memorial Sloan Kettering Cancer Center showed that survival at 5 years was 83 % in patients without nodal invasion and was 56 % in those with positive nodes [2]. A recent publication from Johns Hopkins reported that 5-year survival was 68 % in patients without lymphadenopathy versus 58 % in those with 1–3 positive nodes and 17 % in patients with ≥4 positive nodes [3]. In summary, lymph node involvement is again considered a significant prognostic factor, and EUS/FNA has the ability to provide this information.

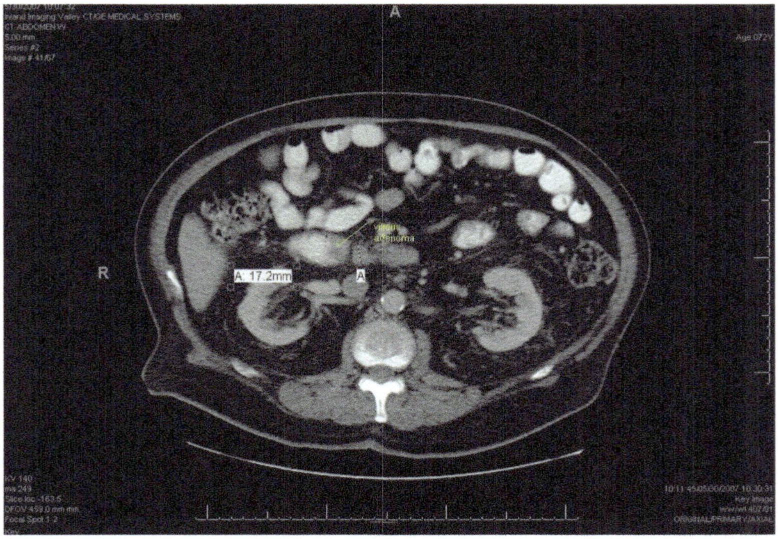

Fig. 4.1 This computed tomography scan shows a duodenal mass with an adjacent lymph node (retrospectively identified as such following the endoscopic ultrasound)

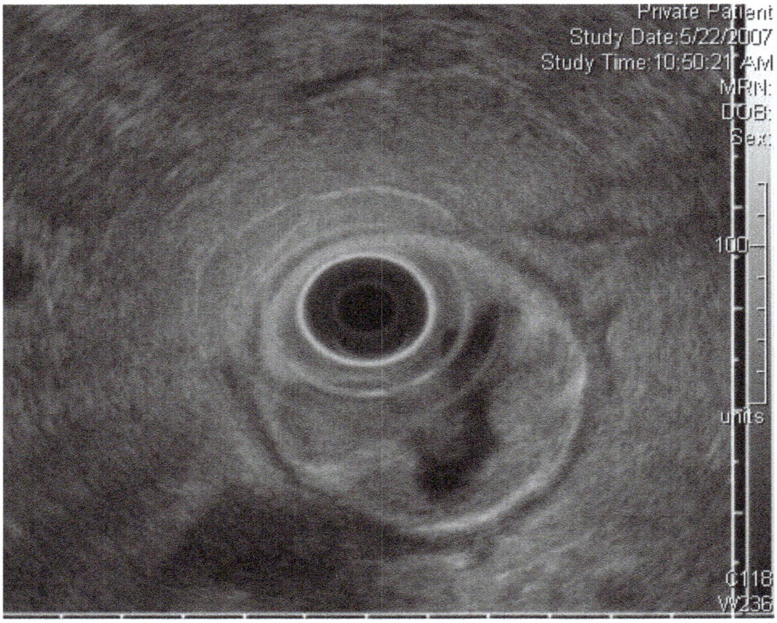

Fig. 4.2 This is the villous-appearing lesion in the duodenum. Endoscopic surface biopsies showed only villous adenoma, and the lesion appears to be confined to the mucosa/submucosa

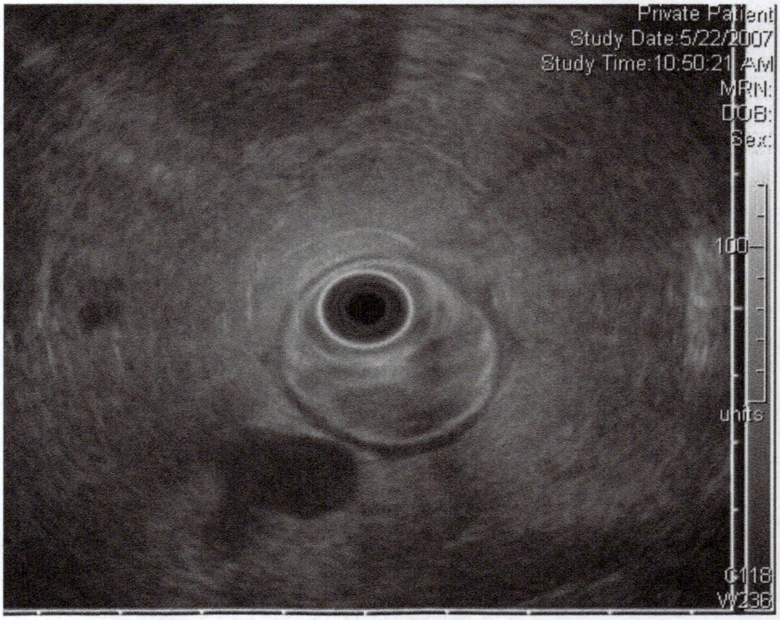

Fig. 4.3 In addition to the villous lesion in the duodenal lumen, a hypoechoic adjacent lymph-node-like structure can be seen

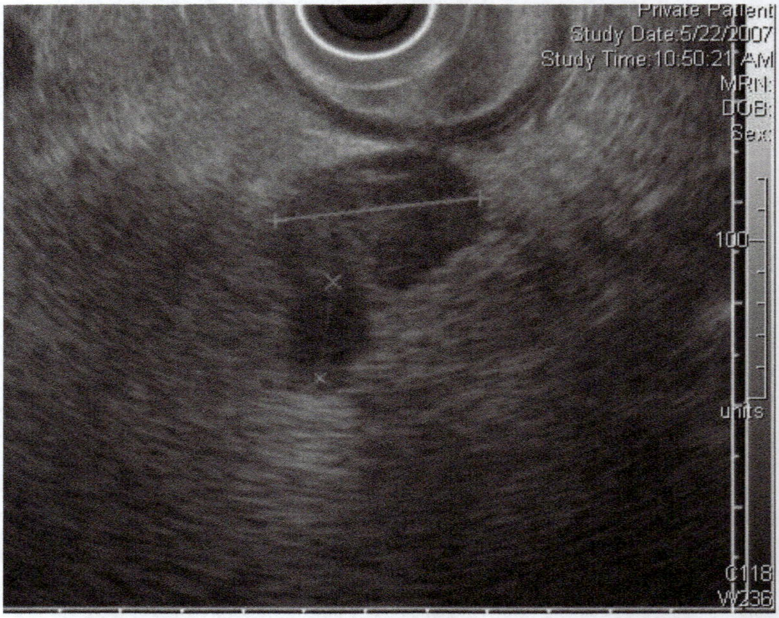

Fig. 4.4 This radial endoscopic ultrasound (EUS) image shows a close-up of the periduodenal lymph node. EUS-guided fine-needle aspiration revealed adenocarcinoma

4.2.2 Duodenal Diverticulum

Duodenal diverticula can be mistaken for cystic pancreatic abnormalities on cross-sectional imaging, especially when they are not filled with air or contrast but fluid [4]. These are two patients in whom periampullary duodenal diverticula and the absence of pancreatic cystic lesions were nicely demonstrated during EUS.

Duodenal diverticula are common in the periampullary area. The presence of these diverticula can limit the evaluation of the distal common bile duct (CBD) or periampullary region on standard imaging studies. Diverticula can contain debris, and they usually fill with air during standard endoscopy. Careful endoscopic visualization of this area is important to avoid false EUS interpretations, particularly if scanning from the duodenal bulb. In these cases filling the diverticulum with water provides appropriate ultrasound wave transmission and allows for a reliable interpretation of adjacent structures.

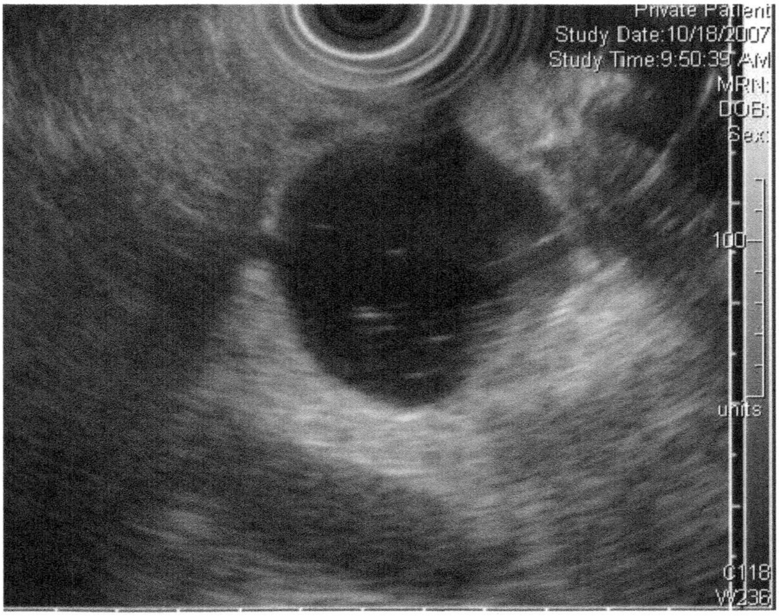

Fig. 4.5 This is a water-filled periampullary duodenal diverticulum that mimicked a hypodense lesion on a computed tomography scan of the pancreas

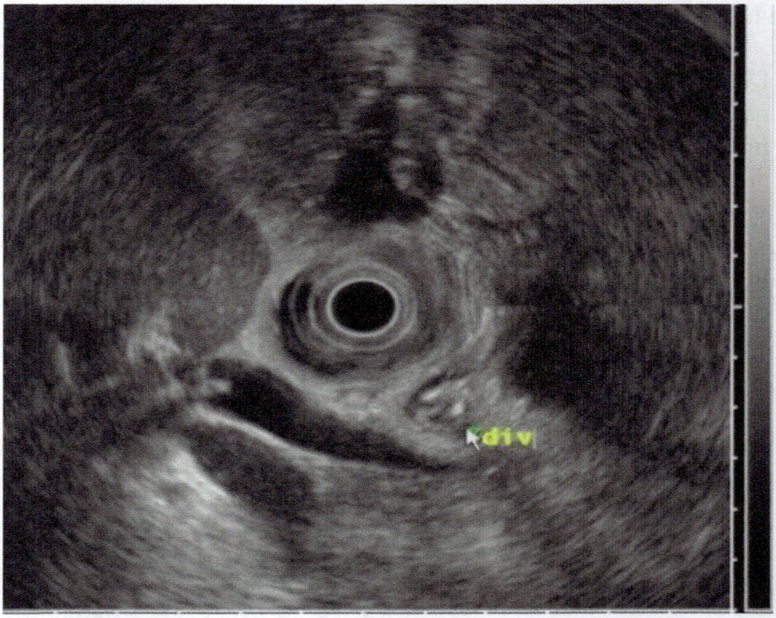

Fig. 4.6 This is another periampullary diverticulum (*div*), which contains debris

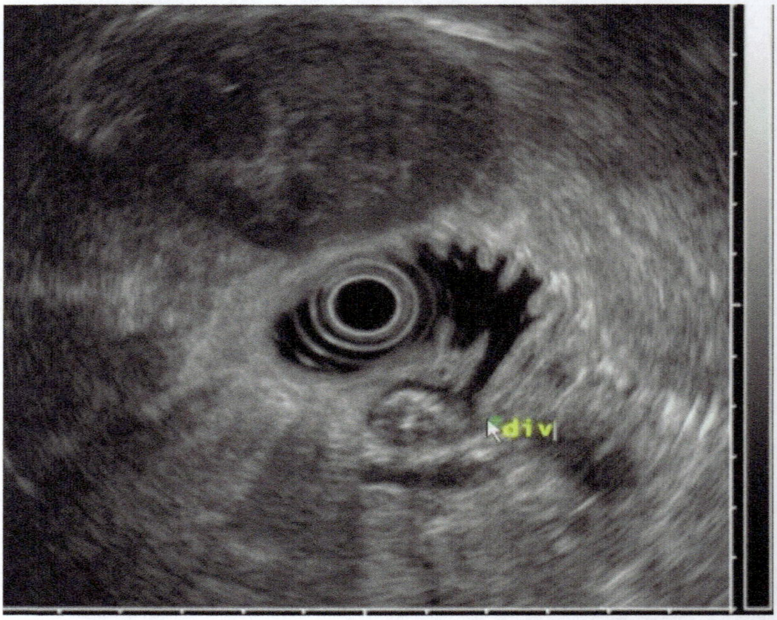

Fig. 4.7 This image reveals the connection to the duodenal lumen. (*div*) diverticulum

4.2.3 Duodenal Perforation by Foreign Body

A 65-year-old woman presented with abdominal pain, weight loss, and fever. A computed tomography (CT) scan of the abdomen showed a retroperitoneal abscess. A duodenal perforation was suspected. The initial upper endoscopy was reportedly unremarkable. The patient was referred for EUS evaluation. Surface endoscopy during EUS showed a duodenal microperforation. EUS showed an echogenic shadowing structure (not air) directly behind the perforation site. Since nothing was seen on the CT scan in this location, a toothpick or a fish bone were the prime suspects. The patient was treated with percutaneous drainage and long-term antibiotics. Eight weeks after the initial presentation she developed portal vein thrombosis, probably related to the presence of the abscess.

Metallic objects (except aluminum), most animal bones, and all glass foreign bodies are opaque on radiographs. Most plastic and wooden foreign bodies and most fish bones are not opaque on radiographs. These can be missed occasionally by CT scan [6], as shown in this case. Ultrasound techniques are helpful in the detection of wooden foreign bodies as small as 2.5 mm long, as shown in multiple reports [7–9].

A systematic review of injuries related to toothpick ingestion reported between 1966 and 2000 [10] found that most patients (70 %) present with abdominal pain, and most commonly reported complications include perforation, bleeding, peritonitis, abscess, or obstruction. However, only a minority (12 %) of patients remembered swallowing a toothpick. The most common site of injury is the duodenum (25 %), although this can occur throughout the entire gastrointestinal tract, and the toothpicks can migrate to the pleura, pericardium, peritoneum, ureter, or bladder. Major vessel involvement can also occur. Therefore, it is important to define the exact location of the entire toothpick before attempting endoscopic removal, which is contraindicated in patients with peritonitis or vessel penetration [11].

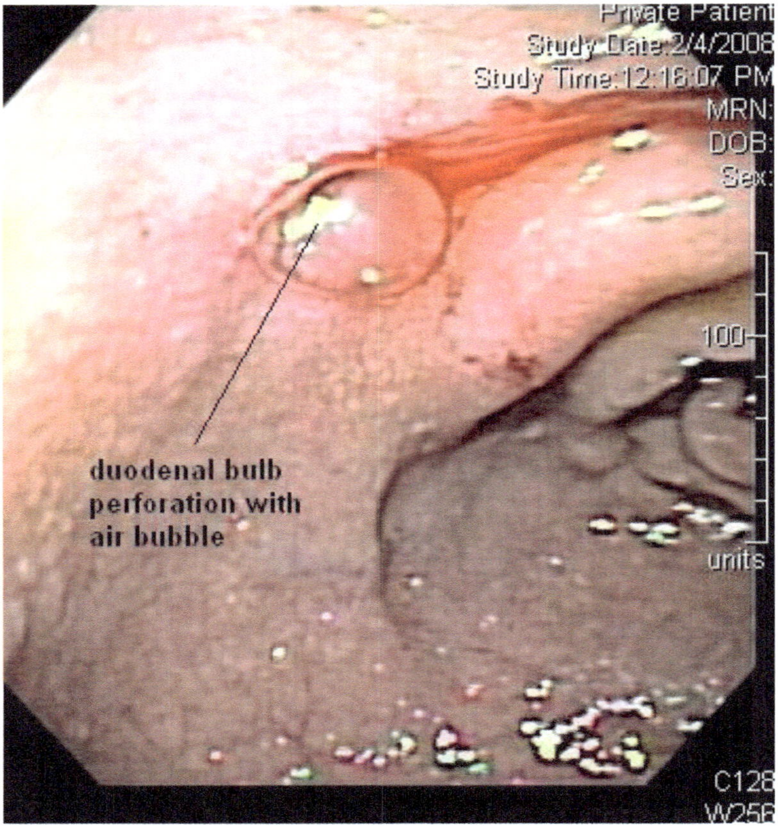

Fig. 4.8 A small 3- to 4-mm-diameter perforation is visible in the duodenal bulb on this esophagogastroduodenoscopy

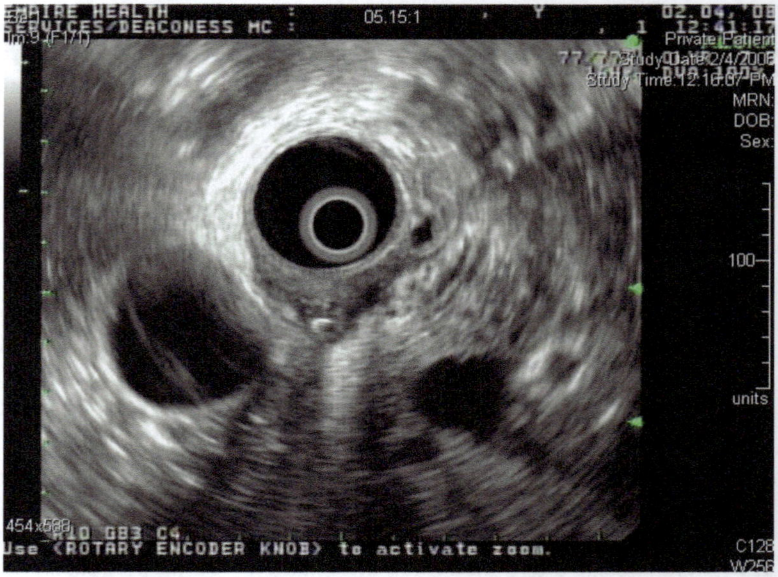

Fig. 4.9 Endoscopic ultrasound shows an echogenic round shadowing structure immediately adjacent to the perforation site

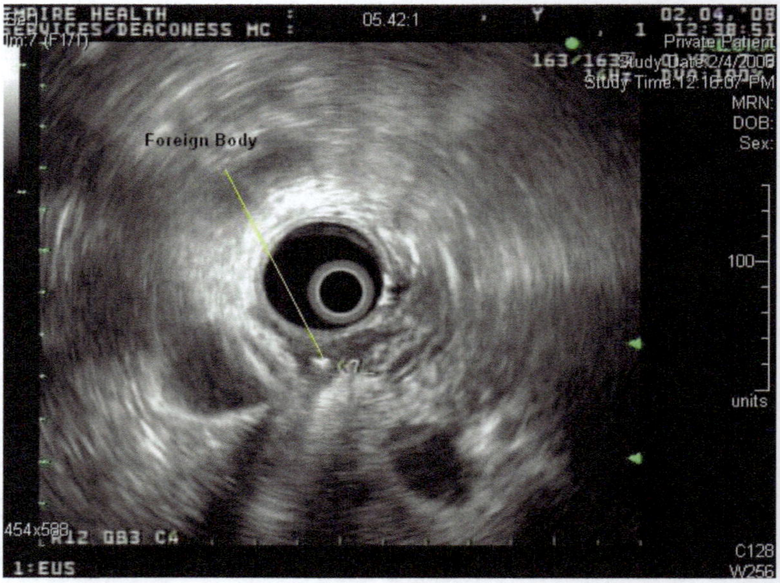

Fig. 4.10 The nature of this foreign body is unclear. A broken-off tooth pick or a fish bone are considerations

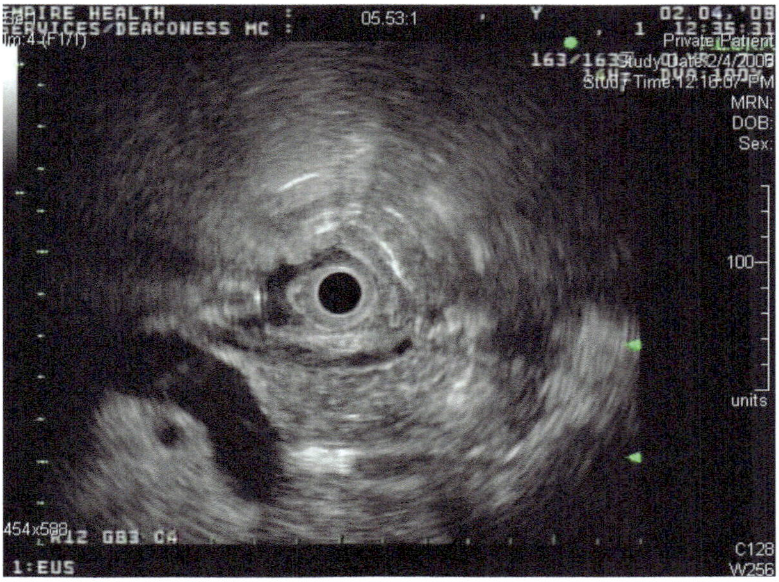

Fig. 4.11 The portal vein appeared normal at initial presentation

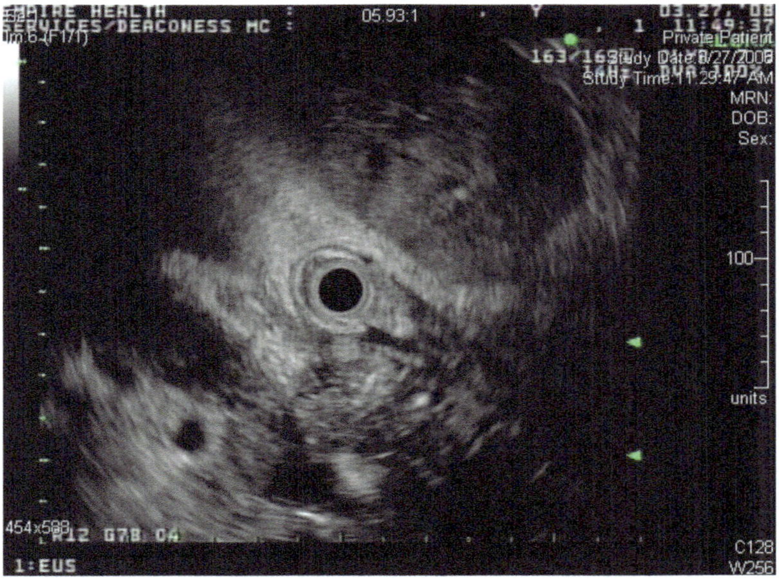

Fig. 4.12 The abscess was managed with percutaneous drainage and antibiotics. This endoscopic ultrasound 8 weeks later shows a portal vein thrombosis adjacent to the abscess

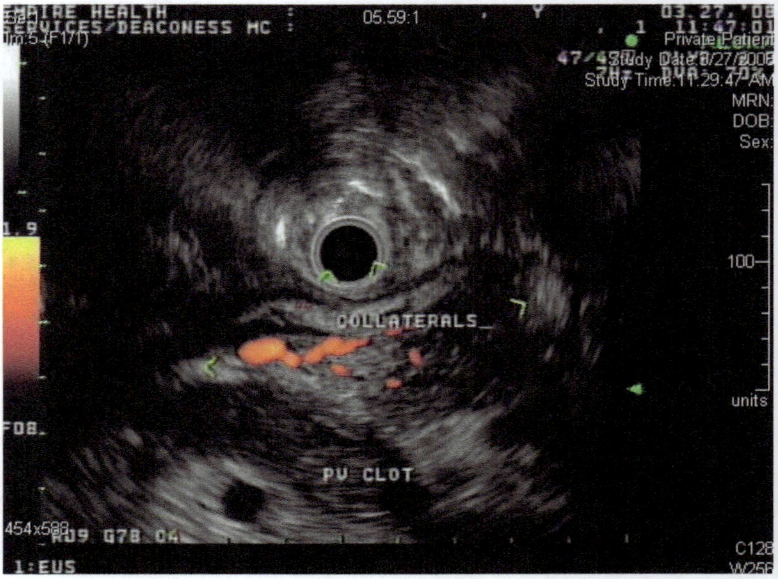

Fig. 4.13 This endoscopic ultrasound shows venous collaterals bypassing the completely clotted portal vein

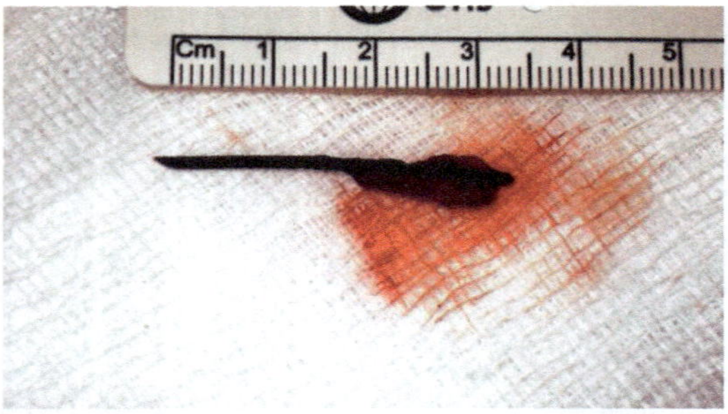

Fig. 4.14 A toothpick after laparoscopic extraction from a different patient (From Al-Khyatt et al. [5])

4.2.4 Duodenal Pseudocyst

This is a 42-year-old man with a drug and alcohol problem who was admitted to the hospital with intractable abdominal pain and because a CT scan had shown a paraduodenal mass. An EUS was requested for further evaluation of multiple abnormalities seen on CT. The EUS showed that there was actually a smaller cyst within the duodenal wall and another larger one, characteristic of a pseudocyst, adjacent to it. The small cyst, if it had been isolated, would have probably been called a duplication cyst. However, the clinical context and the fact that it had resolved 6 months later make it much more likely that this is a duodenal wall intramural pseudocyst.

Pseudocysts that migrate into the wall of the duodenum or elsewhere in the gastrointestinal tract, including the stomach and colon, have been reported [12], but awareness of this phenomenon is limited in the medical community. Duodenal pseudocysts are found between the muscularis propria and the mucosa or between serosa and muscularis propria. The surface of the posterior wall of the duodenum is in direct contact with the head of the pancreas, without a clear barrier to the disruptive effect of pancreatitis and pseudocysts. Complications of these lesions include perforation or duodenal obstruction. EUS allows for the detection of these cystic-appearing lesions, which can be confirmed by aspiration of fluid rich in amylase [13].

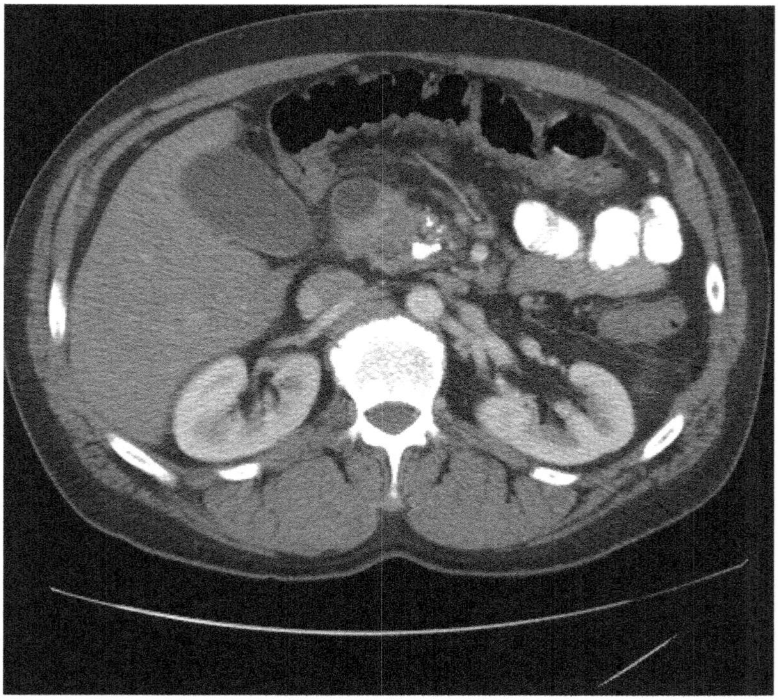

Fig. 4.15 A duodenal cyst on a computed tomography scan of the abdomen

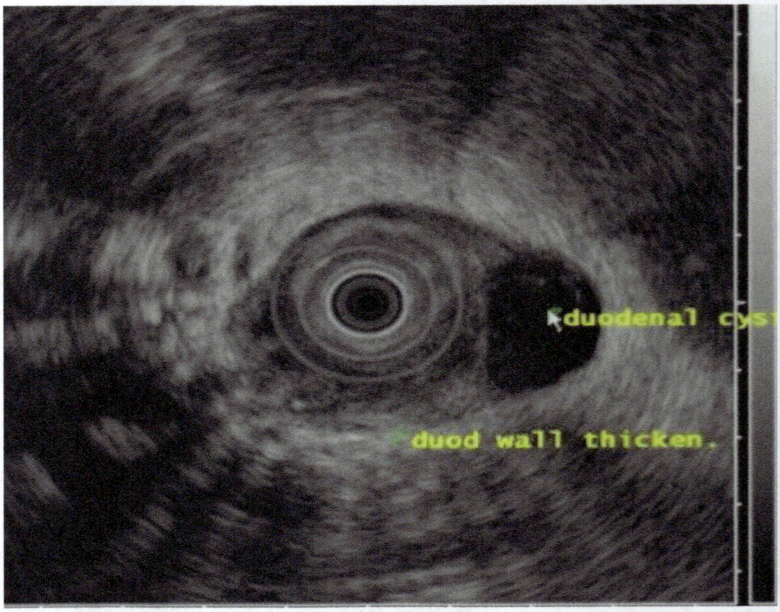

Fig. 4.16 The same duodenal cyst as seen on endoscopic ultrasound

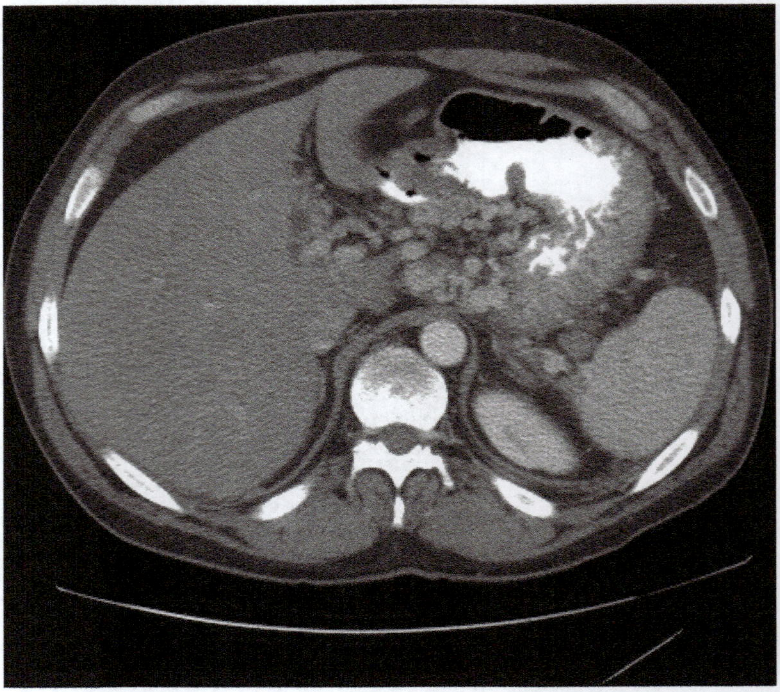

Fig. 4.17 Extensive collateral circulation on computed tomography secondary to splenic vein thrombosis

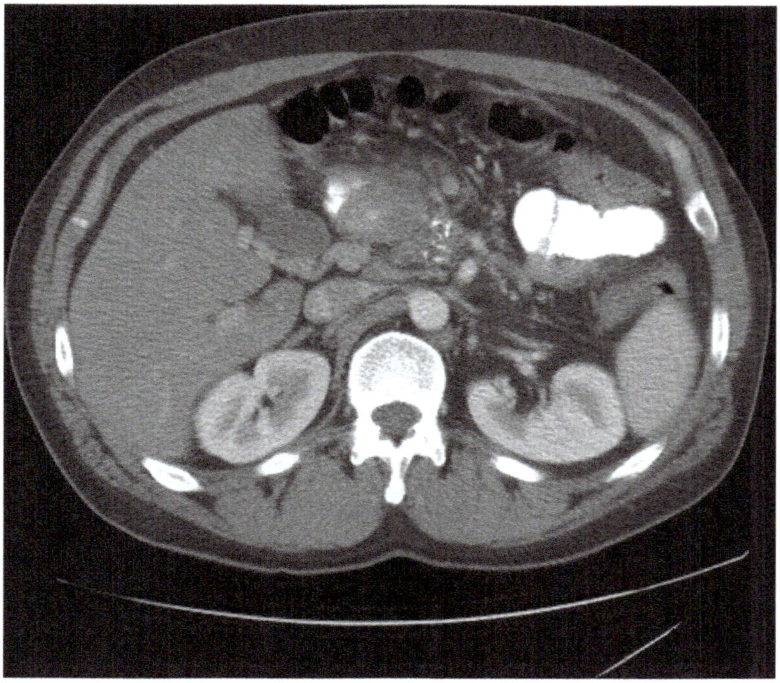

Fig. 4.18 A periduodenal mass as seen on computed tomography

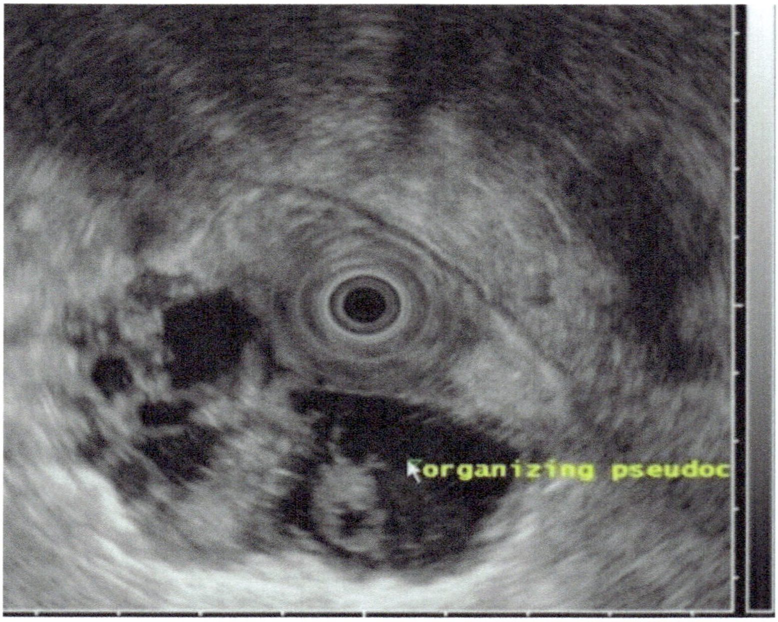

Fig. 4.19 The periduodenal mass is shown to be a septated pseudocyst on this endoscopic ultrasound

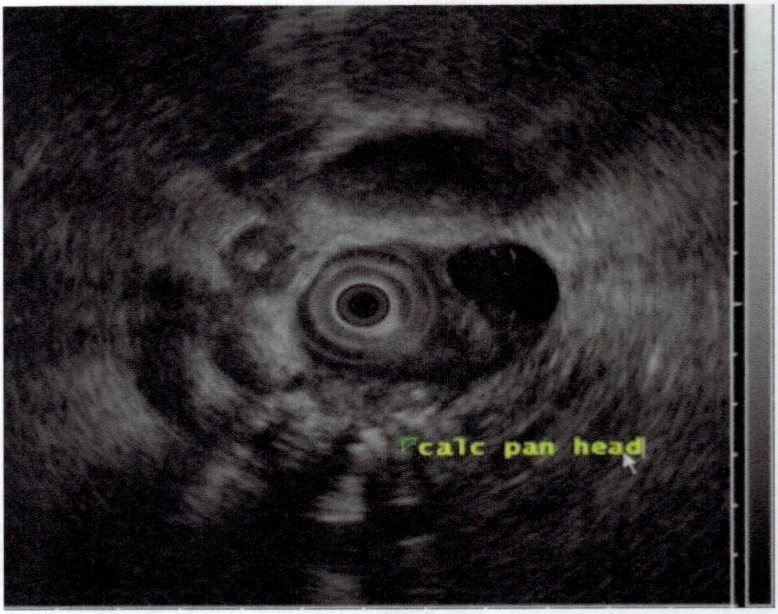

Fig. 4.20 Changes of severe chronic pancreatitis with calcifications are seen

4.2.5 Ampullary Carcinoma

This is a 58-year-old man who presented with a mildly dilated (CBD) and abnormal liver tests 9 months earlier. He underwent several endoscopic retrograde cholangiopancreatography (ERCP) evaluations, had a biliary sphincterotomy, and had bile duct stents placed for presumed benign sphincter stenosis. After his most recent (ERCP) he was referred for EUS evaluation. The study showed a hypoechoic cap or plug obstructing the biliary and pancreatic orifices. Biopsies of the cut surface of the papilla revealed adenocarcinoma.

EUS has become an important diagnostic and staging tool in the evaluation of patients with ampullary lesions. The goal of this procedure is to estimate the depth of invasion into periduodenal wall layers, the pancreas, the bile duct, or the pancreatic duct. T staging by EUS is more reliable than other diagnostic techniques, including CT or magnetic resonance imaging (MRI), although it is not as sensitive for locoregional lymph node invasion [14].

Standard endoscopic biopsies of ampullary tumors are highly specific but not sensitive enough and can be falsely negative in patients with adenocarcinoma, even after sphincterotomy [15]. EUS similarly cannot exclude focal adenocarcinoma in patients with superficial, minimally invasive lesions. In patients without evidence of deep invasion (duodenal wall, biliary or pancreatic ducts, or pancreatic parenchyma) an endoscopic ampullectomy can be performed.

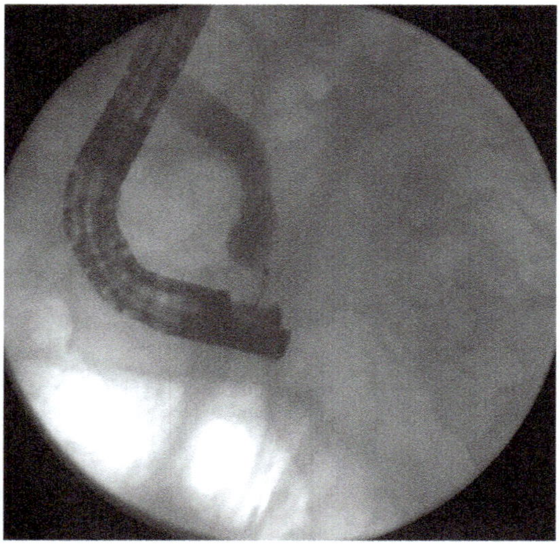

Fig. 4.21 Plump appearance of the termination of the distal (CBD)

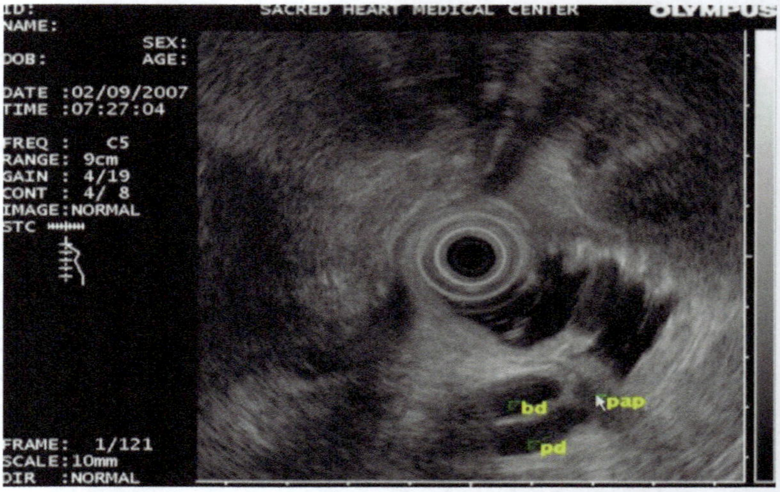

Fig. 4.22 Endoscopic ultrasound shows a hypoechoic cap at the ampulla, *bd* bile duct, *pd* pancreatic duct, *pap* papilla

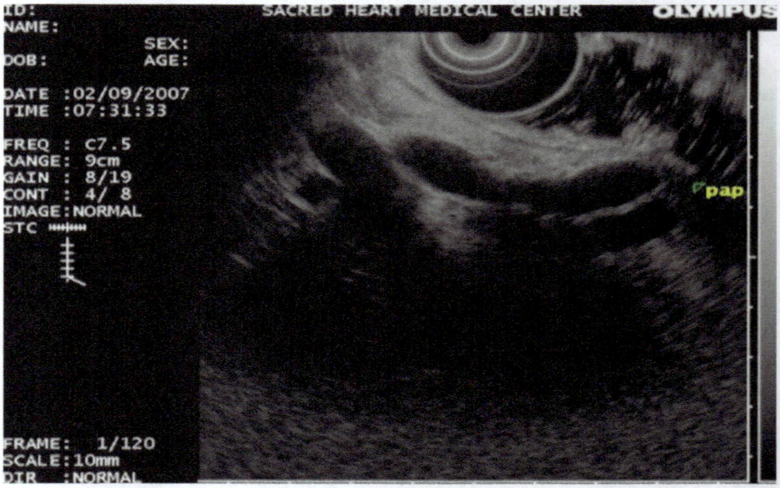

Fig. 4.23 Another view of the hypoechoic "cap" over the biliary and pancreatic duct orifice on endoscopic ultrasound, *pap* papilla

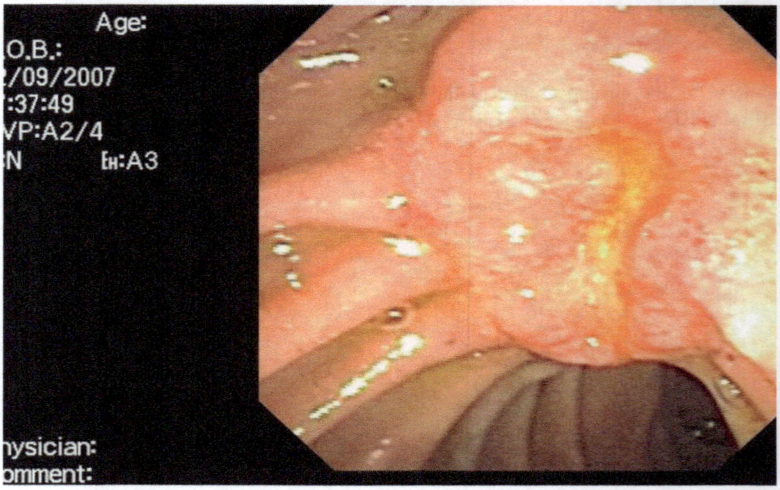

Fig. 4.24 An irregular appearance of the cut surface of the papilla is visible on surface endoscopy

4.2.6 Familial Adenomatous Polyposis

This is a 25-year-old patient with familial adenomatous polyposis (FAP). Six years earlier he had undergone a total colectomy. Since that time he had done well in general except for two episodes of pancreatitis, one of which was associated with the formation of a pseudocyst, which resolved. His last endoscopy was 3 years before the referral for this EUS, which was done for the evaluation of mild bile duct dilation. A normal papilla was described on his previous esophagogastroduodenoscopy (3 years ago). The current images show a villous lesion bulging into the main pancreatic duct. There was no evidence of invasive cancer during surgical duodenotomy.

In patients with FAP the second portion of the duodenum, especially the periampullary area, is particularly prone to adenomatous transformation. Periampullary and duodenal adenomas develop in up to 80 % of patients with FAP. About 5–8 % of patients with FAP eventually develop duodenal or periampullary cancers. The relative risk of periampullary cancer is 124-fold greater than in the general population, as shown in a study from the Johns Hopkins Registry [16].

A sequence of progression from adenoma to carcinoma is believed to occur in most of these patients, offering an opportunity for endoscopic surveillance and detection of early lesions, although the efficacy of this approach has not been proven. A surveillance program starting at age 20–25 has been recommended and includes forward and side-view visualization and biopsies of the major papilla and a follow-up interval of at least 3 years for patients with FAP and normal-appearing papilla. Adenoma has been found in up to 54 % of biopsies obtained from FAP patients with normal-appearing papilla [17]. Patients who have already developed duodenal adenomas are expected to be at higher risk of cancer and should undergo closer surveillance.

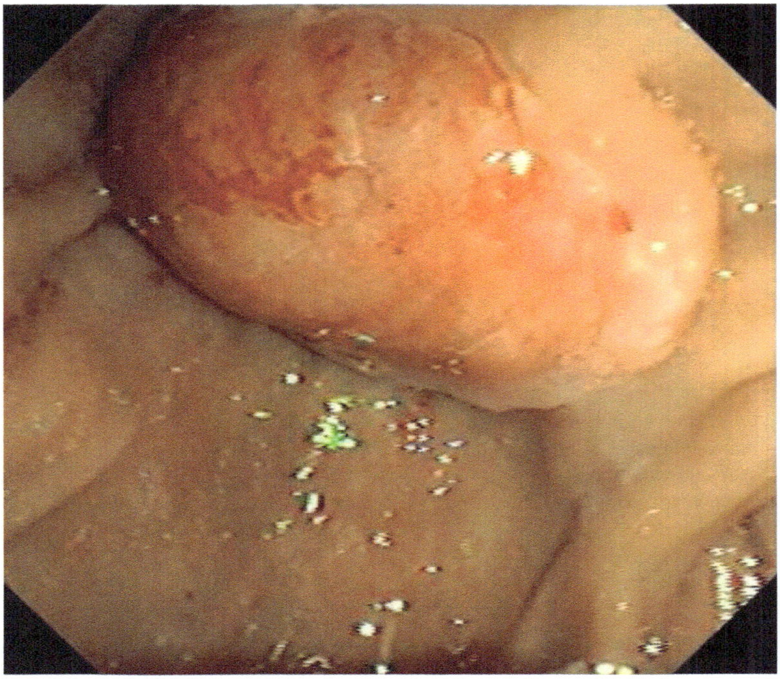

Fig. 4.25 This is an endoscopy image of an ampullary tumor that appears to be relatively small in a 25-year-old with familial adenomatous polyposis

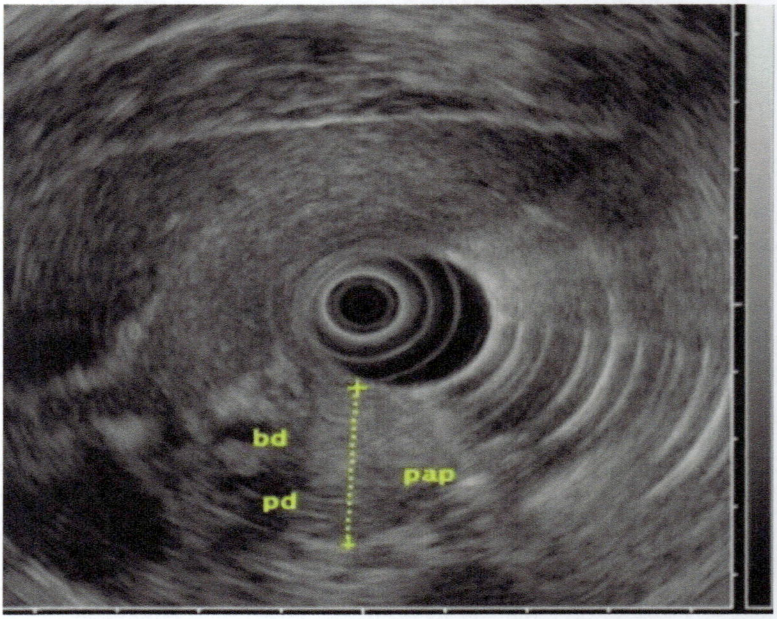

Fig. 4.26 This radial endoscopic ultrasound image shows that the tumor actually measures 2.4 cm in diameter and is not so small after all. *pd* pancreatic duct; *bd* bile duct, *pap* papilla

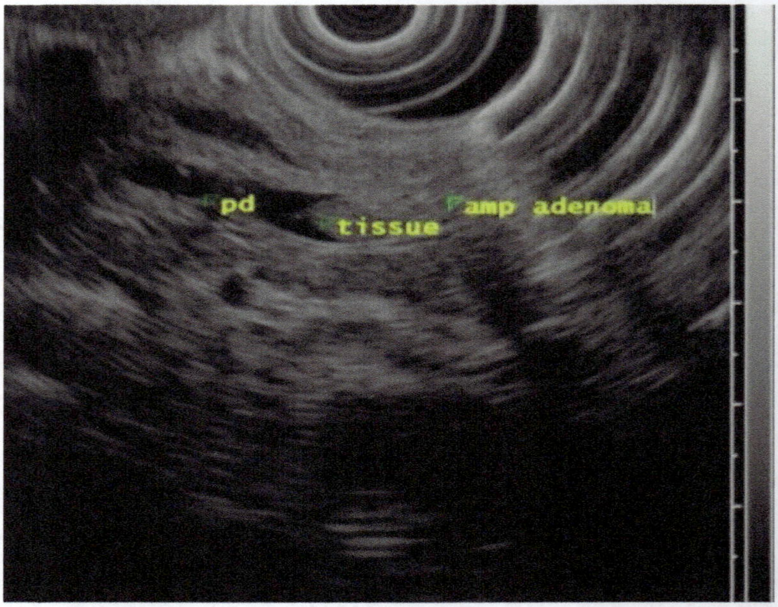

Fig. 4.27 This endoscopic ultrasound image shows tissue ingrowth into the *pd* pancreatic duct; *amp adenoma* ampullary adenoma

4.2.7 Periduodenal Collaterals

This is a 58-year-old patient with back pain. A CT scan showed hypodense areas and parenchymal calcifications thought to represent chronic pancreatitis. To be sure, an EUS evaluation was requested. The first abnormality that caught our attention was the presence of periduodenal collaterals. After a careful search for a mass lesion, one was indeed found in the body region of the pancreas.

As shown in this case, the presence of periduodenal collateral veins should raise suspicion of carcinomatous involvement of the portal circulation. In a study of 338 patients who underwent EUS for the evaluation of pancreatobiliary disorders, periduodenal collaterals were detected in 22 patients. CT detected these collaterals in only 2 of 22 patients (9.1 %). Twenty-one of these had pancreatic cancer; unfortunately the presence of these collaterals did not allow transduodenal FNA in 9 of the 22 patients (41 %) [18].

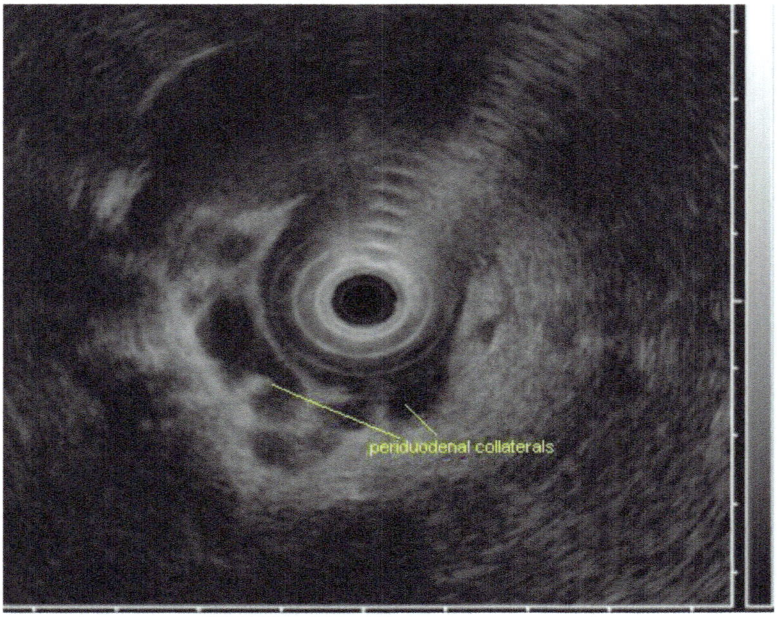

Fig. 4.28 Periduodenal venous collaterals are frequently associated with pancreatic cancers

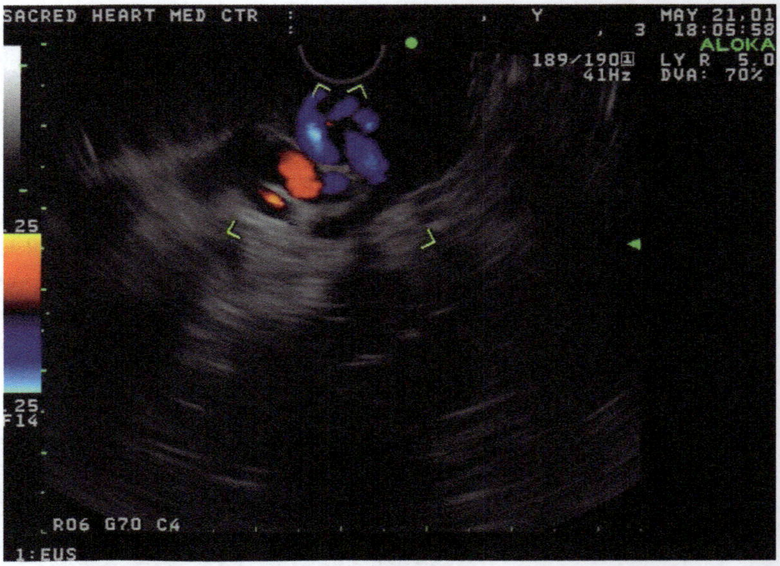

Fig. 4.29 The same collaterals as seen by linear endoscopic ultrasound with color Doppler

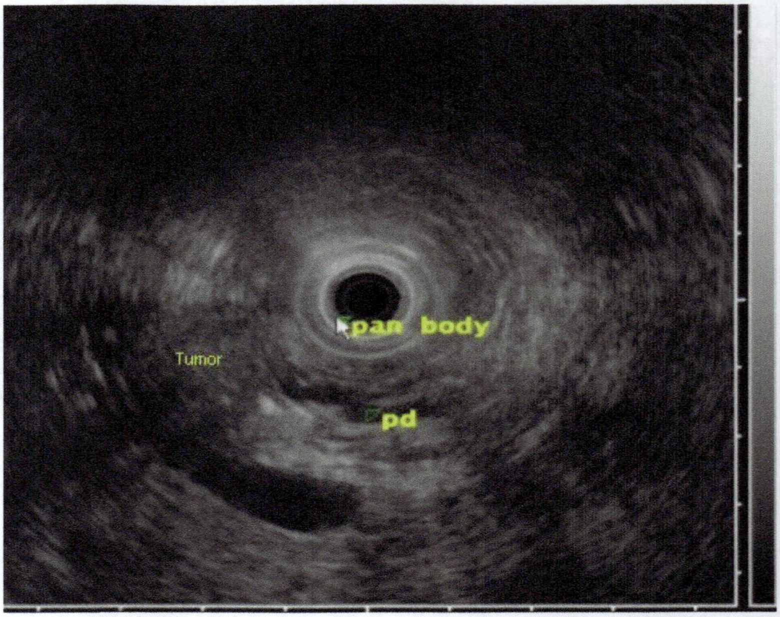

Fig. 4.30 This is a pancreatic body mass (pan body) on radial endoscopic ultrasound (EUS), which can be seen more clearly on linear EUS. *pd* pancreatic duct

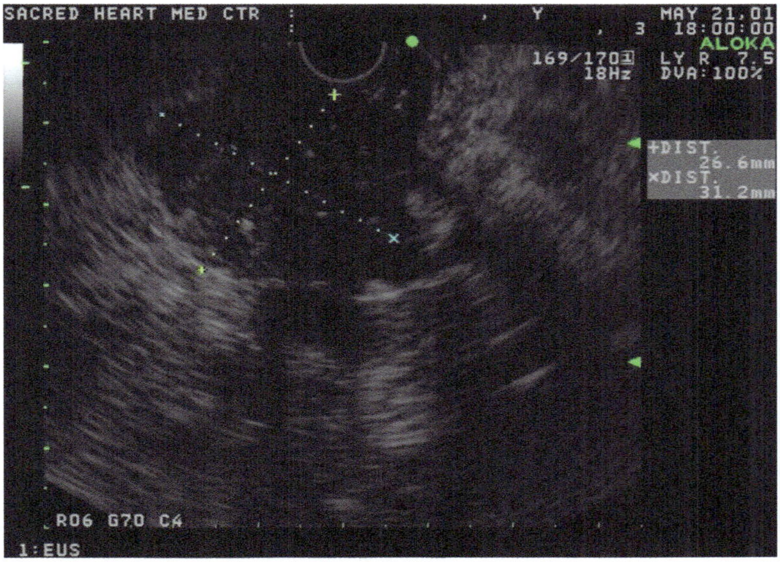

Fig. 4.31 The same tumor seen with the linear array endoscopic ultrasound scope before biopsy

4.2.8 Primary Duodenal Non-Hodgkin's Lymphoma

This is a 61-year-old woman with early satiety who underwent endoscopy and was found to have a duodenal B-cell non-Hodgkin's lymphoma. Metastatic lesions were seen in the liver. EUS was requested to evaluate the duodenum for transmural involvement.

Primary small intestinal lymphoma is uncommon and primary duodenal lymphomas are rare. Most of these patients present with abdominal pain; other clinical manifestations may include weight loss, ileus, bleeding, perforation, or palpable mass [19]. Two reported series of duodenal lymphoma have shown predominantly advanced disease at the time of diagnosis [20, 21]. EUS typically reveals loss of the layer structure of the duodenal wall but may also show areas of focal/multifocal tumor growth and regional lymphadenopathy. Surgery may play a role in metastatic cases because transmural involvement may lead to intestinal obstruction or perforation during treatment.

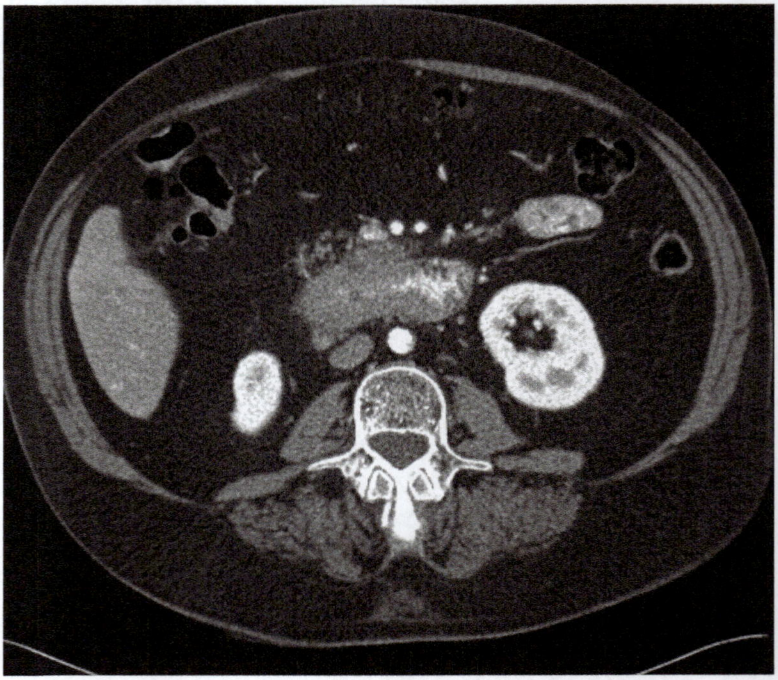

Fig. 4.32 A duodenal non-Hodgkin's lymphoma on computed tomography scan

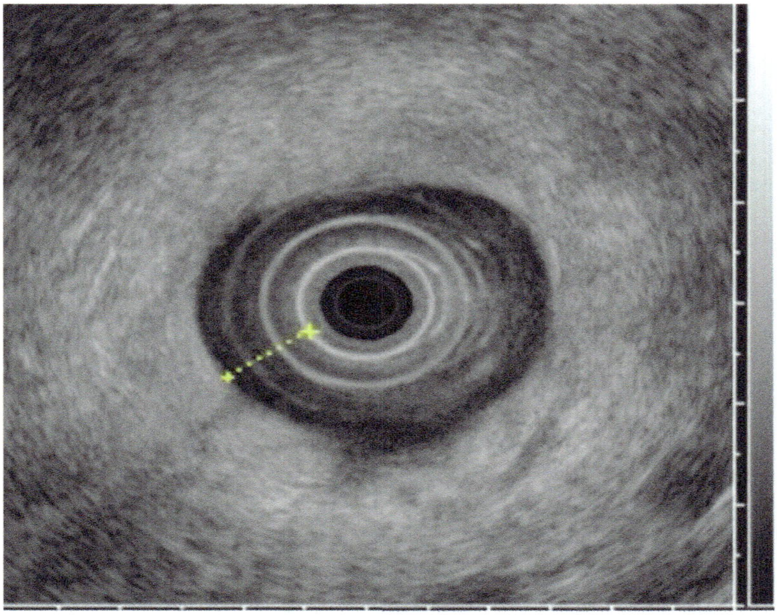

Fig. 4.33 Duodenal lymphoma on endoscopic ultrasound

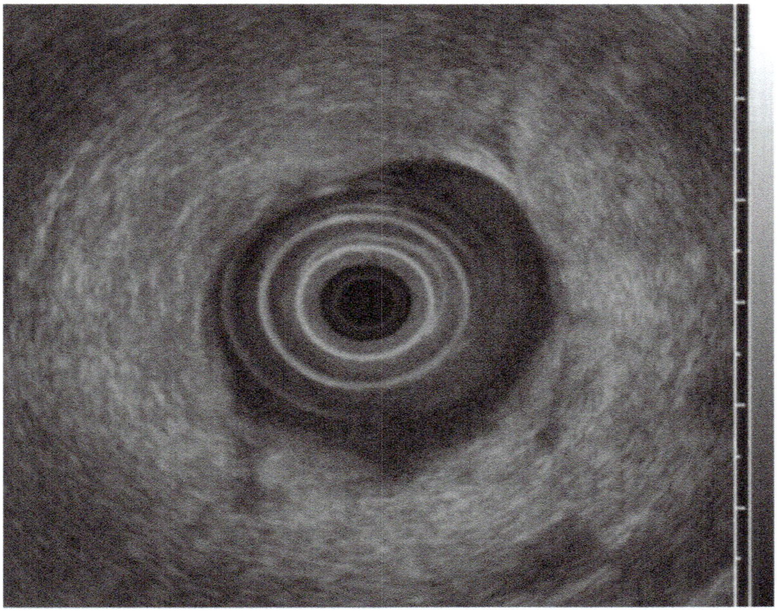

Fig. 4.34 Duodenal non-Hodgkin's lymphoma with endoscopic ultrasound showing full-thickness involvement

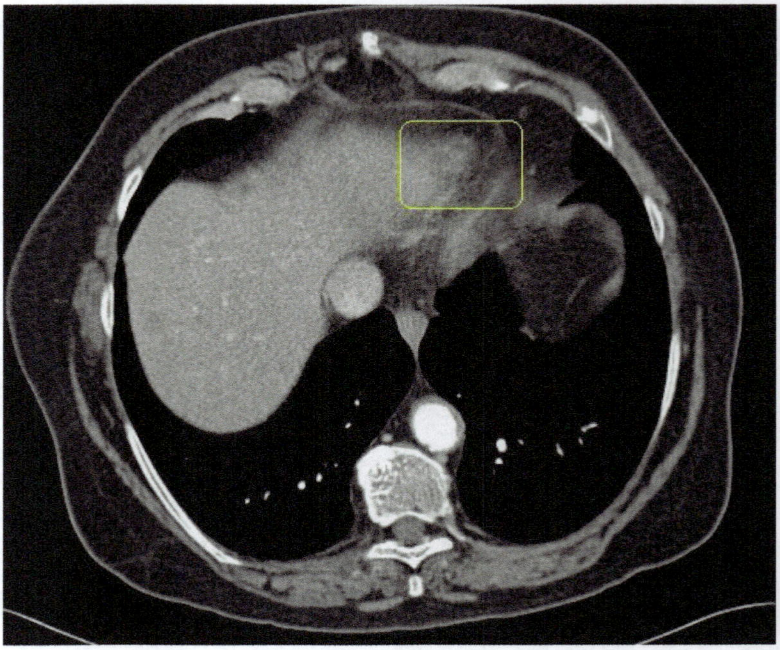

Fig. 4.35 Metastatic lesions in the tip of the left lobe of the liver (*yellow square*)

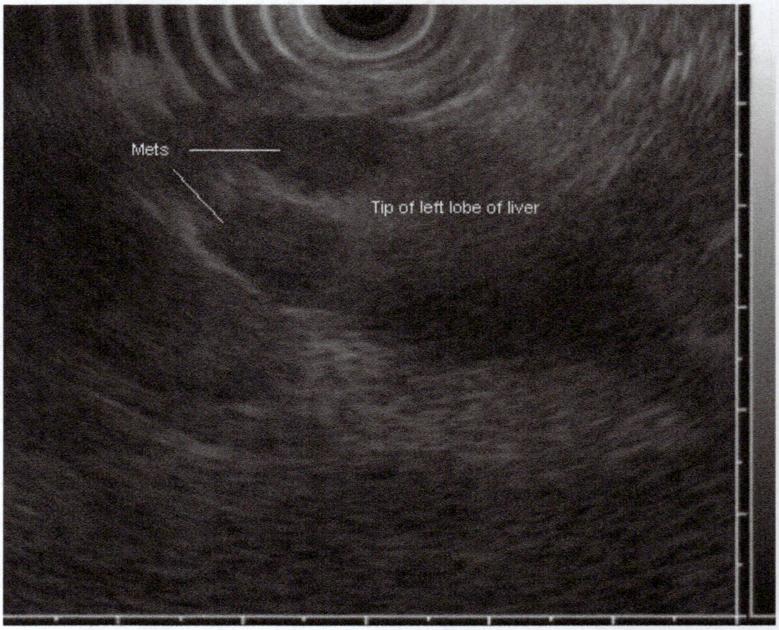

Fig. 4.36 Group of two lymphoma metastases (*mets*) in the liver

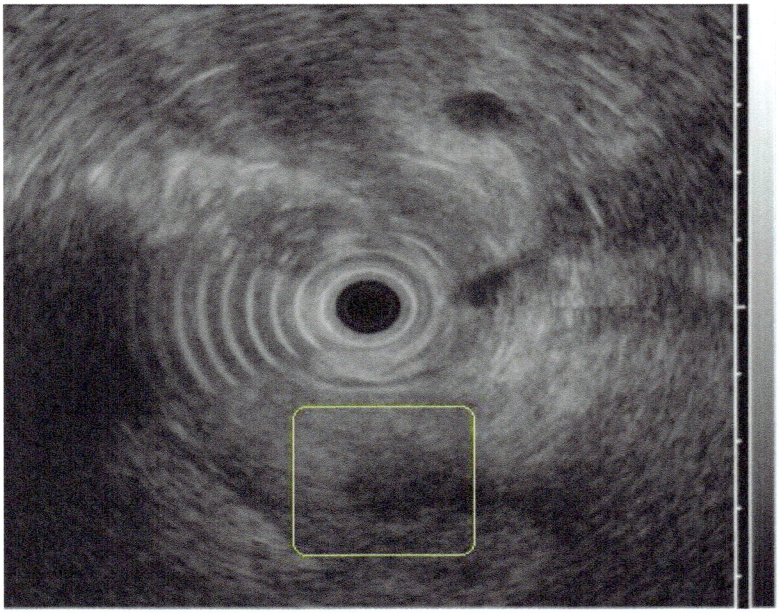

Fig. 4.37 Single metastatic nodule of non-Hodgkin's lymphoma of the duodenum in the left lobe of the liver (*yellow square*)

4.2.9 Transduodenal Abscess Drainage

This is a 62-year-old patient who presented with fever and abdominal pain. A CT scan of the abdomen showed three abdominal abscesses of unclear etiology in a perihepatic and periduodenal location. The clinical history regarding the possible nature and etiology of the abscesses was unrevealing. Two of these abscesses were successfully managed by percutaneous drainage. Cultures grew streptococcus viridans. The third abscess was difficult to approach percutaneously, and endoscopic transduodenal drainage was requested. We anticipated dense debris and were prepared to perform a transduodenal necrosectomy. Ultimately the contents of the abscess were much more liquid and little debridement was required. The details of the procedural approach are outlined in the legends of Figs. 4.38–4.49.

EUS provides access to anatomic areas adjacent to the esophagus, stomach, duodenum, and rectosigmoid. Multiple reports of successful EUS-guided drainage of abscesses in these locations are now available. Additional outcome-oriented prospective trials are necessary to define the role of EUS compared with alternative approaches including percutaneous or surgical drainage. In cases where a percutaneous or surgical approach is not safe or desired, EUS certainly can be considered if the imaging studies demonstrate a close proximity between the abscess and the lumen, a large-diameter single cavity (ideally >4 cm), and a mature wall [22].

The principles of the procedure are to access the cavity with a 19Fr-gauge FNA needle under EUS; place a guidewire at the cavity with EUS and fluoroscopic guidance; expand the mural track over the wire (alternatives include use of a needle knife, balloon dilators, or a commercially available cystotome); and place stents. A nasocystic drainage catheter can also be placed for irrigation and the management of residual abscess content. An excellent discussion of the alternatives and technical details of this procedures has been published by Prasad and Varadarajulu [22].

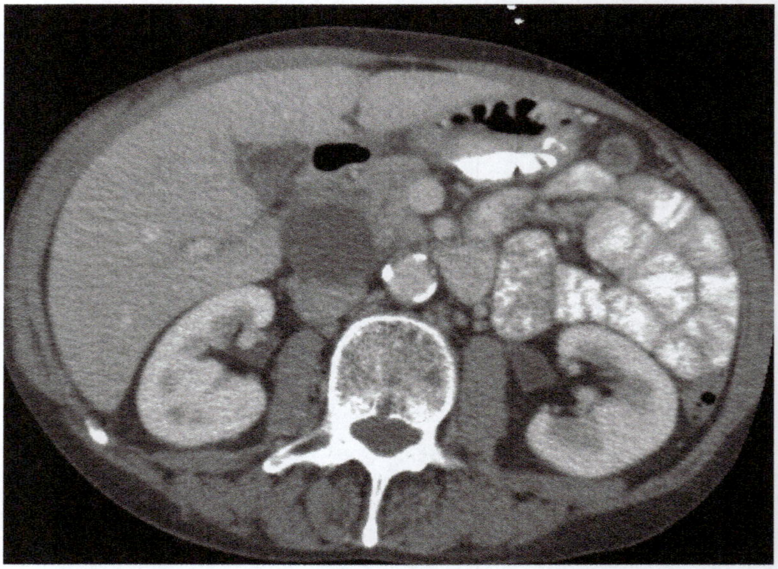

Fig. 4.38 This computed tomography scan shows a 3.6-cm periduodenal abscess

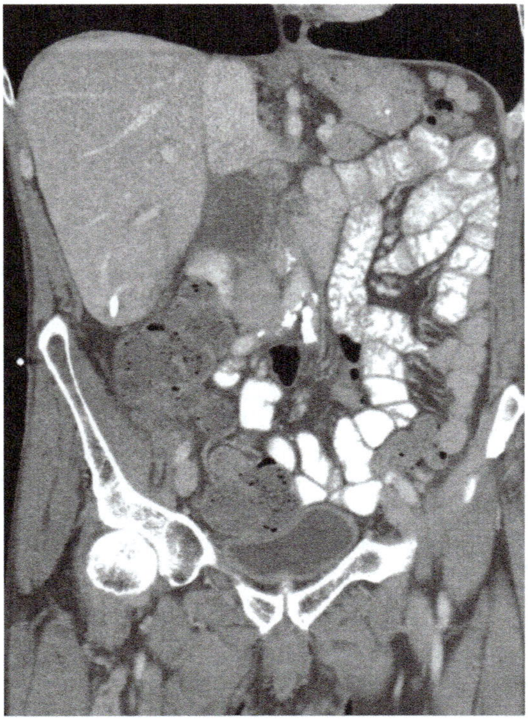

Fig. 4.39 This is a coronal computed tomography reconstruction showing the abscess

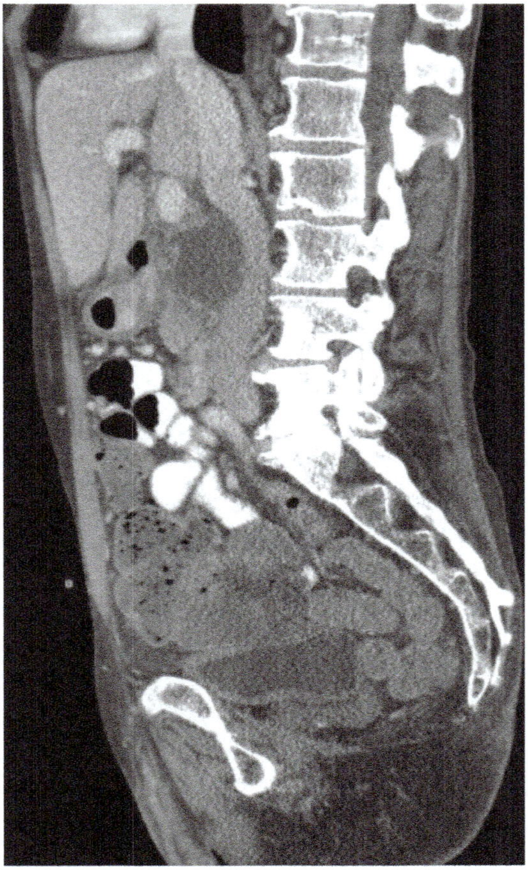

Fig. 4.40 This sagittal computed tomography reconstruction shows how the abscess compresses the inferior vena cava

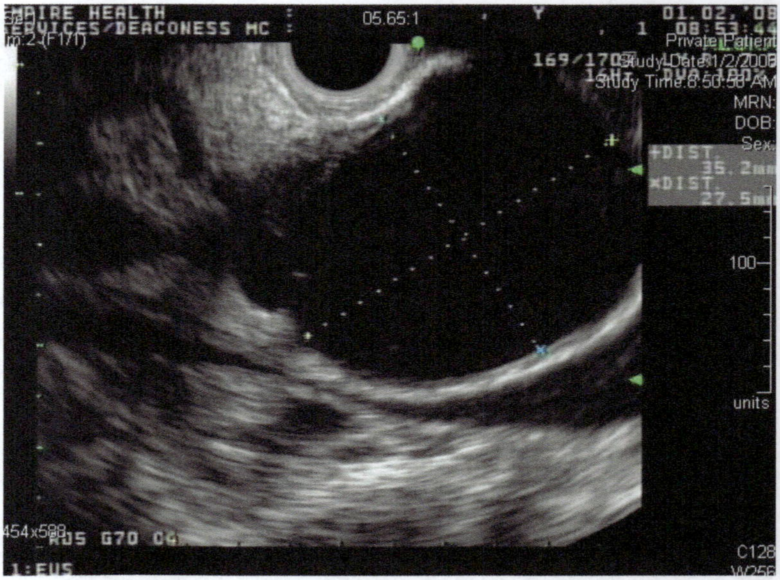

Fig. 4.41 This endoscopic ultrasound with the GF-UC140P shows the dimensions of the abscess. The contents appear to be mostly fluid

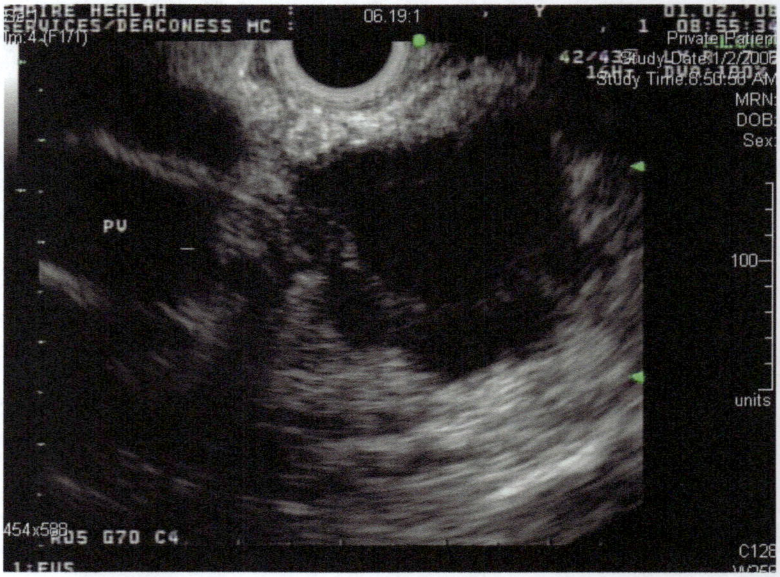

Fig. 4.42 A different view shows the solid components of the abscess cavity that are adherent to the wall

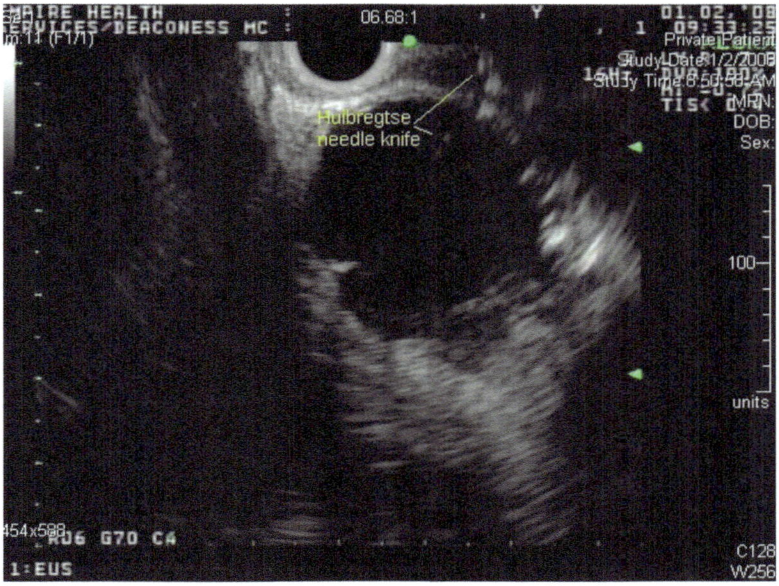

Fig. 4.43 A Huibregtse needle knife was advanced through the working channel of the linear endoscopic ultrasound instrument, and the abscess cavity was punctured using cautery current

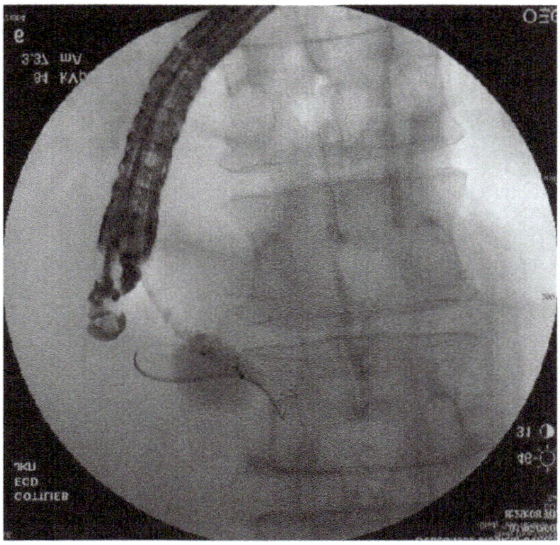

Fig. 4.44 A 0.035 inch guidewire was advanced through the needle knife catheter and curled up in the cyst cavity. A small amount of contrast starts outlining the cyst

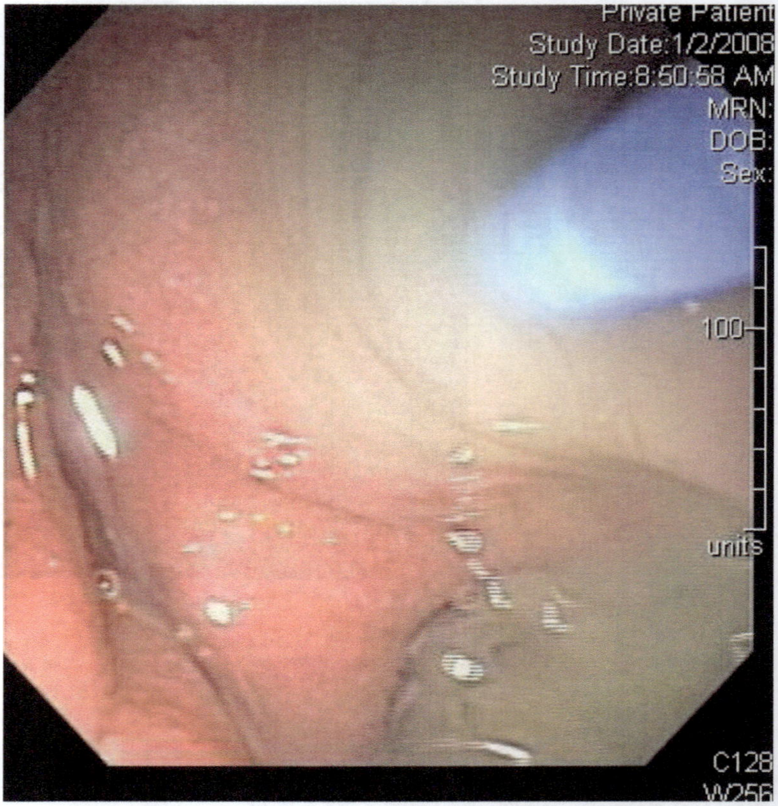

Fig. 4.45 This endoscopic view shows pus exiting from the abscess into the duodenum at the needle knife puncture site. Radial extensions of the cut were made carefully

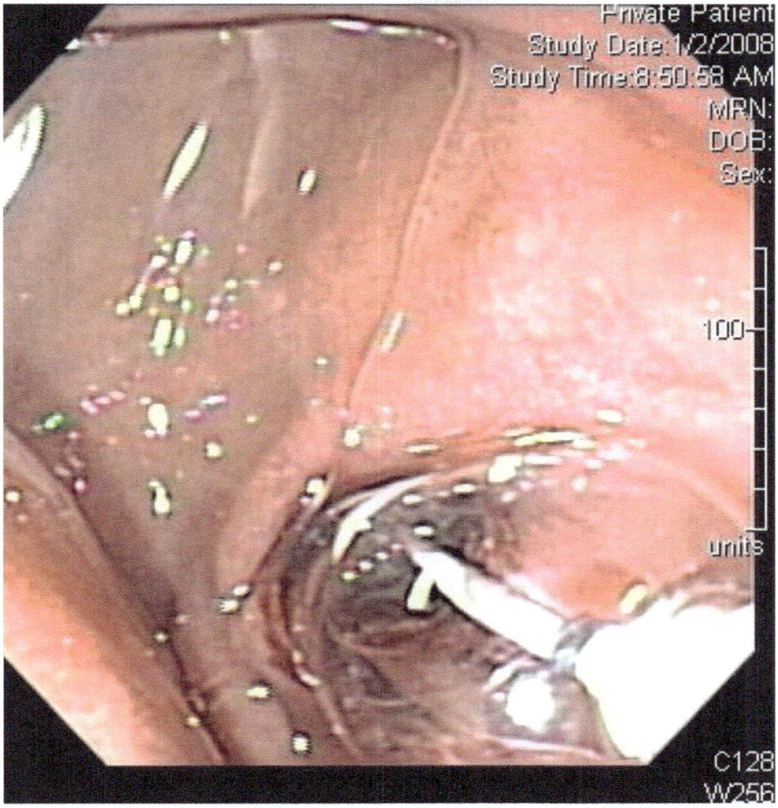

Fig. 4.46 The initial dilation of the needle knife tract was done through the endoscopic ultrasound scope using an 8-mm final diameter Hurricane biliary balloon (Boston-Scientific). Subsequent dilations were done using a duodenoscope and controlled radial expansion (CRE) balloons with diameters of 8–10 and 10–12 mm

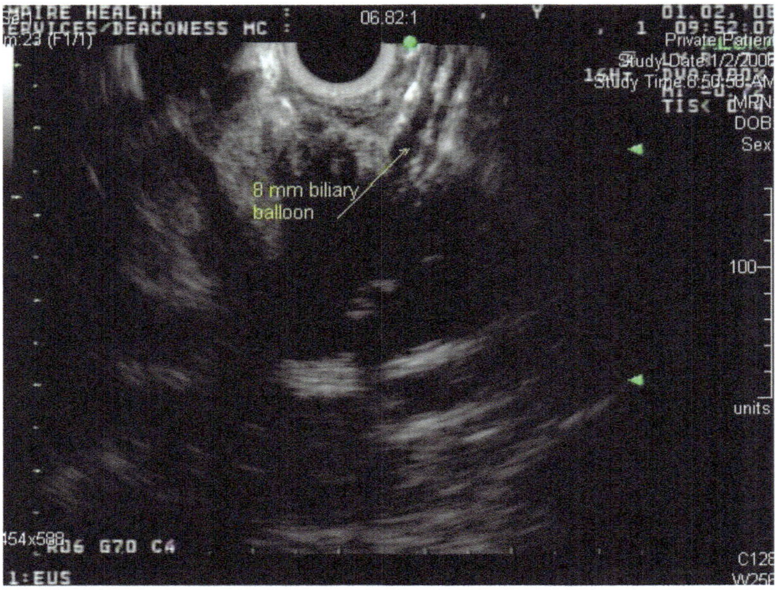

Fig. 4.47 This endoscopic ultrasound image shows the 8-mm biliary balloon in position

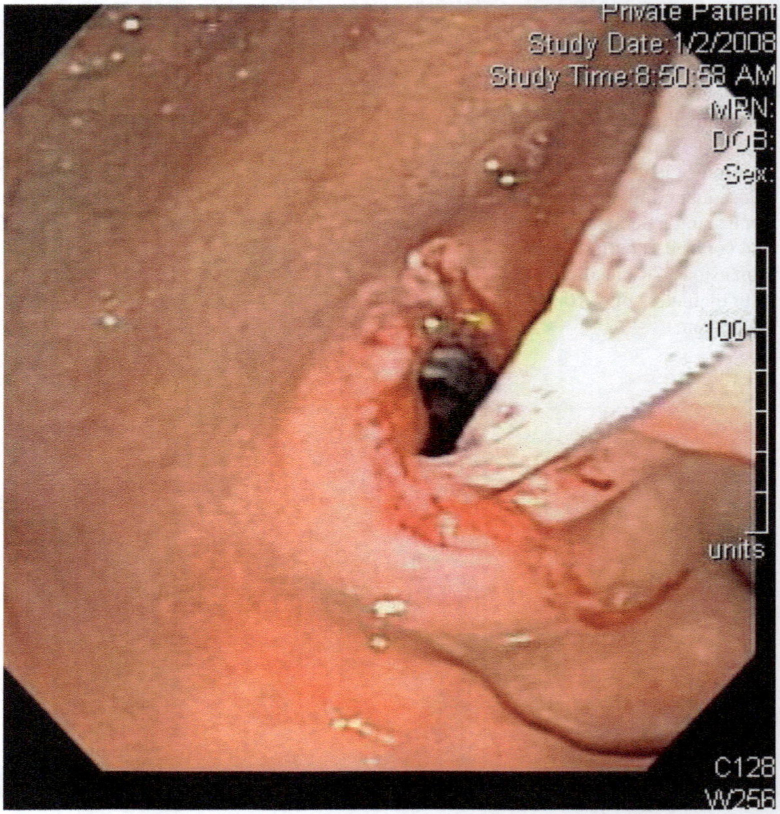

Fig. 4.48 This endoscopic image shows the results of the successive dilations to a final diameter of 12 mm

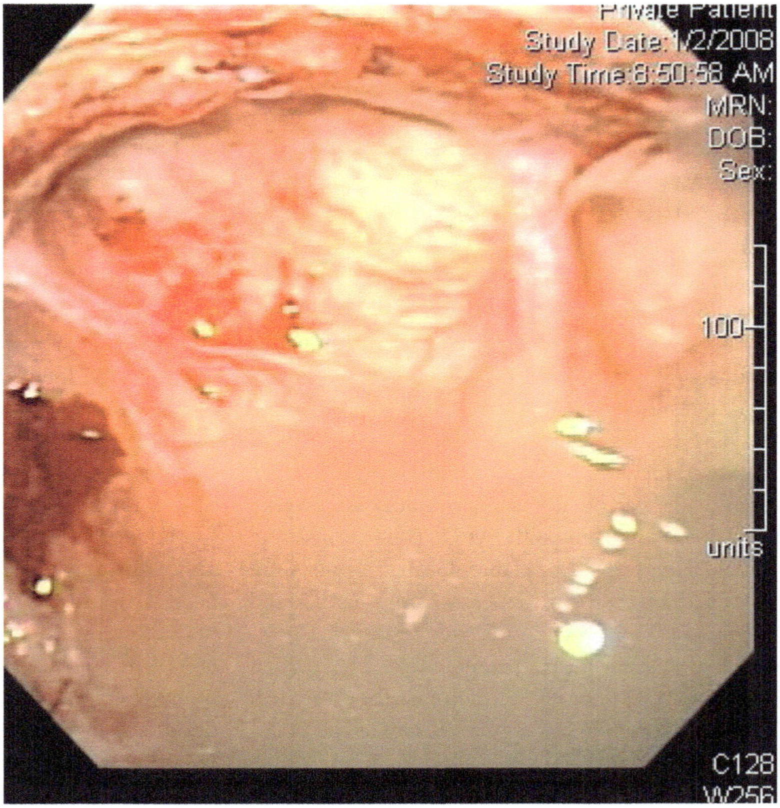

Fig. 4.49 This is an endoscopic view of the abscess cavity after it had been irrigated and cleaned out. Some pus is layering in a dependent position

4.2.10 Zollinger-Ellison Syndrome: An Imaging Odyssey

This is a 55-year-old female patient who complained of abdominal pain and weight loss of 70 lb. An upper endoscopy showed reflux esophagitis and several small duodenal ulcerations. A CT scan was interpreted as showing thickening of the duodenum and portions of the jejunum. No other findings were reported on the CT scan. Lymphoma was suspected but biopsies during endoscopy showed only inflammation. A surgeon was consulted for a full-thickness laparoscopic biopsy, before which an MRI was requested. Again, thickening of the duodenum was noted. A significant periduodenal abnormality apparently was not recognized on the MRI. The laparoscopic biopsies were unremarkable. Gastrin levels were obtained on two different occasions and found to be 4,000 and 500 pg/ml , suggesting the presence of a gastrin-producing tumor. The patient was referred to an endocrinologist. Serum chromogranin levels were mildly elevated. The endocrinologist requested an octreotide scan, which was positive. The octreotide scan was, however, interpreted as showing an adrenal tumor consistent with a pheochromocytoma. The endocrinologist then requested an EUS evaluation. The EUS showed a 2.5-cm lesion located in the "gastrinoma triangle" adjacent to the duodenum. FNA biopsies were obtained. The immunohistochemistry on the FNA cell block shows a neuroendocrine tumor without features of a pheochromocytoma. The patient had surgery, at which time the mass that was previously biopsied with EUS guided FNA was identified as a metastatic lymph node. The primary tumor was actually a small nodule in the duodenal wall not seen on EUS or with any of the other imaging modalities. One of six periportal lymph nodes also was involved by the gastrin-producing metastatic neuroendocrine tumor.

The detection of gastrointestinal neuroendocrine tumors (NETs) of the small bowel has increased by 300–500 % during the past 35 years [23, 24]. Approximately 20 % of the small-bowel NETs are located in the duodenum [25]. Duodenal NETs are mostly found incidentally and are nonfunctional, small tumors (<10 mm) limited to the duodenal wall.

About 10 % of duodenal NETs present with Zollinger-Ellison syndrome [25]. In general, gastrinomas have been found mostly in the duodenum and, less commonly, in the pancreas [26]. Approximately 80 % of gastrinomas are located in the gastrinoma triangle, which is defined superiorly by the junction of the cystic and (CBD) inferiorly by the junction of the second and third portions of the duodenum, and medially by the junction of the neck and body of the pancreas [27].

These tumors behave aggressively, and most of them have lymph node metastases at the time of diagnosis [28], even gastrinomas <10 mm, although lymph node metastases do not seem to have a significant effect on survival in patients undergoing surgical resection. Patients with liver metastases have a poor prognosis. It has been recommended that serum gastrin, serum chromogranin-A, and gastric fluid pH (or gastric acid output if appropriate) be checked in all patients with duodenal neuroendocrine tumors to evaluate for Zollinger-Ellison syndrome [25].

EUS allows determination of the size of the tumor, layer of origin, and depth of involvement in the duodenal wall and permits the evaluation of regional lymphadenopathy or a coexisting pancreatic tumor. Patients with gastrinomas associated with multiple endocrine neoplasia type 1 (MEN1) frequently have multiple tumors, and a careful visual and sonographic inspection should be done to detect additional gastronomic foci. The size of pancreatic gastrinomas has been demonstrated to correlate with the risk of developing hepatic metastases in patients with MEN1: 4 % in those with gastrinomas <1 cm, 28 % in those with tumors 1–3 cm, and 61 % in gastrinomas >3 cm [29].

Surgical resection with lymphadenectomy is the standard therapy for sporadic duodenal gastrinoma but not for carcinomas related to MEN1. The latter are not usually not considered to be curable by surgery [29, 30].

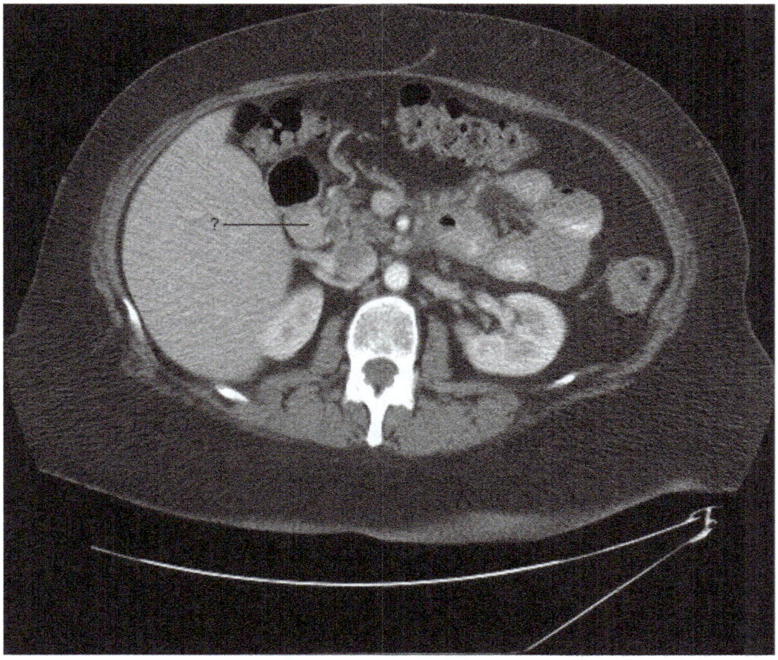

Fig. 4.50 Computed tomography scan shows a tumor adjacent to the duodenum

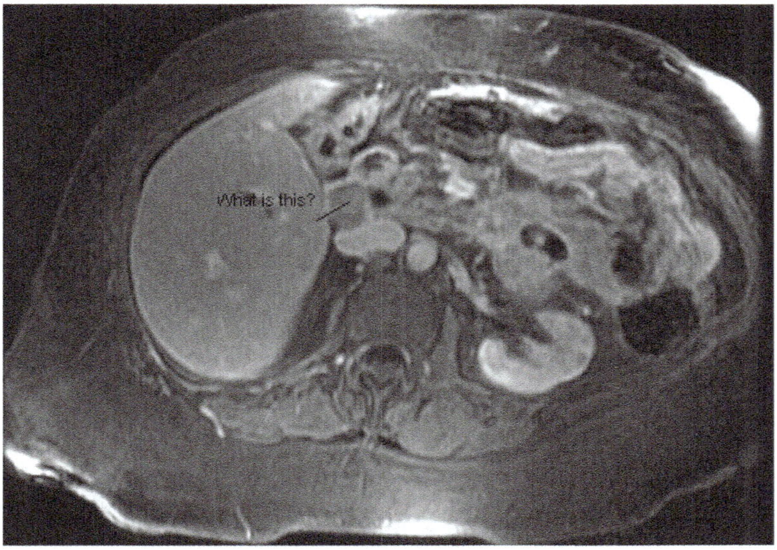

Fig. 4.51 T1-weighted magnetic resonance imaging shows a tumor adjacent to the duodenum

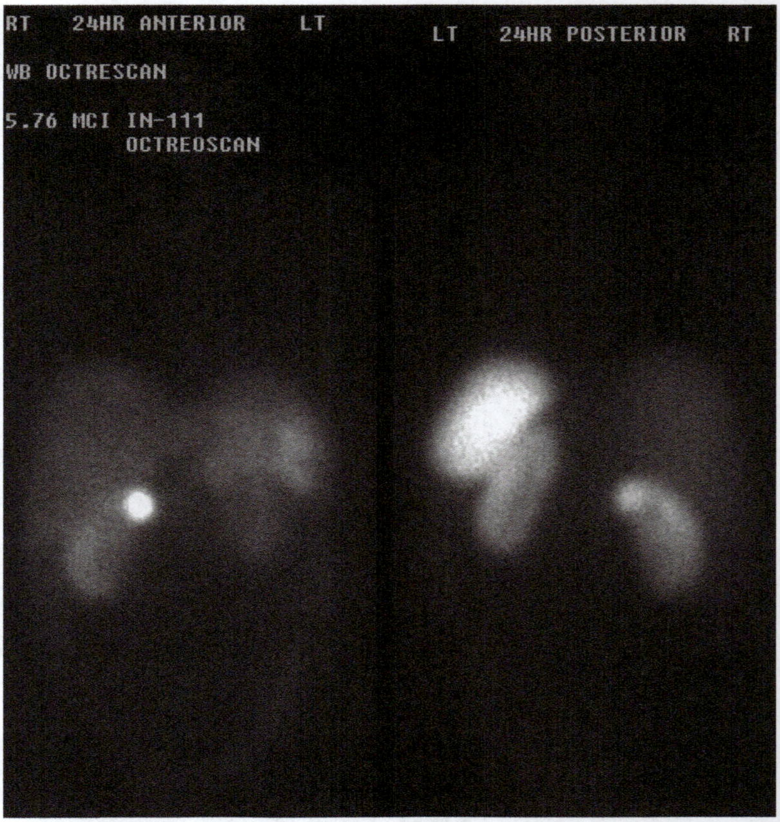

Fig. 4.52 Octreotide scan of the neuroendocrine tumor

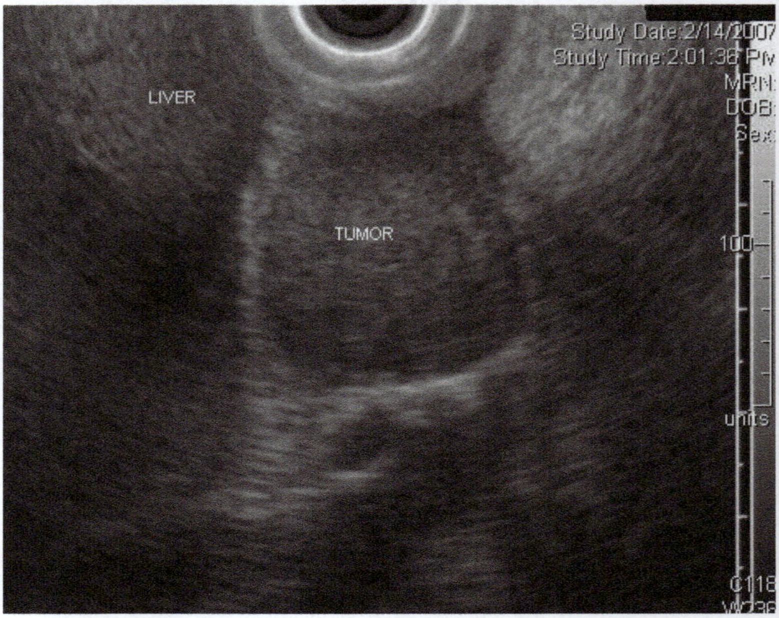

Fig. 4.53 Appearance of the suspected gastrinoma on endoscopic ultrasound

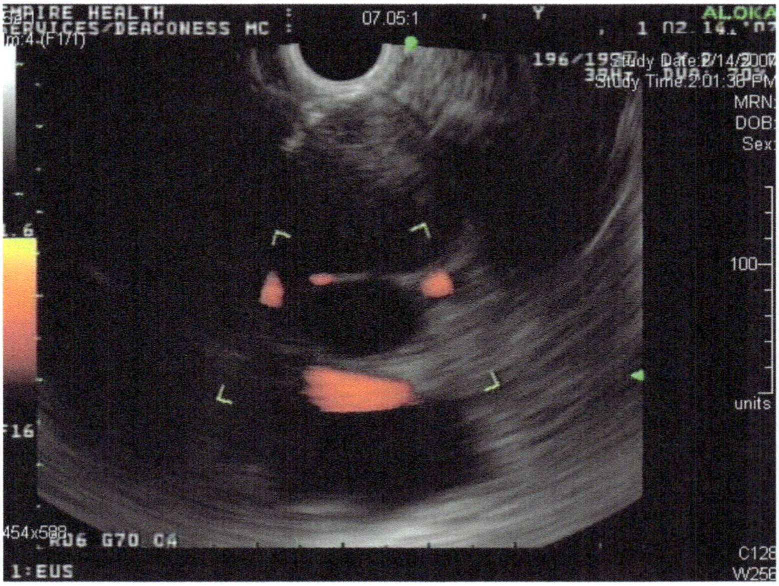

Fig. 4.54 Tumor as seen with linear endoscopic ultrasound before biopsy

References

1. Ryder NM, Ko CY, Hines OJ, Gloor B, Reber HA. Primary duodenal adenocarcinoma: a 40-year experience. Arch Surg. 2000;135(9):1070–4, discussion 1074–5.
2. Sarela AI, Brennan MF, Karpeh MS, Klimstra D, Conlon KCP. Adenocarcinoma of the duodenum: importance of accurate lymph node staging and similarity in outcome to gastric cancer. Ann Surg Oncol. 2004;11(4):380–6.
3. Poultsides GA, Huang LC, Cameron JL, Tuli R, Lan L, Hruban RH, et al. Duodenal adenocarcinoma: clinicopathologic analysis and implications for treatment. Ann Surg Oncol. 2012;19(6):1928–35.
4. Macari M, Lazarus D, Israel G, Megibow A. Duodenal diverticula mimicking cystic neoplasms of the pancreas: CT and MR imaging findings in seven patients. AJR Am J Roentgenol. 2003;180(1):195–9.
5. Al-Khyatt W, Rashid F, Iftikhar SY. Accidental finding of a toothpick in the porta hepatis during laparoscopic cholecystectomy: a case report. J Med Case Rep. 2011;5(1):1–3.
6. Pattamapaspong N, Srisuwan T, Sivasomboon C, Nasuto M, Suwannahoy P, Settakorn J, et al. Accuracy of radiography, computed tomography and magnetic resonance imaging in diagnosing foreign bodies in the foot. Radiol Med. 2013;118(2):303–10.
7. Jacobson JA, Powell A, Craig JG, Bouffard JA, van Holsbeeck MT. Wooden foreign bodies in soft tissue: detection at US. Radiology. 1998;206(1):45–8.
8. Orlinsky M, Knittel P, Feit T, Chan L, Mandavia D. The comparative accuracy of radiolucent foreign body detection using ultrasonography. Am J Emerg Med. 2000;18(4):401–3.
9. Graham Jr DD. Ultrasound in the emergency department: detection of wooden foreign bodies in the soft tissues. J Emerg Med. 2002;22(1):75–9.
10. Li SF, Ender K. Toothpick injury mimicking renal colic: case report and systematic review. J Emerg Med. 2002;23(1):35–8.
11. Robert B, Bartoli E, Fumery M, Eoche M, Chivot C, Demasure F, et al. Duodenal perforation due to toothpick perforation, an uncommon cause of chronic abdominal pain. Endoscopy. 2012;44(Suppl 2 UCTN):E27–8.
12. Bellon EM, George CR, Schreiber H, Marshall JB. Pancreatic pseudocysts of the duodenum. AJR Am J Roentgenol. 1979;133(5):827–31.
13. Sugiura T, Uesaka K, Kanomata H, Sasaki K, Kanemoto H, Mizuno T. Intramural pseudocyst of the duodenum caused by pancreatic head cancer: report of a case. Surg Today. 2012;42(8):805–7.
14. El Hajj II, Coté GA. Endoscopic diagnosis and management of ampullary lesions. Gastrointest Endosc Clin N Am. 2013;23(1):95–109.
15. Menzel J, Poremba C, Dietl KH, Böcker W, Domschke W. Tumors of the papilla of Vater–inadequate diagnostic impact of endoscopic forceps biopsies taken prior to and following sphincterotomy. Ann Oncol. 1999;10(10):1227–31.
16. Offerhaus GJ, Giardiello FM, Krush AJ, Booker SV, Tersmette AC, Kelley NC, et al. The risk of upper

gastrointestinal cancer in familial adenomatous polyposis. Gastroenterology. 1992;102(6):1980–2.
17. Burke CA, Beck GJ, Church JM, van Stolk RU. The natural history of untreated duodenal and ampullary adenomas in patients with familial adenomatous polyposis followed in an endoscopic surveillance program. Gastrointest Endosc. 1999;49(3 Pt 1):358–64.
18. Eloubeidi MA, Iseman DT, Chen VK, Vickers SM, Wilcox CM. Prevalence and significance of periduodenal venous collaterals in patients evaluated for pancreaticobiliary disorders by endosonography. Endoscopy. 2003;35(12):1015–9.
19. Beaton C, Davies M, Beynon J. The management of primary small bowel and colon lymphoma – a review. Int J Colorectal Dis. 2012;27(5):555–63.
20. Sarkhosh K, Bathe OF, Stewart DA, Mack LA. The role of surgical intervention in the management of duodenal lymphoma. J Surg Oncol. 2009;99(7):428–32.
21. Chestovich PJ, Schiller G, Sasu S, Hiatt JR. Duodenal lymphoma: a rare and morbid tumor. Am Surg. 2007;73(10):1057–62.
22. Prasad GA, Varadarajulu S. Endoscopic ultrasound-guided abscess drainage. Gastrointest Endosc Clin N Am. 2012;22(2):281–90, ix.
23. Modlin IM, Oberg K, Chung DC, Jensen RT, de Herder WW, Thakker RV, et al. Gastroenteropancreatic neuroendocrine tumours. Lancet Oncol. 2008;9(1):61–72.
24. Yao JC, Hassan M, Phan A, Dagohoy C, Leary C, Mares JE, et al. One hundred years after "carcinoid": epidemiology of and prognostic factors for neuroendocrine tumors in 35,825 cases in the United States. J Clin Oncol. 2008;26(18):3063–72.
25. Scherübl H, Jensen RT, Cadiot G, Stölzel U, Klöppel G. Neuroendocrine tumors of the small bowels are on the rise: early aspects and management. World J Gastrointest Endosc. 2010;2(10):325–34.
26. Klöppel G, Rindi G, Anlauf M, Perren A, Komminoth P. Site-specific biology and pathology of gastroenteropancreatic neuroendocrine tumors. Virchows Arch. 2007;451 Suppl 1:S9–27.
27. Stabile BE, Morrow DJ, Passaro Jr E. The gastrinoma triangle: operative implications. Am J Surg. 1984;147(1):25–31.
28. Jensen RT, Niederle B, Mitry E, Ramage JK, Steinmuller T, Lewington V, et al. Gastrinoma (duodenal and pancreatic). Neuroendocrinology. 2006;84(3): 173–82.
29. Morrow EH, Norton JA. Surgical management of Zollinger-Ellison syndrome; state of the art. Surg Clin North Am. 2009;89(5):1091–103.
30. Norton JA, Fraker DL, Alexander HR, Venzon DJ, Doppman JL, Serrano J, et al. Surgery to cure the Zollinger-Ellison syndrome. N Engl J Med. 1999; 341(9):635–44.

Gallbladder, Liver, and Bile Ducts

5

Contents

5.1 **General Principles** ... 235

5.2 **Cases and Discussions** ... 237
5.2.1 Gallbladder ... 237
5.2.1.1 Cholecystitis and Cholelithiasis ... 237
5.2.1.2 Gallbladder Carcinoma ... 240
5.2.1.3 Gallbladder Cysts ... 244
5.2.1.4 Courvoisier's Sign ... 245
5.2.1.5 Heister Valves ... 246
5.2.2 Liver ... 248
5.2.2.1 A Growing Subhepatic Cyst ... 248
5.2.2.2 Hemangioma ... 251
5.2.2.3 Hepatoma ... 253
5.2.2.4 Hepatic Lymph Nodes ... 257
5.2.2.5 Portal Vein and Hepatic Vein Branches ... 260
5.2.2.6 Cavernous Transformation of the Portal Vein ... 262
5.2.3 Bile Ducts ... 265
5.2.3.1 Isolated Bile Duct Dilation, Normal Liver Tests ... 265
5.2.3.2 Bile Duct Dilation Caused by a Crossing Vessel ... 268
5.2.3.3 Common Bile Duct Stone ... 270
5.2.3.4 Bile Duct Stone Missed by EUS and ERCP ... 272
5.2.3.5 Possible "Narcotic Bile Duct" ... 275
5.2.3.6 Primary Sclerosing Cholangitis ... 277
5.2.3.7 Malignant Bile Duct Stricture ... 280
5.2.3.8 Type II (Todani) Choledochal Cyst ... 284
5.2.3.9 Extrinsic Compression of the Bile Duct by Metastatic Melanoma ... 287
5.2.3.10 Eccentric Filling Defect in the Common Hepatic Duct ... 290
5.2.3.11 Choledochocele vs. Bile Duct Web ... 292
5.2.3.12 Villous Lesions of the Distal Common Bile Duct ... 294

References ... 296

5.1 General Principles

Endoscopic ultrasound (EUS) is one of the best modalities for imaging the gallbladder and bile ducts. Substantial portions of the liver can also be examined by EUS as the instrument is advanced through the esophagus, stomach, and duodenum.

The number of differential diagnostic possibilities for abnormalities of the gallbladder and bile ducts is limited. In contrast, there are many liver lesions that have a similar appearance on ultrasound but different clinical implications. Fortunately, it is not too difficult to acquire a working knowledge of liver diagnostic ultrasound by using online resources such as the World Health Organization's *Manual of Diagnostic Ultrasound* [1] (see Box 5.1). Careful scrutiny of the liver needs to be a routine part of any staging of tumors in the upper gastrointestinal tract.

While the gallbladder can easily be found in the upper gastrointestinal tract from the antrum and duodenum during an EUS exam, a cursory exam is not recommended. Small stones can easily be missed unless the gallbladder is evaluated in a protocol-driven fashion. As previously stated, endosonographers need to be familiar with the basics of conventional abdominal ultrasound anatomy. The thickness of the normal gallbladder wall measured by ultrasound has been found to be 2.1 ± 0.06 mm [2]. A value greater than 3 mm is considered abnormal. It is important to keep in mind that cirrhosis or hepatitis

K. Gottlieb, G. Marino, *Diagnostic Endosonography*,
DOI 10.1007/978-3-642-39118-7_5, © Springer-Verlag Berlin Heidelberg 2014

without intrinsic gallbladder pathology can increase this thickness.

A quick review of the basics can be accomplished by watching the videos listed in Box 5.1. The most common gallbladder finding are stones and polyps, which, when less than 10 mm in size, are almost never malignant. An excellent tutorial about the portal venous anatomy was published in the new open access journal *Endoscopic Ultrasound* (see Box 5.1), and we will describe some cases illustrating portal vein pathology.

EUS is particularly strong in the evaluation of the extrahepatic bile duct and, as the cases in this chapter illustrate, is often instrumental in establishing a diagnosis or change in the management plan.

Box 5.1: Free Online Resources

- *Manual of Diagnostic Ultrasound* (World Health Organization, 2011) http://is.gd/ioA6rH
- Three-part instructional video about gallbladder ultrasound provided by Sonosite (www.sonosite.com)
  - Part 1 http://is.gd/60NQXD
  - Part 2 http://is.gd/83oiJH
  - Part 3 http://is.gd/E5clEx
- A seven-part instructional video about liver ultrasound provided by SonoWorld (www.sonoworld.com)
- A seven-part CME video course about liver sonography provided by SonoWorld (www.sonoworld.com) at http://is.gd/pWFqJm also available on YouTube (no CME credit) at http://is.gd/h2tCAR
- Portal venous system and its tributaries: a radial endosonographic assessment (Spring Publishing) http://is.gd/kpCjxu
- Gallbladder lesions identified on ultrasound. Lessons from the last 10 years (*J Gastrointest Surg*, 2011) http://is.gd/rUchI6
- Stage information for extrahepatic bile duct cancer (National Cancer Institute) http://is.gd/cXDq09
- Stage information for gallbladder cancer (National Cancer Institute) http://is.gd/UbIDBf
- Stage information for adult primary liver cancer (National Cancer Institute) http://is.gd/GFX2Qp
- *Endoscopic Ultrasound* (journal) http://www.eusjournal.com

5.2 Cases and Discussions

5.2.1 Gallbladder

5.2.1.1 Cholecystitis and Cholelithiasis

This is a 59-year-old patient with widely metastatic breast cancer who developed severe abdominal pain. A computed tomography (CT) scan of the abdomen shows a stone impacted in the cystic duct. A hepatobiliary iminodiacetic acid (HIDA) scan revealed nonfilling of the gallbladder. Magnetic resonance cholangiopancreatography (MRCP) was performed to rule out a common bile duct stone because the patient's bilirubin level was mildly elevated. No stone was seen in the common bile duct. The interesting abnormality in the distal common bile duct (choledochocele vs. web) is discussed in the Liver section of this chapter. The EUS images (Fig. 5.5) show echogenic bile and a thickened gallbladder wall but no pericholecystic fluid and no stones in the gallbladder itself. During surgery the gallbladder was densely adherent to the liver and filled with pus. A stone was stuck in the cystic duct.

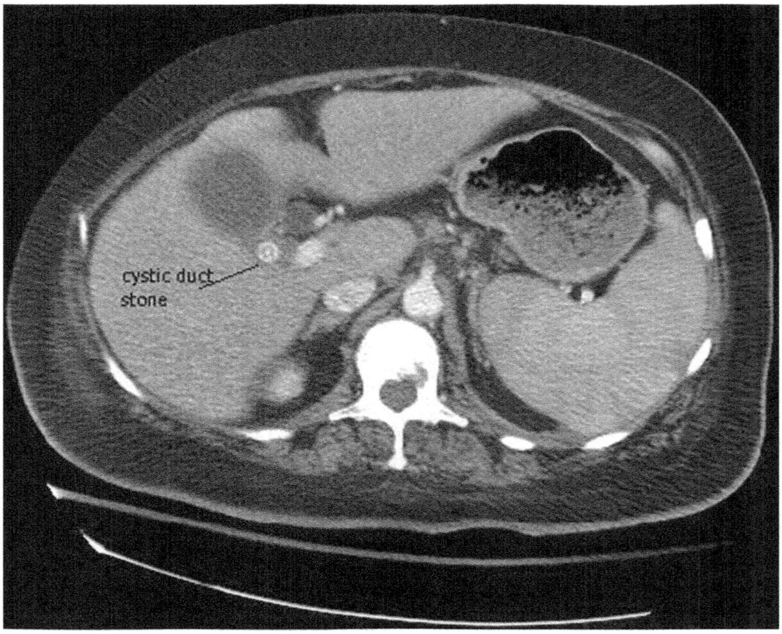

Fig. 5.1 This computed tomography scan shows a stone obstructing the cystic duct

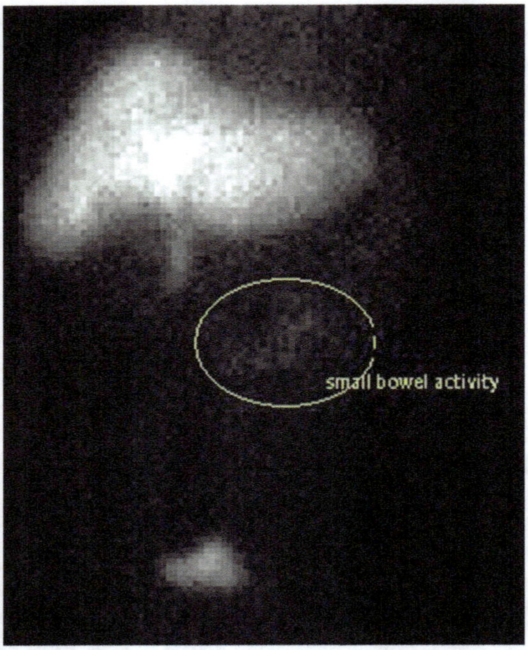

Fig. 5.2 This HIDA scan shows activity in the small intestine and urinary bladder but not in the gallbladder

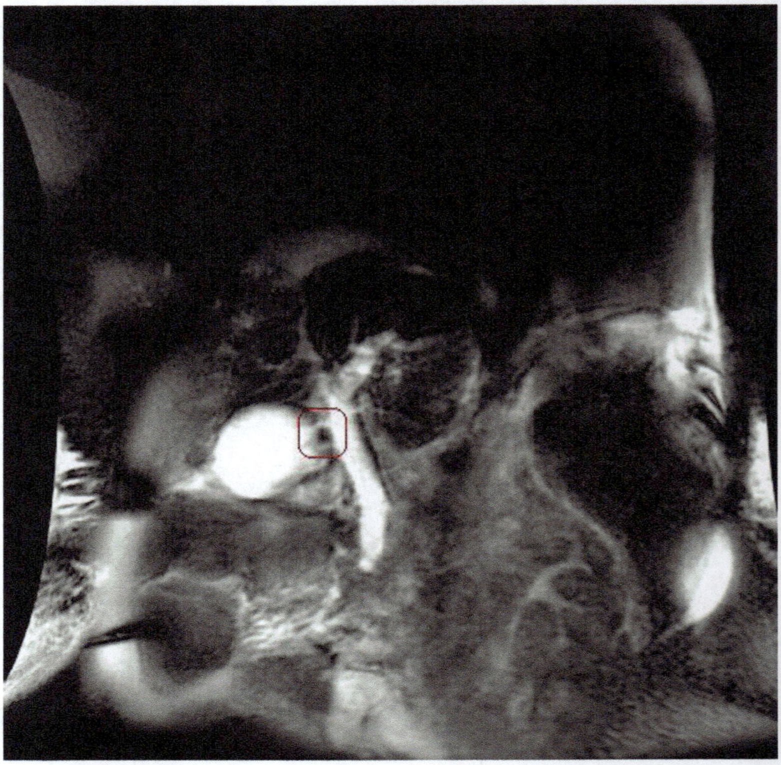

Fig. 5.3 Magnetic resonance cholangiopancreatography shows a stone in the cystic duct and an abnormality of the distal common bile duct

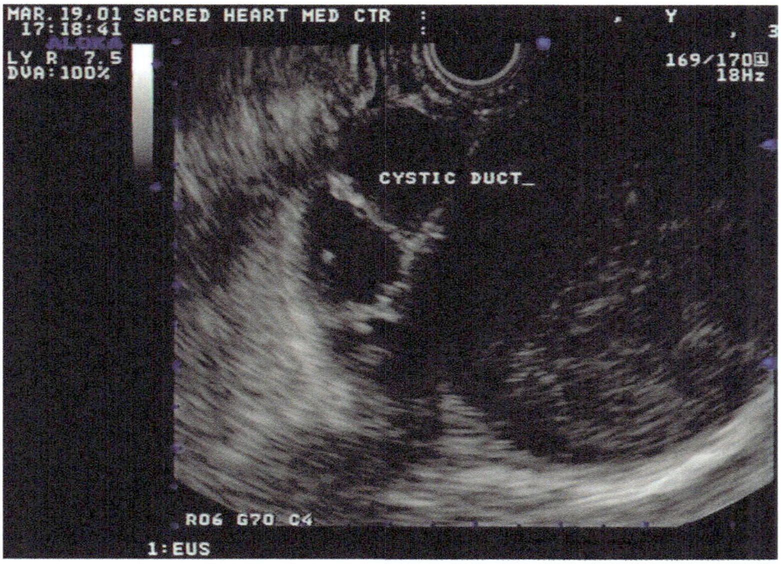

Fig. 5.4 Endoscopic ultrasound shows a greatly dilated cystic duct, consistent with obstruction

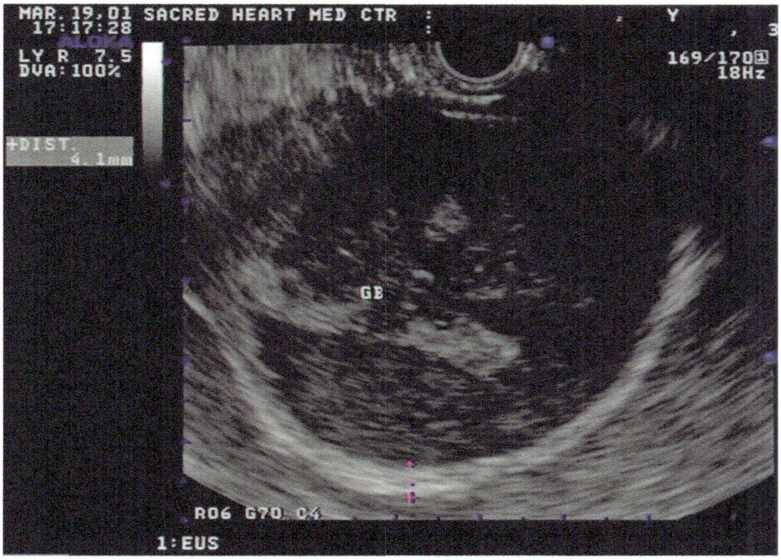

Fig. 5.5 Endoscopic ultrasound showing the gallbladder (*GB*) filled with echogenic bile. During surgery it was found to contain pus. Note the thickening of the gallbladder wall

5.2.1.2 Gallbladder Carcinoma

When diagnosed incidentally during cholecystectomy, surgical resection can be curative. However, most often the tumor is unresectable at the initial presentation of the patient. Fortunately, gallbladder cancer is rare in North America. The highest incidence of gallbladder cancer is found among Andean populations, North American Indians, and Mexican Americans [3]. Early diagnosis could improve the clinical outcome and cure rate. However, conventional imaging modalities such as transcutaneous abdominal ultrasound and CT can be difficult to interpret, as this case shows. This is an 84-year-old patient who initially presented with obstructive jaundice. Endoscopic retrograde cholangiopancreatography (ERCP) performed by a different examiner revealed a stricture of the common hepatic duct, which was stented. The gallbladder did not fill. The abnormalities on the CT scan suggesting a gallbladder mass were initially not appreciated, presumably because there were other more impressive things to be seen, such as a large pseudocyst. A HIDA scan was ordered and showed nonfilling of the gallbladder. Cholecystitis was suspected and, because of the patient's debilitated state, arrangements were made for the placement of a cholecystotomy tube. Fortunately, an EUS also was requested and showed an obvious gallbladder cancer. The cholecystomy tube was not placed.

EUS typically uses higher scanning frequencies than transcutaneous abdominal ultrasound (5–10 vs. 2–5 MHz) and can visualize the gallbladder from a closer distance (from the antrum or duodenal bulb), providing more detailed views of gallbladder abnormalities, including a double-layer wall ultrasound pattern [4]. A gallbladder wall thicker than 10 mm, disruption of the normal two layers of the gallbladder wall, hypoechoic internal echogenicity, and the absence of gallstones were found to correlate with gallbladder neoplasia [4].

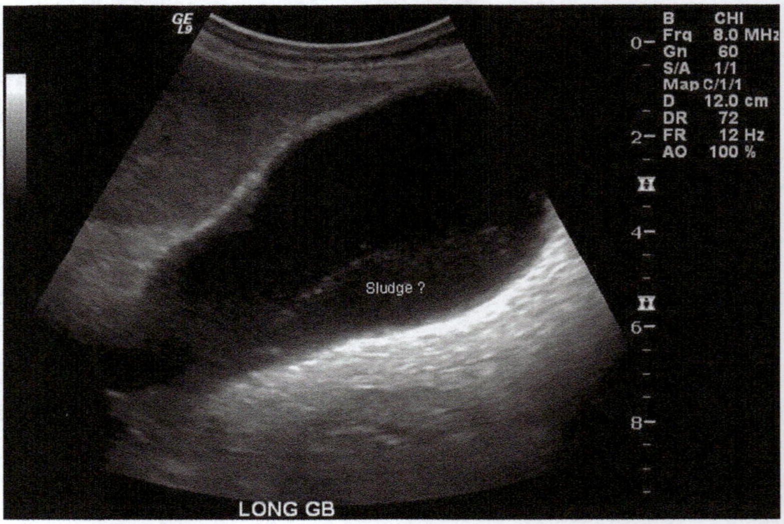

Fig. 5.6 This transabdominal ultrasound shows "sludge" that is somewhat lumpy and does not seem to layer well in a dependent position. *GB* gallbladder

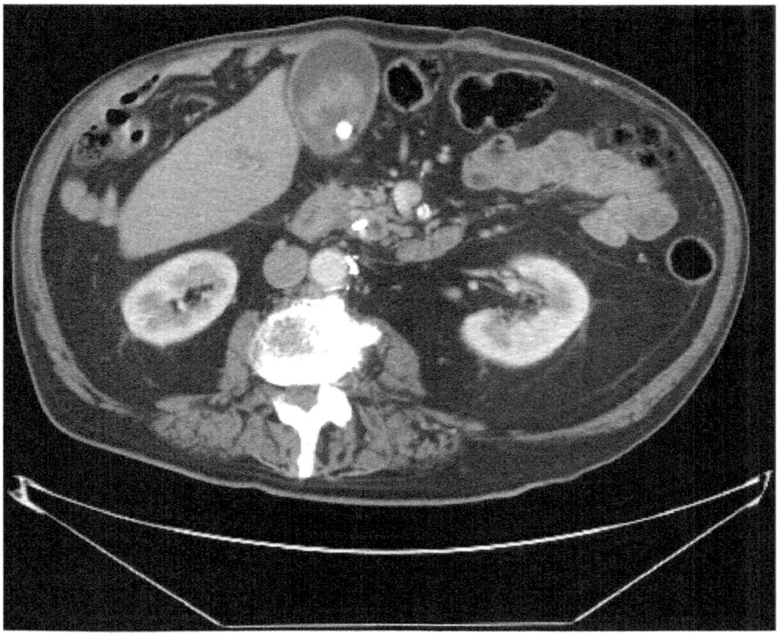

Fig. 5.7 A stone in the gallbladder and intraluminal tissue that enhances with intravenous contrast is seen on this computed tomography scan. However, these were not initially reported

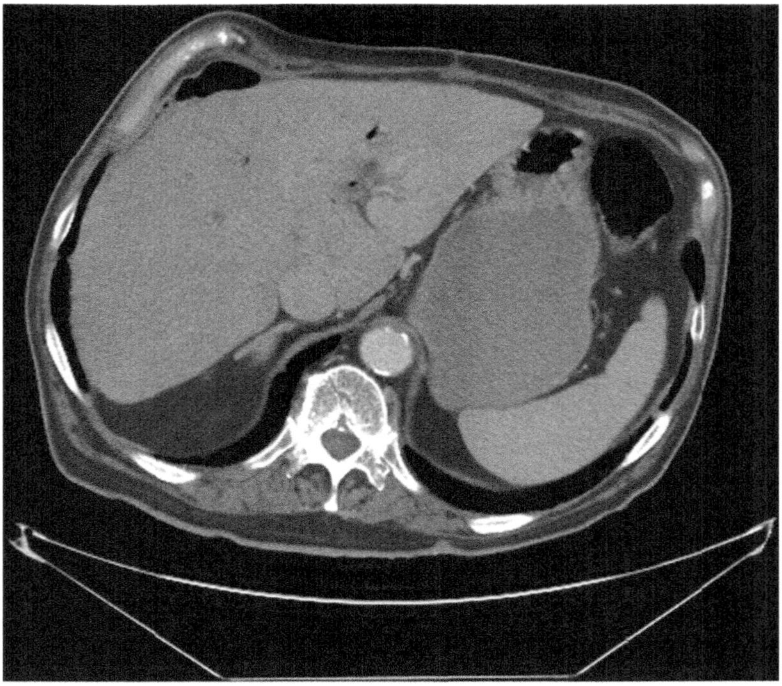

Fig. 5.8 This large pseudocyst diverted attention from the gallbladder

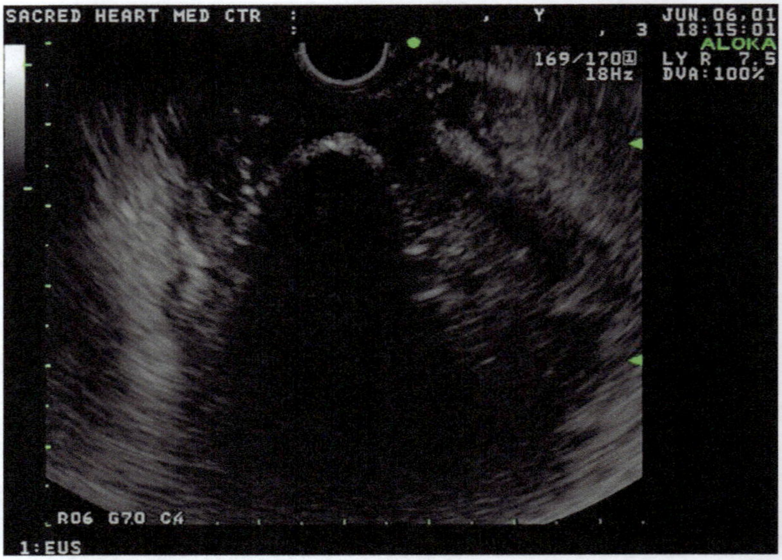

Fig. 5.9 This linear endoscopic ultrasound image shows the gallbladder stone (casting a *large shadow*) surrounded by hypoechoic tissue

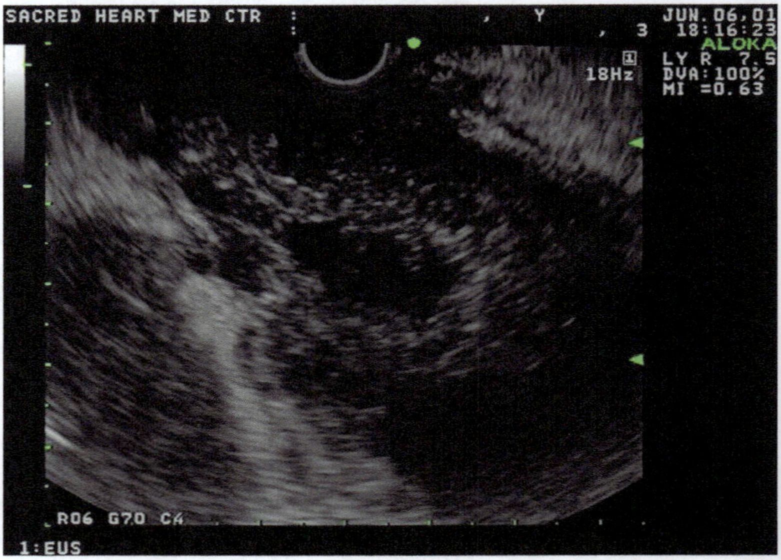

Fig. 5.10 This linear endoscopic ultrasound image shows that the entire gallbladder is filled with tumor tissue

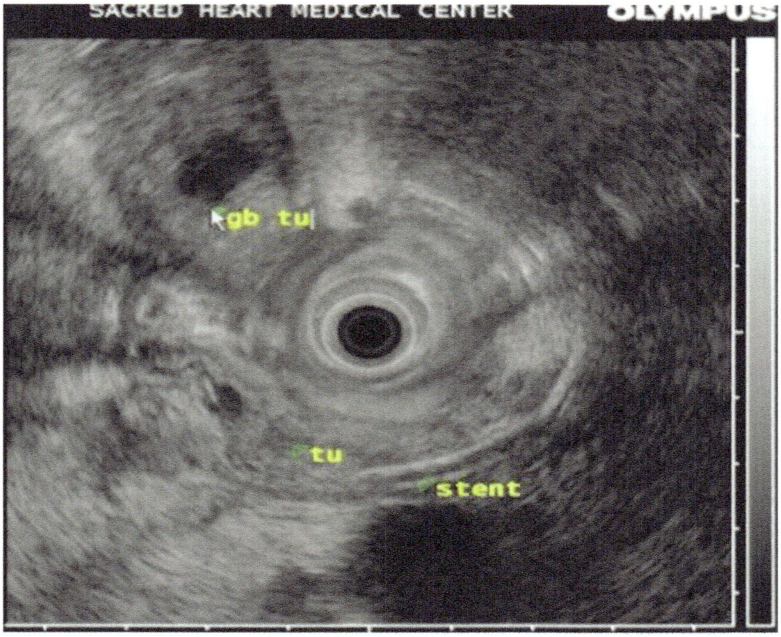

Fig. 5.11 This radial endoscopic ultrasound image shows that the gallbladder tumor (*gb tu*) extends from the gallbladder to the extrahepatic bile ducts

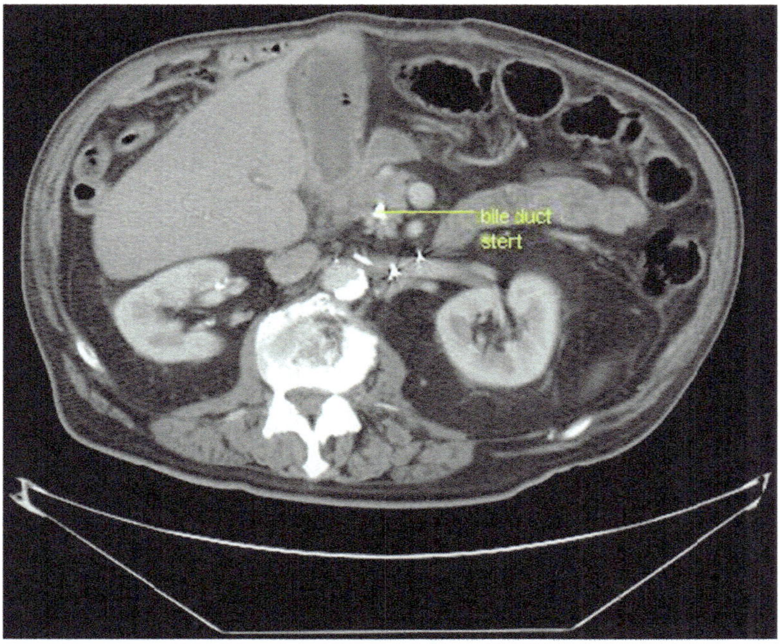

Fig. 5.12 This computed tomography scan shows the bile duct stent surrounded by tumor

5.2.1.3 Gallbladder Cysts

Intramural cysts of the gallbladder are rare; according to one case report only 13 cases have been reported in the world literature up to 2002 [4]. Here we present is an elderly patient who was sent to us for EUS evaluation of a dilated main pancreatic duct. The pancreas was otherwise normal. The cystic lesion in the gallbladder was incidentally found. The EUS clearly shows the epithelial origin of the cyst.

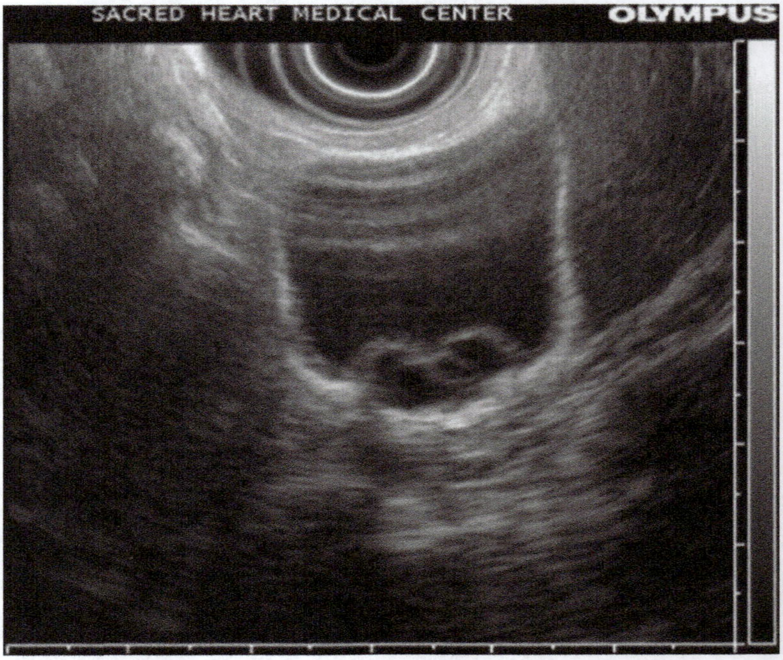

Fig. 5.13 Transverse section through the gallbladder showing the epithelial cyst

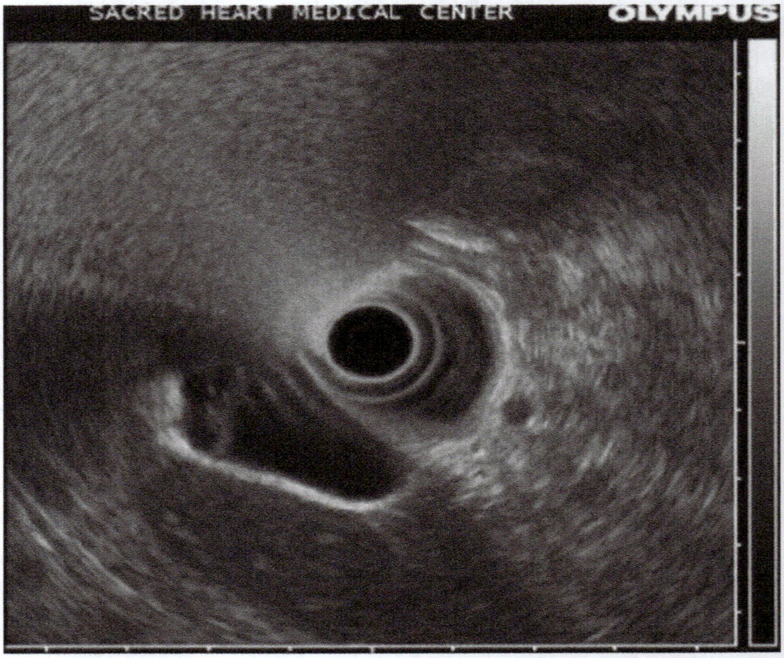

Fig. 5.14 The same gallbladder cyst as in Fig. 5.13 seen in a longitudinal section

5.2.1.4 Courvoisier's Sign

Courvoisier's law states that in the presence of a palpable gallbladder, jaundice is unlikely to be caused by gallstones. However, Courvoisier was not quite as dogmatic. Here is what he actually wrote in his Treatise on the Pathology and Surgery of the Biliary Passages (translated from the German) [5]:

> Obstruction by stone is supported by
>
> 1. prior (self-limited) jaundice attacks
> 2. continuing but fluctuating jaundice
> 3. jaundice present for years
> 4. prior typical biliary colic attacks, especially if they were associated with jaundice
> 5. previous passage of gallstones
> 6. no or only mild distention of the gallbladder
> 7. fever with more or less intermittent character
>
> Obstructions of other types are indicated by the lack of these characteristics and most importantly by the presence and considerable size of a distended gallbladder [5].

This is a 61-year-old patient with obstructive jaundice secondary to cancer of the pancreatic head who has a very dilated gallbladder.

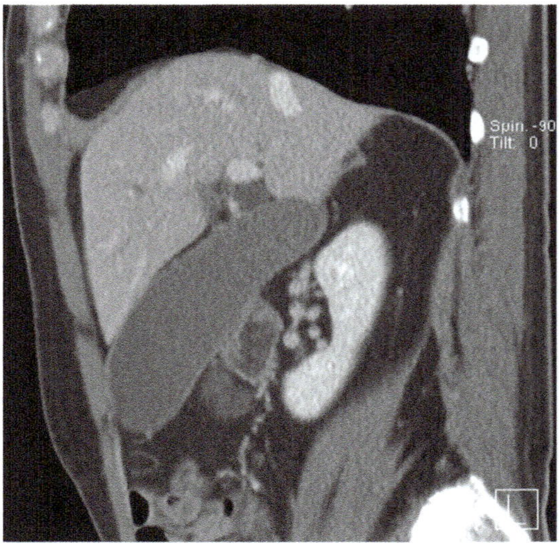

Fig. 5.15 Sagittal reconstruction of a computed tomography scan of a patient with an obstruction of the distal common bile duct caused by a pancreatic cancer and a typical Courvoisier gallbladder

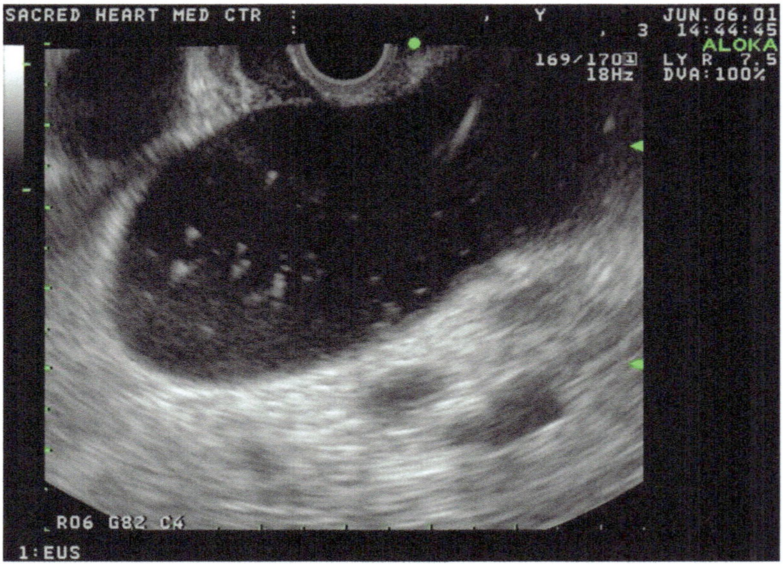

Fig. 5.16 The same distended Courvoisier gallbladder as in Fig. 5.15, seen with a linear array echoendoscope. Note the microcrystals

5.2.1.5 Heister Valves

The function of the spiral mucosal folds seen in the cystic duct are unknown. The duct and spiral folds contain muscle fibers that apparently respond to a variety of stimuli but there is no discrete muscular sphincter. It is speculated that the spiral valves are mechanical devices that keep the tortuous cystic duct patent. During endosonography the Heister valves can sometimes be demonstrated.

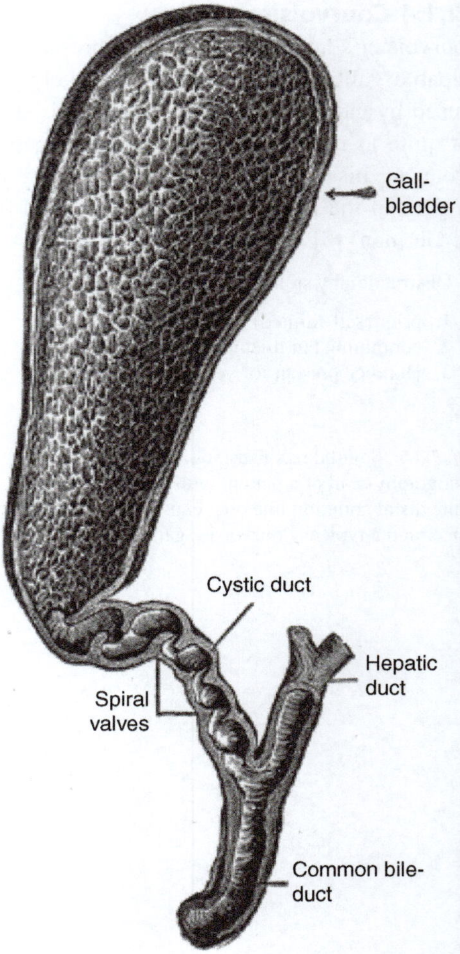

Fig. 5.17 This image shows the Heister or spiral valves in the cystic duct (From Wikimedia Commons)

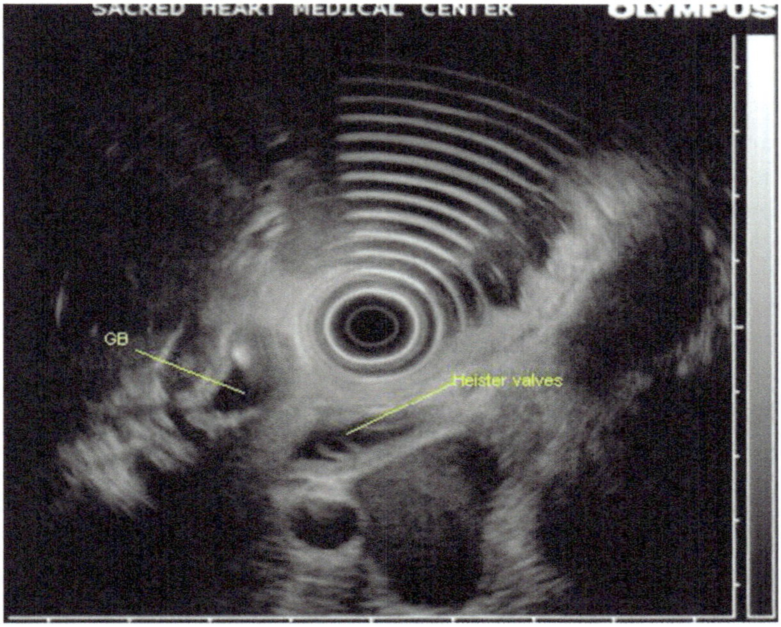

Fig. 5.18 Heister valves in an unusually prominent cystic duct. *GB* gallbladder

5.2.2 Liver

5.2.2.1 A Growing Subhepatic Cyst

This is a 40-year-old woman with a symptomatic subhepatic cyst initially believed to be a choledochalcyst. The size of the cyst increased significantly over the course of 2 years and the patient eventually became deeply jaundiced. A preoperative CT scan surprisingly showed no connection to the biliary system, but the cyst caused extrinsic compression of the biliary tree. The excised cyst was lined by a squamous epithelium, an unusual feature, but contained no malignancy. Choledochal cysts are lined by a biliary-type epithelium but often have focal or extensive squamous metaplasia in response to chronic inflammation. The exact taxonomy of this cyst remains unclear but is does not appear to derive from the biliary tree. There are several reviews about common presentations, diagnostic methods, and treatment of congenital and acquired liver cysts [6, 7].

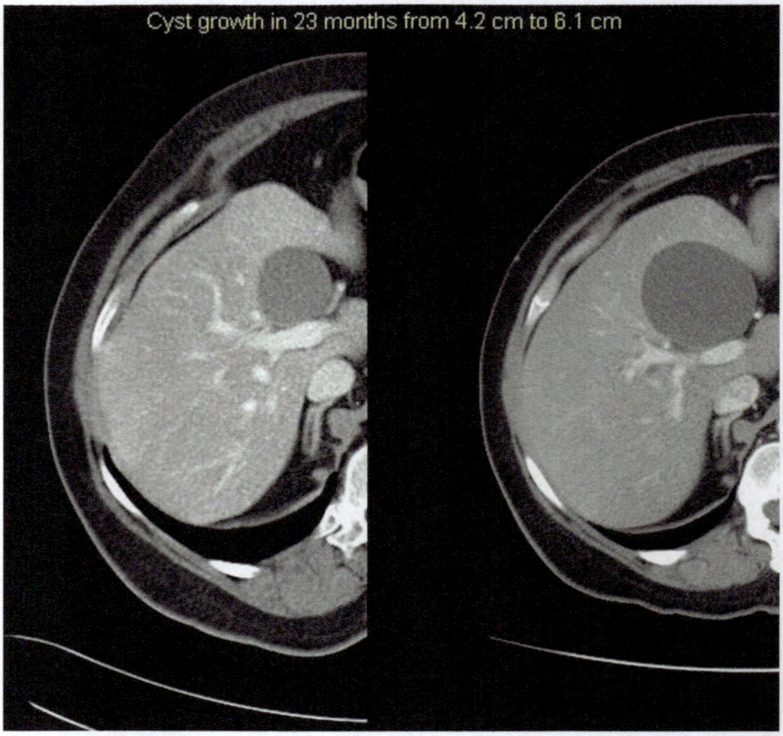

Fig. 5.19 These computed tomography scans show a growing subhepatic cyst, from baseline (*left*) to 23 months later (*right*)

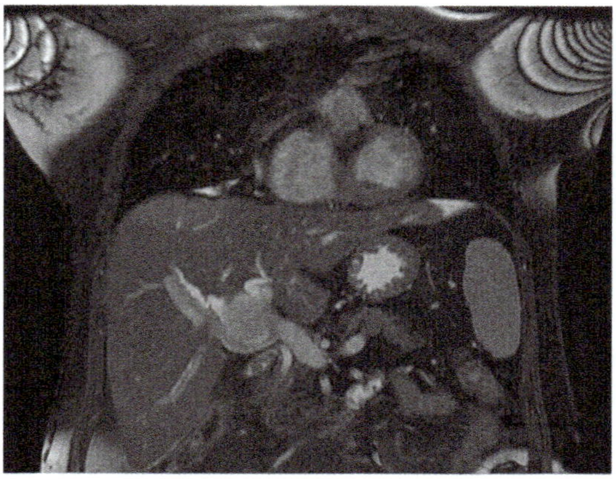

Fig. 5.20 This coronal magnetic resonance imaging section appears to show displacement of the right hepatic duct

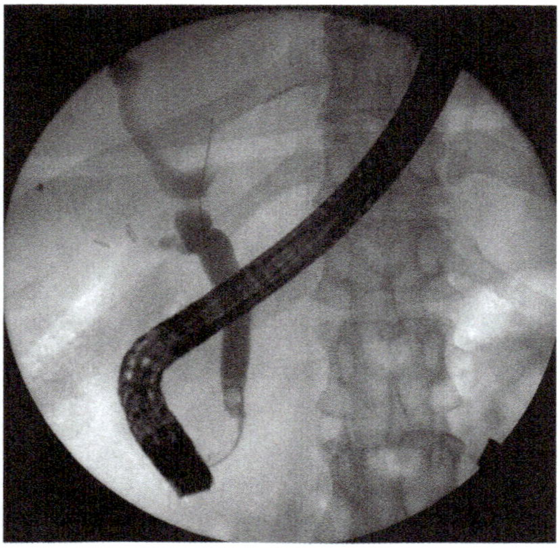

Fig. 5.21 The compression of the right hepatic duct by the cyst can be seen during the initial stages of dye injection. Air bubbles are present in the distal common bile duct

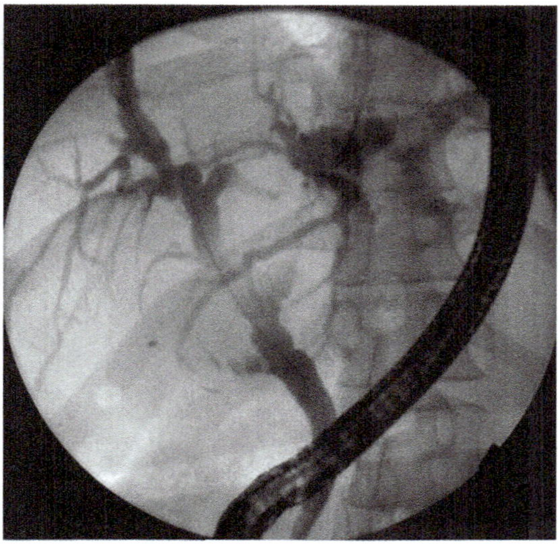

Fig. 5.22 After complete filling, a mass effect on the hilar structures is still apparent; more important is that the cystic structure does not fill with dye, indicating that there is no communication with the biliary system

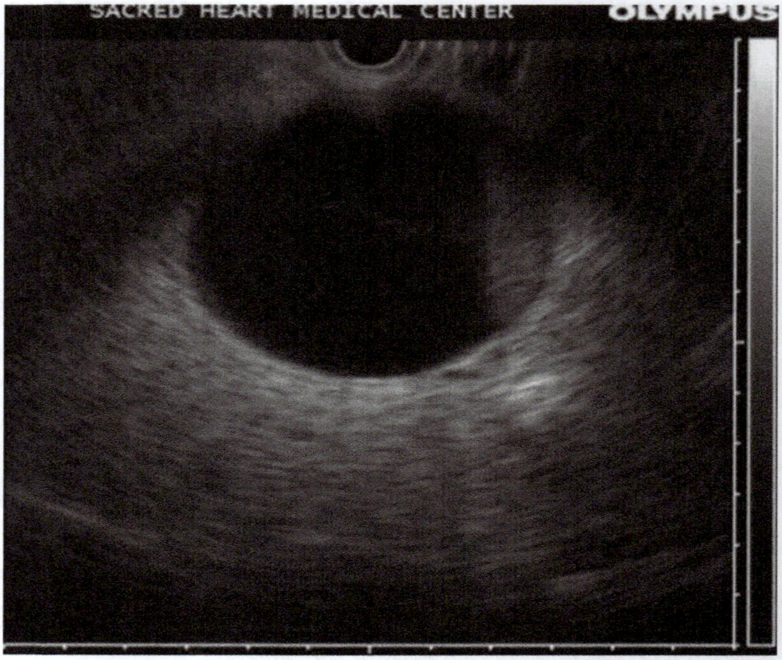

Fig. 5.23 Endoscopic ultrasound shows a cyst with typical posterior enhancement, layering sludge, and a faint central filamentous structure (horizontally in the middle of the cyst)

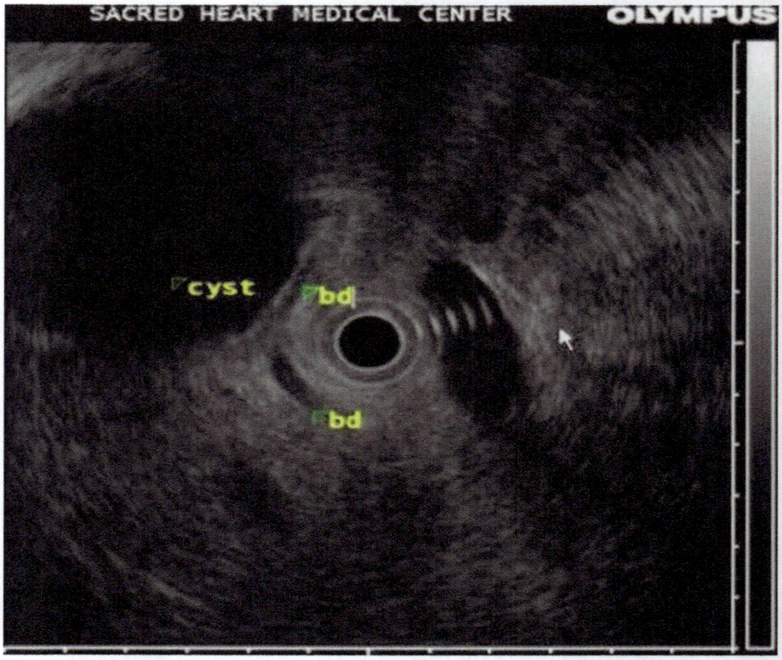

Fig. 5.24 The bile duct (*bd*) is intimately associated with the cyst and compressed

5.2.2.2 Hemangioma

Typical ultrasound features of hepatic hemangiomas are their small size, uniform hyperechogenicity, well-defined margins, and posterior echo enhancement. These typical characteristics are modified as the hemangioma grows larger.

Not all hemangiomas are hyperechoic. In one recent large series, hepatic hemangiomas diagnosed with contrast-enhanced CT were classified by internal echo pattern as homogeneous hyperechoic (35.0 %), homogeneous hypoechoic (22.9 %), isoechoic (5.2 %), mixed hyperechoic (22.1 %), or mixed hypoechoic (14.8 %) [8].

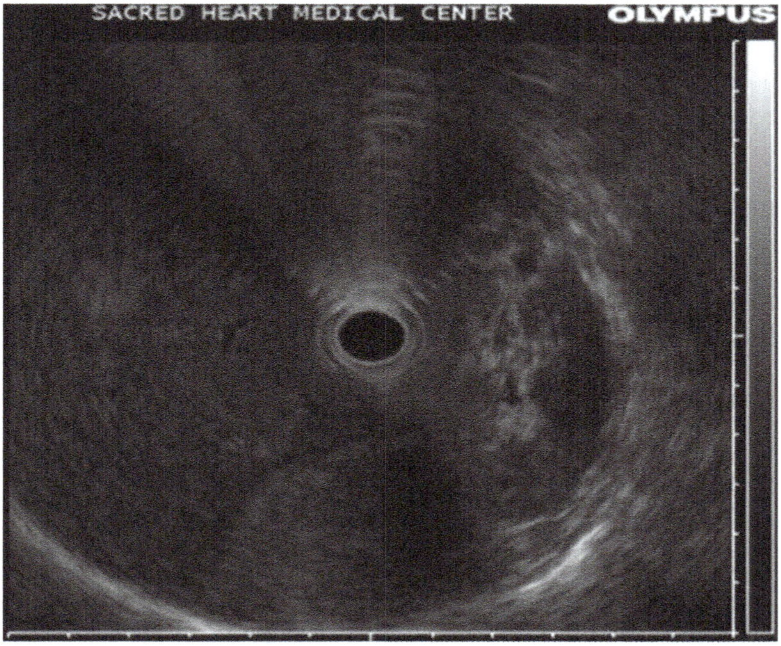

Fig. 5.25 This image, taken with the GF-UM160 echoinstrument, shows two hemangiomas: a small one and a large one located in the periphery

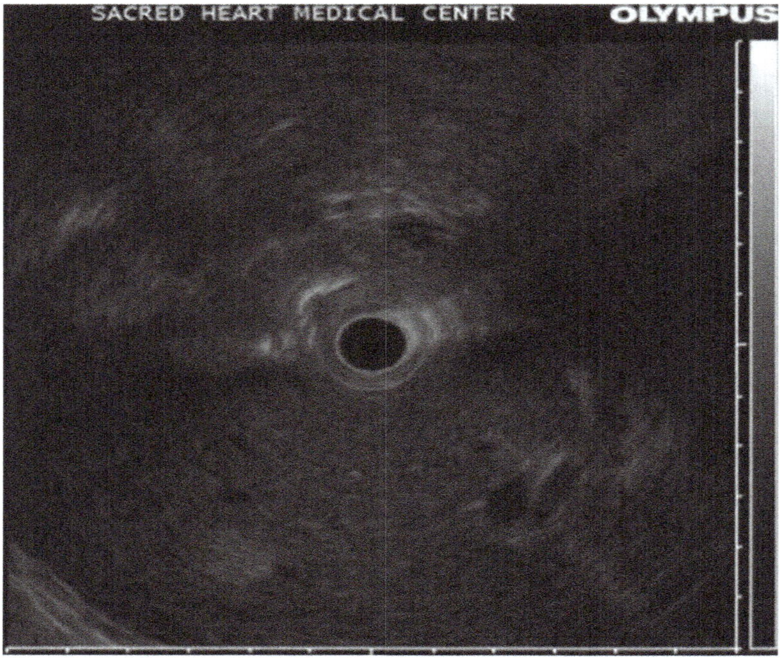

Fig. 5.26 This image puts the smaller of the two lesions into focus. Hemangiomas are sharply demarcated, round, echogenic lesions that typically measure from 1 to 3 cm in diameter

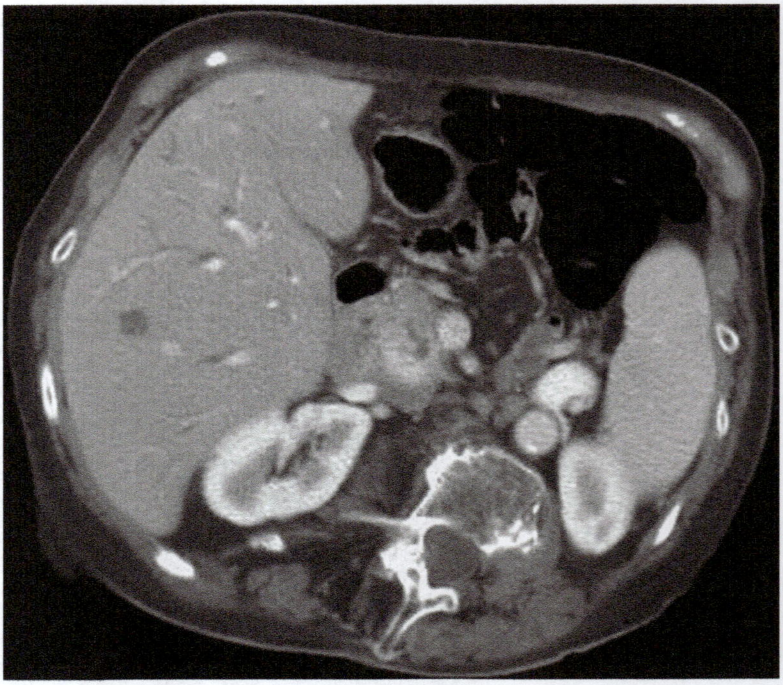

Fig. 5.27 This computed tomography scan shows the smaller of the two hemangiomas

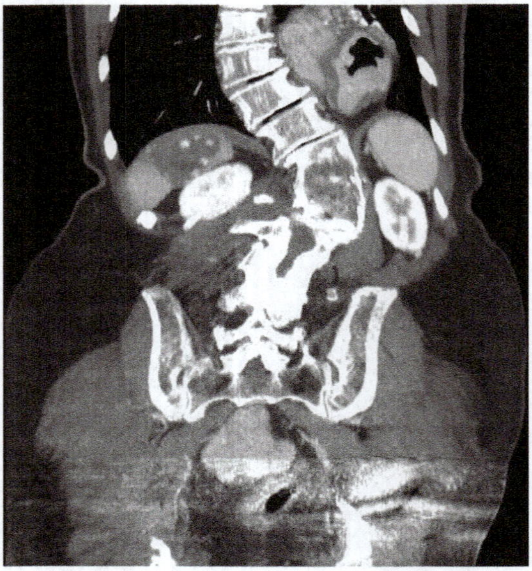

Fig. 5.28 This coronal reconstruction reveals calcifications in a large peripheral hemangioma

5.2.2.3 Hepatoma

Hepatomas, especially small ones, are difficult to diagnose or biopsy. Obviously, some segments of the liver are not accessible by EUS. Nevertheless, EUS should be considered when the lesions are within the reach of the echoendoscope. The valuable role EUS can play in the detection and biopsy of small hepatomas that are not well visualized or would be difficult to access by percutaneous ultrasound is increasingly being recognized [9]. According to published retrospective series, EUS-guided FNA provides adequate tissue for diagnosis and with minimal risk of complications [10]. Moreover, metastatic lesions, especially to lymph nodes, can also easily be biopsied as this next case and others show [11]. This patient is a 51-year-old man with a history of chronic liver disease who had increasing alpha-fetoprotein levels and large bilateral adrenal masses without known liver lesions. An initial EUS-guided fine-needle aspiration (FNA) could not be completed because of problems during sedation. The study did, however, show liver lesions suspicious for hepatoma that were not previously recognized by CT. Magnetic resonance imaging also demonstrated the lesions seen during EUS. During a subsequent EUS with anesthesia support, FNA biopsies or aspirates were obtained from two liver lesions (showing hepatoma), ascites (negative), the left adrenal lymph node (benign), and two small perigastric lymph nodes (metastatic hepatoma).

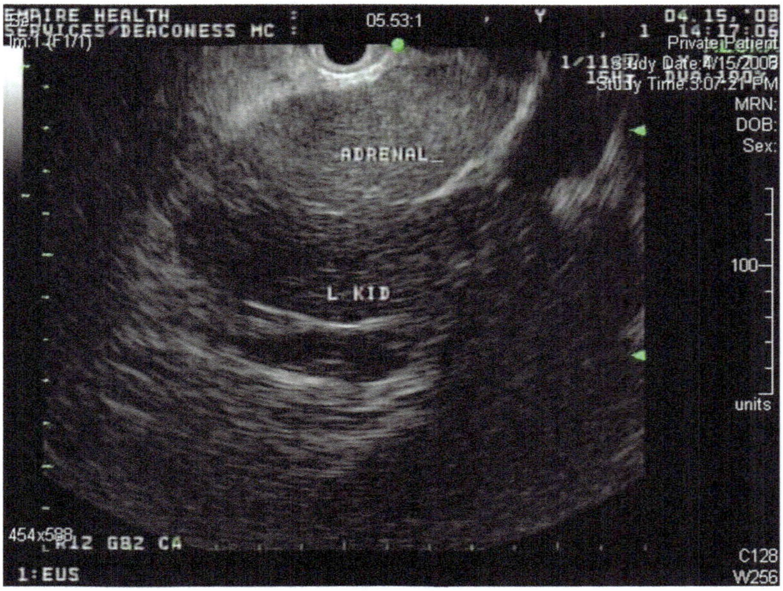

Fig. 5.29 This large left adrenal mass was biopsied but only bland adrenocortical type cells were seen. *L KID* left kidney

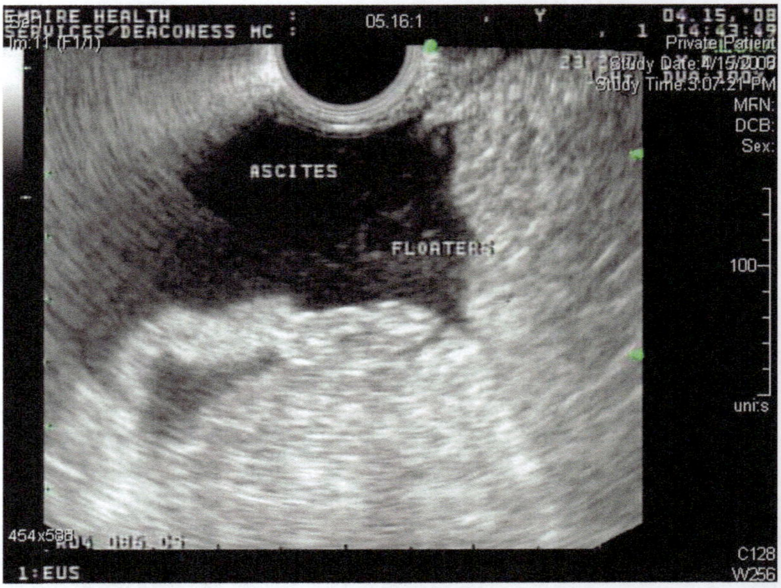

Fig. 5.30 There was a moderate amount of ascites with negative cytology

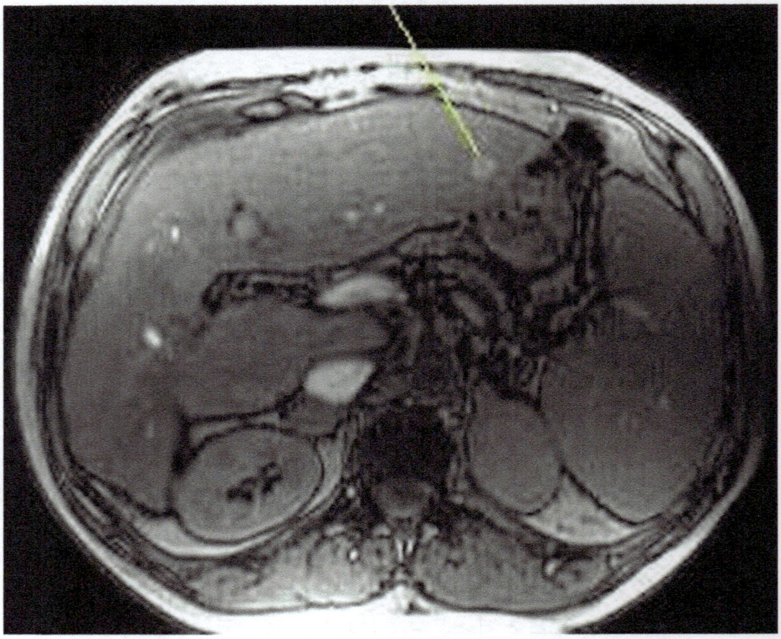

Fig. 5.31 Magnetic resonance imaging obtained after endoscopic ultrasound suggested the presence of small hepatomas, showing several small lesions like the one seen in this image. In view of the high alpha-fetoprotein values, this was suspicious for hepatocellular carcinoma

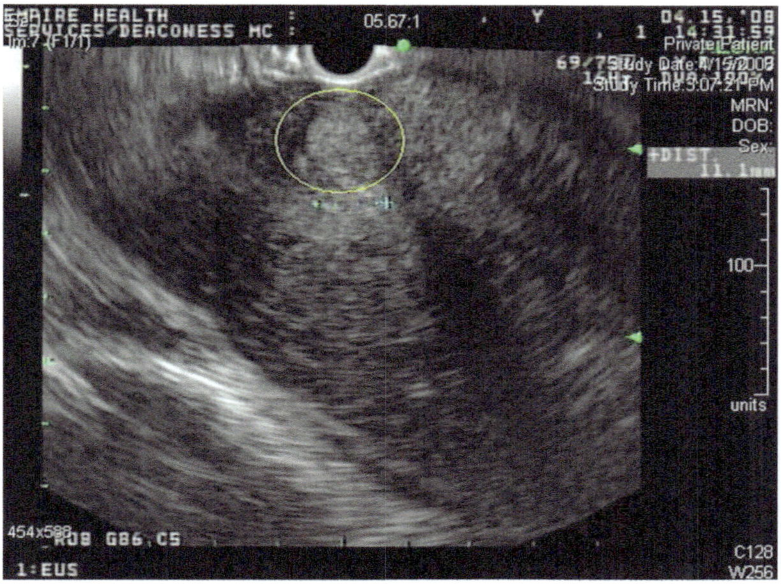

Fig. 5.32 This is the endoscopic ultrasound appearance of the mass shown on magnetic resonance imaging

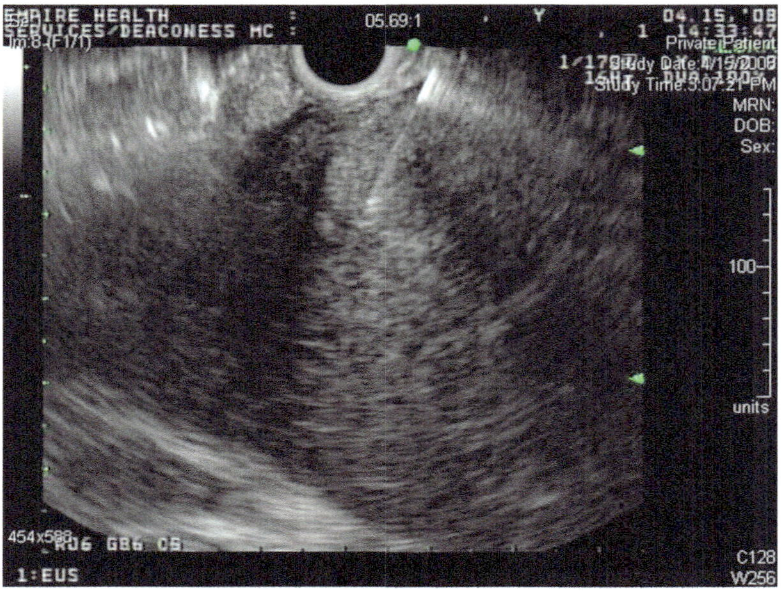

Fig. 5.33 Biopsies of this 11-mm-diameter nodule and another one like it showed hepatoma

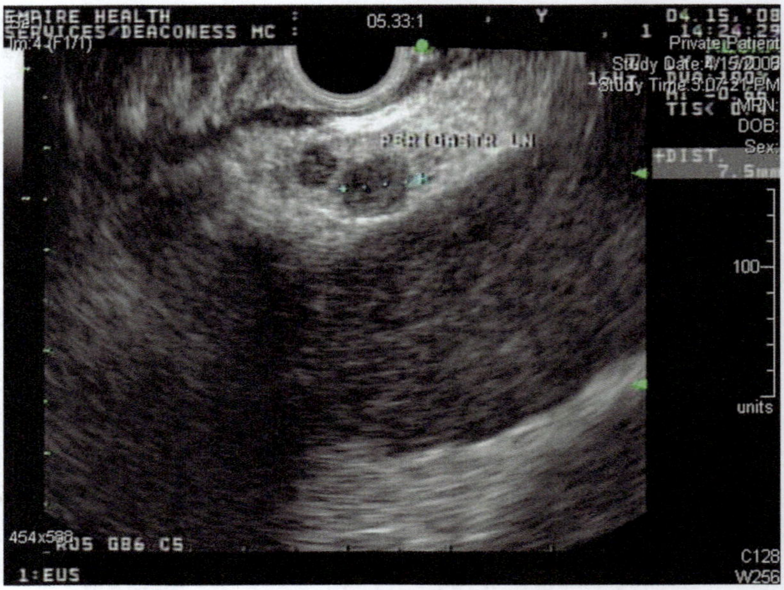

Fig. 5.34 Unfortunately, endoscopic ultrasound–guided fine-needle aspiration of these small (7 mm) perigastric lymph nodes (*LN*) revealed metastatic hepatoma

5.2.2.4 Hepatic Lymph Nodes

The most important pathway for lymphatic drainage of the liver goes through the hepatic hilum and the retropancreatic area and along the hepatic artery and the celiac axis. The first lymph node stations are nodes of the hepatoduodenal ligament and the retropancreatic area then the hepatic artery and celiac axis. The size of normal hepatic lymph nodes is quite variable; they tend to be larger than lymph nodes in other regions of the body. They are frequently enlarged in patients with chronic hepatitis [12]. Normal lymph nodes are described sonographically as hypoechoic, oval/flattened structures that can have a hyperechoic zone at the hilum due to the presence of fat and in some cases hilar vascularity, although the majority of them are hypovascular [13]. This patient had an unusually interesting lymph node with a clear difference of echogenicity of the cortex and medulla and a hilar vessel that could be interrogated by spectral Doppler.

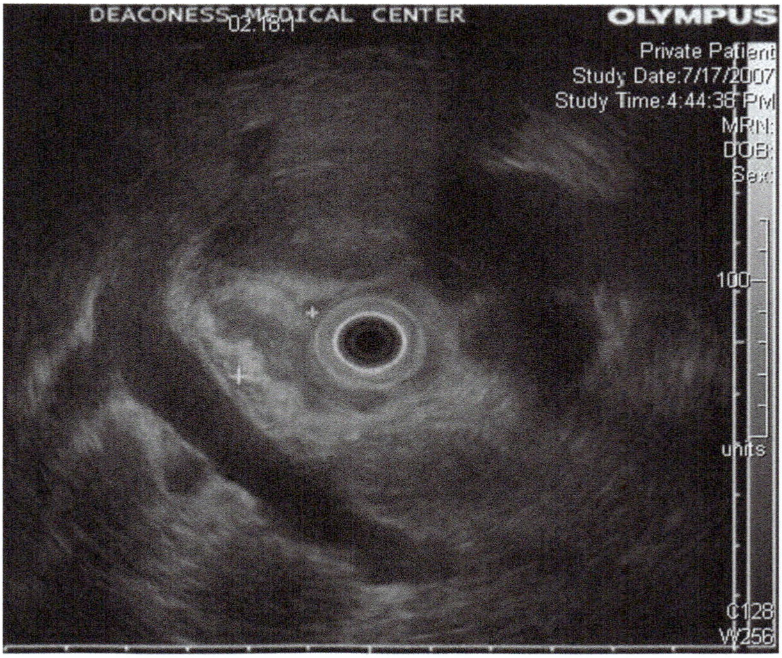

Fig. 5.35 This radial endoscopic ultrasound image shows a hepatoduodenal ligament (periportal, hepatic) lymph node that has an unusual prominent echogenic cortex with a hypoechoic medulla

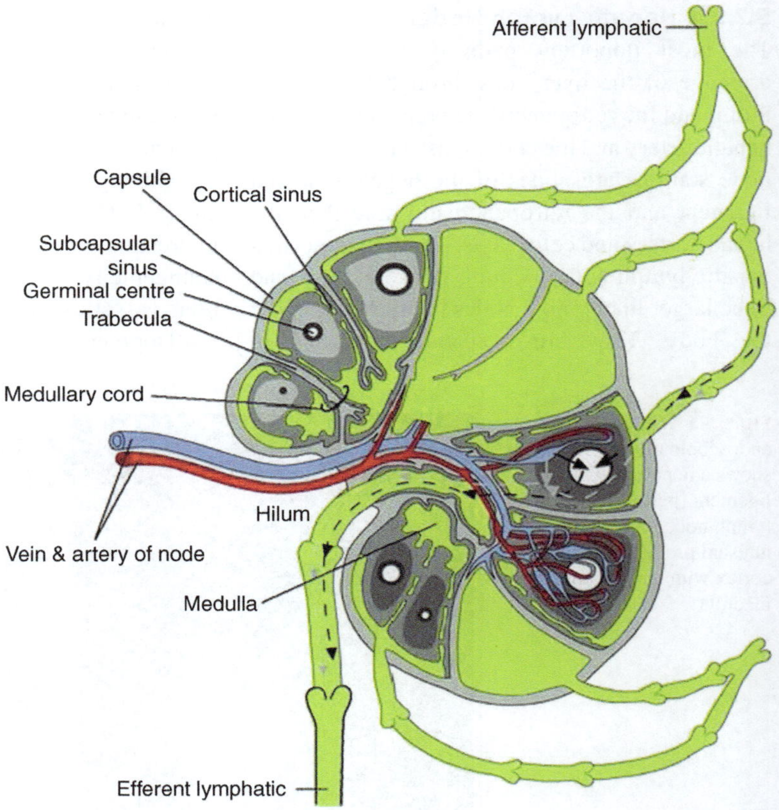

Fig. 5.36 Typical lymph node anatomy (From Ying et al. [14])

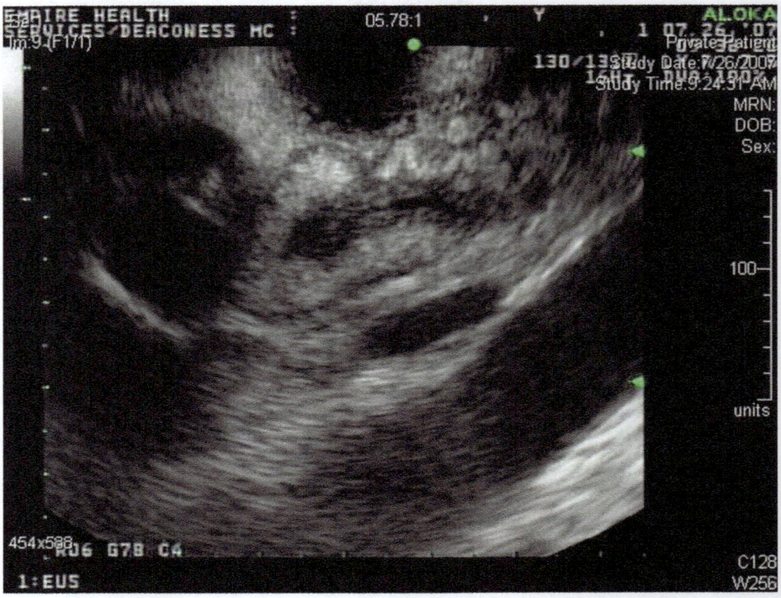

Fig. 5.37 This linear endoscopic ultrasound image shows more details of the periportal lymph node

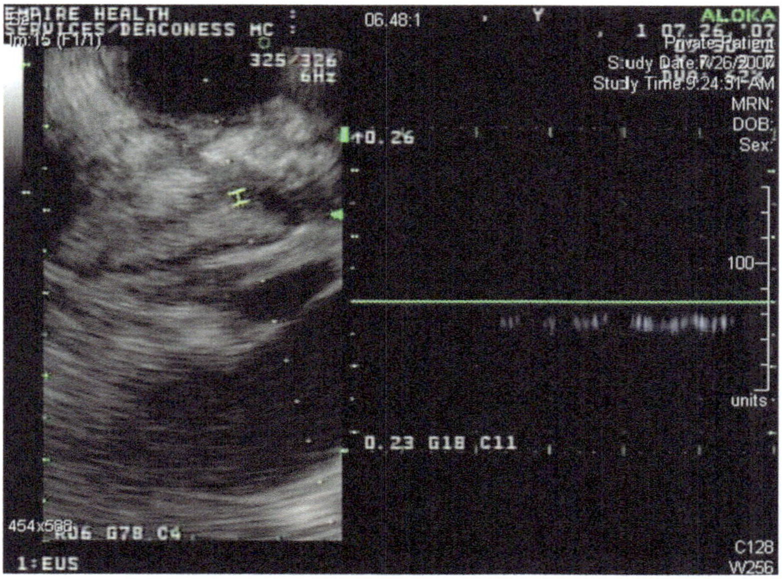

Fig. 5.38 Spectral Doppler in the center of the lymph node shows a faint venous signature

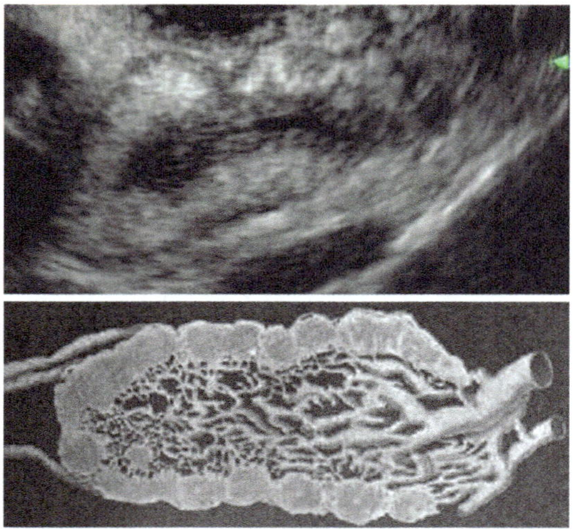

Fig. 5.39 This image juxtaposes the endoscopic ultrasound image of the lymph node (*top*) with an anatomical illustration more than 100 years old (*bottom*)

5.2.2.5 Portal Vein and Hepatic Vein Branches

Although endosonographers cannot visualize the entire liver, they often encounter hepatic pathology that they should be able to recognize and, if appropriate, biopsy. A prerequisite for this is a good understanding of liver ultrasound, including vascular anatomy. Differentiating between hepatic vein and portal vein branches is accomplished relatively easily, even without Doppler. The hepatic vein branches come from the periphery and converge toward the level of the diaphragm in a generally craniocaudal direction. They have anechoic walls, run a relatively straight course, and do not branch as often as the portal vein. In contrast the branches of the portal vein run principally in a sagittal plane, diverge from the portahepatis toward the periphery, branch more frequently, and have highly echogenic walls.

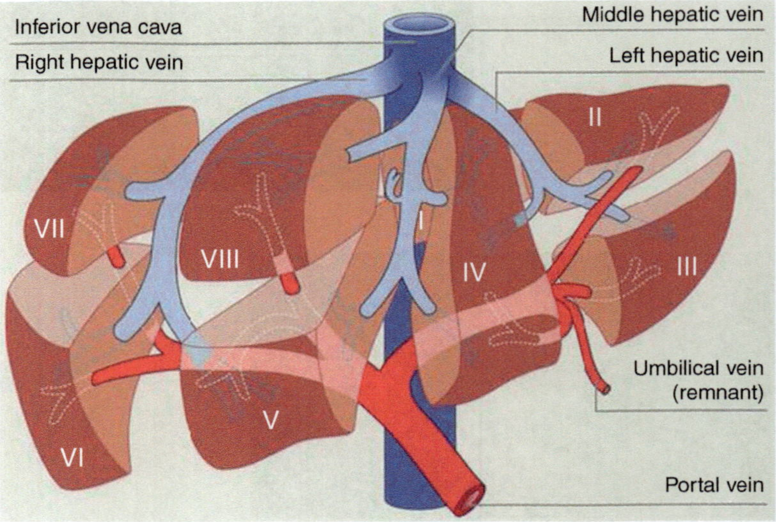

Fig. 5.40 The general course of hepatic veins and portal vein branches (From Dancygier [15])

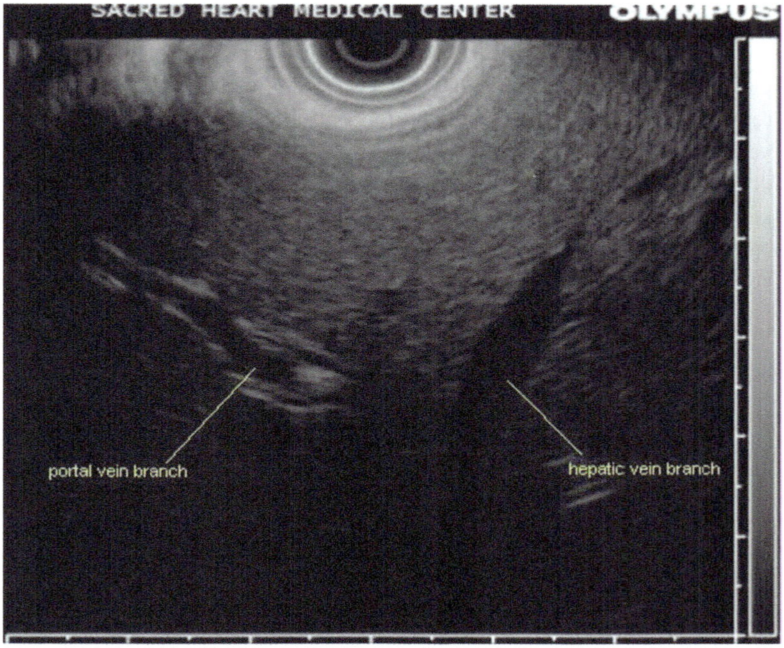

Fig. 5.41 This endoscopic ultrasound image illustrates the points made in the narrative, especially the striking difference in the echogenicity of the vessel wall

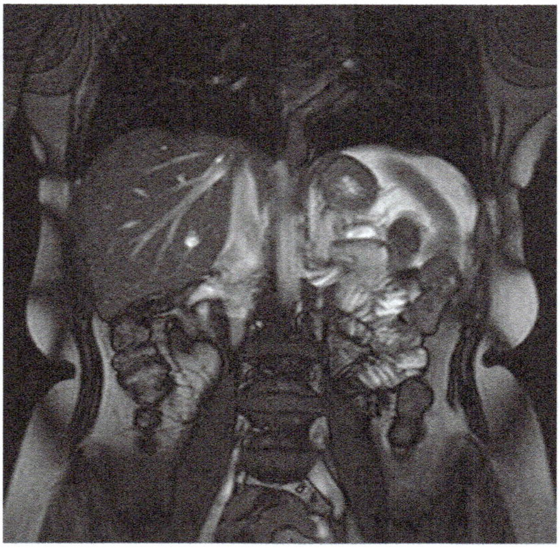

Fig. 5.42 The general course of the hepatic veins on a native magnetic resonance image

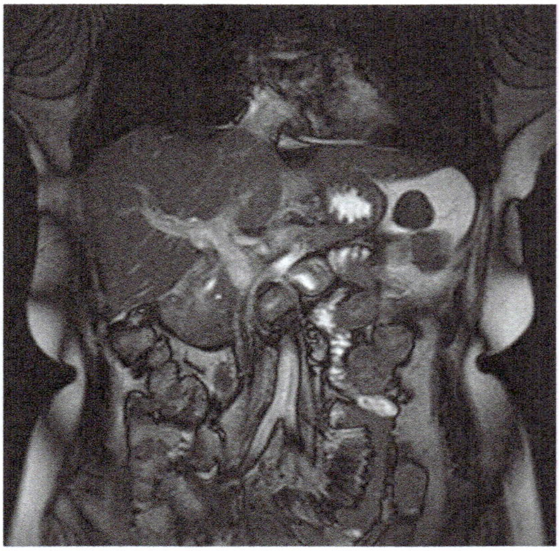

Fig. 5.43 The course of the portal vein with left and right branches

5.2.2.6 Cavernous Transformation of the Portal Vein

Cavernous transformation of the portal vein refers to the enlargement of the normally minute veins that accompany the portal vein when it is occluded. Small, tubular, serpiginous venous collaterals running along the occluded portal vein can be visualized on color Doppler ultrasound or contrast-enhanced CT. This is a 57-year-old patient who 2 years ago was diagnosed with ovarian cancer. At that time EUS showed a 3-cm mass in the porta hepatis that was compressing the portal vein. In the interim, the metastasis has invaded the portal vein, occluding it completely but with a tangle of small collaterals bypassing the obstruction. The mass has recently started obstructing the common hepatic duct, causing jaundice. During ERCP a metal stent was placed across the biliary stricture, draining the right hepatic system; the jaundice resolved.

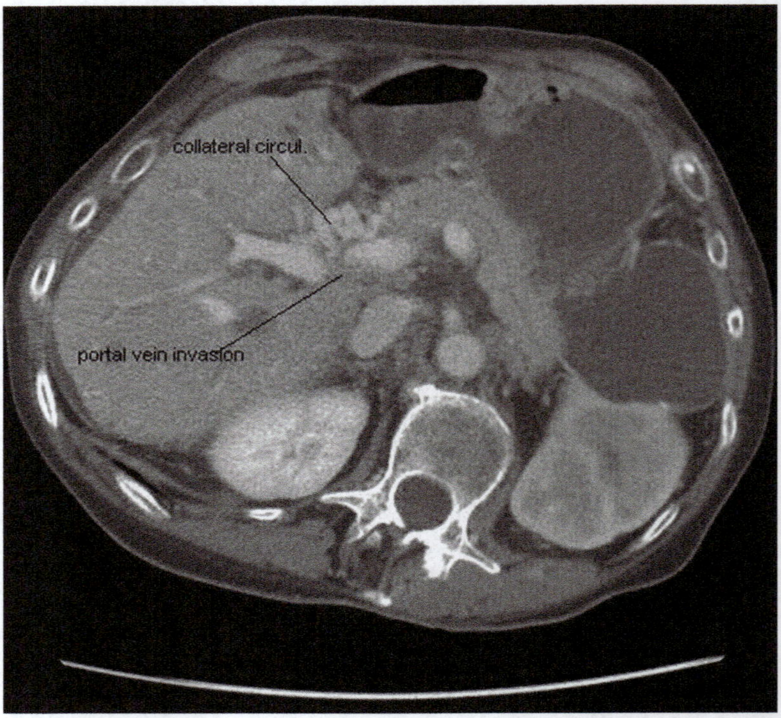

Fig. 5.44 This computed tomography scan shows tumor invading into the portal vein with complete occlusion and a tangle of collaterals bypassing the obstruction

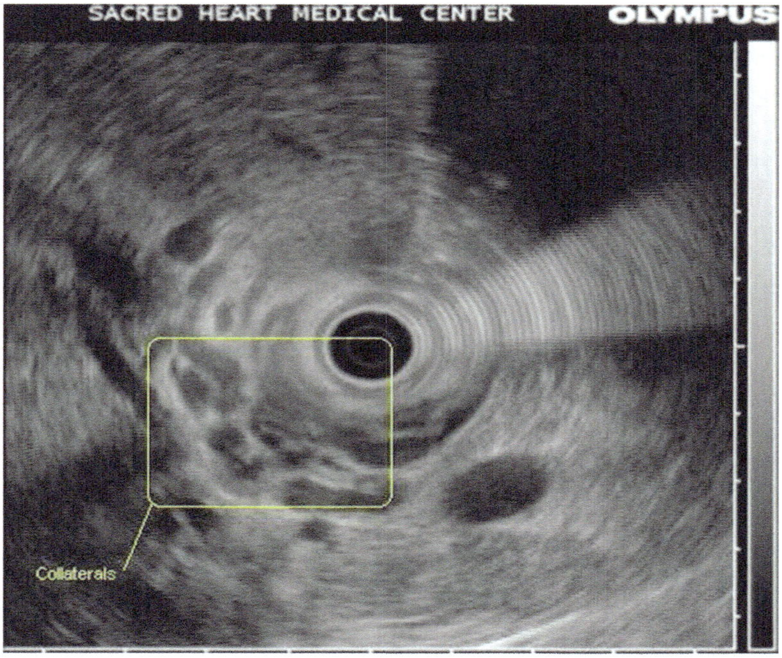

Fig. 5.45 Numerous collaterals, mostly in cross section, can be appreciated on this radial endoscopic ultrasound image

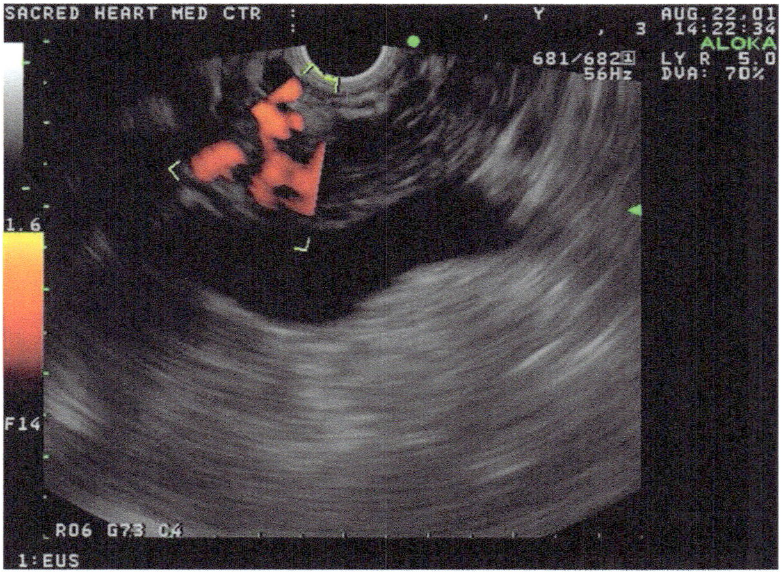

Fig. 5.46 This linear endoscopic ultrasound image shows the collaterals, which are highlighted with power Doppler

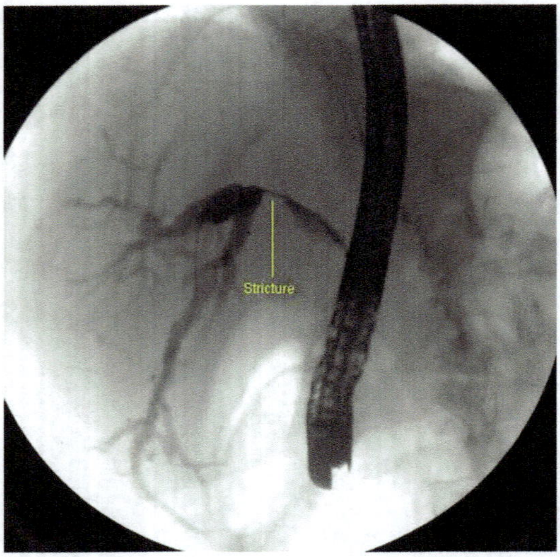

Fig. 5.47 Endoscopic retrograde cholangiopancreatography shows a high-grade hilar stricture

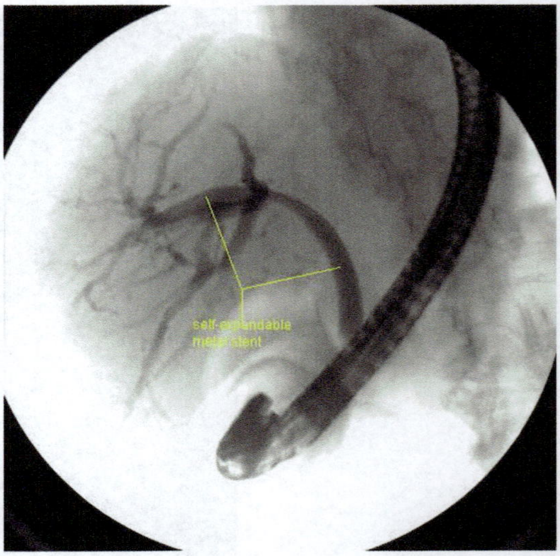

Fig. 5.48 A 6-cm-long, 10-mm-diameter, self-expandable metal stent was placed across the stricture. Note the waistline. The jaundice resolved

5.2.3 Bile Ducts

5.2.3.1 Isolated Bile Duct Dilation, Normal Liver Tests

There are numerous occasions when imaging studies show isolated bile duct dilation in patients who are either asymptomatic, have normal liver tests, or both. If the latter is the case (i.e., good-quality routine imaging shows no pathology), many experts feel that no further investigations are warranted [16]. Nevertheless, EUS can be reassuring. This is such a case: an 84-year-old woman with severe chronic obstructive pulmonary disease and a prior cholecystectomy years ago presented with right upper quadrant abdominal pain. Her liver tests remained within normal limits throughout this episode and her pain resolved. EUS showed a dilated bile duct, 12 mm in diameter, with dilation of the right and left hepatic duct but no other abnormalities. The pancreatic duct was normal. Good-quality images of the region of the papilla of Vater were obtained. She has remained asymptomatic over 6 months of follow-up. Without the availability of EUS this patient may have been subjected to ERCP, risking significant procedure-related morbidity.

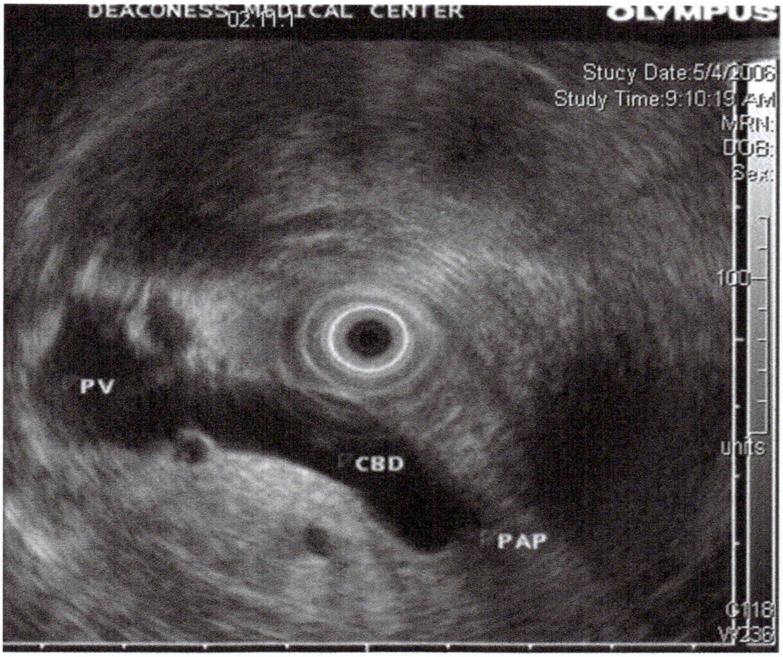

Fig. 5.49 This radial endoscopic ultrasound image shows uniform dilation of the extrahepatic biliary system. *CBD* common bile duct, *PAP* papilla of vater, *PV* portal vein

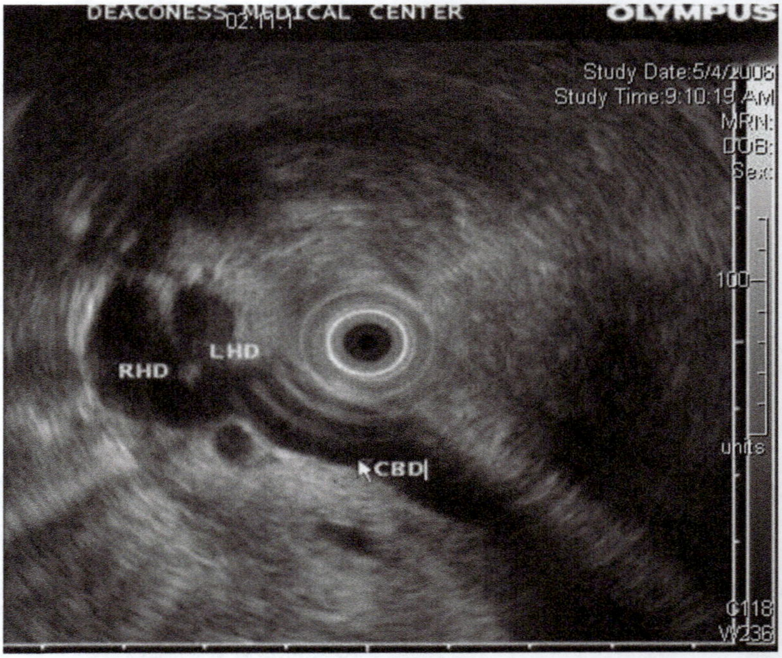

Fig. 5.50 Dilated right (*RHD*) and left hepatic ducts (*LHD*) are shown. *CBD* common bile duct

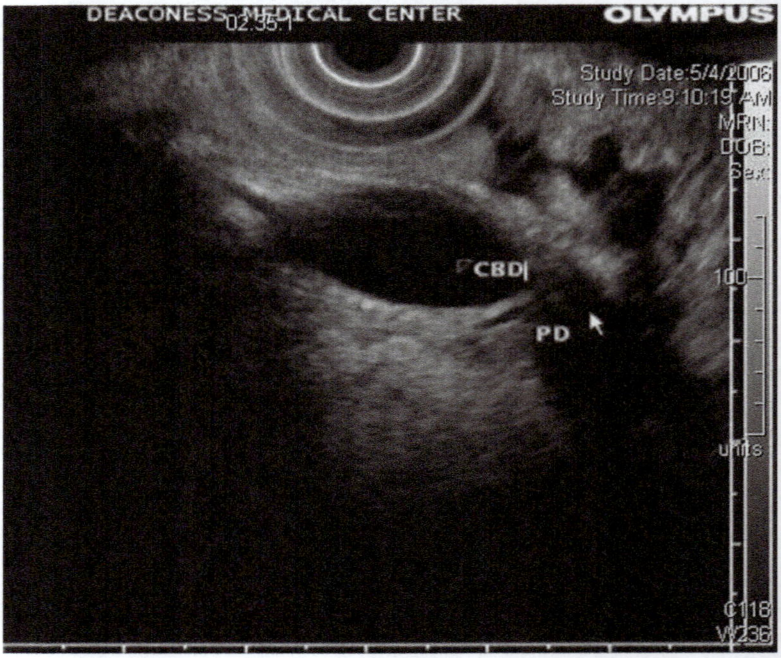

Fig. 5.51 The periampullary region was unremarkable; the *shadow* is an artifact. The main pancreatic duct (*PD*) is visible and appears slender. *CBD* common bile duct

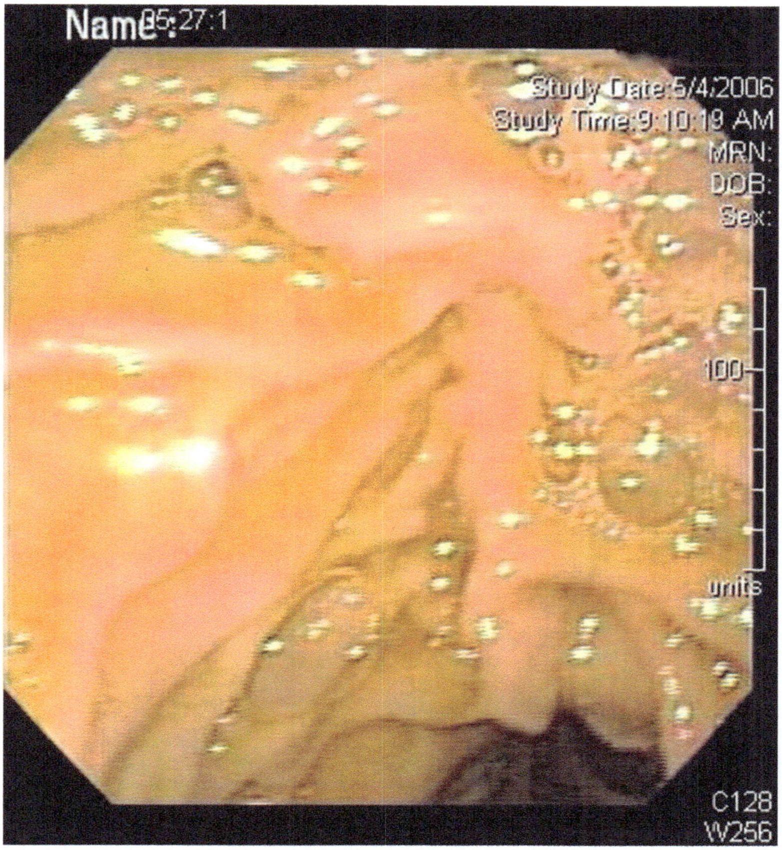

Fig. 5.52 An endoscopic view of the papilla shows no abnormalities

5.2.3.2 Bile Duct Dilation Caused by a Crossing Vessel

This case is similar to another one described in this chapter (right hepatic artery syndrome), but the imaging features in this patient are even more instructive. Imaging abnormalities involving the hepatic duct may be related to stones, Mirizzi syndrome, polyps, strictures, cholangiocarcinoma, or metastatic lymph nodes, and, as this case demonstrates, compression by vascular structures. Clinically relevant common hepatic duct compression caused by the right hepatic artery is an extremely rare condition. When jaundice is present, the compression is often associated with a hepatic artery aneurysm or aberrant anatomy. However, asymptomatic common duct compression by the right hepatic artery is increasingly recognized on magnetic resonance cholangiography as an incidental finding [17]. In this case a 67-year-old woman was referred to us for EUS evaluation of a dilated bile duct seen on a CT scan. EUS demonstrated a caliber step-up associated with a crossing right hepatic artery.

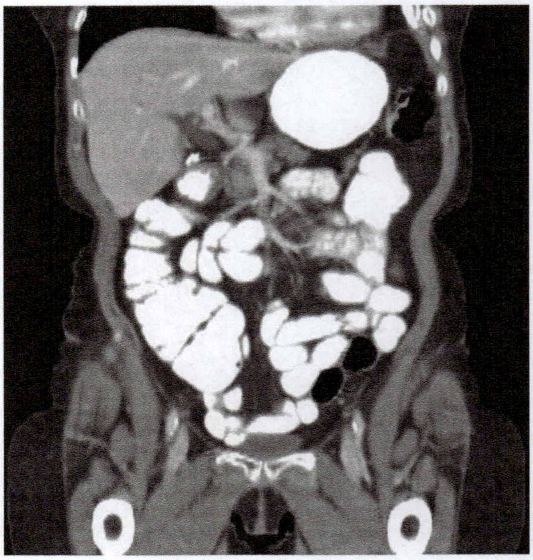

Fig. 5.53 This coronal reconstruction shows an arterial vessel crossing anterior to a dilated appearing bile duct

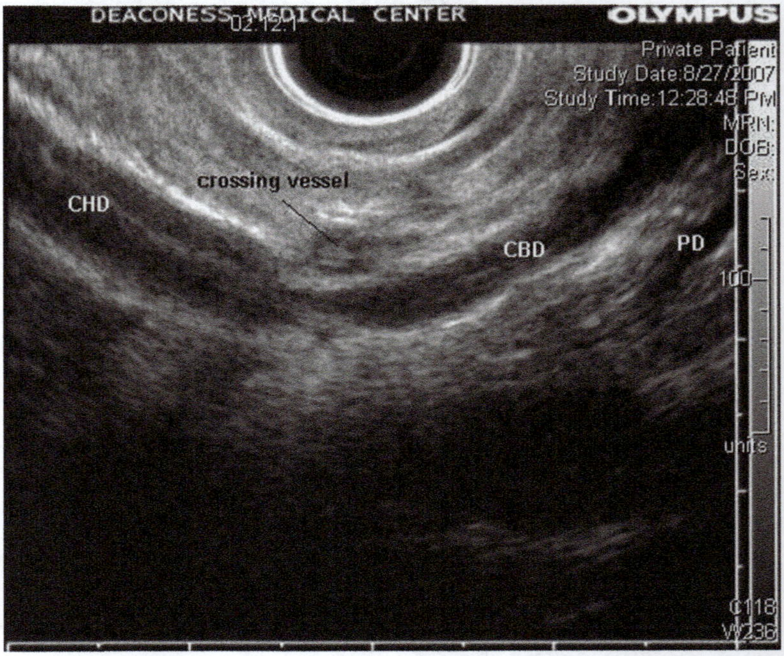

Fig. 5.54 This radial endoscopic ultrasound image shows the cross section of a vessel traversing the common bile duct (*CBD*) at the location of the caliber change. *CHD* common hepatic duct, *PD* pancreatic duct

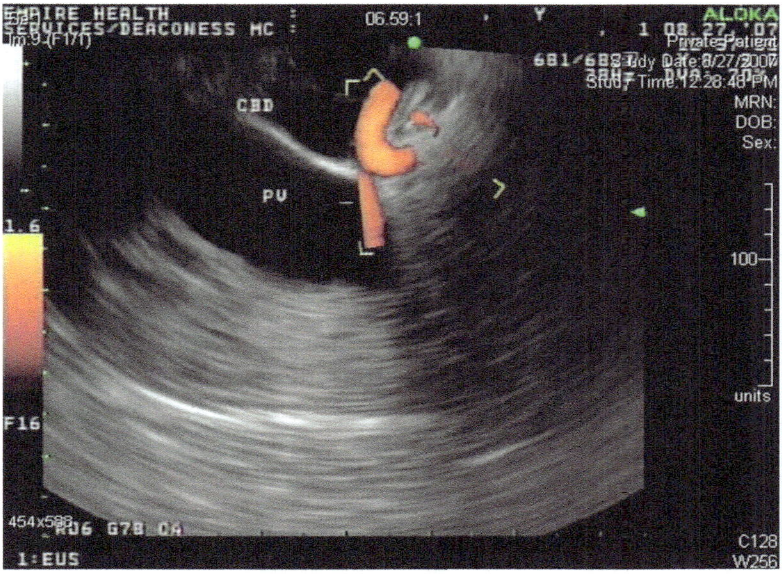

Fig. 5.55 This power Doppler endoscopic ultrasound study shows a dilated common bile duct (*CBD*) upstream from (or proximal to) an artery compressing it. *PV* portal vein

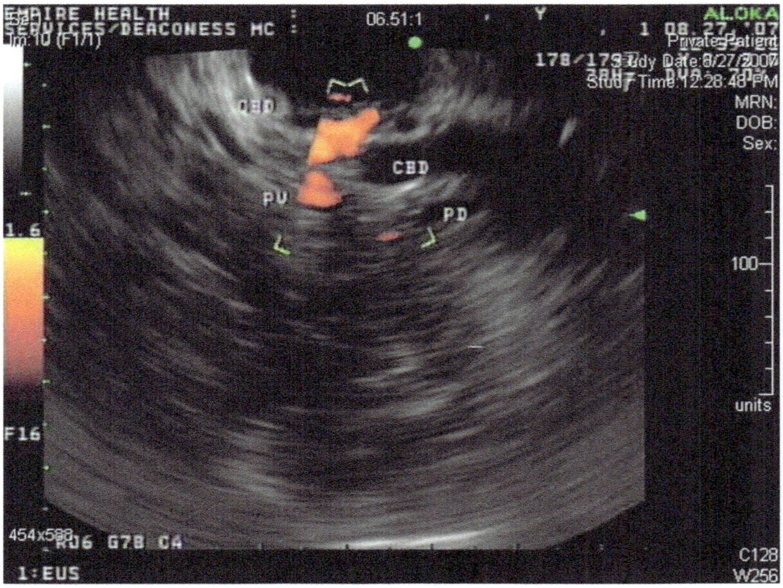

Fig. 5.56 This corresponding Doppler study shows a normal caliber common bile duct (*CBD*) distal to (downstream from) the crossing artery. *PD* pancreatic duct, *PV* portal vein

5.2.3.3 Common Bile Duct Stone

Both MRCP and EUS have been evaluated for the detection of stones in the common bile duct, using ERCP as the reference standard. The sensitivity and specificity of these techniques exceed 90 % when compared with ERCP [18]. We think that EUS is often a better choice than MRCP in patients with a low or intermediate probability of having a stone in the common bile duct, especially if they have significant comorbidities. Although MRCP is entirely noninvasive, the sickest patients are the least likely to cooperate, and motion artifacts frequently deteriorate the image quality so that no decisions can be made. Many units are now set up to follow an EUS that shows a stone in the common bile duct, using ERCP for removal. This is a 71-year-old patient with an abnormality in the distal common bile duct who was referred for EUS evaluation. A large stone in the common bile duct was seen and was removed during subsequent ERCP. In addition, see the case of an MRCP that showed an abnormality requiring EUS for clarification (Cholodochocele vs. Bile Duct Web).

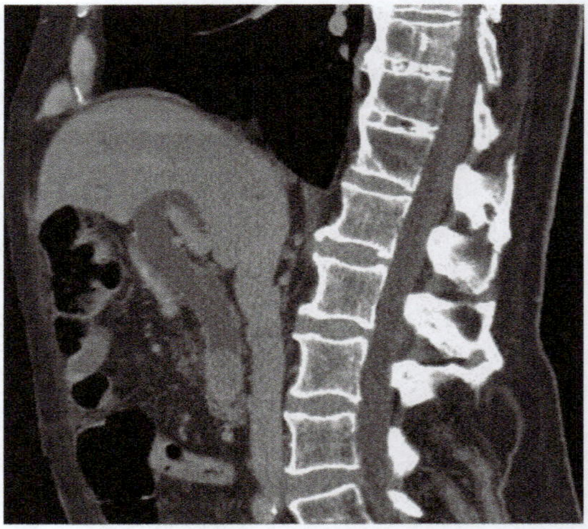

Fig. 5.57 This is a sagittal reconstruction of the computed tomography. While a large stone was the most likely diagnosis, the radiologist offered a tumor mass as differential diagnosis

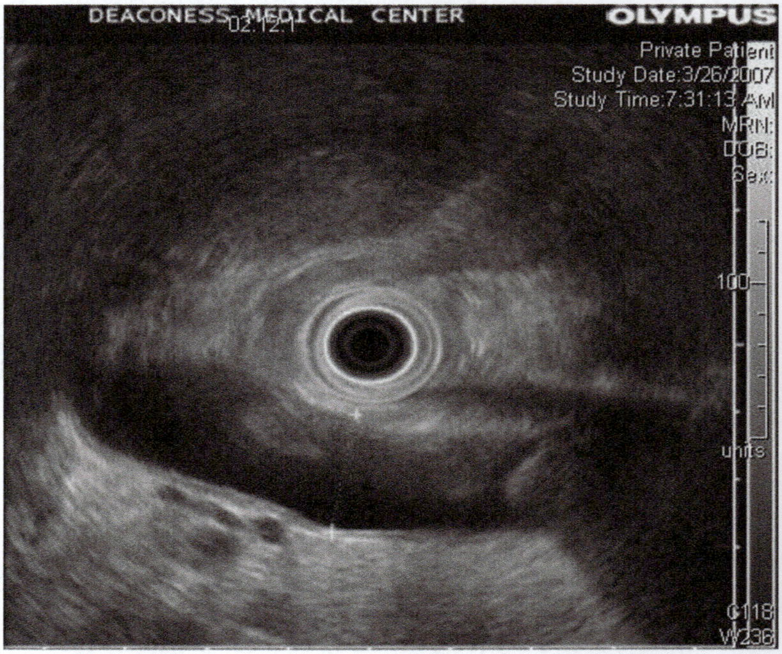

Fig. 5.58 A large stone with typical posterior shadowing was seen in the distal common bile duct on endoscopic ultrasound

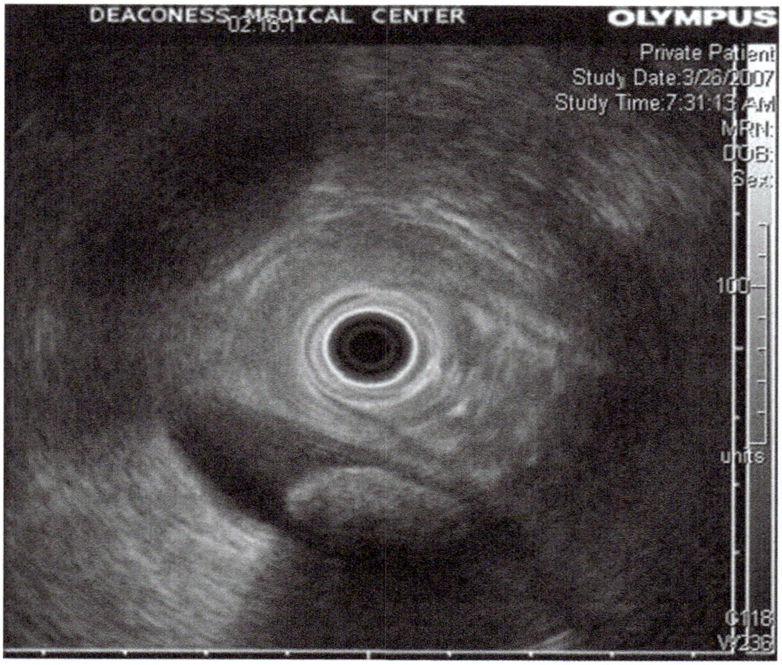

Fig. 5.59 There is no adherence to the bile duct wall or origination from it, so a tumor can be ruled out

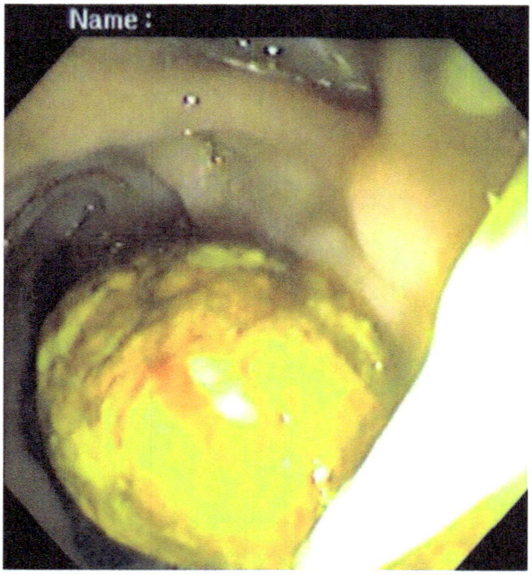

Fig. 5.60 A large stone was removed during endoscopic retrograde cholangiopancreatography

5.2.3.4 Bile Duct Stone Missed by EUS and ERCP

This is a 68-year-old patient who had an attempted laparoscopic cholecystectomy that was converted to an open procedure 15 months before this presentation. He initially did well but lately he has developed symptoms of right upper quadrant pain and was found to have elevated liver tests and a dilated bile duct on imaging studies. Of interest is that the intraoperative cholangiogram at the time of surgery showed abrupt narrowing of the bile duct and some bile duct dilation but no filling defects. A recent CT scan showed a 14-mm hypodense area close to the papilla in the head of the pancreas in addition to dilation of the bile duct (but no dilation of the pancreatic duct). Subsequent EUS did not show any pancreatic mass but revealed a narrow-mouthed but relatively deep periampullary diverticulum, which explains the hypodense area close to the papilla. Briefly, what appeared to be a possible stone was seen but was not reproducible. Type I dysfunction of the sphincter of Oddi was suspected and the patient subsequently had ERCP. No stone was seen during the cholangiogram. A biliary sphincterotomy was performed and to be comprehensive the bile duct was swept with a balloon occlusion catheter. This sweep surprisingly recovered a 4-mm-diameter black stone. The negative predictive value of EUS for bile duct stones in prospective studies has been close to 95 %, but, as this case demonstrates, a degree of skepticism is always appropriate. This case also illustrates the problems duodenal diverticula can cause for cross-sectional imaging: During CT, the duodenal diverticulum could be filled by contrast, air, bile, duodenal or pancreatic juice (body fluids), or food debris. In this case we suspect it was body fluids that gave the appearance of a small pancreatic hypodensity [19].

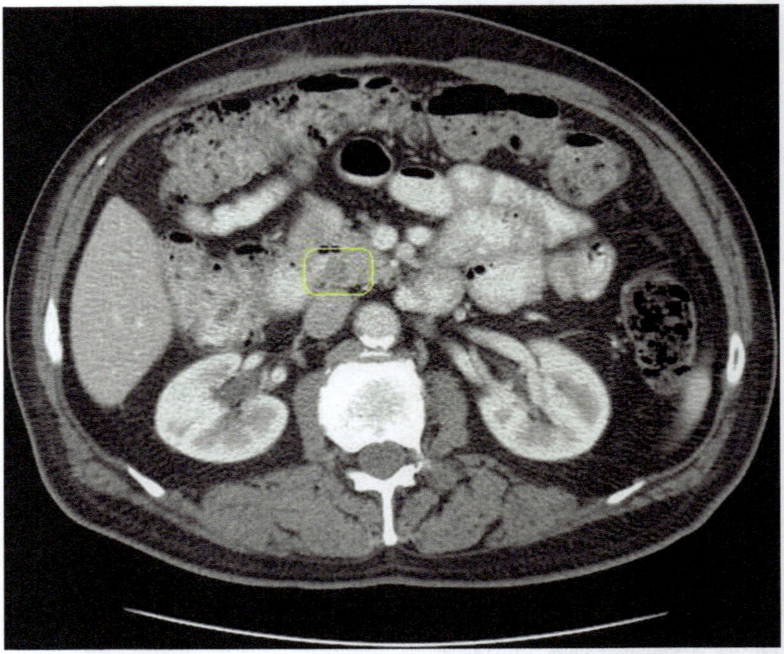

Fig. 5.61 This computed tomography scan shows a small (1.4-cm diameter) hypodense area close to the papilla of Vater, apparently in the pancreas

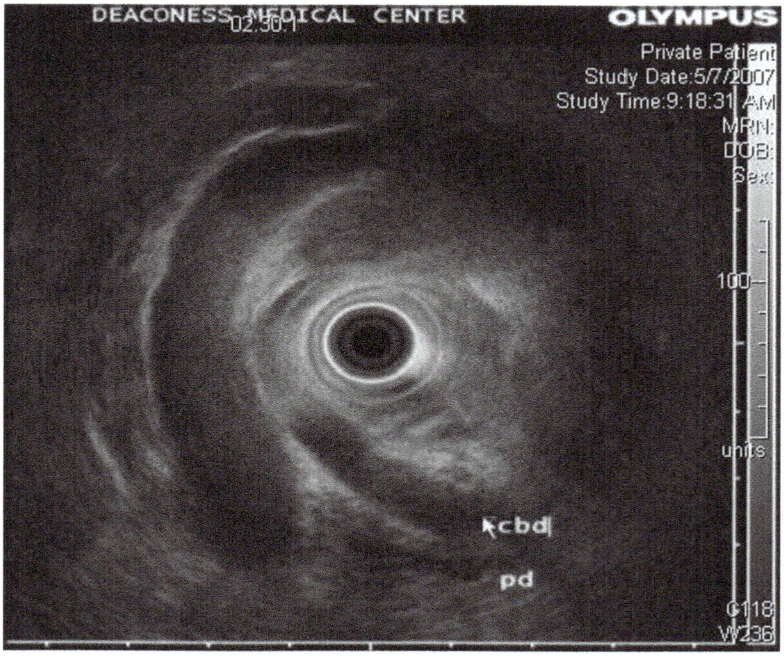

Fig. 5.62 Endoscopic ultrasound shows a mildly dilated common bile duct (*cbd*) but no mass lesion. Briefly, what appeared to be a small shadowing concrement was seen but it could not be demonstrated again. *pd* pancreatic duct

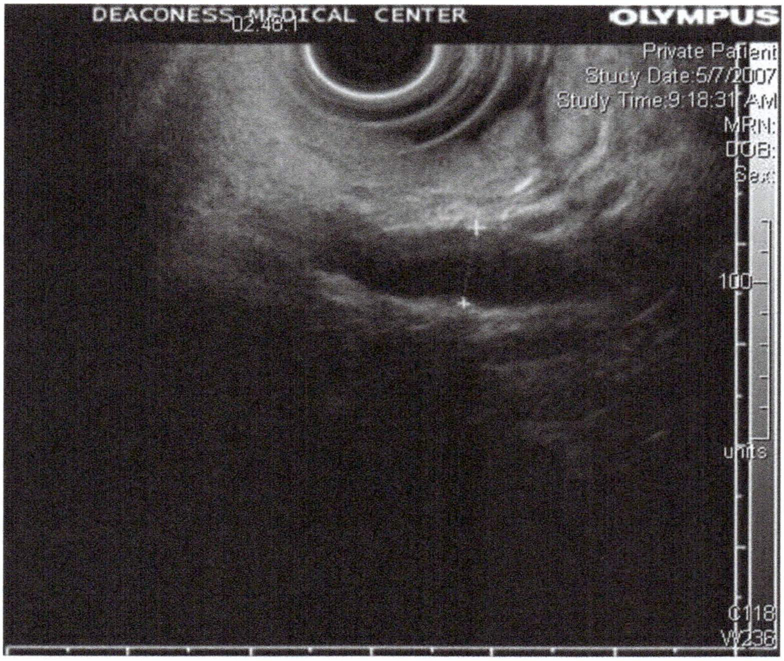

Fig. 5.63 A close-up of the common bile duct and pancreatic duct as they converge toward the level of the papilla shows no mass or lesion

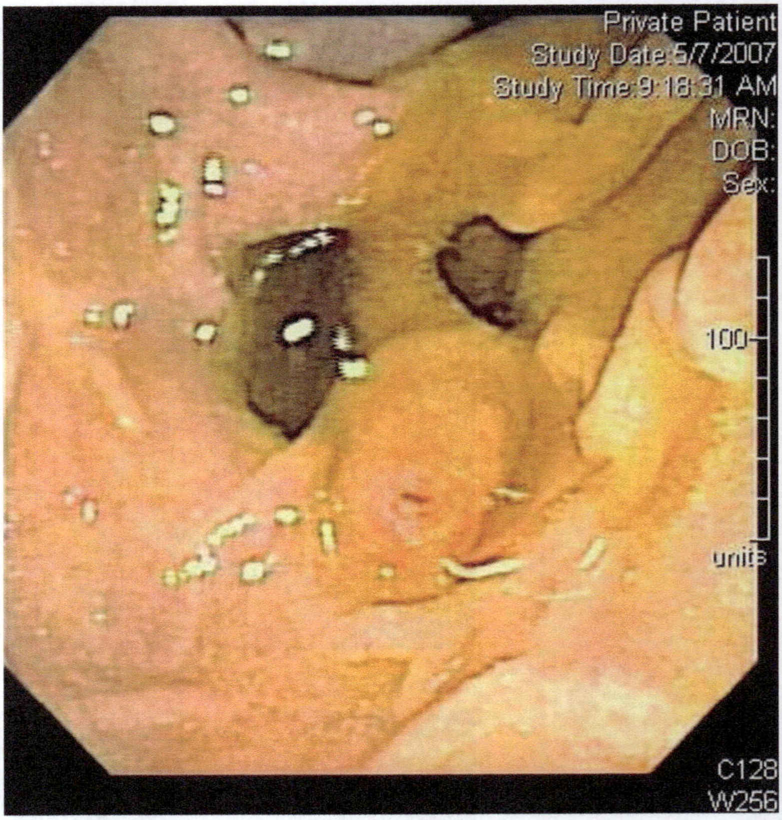

Fig. 5.64 Surface endoscopy shows a narrow-mouthed but relatively deep periampullary diverticulum. As can be seen, this diverticulum is filled with bile. On cross-sectional imaging this could give the impression of a hypodense lesion

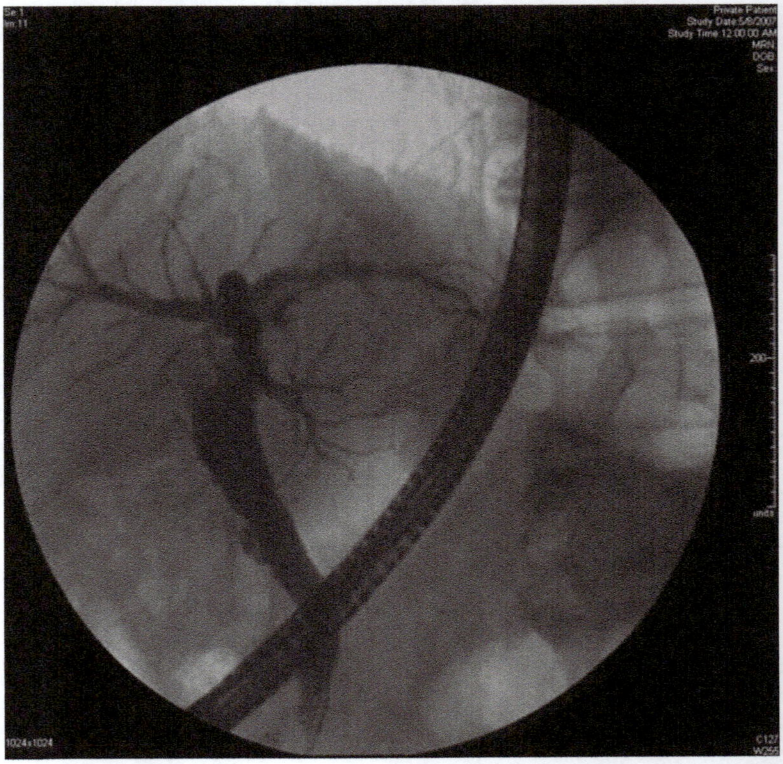

Fig. 5.65 The endoscopic retrograde cholangiopancreatography did not show any filling defects, but a 4-mm-diameter black stone was pulled out of the bile duct after biliary sphincterotomy and a balloon sweep

5.2.3.5 Possible "Narcotic Bile Duct"

There are a number of case series indicating an association between asymptomatic enlargement of the bile duct and chronic narcotic use. A 2007 Iranian study conducted on 110 opium addicts showed a significant association between the length of the addiction and the size of the bile duct even if corrected for age [20]; similar results were reported elsewhere [21]. This is a 45-year-old woman with an at least 10-year history of drug and alcohol problems who complained of chronic mostly left-sided abdominal pain. She is highly focused on obtaining pain medications and has been taking narcotics for years; more recently she also has been using a fentanyl transdermal patch. Imaging studies showed a dilated bile duct, and EUS evaluation was requested. The EUS showed a mildly dilated common bile duct (12 mm) but no other abnormalities. Dilation of the intrapancreatic portion of bile ducts as shown in the EUS images excludes the possibility of alcohol-induced chronic pancreatitis causing extrinsic compression/partial obstruction of the bile ducts.

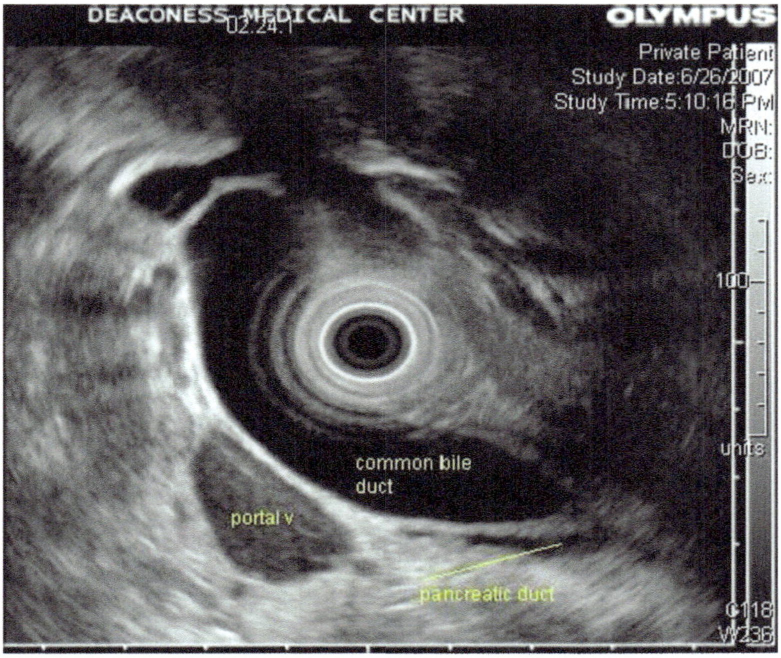

Fig. 5.66 This is a radial endoscopic ultrasound image of a patient who has been taking high doses of narcotics for years

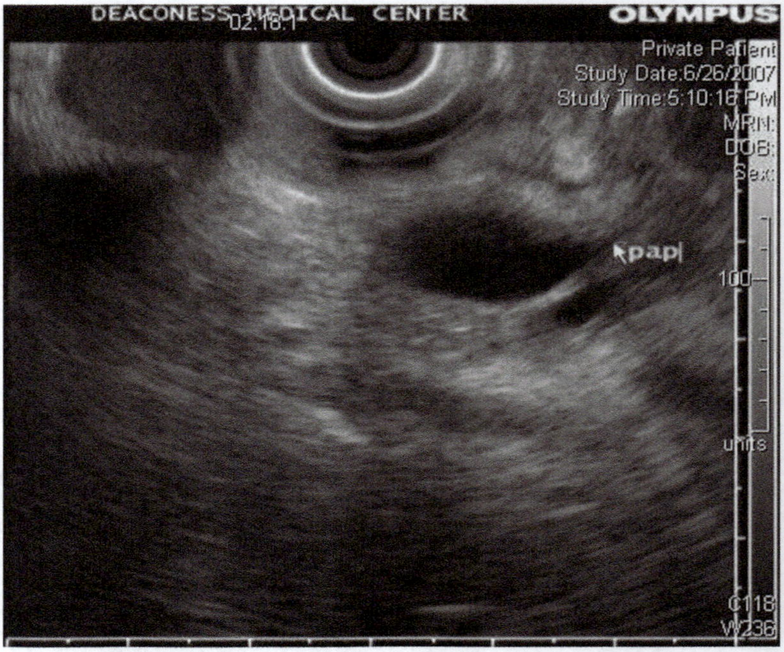

Fig. 5.67 Close views of the papilla showed no abnormalities. It has been speculated that chronic opioid use leads to sphincter dysfunction followed by bile duct dilation

5.2.3.6 Primary Sclerosing Cholangitis

This is an 80-year-old patient with abdominal pain and mildly abnormal liver function tests. A CT scan was unremarkable except for mild dilation of the bile duct. A HIDA scan showed nonfilling of the gallbladder. EUS was requested and the images show marked thickening of the wall of the extrahepatic bile duct with a wrinkled, irregular, wavy, serrated outline. A small shadowing concrement also is present. The cystic duct lymph node was prominent and EUS-guided FNA was performed so we did not miss an opportunity to diagnose cholangiocarcinoma. The cytology showed reactive appearing changes. ERCP evaluation confirmed the classic findings of intra- and extrahepatic primary sclerosing cholangitis (PSC). Bile duct brushings were also negative for carcinoma. The gallbladder did fill. The case is noteworthy for the textbook findings visible on both ERCP and EUS. The onset of PSC varies from childhood (age younger than 10 years) up to elderly patients in the 7th or 8th decade of life; however, PSC mostly affects young men aged 30–40 years [22].

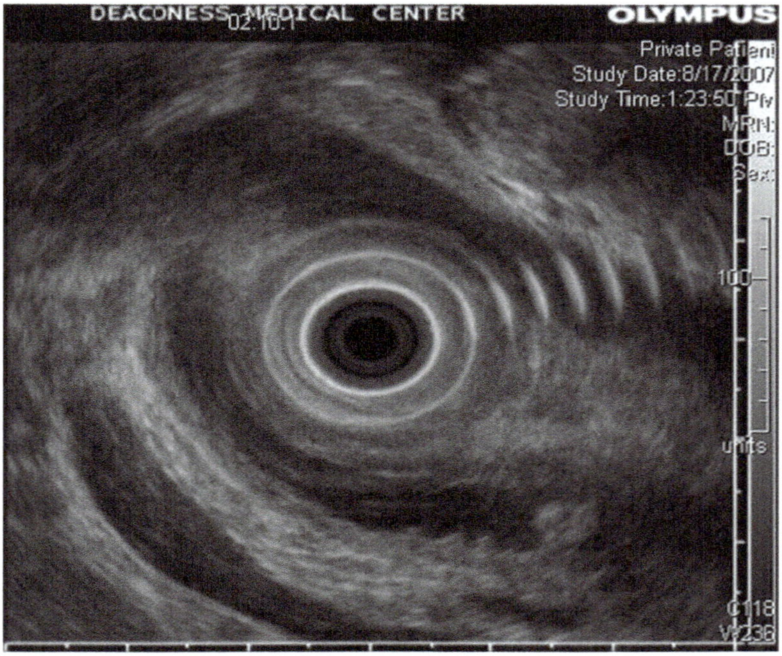

Fig. 5.68 This endoscopic ultrasound image shows a markedly thickened distal common bile duct with crenellations characteristic of primary sclerosing cholangitis. Note the stone

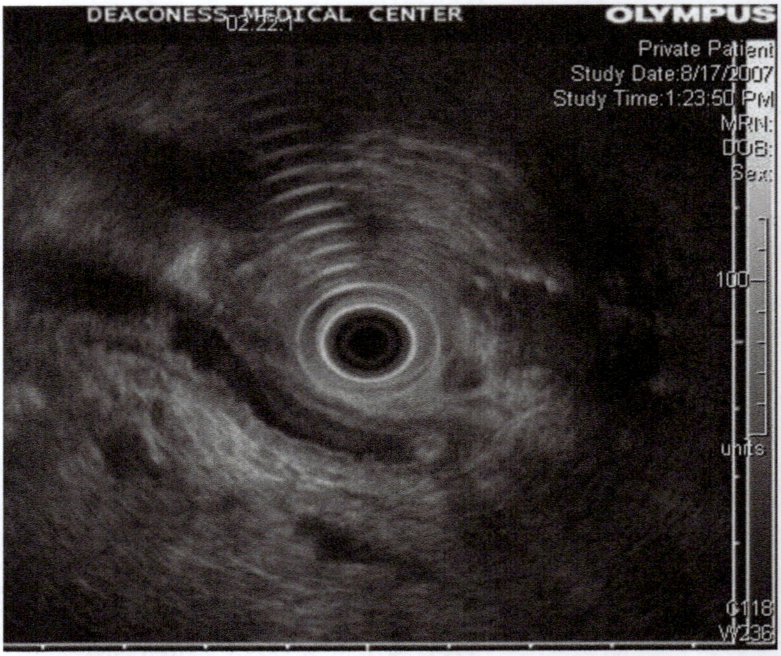

Fig. 5.69 This is another endoscopic ultrasound image featuring the characteristic changes in the bile duct

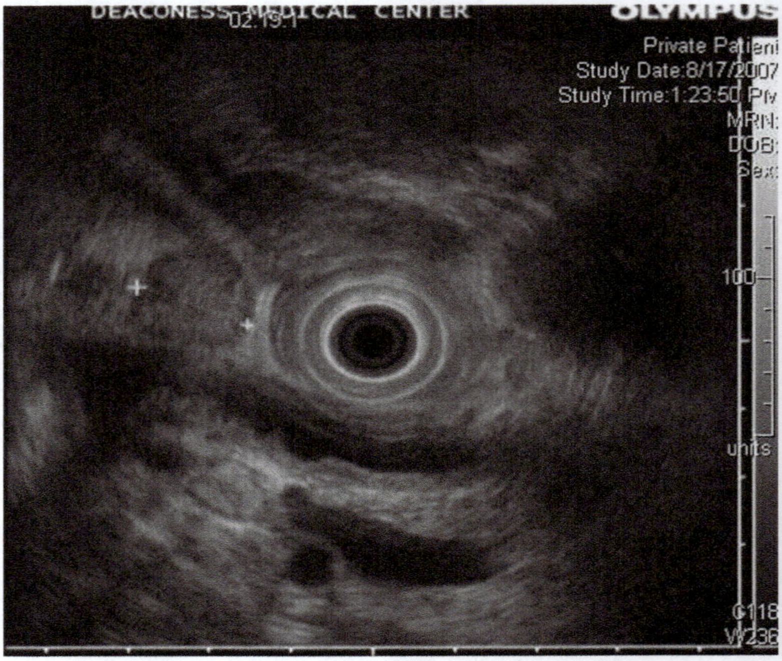

Fig. 5.70 The enlarged-appearing cystic duct lymph node was biopsied. Only reactive changes were seen

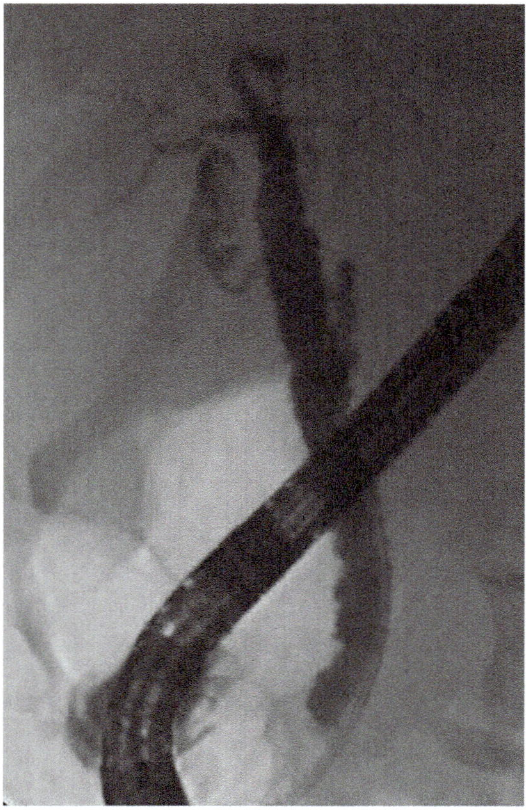

Fig. 5.71 The endoscopic retrograde cholangiopancreatography image shows the characteristic beading of the intrahepatic bile ducts and the crenellation of the extrahepatic bile ducts

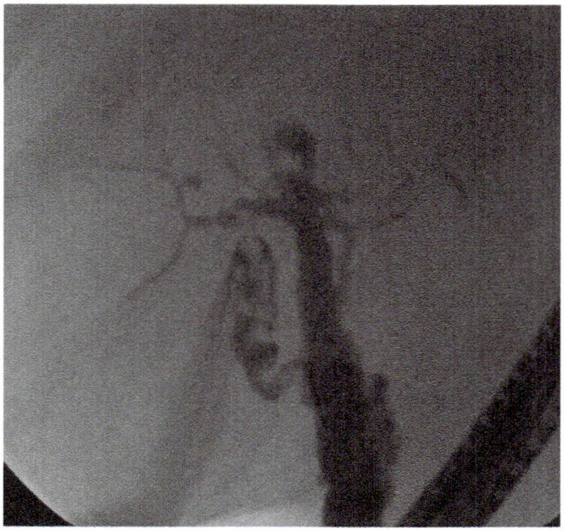

Fig. 5.72 This endoscopic retrograde cholangiopancreatography image shows a close-up of the intrahepatic ducts

5.2.3.7 Malignant Bile Duct Stricture

This is a 72-year-old patient who presented with right upper quadrant pain. Laboratory tests including liver tests were normal except for a minimally elevated alkaline phosphatase. CT was performed and initially interpreted as showing cholecystitis. An attempt at laparoscopic cholecystectomy failed and the procedure had to be converted to an open cholecystectomy. The gallbladder appeared very fibrotic. The pathology of the resected gallbladder revealed adenocarcinoma. ERCP evaluation was requested but the bile duct could not be cannulated by another examiner. The patient was then referred for EUS, which shows a tumor in the extrahepatic bile duct that wraps around the hepatic artery, making this a stage T4 or stage III cancer. In addition, the EUS showed ascites (not shown here). The CT images shown were obtained before the cholecystectomy and interpreted with the benefit of hindsight.

The largest series of cholangiocarcinoma that included preoperative EUS evaluation published to date confirms the superiority of EUS compared with CT and magnetic resonance imaging in detecting both proximal and distal bile duct tumors [23].

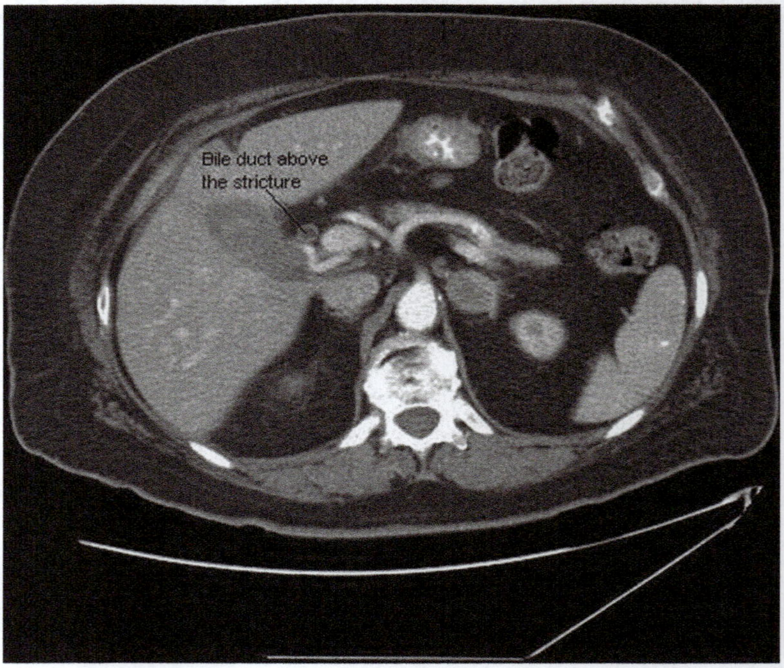

Fig. 5.73 This computed tomography scan shows the common bile duct two cuts above the stricture

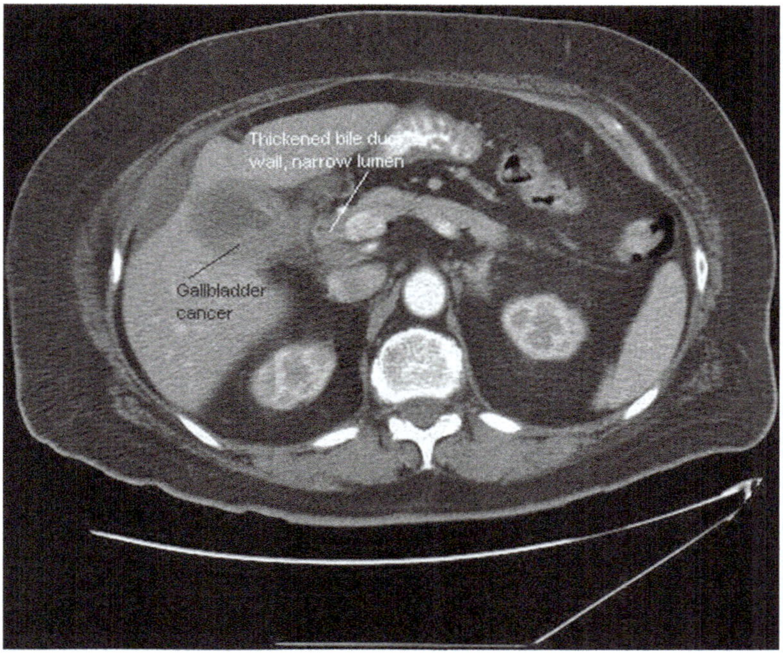

Fig. 5.74 This computed tomography slice shows an irregular filling defect in the gallbladder and a thickened bile duct wall with a small lumen

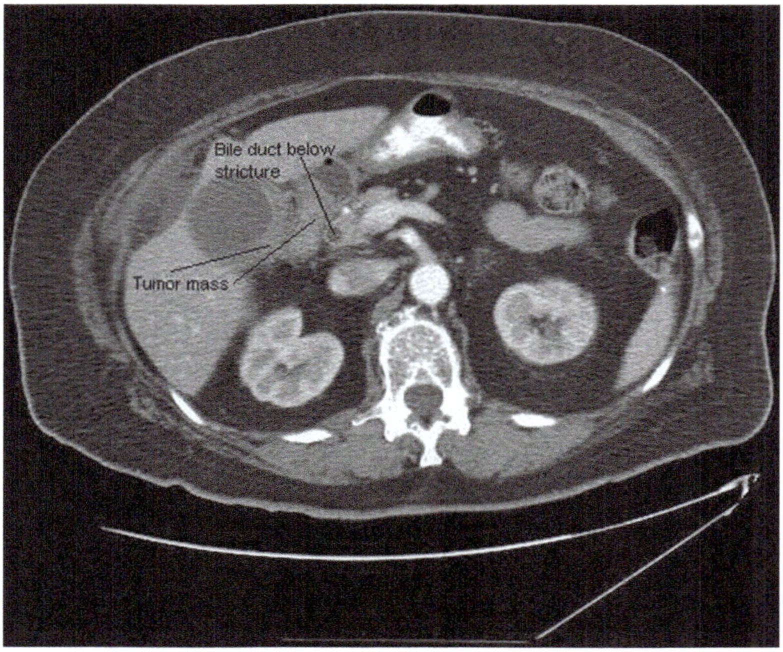

Fig. 5.75 This slice shows the bile duct below the stricture. It is still thickened but the lumen is noticeably larger

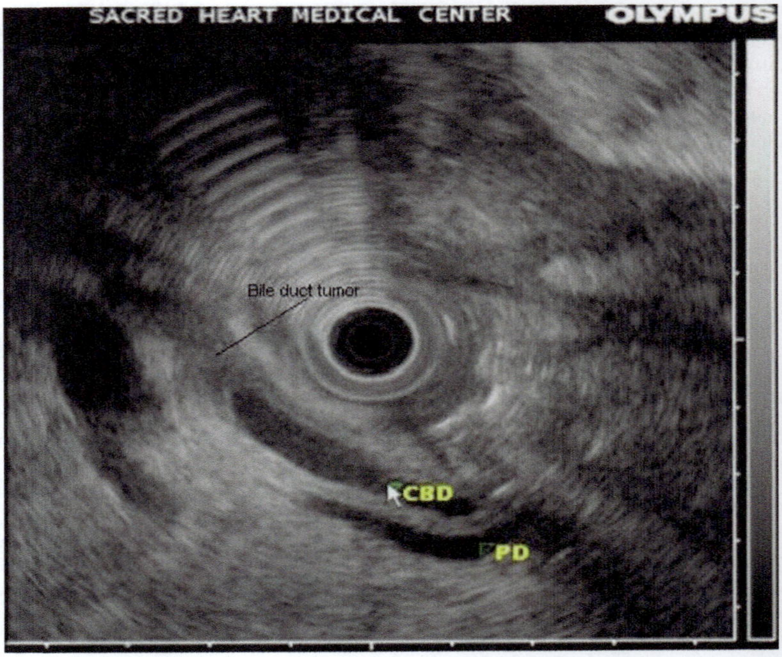

Fig. 5.76 This radial endoscopic ultrasound image shows the bile duct tumor in the mid-common bile duct (*CDB*). The lumen appears obliterated. *PD* pancreatic duct

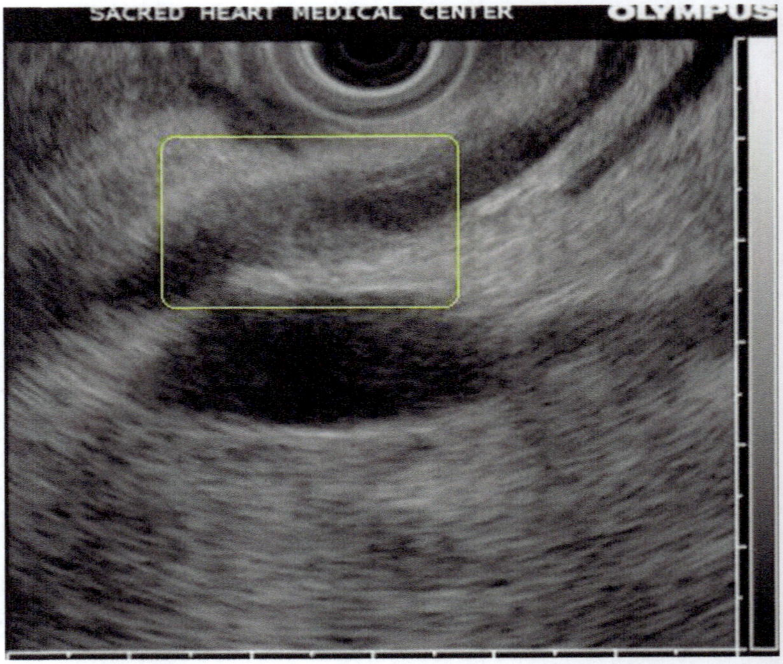

Fig. 5.77 This close-up shows the bile duct tumor in the mid-common bile duct. It is not entirely clear whether the bile duct tumor or the tumor in the gallbladder was the primary lesion

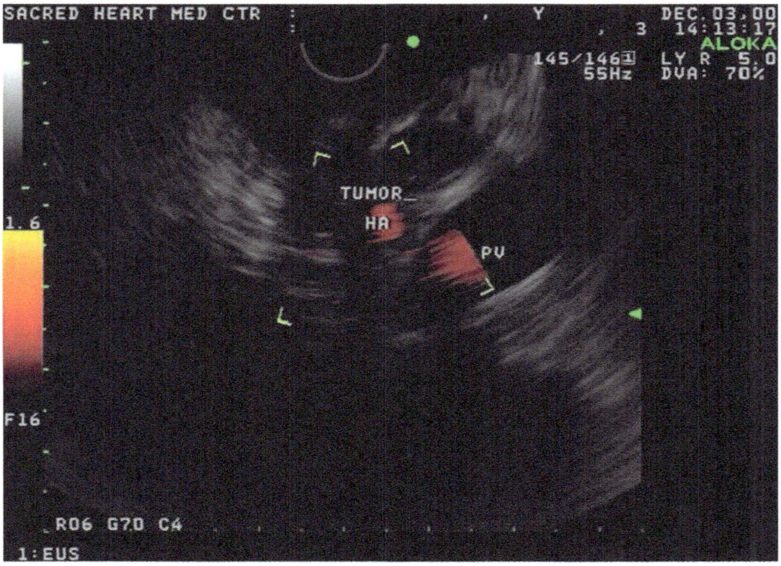

Fig. 5.78 The tumor surrounds the hepatic artery (*HA*). *PV* portal vein

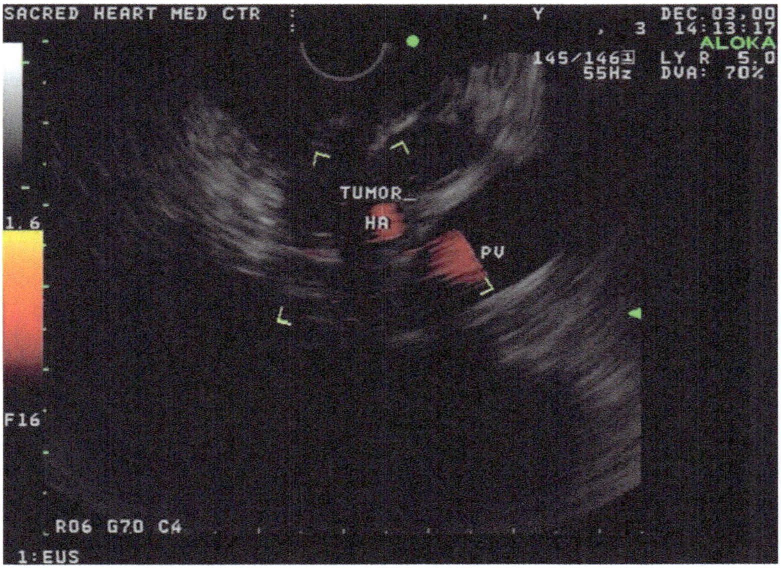

Fig. 5.79 The carcinoma surrounds the hepatic artery (*HA*). *PV* portal vein

5.2.3.8 Type II (Todani) Choledochal Cyst

Choledochal cysts are congenital anomalies of the bile ducts. They consist of cystic dilatations of the extrahepatic biliary tree, intrahepatic biliary radicles, or both. Choledochal cysts are more commonly seen in Asia than in the USA, where reported rates range from 1 case per 2 million live births to 1 case per 100,000–150,000 live births. MRCP is the preferred study to evaluate the anatomy of suspected choledochal cysts. A three-part review about choledochal cysts was recently published in an open-access journal [24–26]. This is a 66-year-old patient with a long history of abnormal liver tests and end-stage cardiomyopathy who was too claustrophobic to undergo MRCP evaluation. A CT scan shows a dilated bile duct. EUS shows a cystic structure originating from the common hepatic duct.

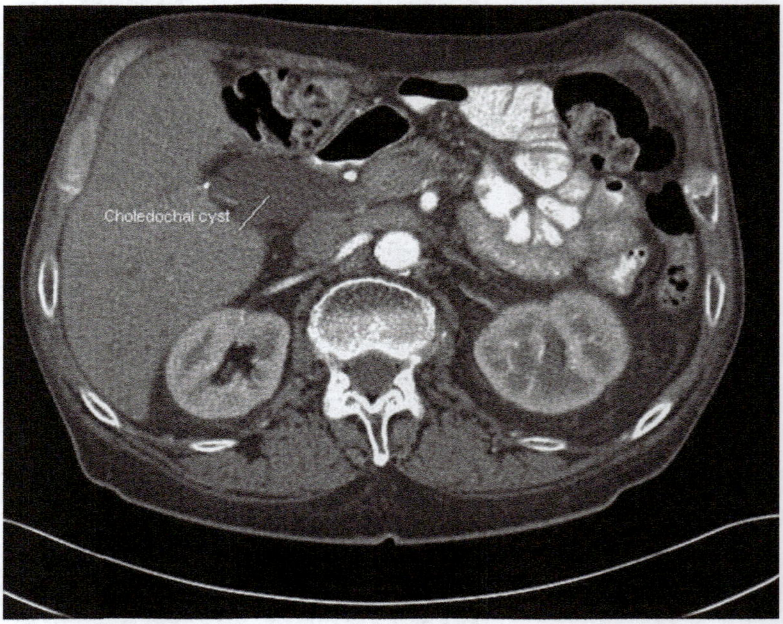

Fig. 5.80 This computed tomography scan was originally interpreted as showing bile duct dilation. A slice-by-slice review makes it clear that this is not uniform bile duct dilation but probably a choledochal cyst

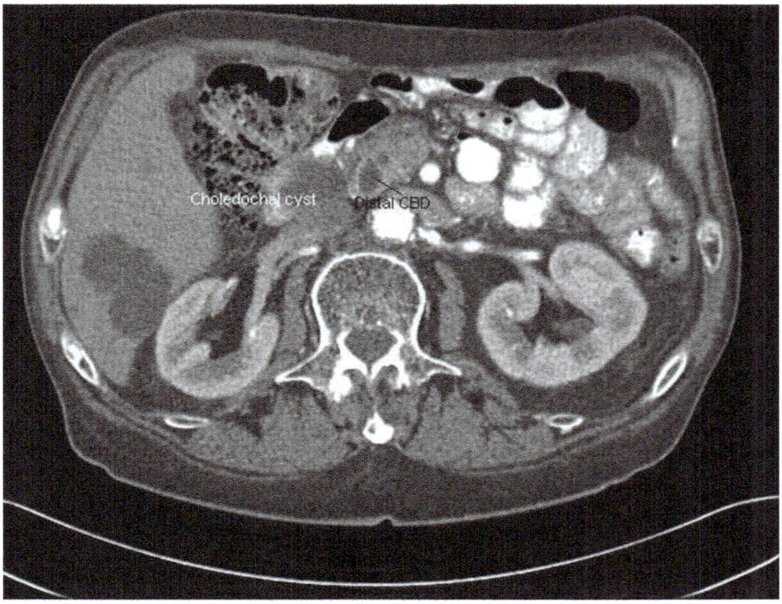

Fig. 5.81 This slice shows the choledochal cyst in relation to the common bile duct (*CBD*)

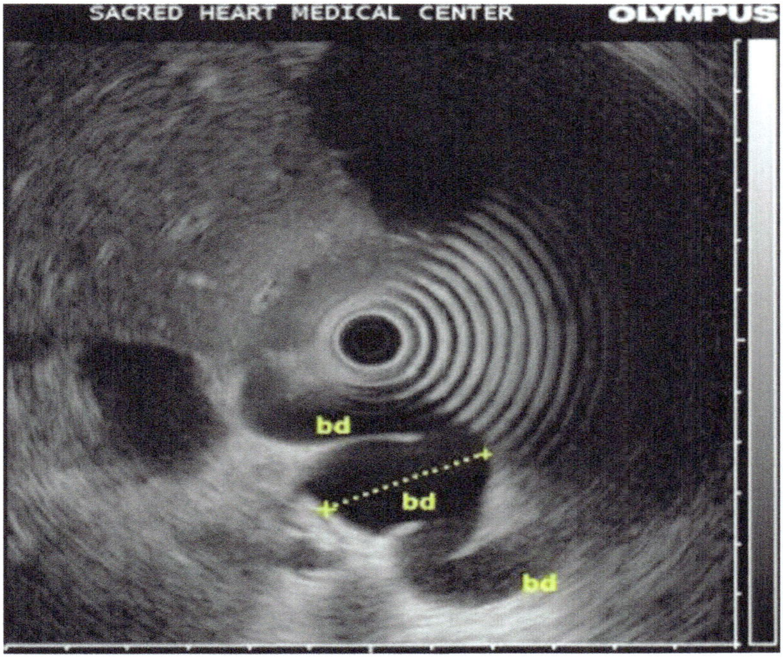

Fig. 5.82 Note the sigmoid-shaped distal common bile duct (*bd*) with the cystic outpouching apparently originating just distal to the bifurcation. According to the Todani classification, this is most consistent with a type II cyst

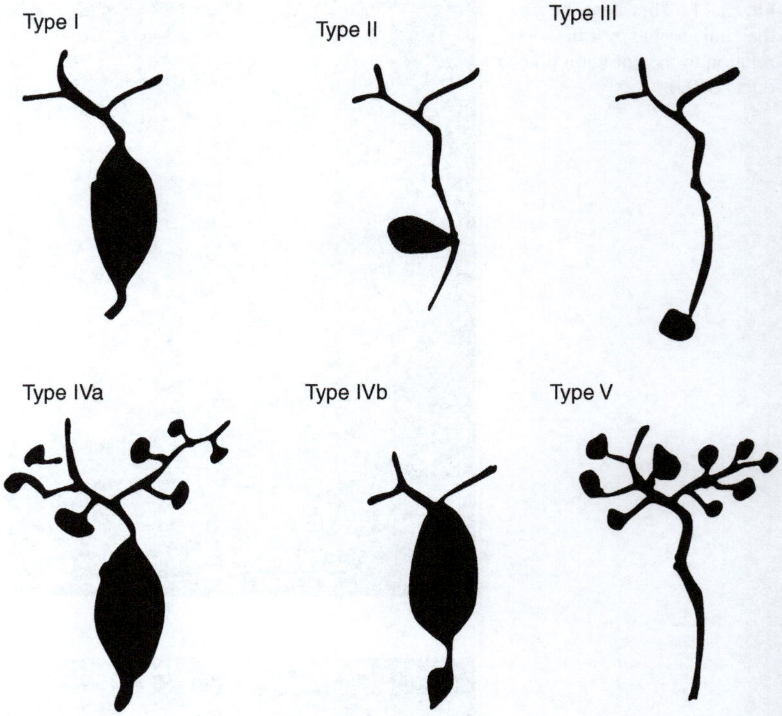

Fig. 5.83 Todani's classification of choledochal cysts: *type I* extrahepatic cyst (single), *type II* extrahepatic diverticulum, *type III* choledochocele, *type IVa* extrahepatic and intrahepatic cysts, *type IVb* multiple extrahepatic cysts, *type V* multiple intrahepatic cysts (From Shah et al. [27])

5.2.3.9 Extrinsic Compression of the Bile Duct by Metastatic Melanoma

This is a 60-year-old woman with a primary malignant melanoma arising from the paranasal sinus. She developed progressive jaundice, and a diffuse abnormality in the pancreatic head area was seen on CT. EUS-guided FNA revealed melanoma metastatic to peripancreatic and subhepatic lymph nodes, causing bile duct compression.

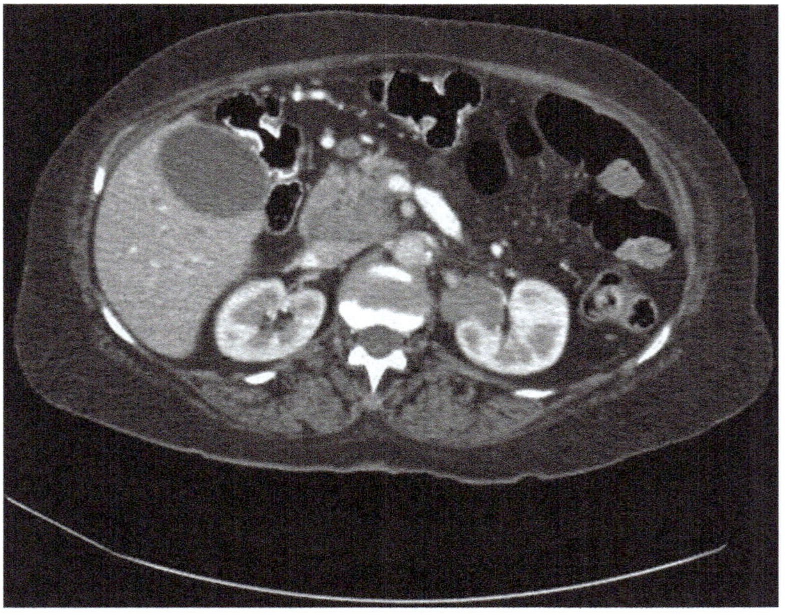

Fig. 5.84 This computed tomography scan of the abdomen shows a diffuse hypodense abnormality in the region of the head of the pancreas

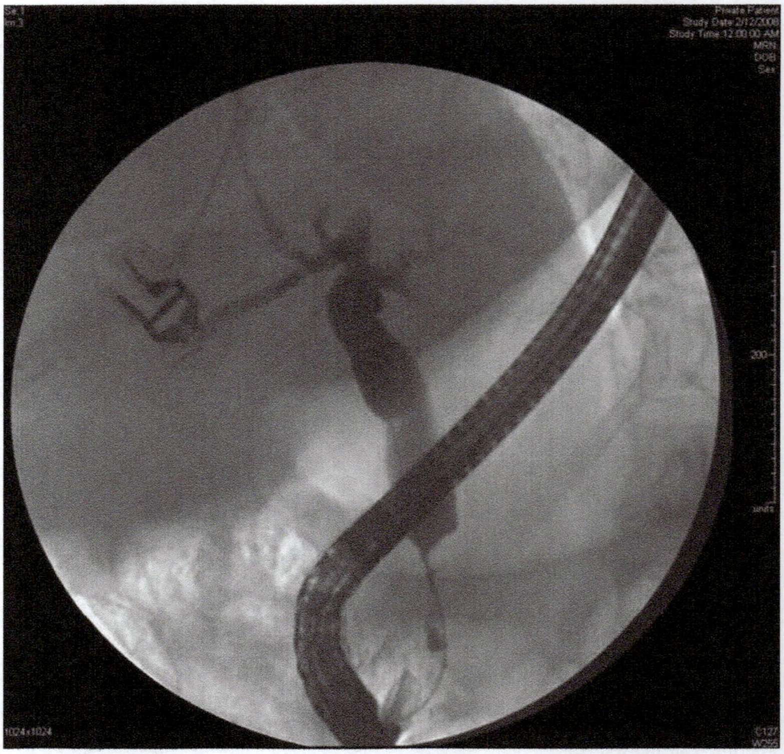

Fig. 5.85 Endoscopic retrograde cholangiopancreatography reveals a high-grade stricture of the distal common bile duct with upstream biliary dilation

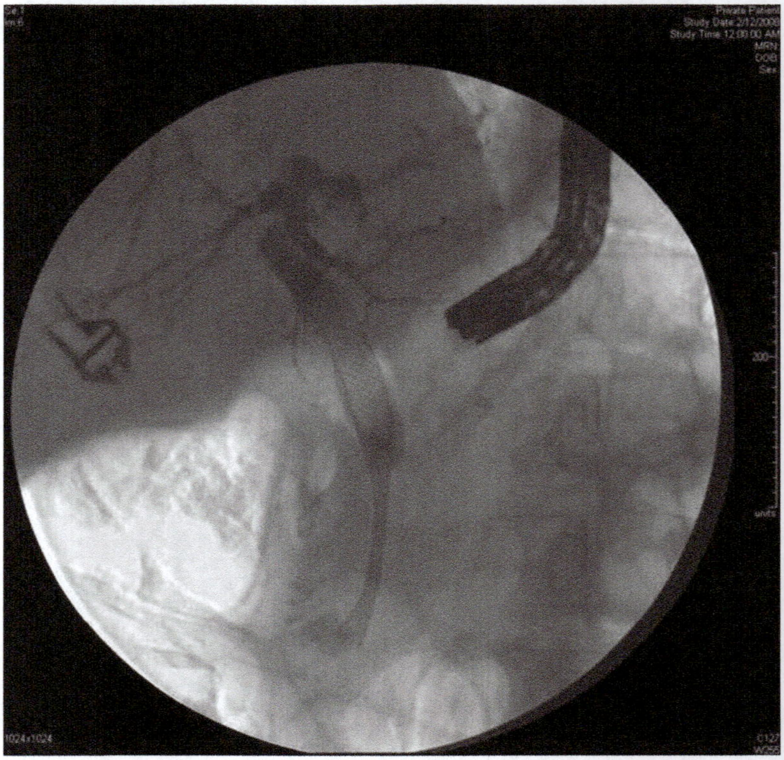

Fig. 5.86 A self-expandable metal stent was placed across the bile duct stricture

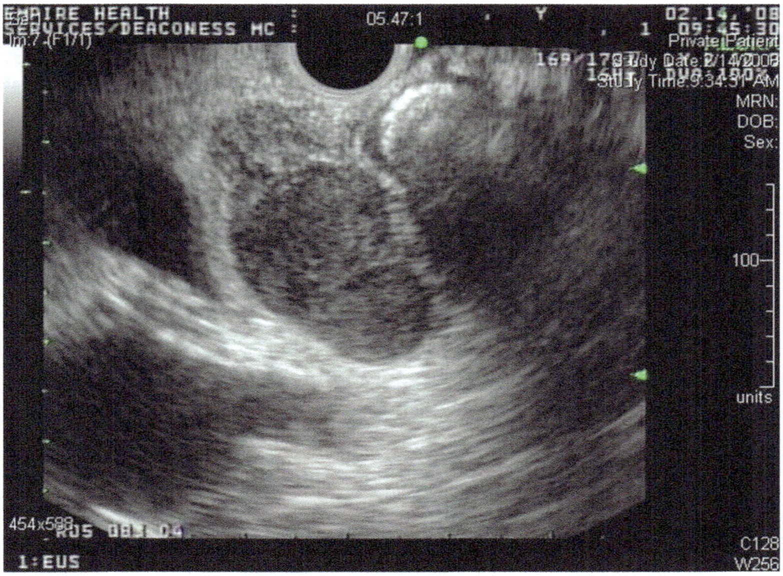

Fig. 5.87 Endoscopic ultrasound reveals the presence of a cluster of neoplastic-appearing lymph nodes that are compressing the bile duct. The metal stent can be seen as a semilunar structure close to the transducer

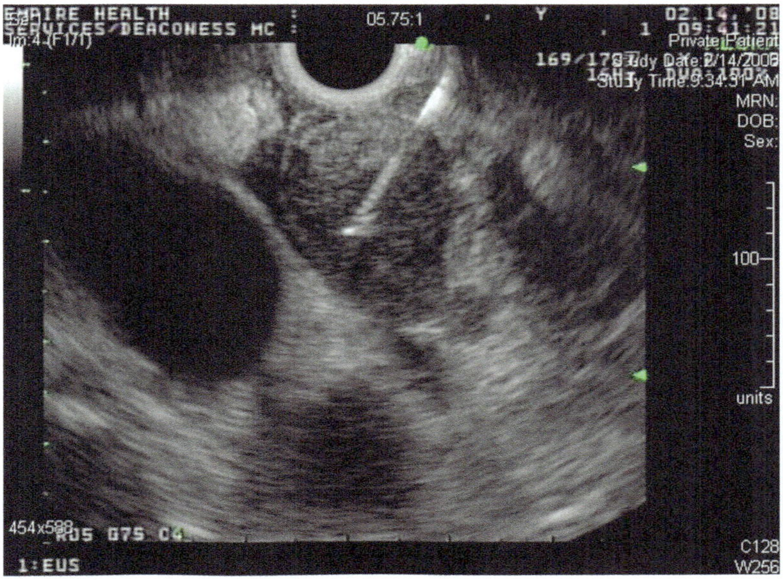

Fig. 5.88 Endoscopic ultrasound–guided fine-needle aspiration of the peripancreatic lymph node revealed metastatic melanoma

5.2.3.10 Eccentric Filling Defect in the Common Hepatic Duct

This is a 57-year-old otherwise healthy patient who had an insurance physical. His laboratory tests were normal except for a markedly elevated gamma-glutamyl transpeptidase level. Subsequent comprehensive liver chemistries and serology were normal except for a minimal elevation of alkaline phosphatase above the normal range. MRCP showed an eccentric filling defect in the common hepatic duct. A differential diagnosis of a crossing vessel, stone, polyp, fold, or neoplasm was offered. EUS with flow and spectral Doppler strongly suggests that it is the right hepatic artery that is causing the compression of the common hepatic duct. A careful reanalysis of prior CT scans and the current magnetic resonance imaging supports this notion. Few cases of compression of the common hepatic duct by the right hepatic artery have been reported [28, 29].

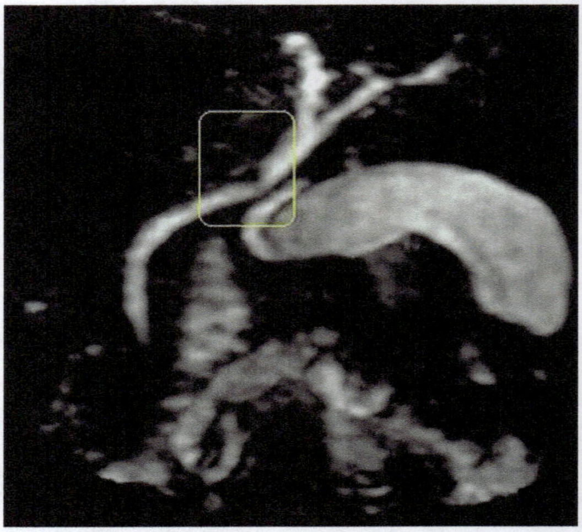

Fig. 5.89 Magnetic resonance cholangiopancreatography shows an eccentric filling defect or notch in the common hepatic duct

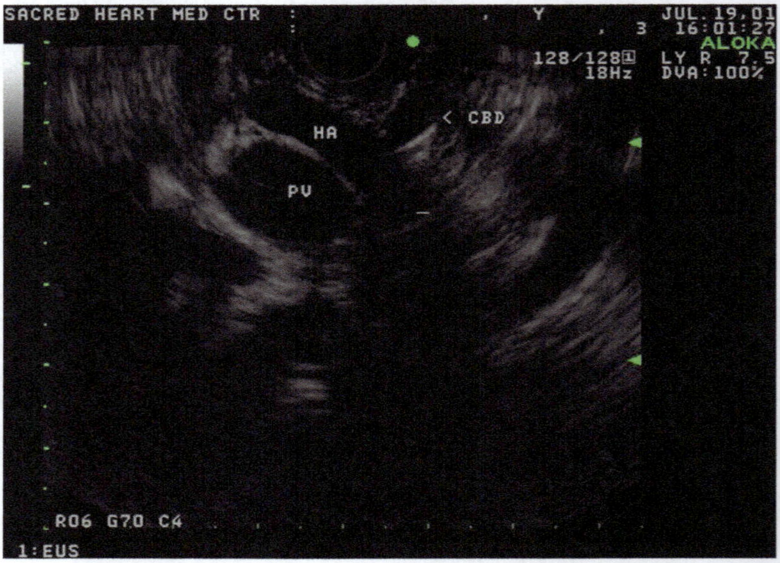

Fig.5.90 This linear endoscopic ultrasound image shows the hepatic artery (*HA*) crossing and compressing the hepatic duct. No other abnormalities were seen. *CBD* common bile duct, *PV* portal vein

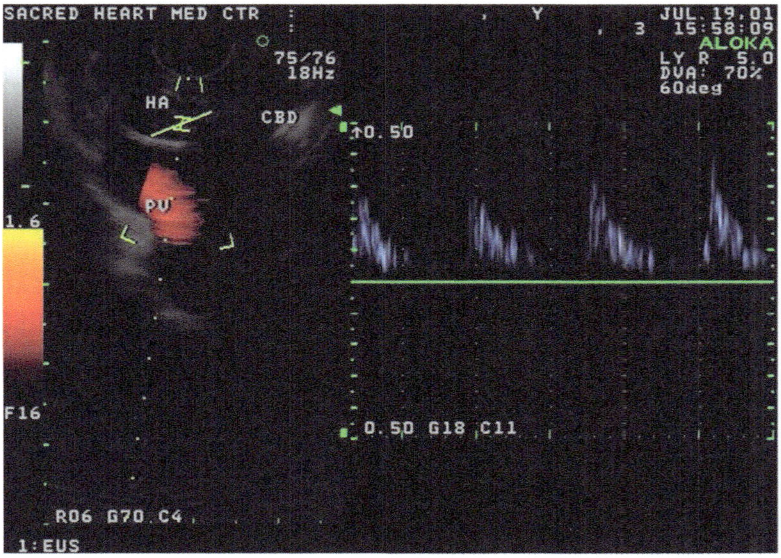

Fig. 5.91 Spectral Doppler study confirms the arterial nature of the crossing vessel. *CBD* common bile duct, *HA* hepatic artery, *PV* portal vein

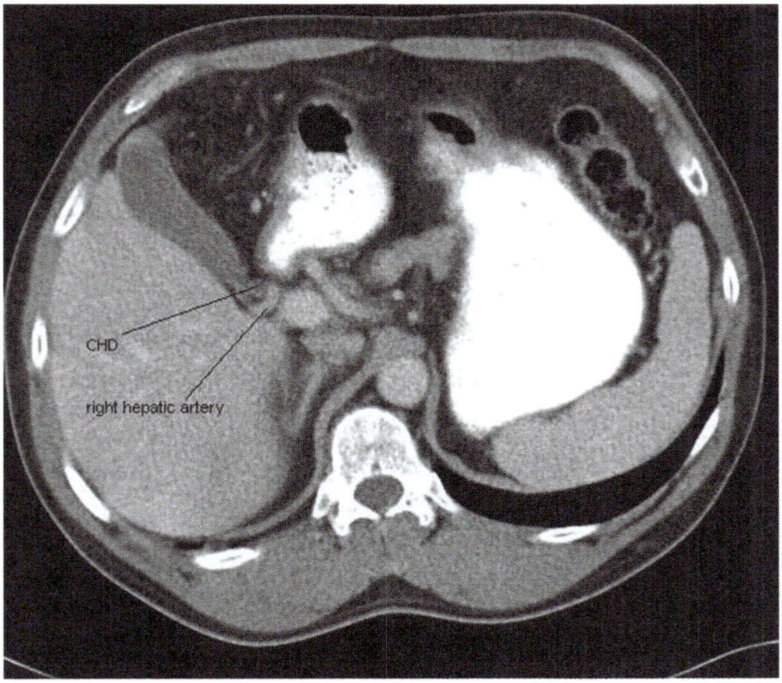

Fig. 5.92 A computed tomography scan obtained several years earlier demonstrates the relationship between the right hepatic artery and the common hepatic duct (*CHD*)

5.2.3.11 Choledochocele vs. Bile Duct Web

This is a 54-year-old patient with metastatic breast cancer and acute cholecystitis. MRCP showed an impacted cystic duct stone and an abnormality in the distal common bile duct close to the papilla, the exact nature of which was unclear. EUS evaluation was requested and the images show a mildly dilated bile duct, which seems to terminate in a saccular structure that was initially interpreted as a choledochocele. However, the EUS also clearly shows normal termination of the pancreatic duct. The majority of choledochal cysts and choledochoceles are associated with an anomalous pancreatobiliary junction. Choledochoceles also typically buckle into the duodenum. This patient appears to have a distal common bile duct web instead. Such webs are rare and may be asymptomatic but sometimes are associated with choledocholithiasis and then come to our attention [30].

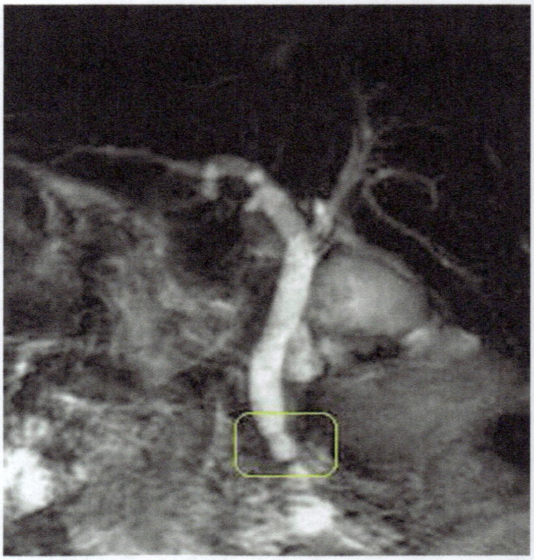

Fig. 5.93 There is a subtle notching in the distal common bile duct (upper half of the *yellow box*). Is this a choledochocele?

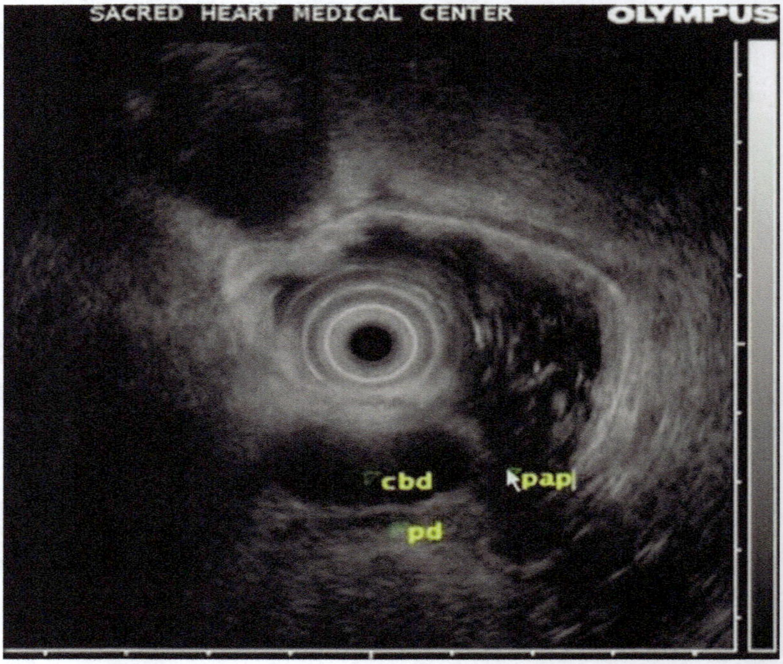

Fig. 5.94 The common bile duct (*cbd*) is prominent but the pancreatobiliary junction is normal, which argues against a choledochocele. *pd* pancreatic duct, *pap* papilla of vater

Fig. 5.95 This is not a choledochocele but rather a web in the distal common bile duct. EUS shows the shelf-like structure in the expected location

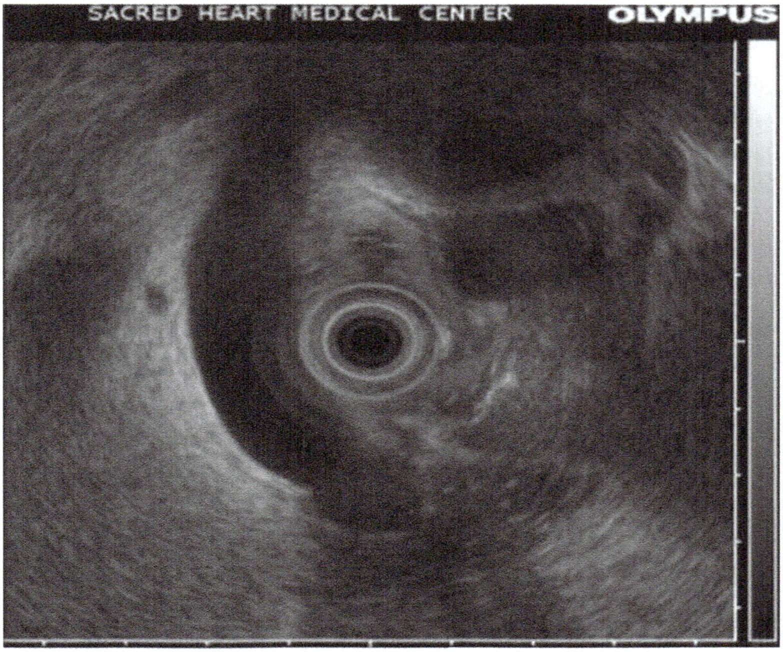

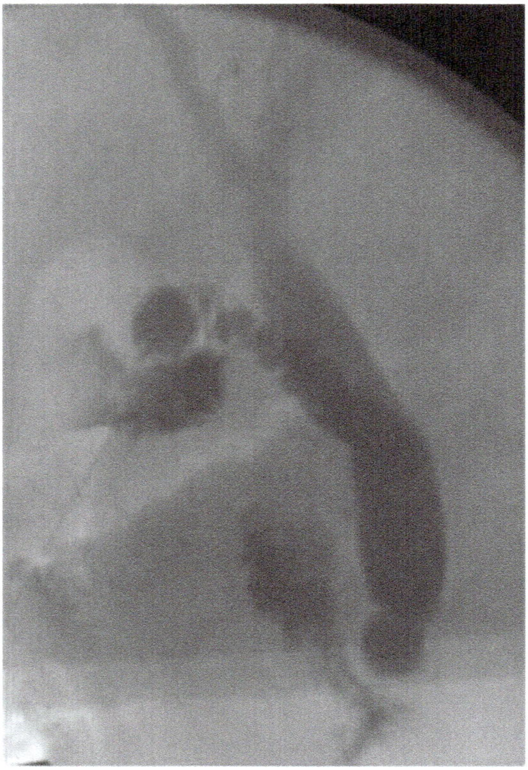

Fig. 5.96 The patient had a laparoscopic cholecystectomy. This intraoperative cholangiogram shows the web nicely. Reflux of contrast into the pancreatic duct, which was not found in this case, is a typical finding in those with an anomalous pancreatobiliary junction

5.2.3.12 Villous Lesions of the Distal Common Bile Duct

Surgical series typically reflect the experience with large (≥3 cm) villous tumors of the duodenum. Even if the initial biopsies are benign, the final surgical pathology shows carcinoma in up to 50 % of cases. The staging of villous tumors of the duodenum by EUS has been described [31] and a more recent pictorial tutorial reviews different imaging modalities [32]. This patient had a large tumor on a short pedicle originating from the periampullary region, with apparent involvement of the bile duct. This information is helpful to the surgeon and patient in planning for the surgery, which in this case would be a Whipple pancreaticoduodenectomy.

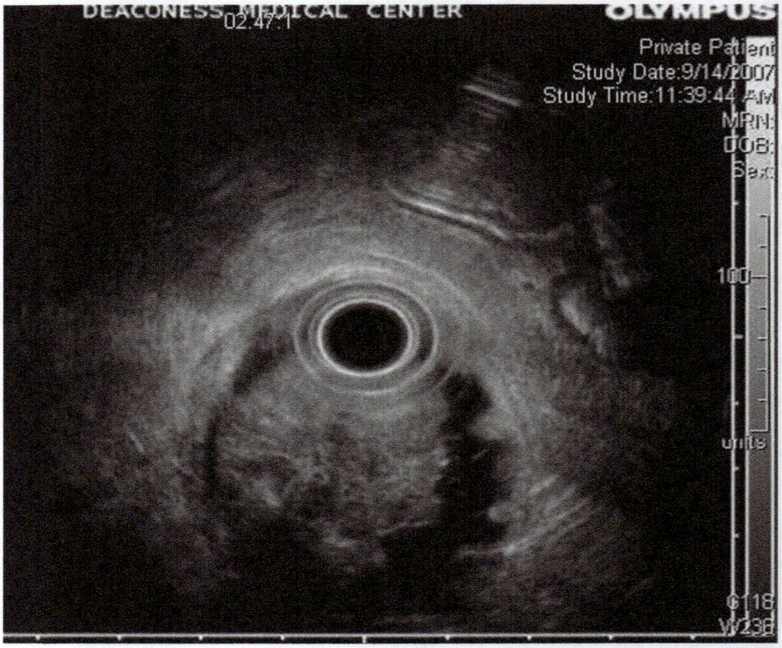

Fig. 5.97 EUS shows a 3-cm-diameter, villous-appearing periampullary duodenal tumor

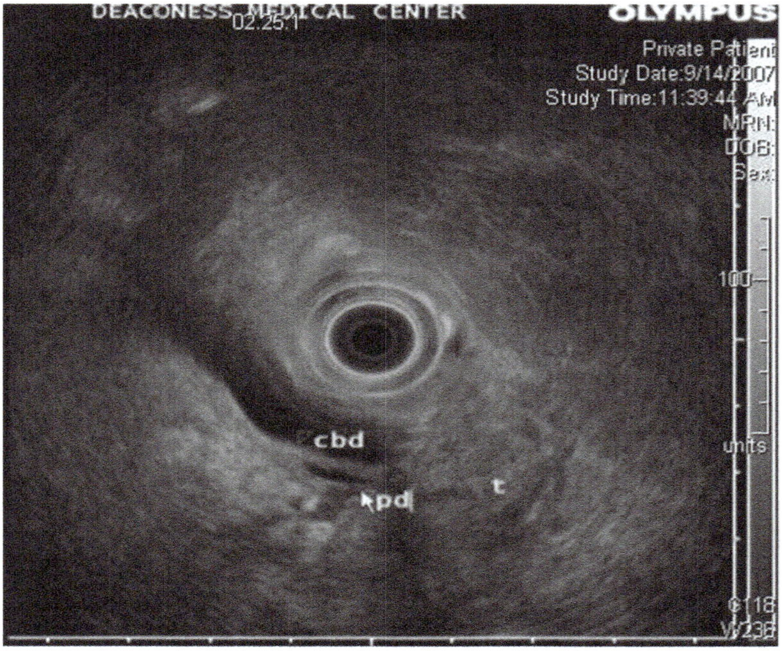

Fig. 5.98 The duodenal tumor (*t*) partially obstructs the common bile duct (*cbd*), which is mildly dilated. *pd* pancreatic duct

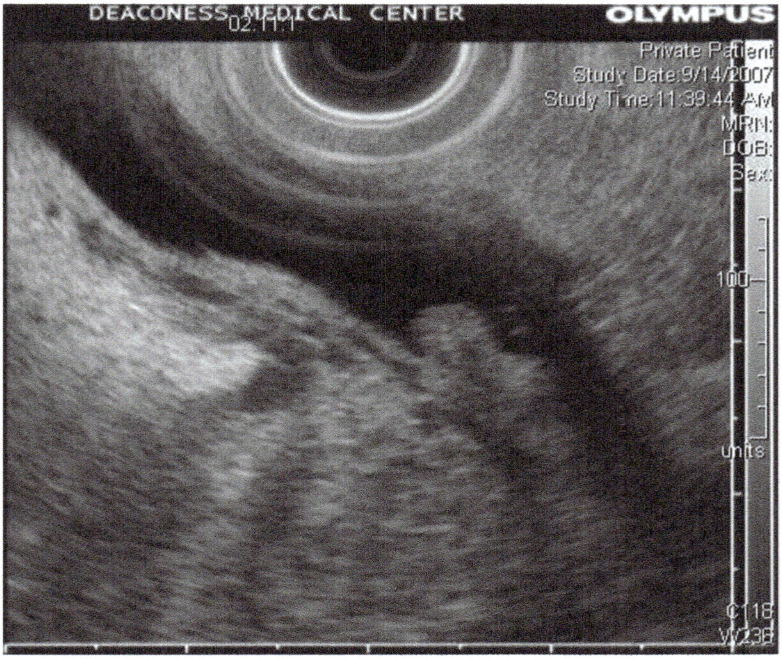

Fig. 5.99 A close-up shows extension of the villous lesion into the bile duct. Note the finely crenelated surface of the growth, differentiating it from sludge in the bile duct, which sometimes has a similar appearance

References

1. Lutz H, Buscarini E. Manual of diagnostic ultrasound. Geneva, Switzerland: World Health Organization; 2011.
2. Loreno M, Travali S, Bucceri AM, Scalisi G, Virgilio C, Brogna A. Ultrasonographic study of gallbladder wall thickness and emptying in cirrhotic patients without gallstones. Gastroenterol Res Pract. 2009;2009:683040.
3. Lazcano-Ponce EC, Miquel JF, Muñoz N, Herrero R, Ferrecio C, Wistuba II, et al. Epidemiology and molecular pathology of gallbladder cancer. CA Cancer J Clin. 2001;51(6):349–64.
4. Matsumoto M, Maruta M, Maeda K, Utsumi T, Sugioka A, Kuroda M. Epithelial cyst of the gallbladder associated with adenocarcinoma. J Hepatobiliary Pancreat Surg. 2002;9(3):389–92.
5. Courvoisier LG. Casuistisch-statistische Beiträge zur Pathologie und Chirurgie der Gallenwege. Leipzig: Vogel; 1890.
6. Cowles RA, Mulholland MW. Solitary hepatic cysts. J Am Coll Surg. 2000;191(3):311–21.
7. Ishikawa H, Uchida S, Yokokura Y, Iwasaki Y, Horiuchi H, Hiraki M, et al. Nonparasitic solitary huge liver cysts causing intracystic hemorrhage or obstructive jaundice. J Hepatobiliary Pancreat Surg. 2002;9(6):764–8.
8. Ito H, Tsujimoto F, Nakajima Y, Igarashi G, Okamura T, Sakurai M, et al. Sonographic characterization of 271 hepatic hemangiomas with typical appearance on CT imaging. J Med Ultrason. 2012;39(2):61–8.
9. Singh P, Erickson RA, Mukhopadhyay P, Gopal S, Kiss A, Khan A, et al. EUS for detection of the hepatocellular carcinoma: results of a prospective study. Gastrointest Endosc. 2007;66(2):265–73.
10. Maheshwari A, Kantsevoy S, Jagannath S, Thuluvath PJ. Endoscopic ultrasound and fine-needle aspiration for the diagnosis of hepatocellular carcinoma. Clin Liver Dis. 2010;14(2):325–32.
11. Kimura H, Matsubayashi H, Fukutomi A, Asakura K, Sasaki K, Yamaguchi Y, et al. Lymph node metastasis diagnosed by EUS-FNA in four cases with hepatocellular carcinoma. Clin Res Hepatol Gastroenterol. 2011;35(3):237–40.
12. Braden B, Faust D, Ignee A, Schreiber D, Hirche T, Dietrich CF. Clinical relevance of perihepatic lymphadenopathy in acute and chronic liver disease. J Clin Gastroenterol. 2008;42(8):931–6.
13. Marchal G, Oyen R, Verschakelen J, Gelin J, Baert AL, Stessens RC. Sonographic appearance of normal lymph nodes. J Ultrasound Med. 1985;4(8):417–9.
14. Ying MTC, Cho CCM, Ahuja AT. Lymph nodes. In: Ultrasound of the thyroid and parathyroid glands. New York: Springer; 2012. p. 211–28.
15. Dancygier H. Gross anatomy. In: Clinical hepatology. Berlin/Heidelberg: Springer; 2010. p. 11–4.
16. Coss A, Enns R. The investigation of unexplained biliary dilatation. Curr Gastroenterol Rep. 2009;11(2): 155–9.
17. Van Hoe L, Mermuys K, Vanhoenacker P. MRCP pitfalls. Abdom Imaging. 2004;29(3):360–87.
18. Cohen S, Bacon BR, Berlin JA, Fleischer D, Hecht GA, Loehrer PJ, et al. National Institutes of Health State-of-the-Science Conference Statement: ERCP for diagnosis and therapy, January 14–16, 2002. Gastrointest Endosc. 2002;56(6):803–9.
19. Coakley FV. Pearls and pitfalls in abdominal imaging: pseudotumors variants and other difficult diagnoses. Cambridge: Cambridge University Press; 2010.
20. Farahmand H, PourGholami M, Fathollah MS. Chronic extrahepatic bile duct dilatation: sonographic screening in the patients with opioid addiction. Korean J Radiol. 2007;8(3):212.
21. Zahedi-Nejad N, Narouei S, Fahimy F. Common Bile Duct (CBD) diameter in opium-addicted men: comparison with non-addict controls. Pol J Radiol. 2010;75(3):20–4.
22. Krones E, Graziadei I, Trauner M, Fickert P. Evolving concepts in primary sclerosing cholangitis. Liver Int. 2012;32(3):352–69.
23. Mohamadnejad M, DeWitt JM, Sherman S, LeBlanc JK, Pitt HA, House MG, et al. Role of EUS for preoperative evaluation of cholangiocarcinoma: a large single-center experience. Gastrointest Endosc. 2011;73(1):71–8.
24. Singham J, Yoshida EM, Scudamore CH. Choledochal cysts. Can J Surg. 2009;52(5):434–40.
25. Singham J, Yoshida EM, Scudamore CH. Choledochal cysts: part 2 of 3: diagnosis. Can J Surg. 2009;52(6): 506–11.
26. Singham J, Yoshida EM, Scudamore CH. Choledochal cysts. Part 3 of 3: management. Can J Surg. 2010; 53(1):51–6.
27. Shah OJ, et al. Choledochal cysts in children and adults with contrasting profiles: 11-year experience at a tertiary care center in Kashmir. World journal of surgery. 2009;33(11):2403–11.
28. Izuishi K, Toyama Y, Wakabayashi H, Usuki H, Maeta H. Compression of the common hepatic duct by the right hepatic artery. Clin Imaging. 2005;29(5): 342–4.
29. Gottlieb K, Brophy MC. Hepatic duct compression syndrome diagnosed by endoscopic ultrasound. J Gastrointestin Liver Dis. 2007;16(3):350–1.
30. Papaziogas B, Lazaridis C, Pavlidis T, Galanis I, Paraskevas G, Papaziogas T. Congenital web of the common bile duct in association with cholelithiasis. J Hepatobiliary Pancreat Surg. 2002;9(2):271–3.
31. Tio TL, Sie LH, Verbeek PC, Wit LTD, Tytgat GN. Endosonography in diagnosing and staging duodenal villous adenoma. Gut. 1992;33(4):567–8.
32. Izgur V, Dass C, Solomides CC. Villous duodenal adenoma1. Radiographics. 2010;30(1):295–9.

Pancreas

6

Contents

6.1 **General Principles** ... 298
6.1.1 Technique ... 298
6.1.2 Endoscopic Ultrasound Probes ... 298
6.1.3 Anatomic Considerations ... 298
6.1.3.1 Ventral and Dorsal Pancreas ... 299

6.2 **Cases and Discussions** ... 301
6.2.1 Acute Pancreatitis with an Edematous Pancreatic Head ... 301
6.2.2 Chronic Pancreatitis ... 306
6.2.2.1 Chronic Pancreatitis with a Stone in the Pancreatic Duct ... 306
6.2.3 Pancreatic Parenchymal Calcifications and Stone in the Pancreatic Duct ... 308
6.2.4 Fatty Infiltration of the Pancreas ... 311
6.2.5 Perivascular Fat Mimicking a Dilated Main Pancreatic Duct ... 314
6.2.6 Vanishing Pancreatic Mass ... 317
6.2.7 Pancreatic Cancer ... 320
6.2.7.1 Stage IV Pancreatic Cancer with Extensive Collaterals ... 320
6.2.8 T2 Adenocarcinoma of the Pancreas ... 323
6.2.9 Pancreatic Tail Mass ... 326
6.2.10 Calcifications in a Hypoechoic Pancreas Tumor ... 328
6.2.11 Chronic Pancreatitis and Pancreatic Cancer ... 329
6.2.12 Small Pancreatic Cancer ... 332
6.2.13 Isodense Pancreatic Cancer ... 334
6.2.14 Large Pancreatic Head in Relation to Body ... 338
6.2.15 Gardner's Syndrome and Pancreatic Cancer ... 341
6.2.16 Missed Pancreatic Cancer ... 344
6.2.17 Ovarian Cancer Metastatic to the Pancreas? ... 348
6.2.18 Characteristic Appearance of a Wallstent on EUS ... 351
6.2.19 FNA Biopsies Through a Wallstent ... 354
6.2.20 Neuroendocrine Tumors ... 355
6.2.20.1 Simultaneous Metastatic Carcinoid and Symptomatic Insulinoma ... 355
6.2.20.2 Cystic Neuroendocrine Tumors of the Pancreas ... 359
6.2.21 Primary Pancreatic Lymphoma ... 361
6.2.22 Mycosis Fungoides Infiltrating the Pancreas ... 364
6.2.23 Pancreatic Cysts ... 367
6.2.23.1 Pancreatic Cyst with Complex Vessel Relationships ... 367
6.2.23.2 Pancreatic Cyst with a Small Polypoid Structure Inside ... 370
6.2.23.3 Pancreatic Pseudocyst ... 373
6.2.23.4 Mucinous Cystic Neoplasm of the Pancreas ... 376
6.2.24 Serous Cystadenoma ... 379

References ... 381

Box 6.1: Resources

- Ian Penman (editor) (eBook)
  Meenan J. EUS: pancreatobiliary. In: Penman I (editor). *Endoscopic Ultrasound*. Wiley-Blackwell and GastroHep.com; 2013 http://www.gastrohep.com/ebooks/ebook.asp?book=1405120819&id=5
- Medical University of South Carolina Digestive Disease Center: EUS Atlas: Normal Anatomy (images) http://www.ddc.musc.edu/professional/education/atlases/EUSatlas/normalAnatomy.cfm

K. Gottlieb, G. Marino, *Diagnostic Endosonography*,
DOI 10.1007/978-3-642-39118-7_6, © Springer-Verlag Berlin Heidelberg 2014

- Medical University of South Carolina Digestive Disease Center: EUS Video Atlas http://www.ddc.musc.edu/professional/education/atlases/EUSvideoAtlas.cfm
- Medical University of South Carolina Digestive Disease Center: Normal pancreas exam during endoscopic ultrasound (used as reference to demonstrate absence of signs of chronic pancreatitis), Drs. G. P. Althal and M. Wallace, Medical University of South Carolina http://www.youtube.com/watch?v=jos33wotYRg
- EUS examination of the pancreas, Dr. Shyam Varadarajulu (uploaded by Boston Scientific) http://www.youtube.com/watch?v=S0UGyD5JGqA
- EUS FNA demonstration of fanning technique, Dr. Shyam Varadarajulu (uploaded by Boston Scientific) http://www.youtube.com/watch?v=RcLhvSdCXtc
- Dave Project – Gastroenterology: Multiple cases demonstrating the use of EUS in pancreatic pathology http://daveproject.org/category/pancreas/
- World Endoscopy Organization: EUS and FNA of a complex pancreatic cystic neuroendocrine tumor by Dr. William R. Brugge, Massachusetts General Hospital http://www.worldendo.org/weo-video-william-brugge.html

6.1 General Principles

6.1.1 Technique

A complete description of the endoscopic technique is available in most textbooks about endoscopic ultrasound (EUS). We recommend study of video recordings to review these techniques and endoscopic maneuvers and develop a systematic approach that goes through the standard EUS stations (body of the stomach, antrum, duodenal bulb, descending duodenum, and third portion of the duodenum), starting at the landmark structures of each station to achieve a complete exam. This systematic approach minimizes the risk of missed lesions or false interpretation of normal variants as abnormalities or masses.

We cannot emphasize enough that to interrogate the pancreas with EUS the endosonographer must have a clear understanding of the normal anatomy of the retroperitoneal region, which provides specific landmarks that allow sonographic recognition of the pancreatic head, body, and tail as well as the surrounding structures.

6.1.2 Endoscopic Ultrasound Probes

Radial and linear scanning echoendoscopes are able to provide complete visualization of the pancreas from different planes of orientation. The preference of endoscope depends on training, experience, and personal preference. Ultrasound waves of lower frequencies (5–7.5 MHz) penetrate deeper, resulting in better visualization of the surrounding anatomy.

6.1.3 Anatomic Considerations

The splenic vein is easily identified from the body of the stomach and provides a good landmark reference given its direct contact with the pancreatic body and tail. This vein is usually found dorsal to the pancreas; it is confirmed and differentiated from other structures such as left renal vein by tracing it from the splenic hilum to the portal confluence. The celiac trunk and superior mesenteric artery allow rapid identification of the pancreatic body during linear EUS because the pancreas lies ventral to the superior mesenteric artery.

The portal vein is a key landmark for the identification of the pancreatic head at the duodenum and can be traced from its confluence to the hepatic hilum. The bile duct can also be identified and followed from the major papilla to the hilum. In the case of biliary obstruction, EUS provides excellent information and allows identification of intraductal lesions or defects, mural thickening, or extrinsic compression and masses. Other important structures that require EUS evaluation from the duodenum include the superior mesenteric artery and vein.

6.1.3.1 Ventral and Dorsal Pancreas

The embryologic pancreas consists of a dorsal bud and a ventral bud or anlage. The dorsal bud arises as a diverticulum of the dorsal aspect of the duodenum (hence the name). The ventral anlage originates as a common diverticulum with the primitive common bile duct (see Fig. 6.1). At 6 weeks the ventral bud rotates 270 degrees to lie posterior and inferior to the dorsal bud (Fig. 6.1b). Fusion of these two buds forms the mature pancreas. In most individuals there are subtle differences in the density on computed tomography (CT), intensity on magnetic resonance imaging (MRI), or echogenicity between these two components, which border each other in the head of the pancreas. The less echogenic ventral pancreas contains less fat than the embryolcgic dorsal pancreas. The difference is noticeable in up to 25 % of normal individuals using abdominal CT or transcutaneous ultrasound [1, 2]. This difference is more frequently detected by EUS; it has been reported in 72 % of patients with normal parenchyma and 29 % of patients with a clear mass or chronic pancreatitis [3]. In the fi-st case below (Acute Pancreatitis with an Edematous Head of Pancreas), a hypodense area of the pancreas was observed (see Fig. 6.2) and the patient was referred for EUS, which showed no mass but the typical differences in echogenicity seen between the ventral and dorsal pancreas. This EUS finding should be easily recognized and not confused with chronic pancreatitis or maligr.ancy.

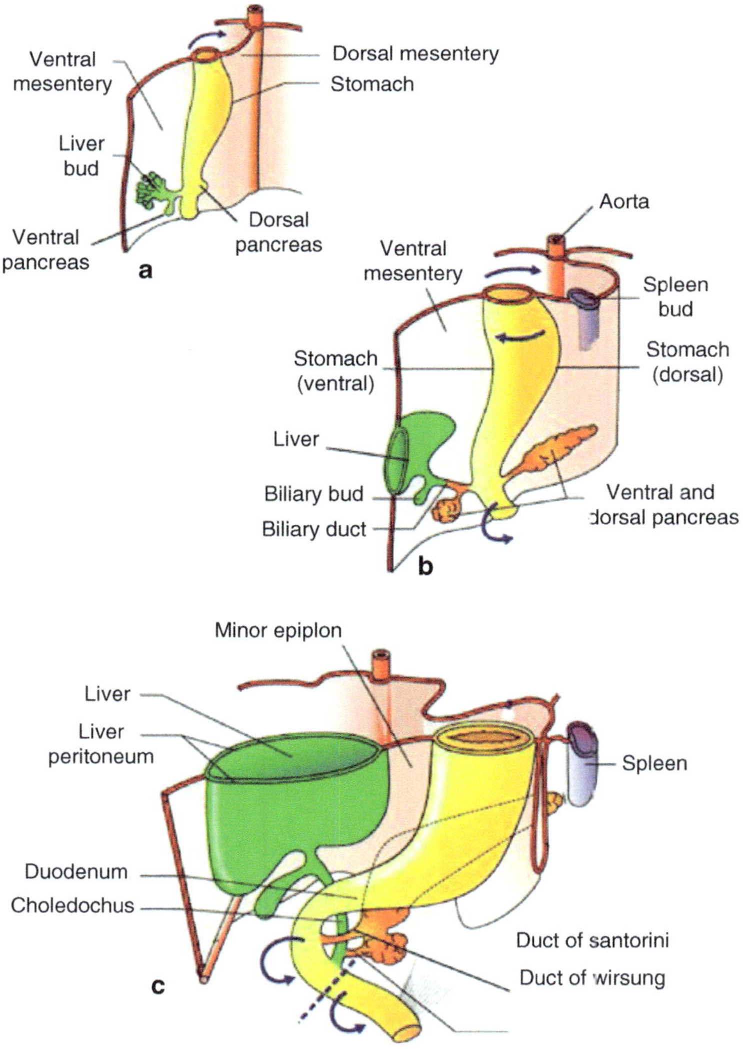

Fig. 6.1 Development of the pancreas in human embryos at 5 (*a*), 6 (*b*), and 7(*c*) weeks. *Arrows* indicate the sense of rotation of the primitive intestine around its longitudinal axis. *Broken line*, limit between foregut and midgut (From Rovasio [4])

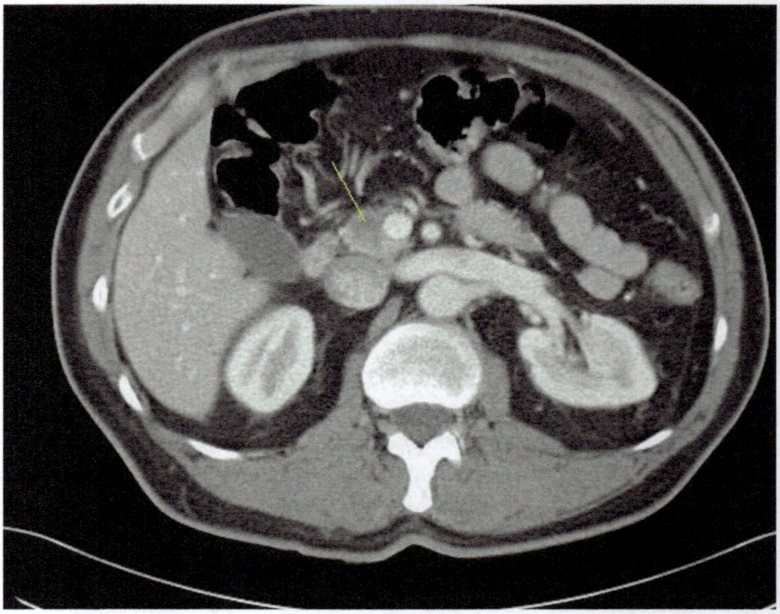

Fig. 6.2 There is a hypodense area in the head of the pancreas (indicated by the *yellow line*)

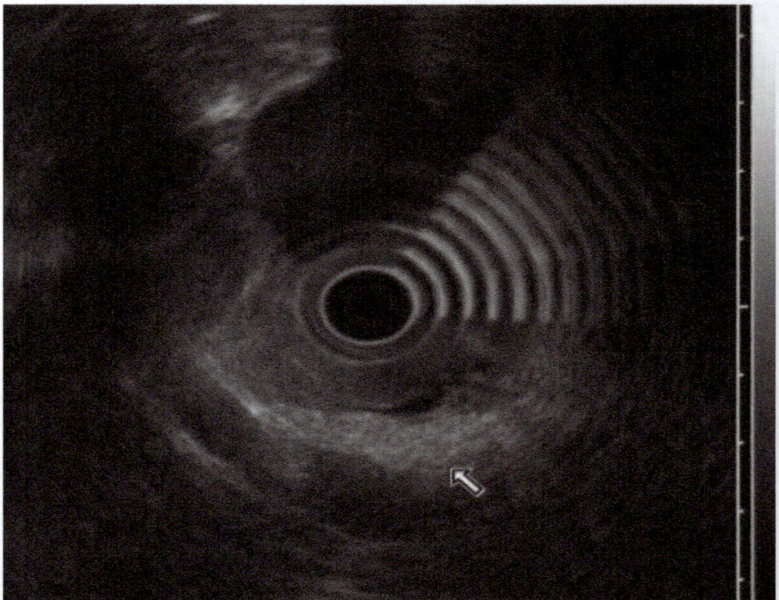

Fig. 6.3 This endoscopic ultrasound image shows a clear demarcation between echo-rich (dorsal, *arrow*) and echo-poor (ventral) pancreas

6.2 Cases and Discussions

6.2.1 Acute Pancreatitis with an Edematous Pancreatic Head

This is a 39-year-old woman admitted to the hospital with acute pancreatitis. At admission her lipase level was 1,238 U/l, but it fell to 210 U/l the following day. She has had a cholecystectomy. An endoscopic retrograde cholangiopancreatography (ERCP) was performed by a different examiner on the day after admission and only the pancreatic duct was injected. The bile duct could not be cannulated. Following the ERCP her lipase level increased from 210 to 7,068 U/l, which his most consistent with pancreatitis after ERCP superimposed on acute spontaneous pancreatitis. An magnetic resonance cholangiopancreatography (MRCP) then was ordered and showed "a dilated tapered common bile duct" but was otherwise unremarkable. Two days later CT was requested to evaluate for pseudocysts. Curiously, the radiologist reported dilation of the bile duct to 2 cm and a "double duct sign" with a dilated pancreatic duct. The clinicians were worried about a pancreatic malignancy and requested clarification by EUS. Performed on the third day after failed ERCP, which had resulted in pancreatitis, EUS showed compression of the intrapancreatic portion of the common bile duct, a normal pancreatic duct, and cystic spaces in the head of the pancreas consistent with acute pancreatitis.

EUS is considered useful in the evaluation of acute pancreatitis of unclear etiology. In experienced hands it can provide excellent views of the extrahepatic bile ducts in more than 95 % of cases [5, 6], and it is frequently performed during the initial phase of pancreatitis to diagnose choledocholithiasis and better select patients who really need therapeutic ERCP, avoiding unnecessary risks. Studies evaluating EUS during an acute attack of pancreatitis have shown a sensitivity of 91–100 % and a specificity of 85–100 % in diagnosing choledocholithiasis [7].

EUS has the potential to detect pancreatic ductal abnormalities during acute pancreatitis, although its role in this setting has not been completely evaluated [7]. The appearance of the pancreas during acute pancreatitis is variable: the size of the gland can be normal or enlarged, and its sonographic pattern is frequently described as hypoechoic but occasionally of normal echogenicity and sometimes hyperechoic or mixed. Small studies have attempted to describe the appearance of pancreatic necrosis as focal hypoechoic areas [8, 9], but these findings require validation in larger studies.

Once the acute attack has subsided, EUS can also be used to evaluate for causes of pancreatitis, including pancreatic and ampullary solid tumors, intraductal papillary mucinous neoplasms, biliary sludge, and pancreas divisum.

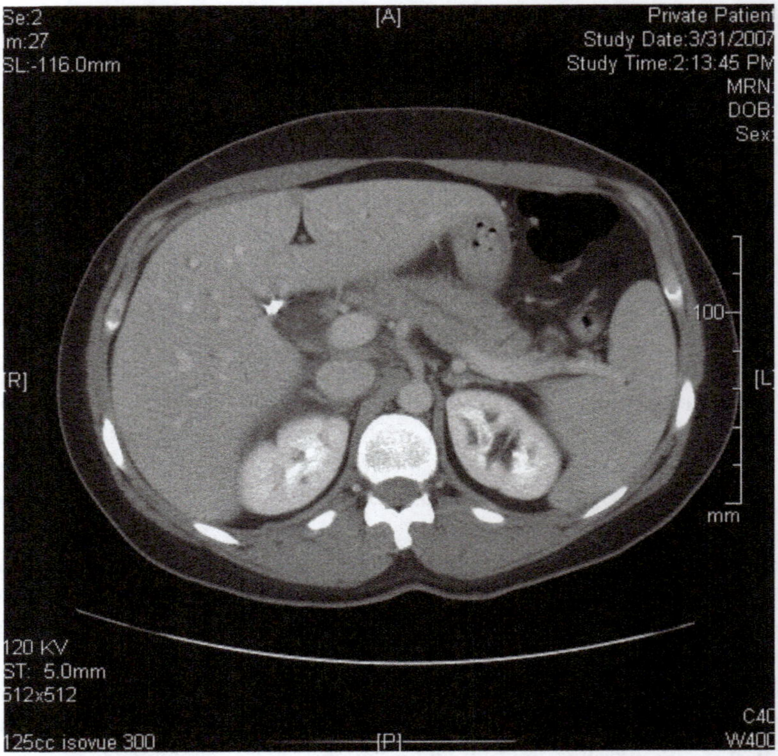

Fig. 6.4 This computed tomography scan seems to show a dilated bile duct (20 mm), but in fact the cystic duct and bile duct are so close together that they were measured as one structure

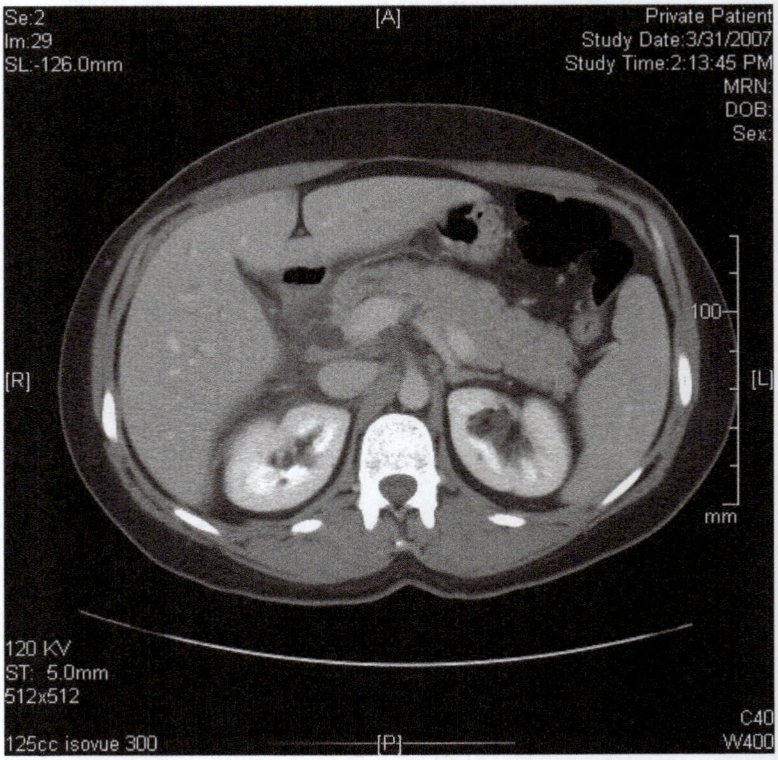

Fig. 6.5 This is the extrapancreatic portion of the bile duct; it is slightly prominent

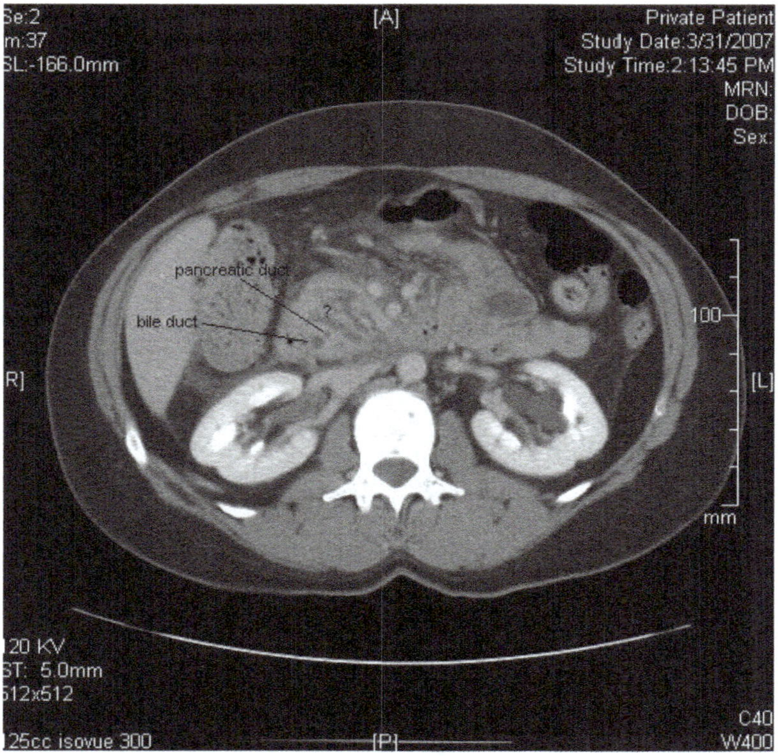

Fig. 6.6 The intrapancreatic segment of the bile duct is slender on this computed tomography scan and the pancreatic duct is certainly not dilated. The area marked by *?* appears to represent intrapancreatic fluid spaces

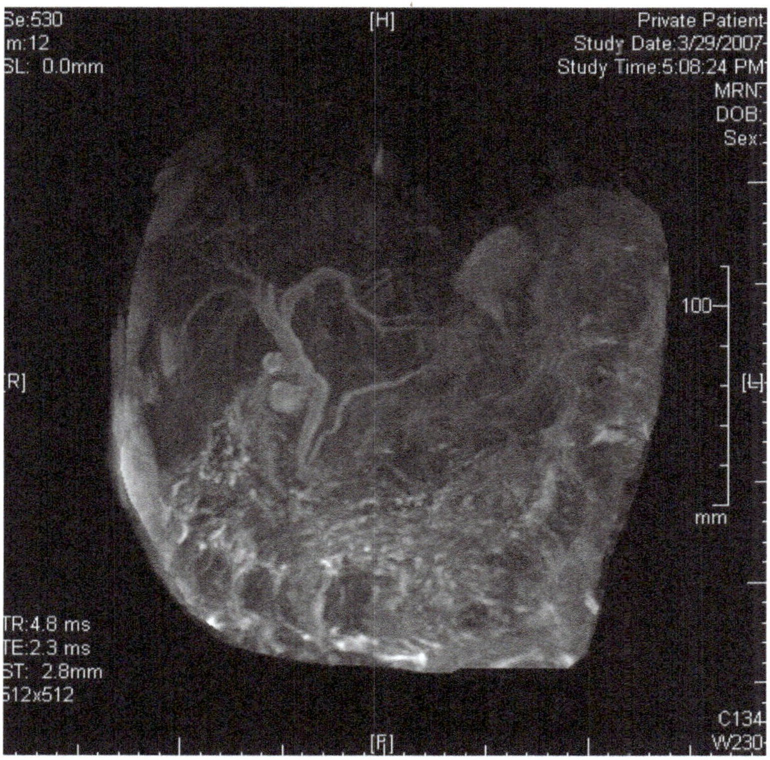

Fig. 6.7 This magnetic resonance cholangiopancreatography image is relatively uninformative: it does not show abnormalities of the pancreatic head or the cause of the mild dilation of the bile duct

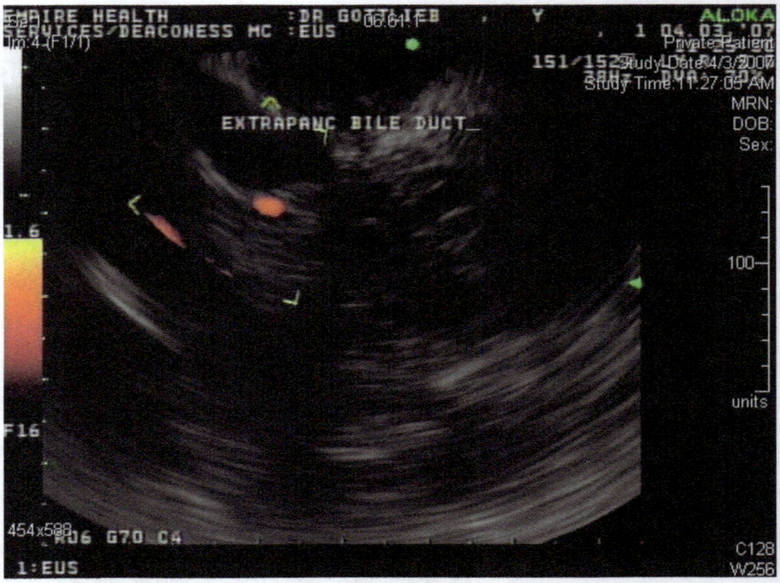

Fig. 6.8 This endoscopic ultrasound image shows a prominent bile duct above the entrance into the pancreas

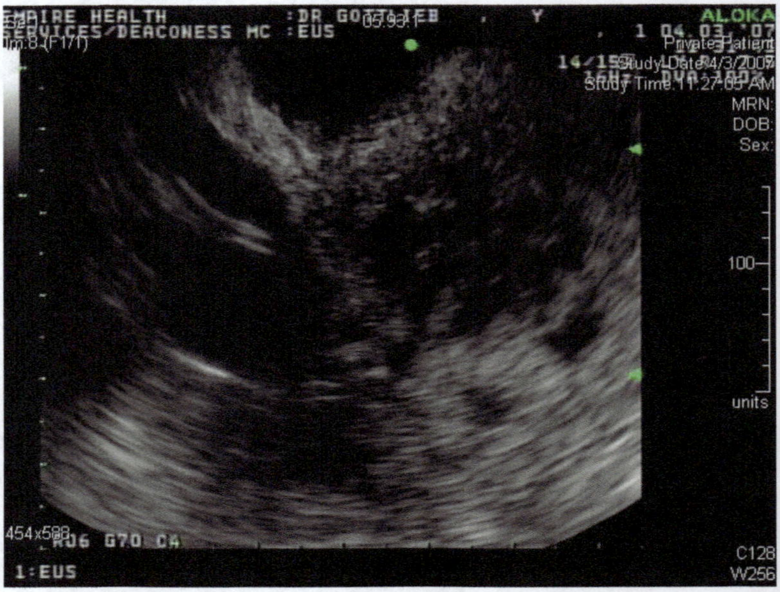

Fig. 6.9 Cystic spaces are seen in the head of the pancreas, which are also visible on the computed tomography scan

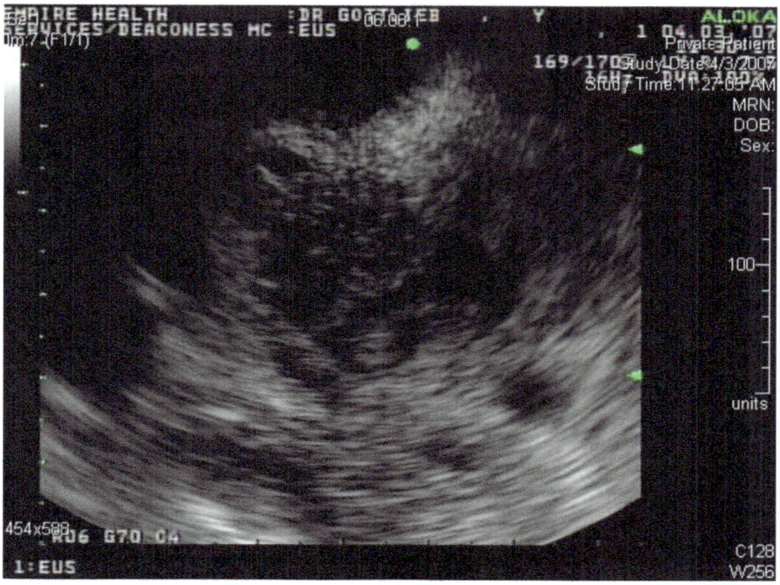

Fig. 6.10 Another image of the cystic areas, which probably represent the sequelae of acute pancreatitis

6.2.2 Chronic Pancreatitis

6.2.2.1 Chronic Pancreatitis with a Stone in the Pancreatic Duct

This is a 45-year-old patient with a history of excess alcohol use and a recent hospitalization for acute pancreatitis. The MRCP suggests a stone but only EUS clearly shows an 8-mm-diameter stone obstructing the main pancreatic duct. The pancreatic duct in the body measured 3.5 mm and had echo-rich borders. The parenchyma of the head area shows the characteristic hyperechoic stranding of chronic pancreatitis. An ERCP was performed. The stone in the pancreatic duct was difficult to discern on the ERCP, underscoring the utility of EUS as imaging modality for pancreatic disease. Also note that the short area of narrowing above the stone can be appreciated both on the EUS and ERCP images. The calculus was successfully removed after a pancreatic sphincterotomy and the use of a balloon occlusion catheter. A temporary pancreatic stent was inserted.

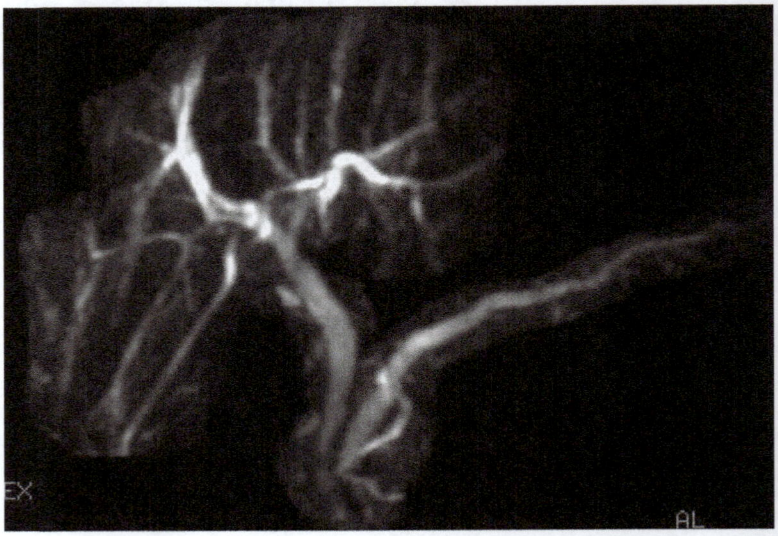

Fig. 6.11 Magnetic resonance cholangiopancreatography was somewhat equivocal about the presence of a stone

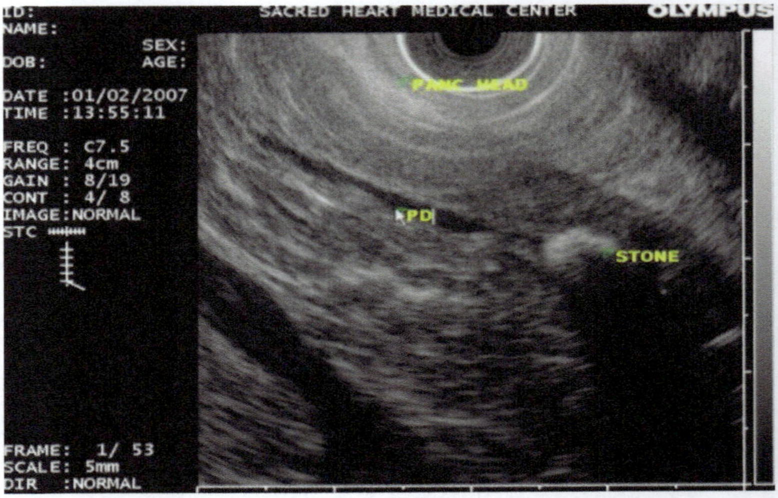

Fig. 6.12 A stone in the pancreatic duct in the head of the pancreas, close to the papilla

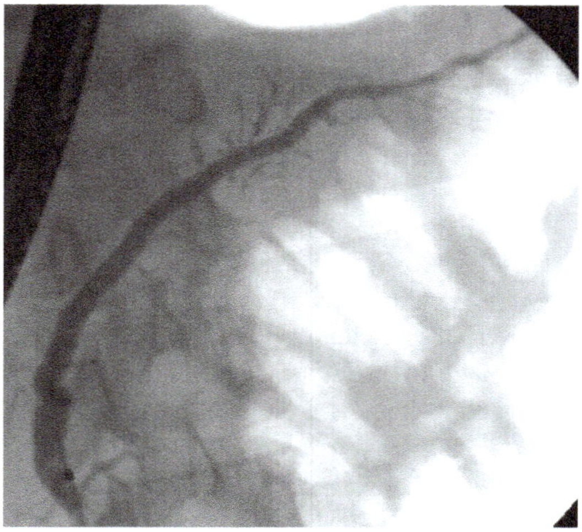

Fig. 6.13 Moderate chronic pancreatitis

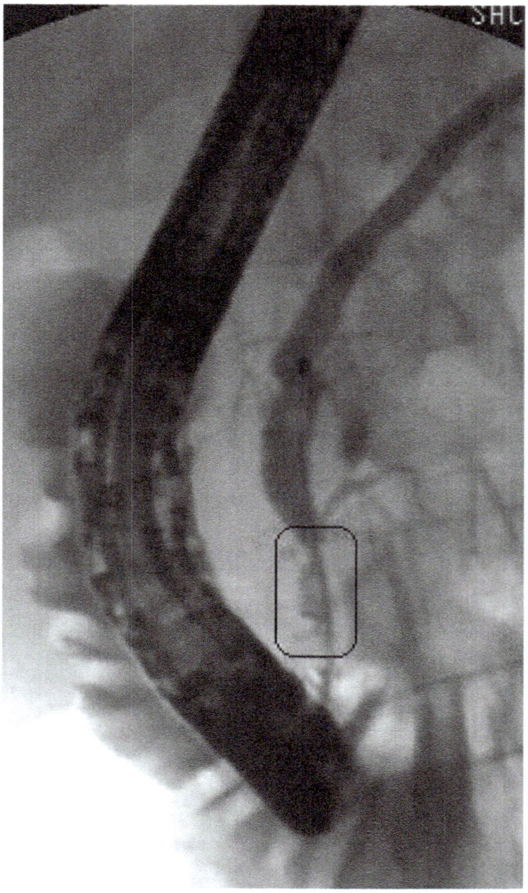

Fig. 6.14 Pancreatic duct stone on endoscopic retrograde cholangiopancreatography

6.2.3 Pancreatic Parenchymal Calcifications and Stone in the Pancreatic Duct

This is a 61-year-old patient with pancreatic parenchymal calcifications and a stone in the main pancreatic duct, which was destroyed with extracorporeal shock wave lithotripsy, leading to significant improvement of her pain.

The diagnosis of chronic pancreatitis can be challenging in patients with inconclusive noninvasive imaging and focal changes that cannot be easily differentiated from pancreatic cancer. ERCP has a low sensitivity in the diagnosis of early chronic pancreatitis, and an abnormal pancreatogram has poor specificity, as confirmed in studies of elderly patients and autopsy studies [10, 11]. CT findings including calcifications and ductal abnormalities are considered specific but not sensitive for mild to moderate disease [12]. One of the most common situations is the presentation of chronic abdominal pain with normal-appearing pancreas on CT or MRI/MRCP in patients with histologic inflammation and fibrosis; this presentation is the so-called minimal-change chronic pancreatitis.

Histologic confirmation is the gold standard for diagnosis but is too invasive and rarely possible. In many patients a diagnosis of chronic pancreatitis can be achieved by EUS and a variety of criteria, such as structural abnormalities of the parenchyma or the pancreatic ducts, or by performing hormone-stimulated pancreatic function tests in conjunction with EUS [13]. In studies comparing EUS and histopathological diagnosis of chronic pancreatitis, the sensitivity of EUS has been reported between 75 and 90 % and the specificity between 80 and 100 % [13–15]. Albashir et al. [13] have reported that combining EUS and secretin-stimulated pancreatic function tests can increase the sensitivity to 100 % (95 % confidence interval, 63–100).

Parenchymal EUS criteria include hyperechoic foci, hyperechoic strands, cysts, lobularity, and calcifications. Ductal EUS criteria include a hyperechoic duct wall, visible side branches, dilatation of the main pancreatic duct, and irregularity of the main pancreatic duct [16]. These criteria have been used without accounting for the greater diagnostic weight of some of them, such as calcifications/stones; a threshold of three to five criteria has been used to establish the diagnosis of chronic pancreatitis by different authors; it is obvious that a greater number will maximize specificity and a lower number will maximize sensitivity. Some of the criteria, particularly hyperechoic strands, hyperechoic foci, irregularity of the main duct, and visible side branches, have a significant degree of interobserver variability ($\kappa < 0.4$) [17, 18].

Given these limitations, a consensus-based, weight-adjusted scoring system, called the Rosemont criteria, was developed in 2007 by a group of experts [19]. This system assigns a greater diagnostic value to pancreatic duct calculi, hyperechoic foci with shadowing, and lobularity with honeycombing. The Rosemont criteria still require validation before it can be implemented in standard EUS practice. A clear definition of EUS features of chronic pancreatitis was established by this group of experts as follows [19]:

- Hyperechoic foci with shadowing: echogenic structures ≥2 mm in length and width that shadow
- Hyperechoic foci without shadowing: echogenic structures ≥2 mm in both length and width with no shadowing
- Lobularity: well-circumscribed structures ≥5 mm in size with an enhancing rim and relatively echo-poor center
- Honeycombing: more than three contiguous lobules
- Cysts: anechoic, rounded/elliptical structures with or without septations
- Stranding: hyperechoic lines of ≥3 mm in length in at least two different directions with respect to the imaged plane
- Main pancreatic duct calculi: echogenic structure(s) within main pancreatic duct with acoustic shadowing
- Irregular main pancreatic duct contour: uneven or irregular outline and ectatic course
- Dilated side branches: three or more tubular anechoic structures each measuring ≥1 mm in width and budding from the main pancreatic duct
- Main pancreatic duct dilation: ≥3.5-mm body or >1.5-mm tail
- Hyperechoic main duct margin: echogenic, distinct structure greater than 50 % of the entire main pancreatic duct in the body and tail of the pancreas

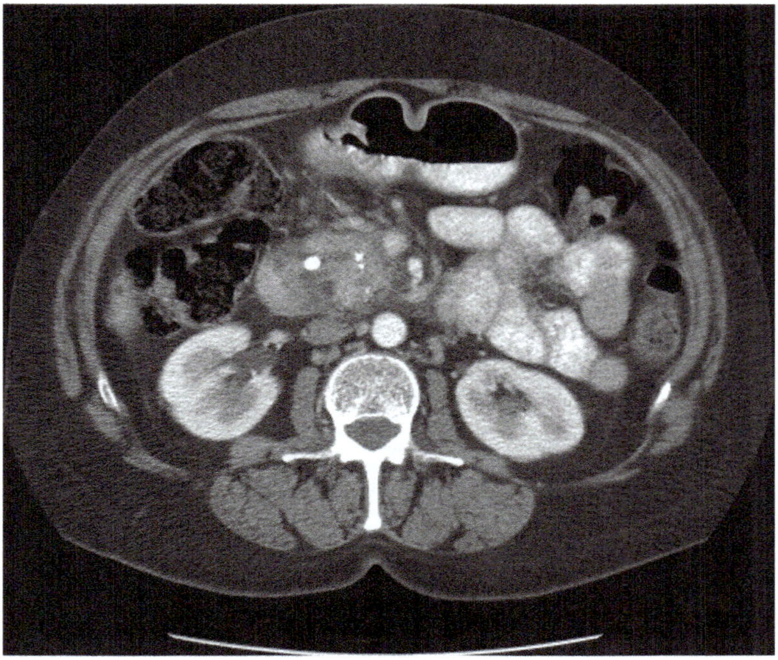

Fig. 6.15 Computed tomography scan showing pancreatic calcifications

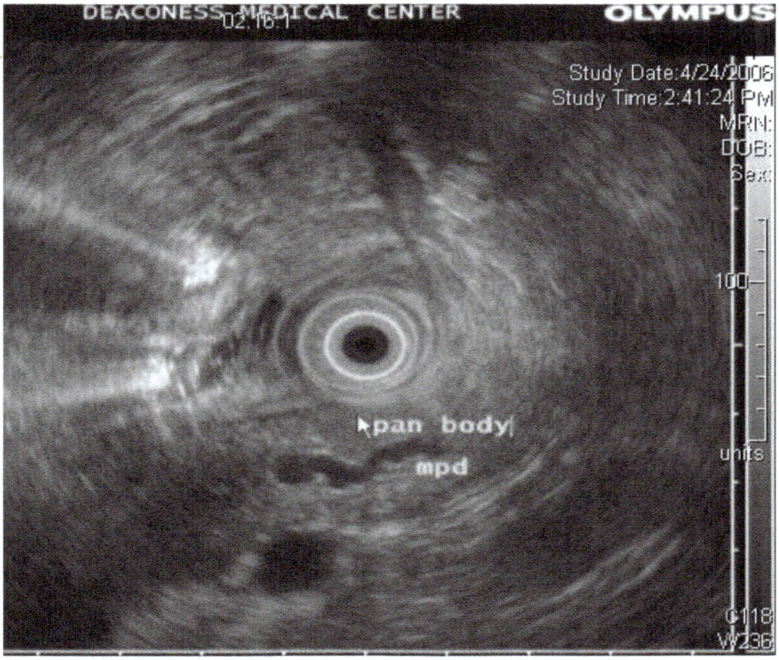

Fig. 6.16 Dilated main pancreatic duct on endoscopic ultrasound

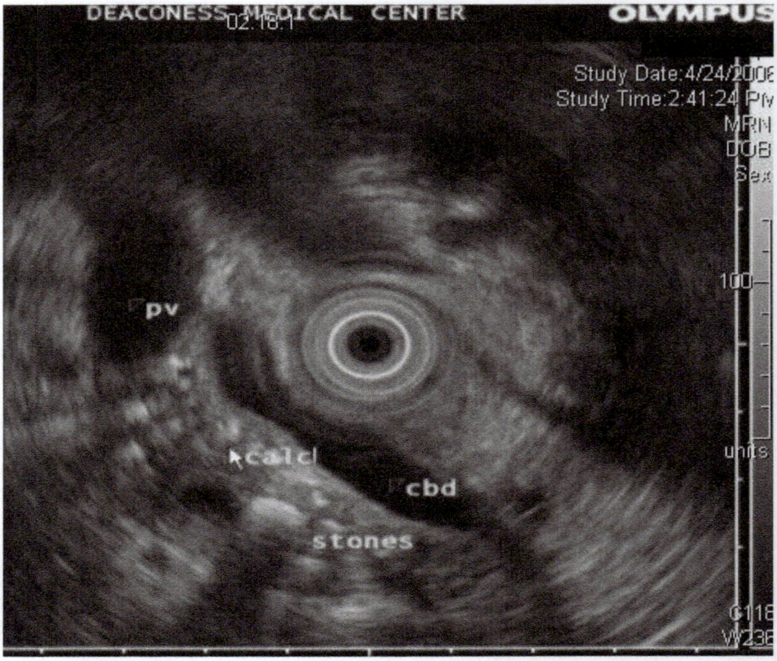

Fig. 6.17 Severe calcific pancreatitis with both intraparenchymal calcifications and a stone in the pancreatic duct

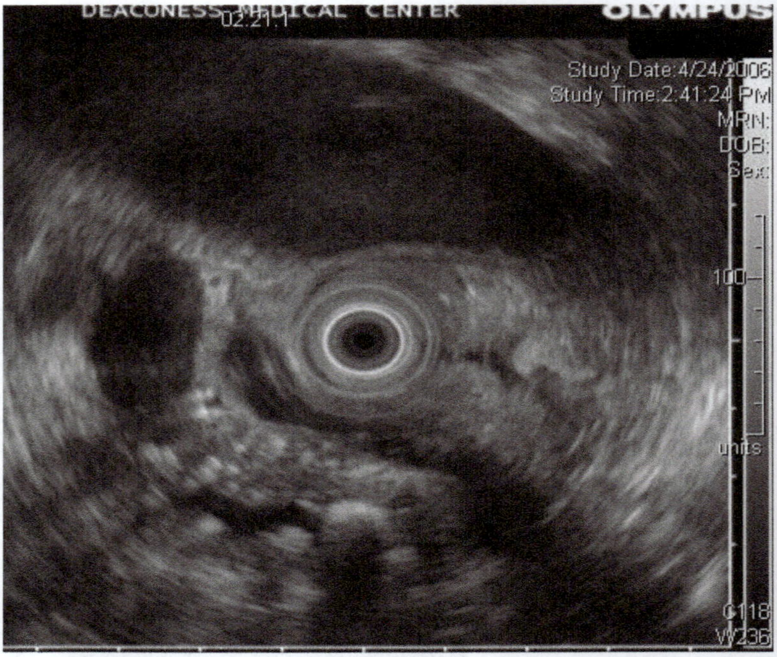

Fig. 6.18 A stone in the pancreatic duct

6.2.4 Fatty Infiltration of the Pancreas

Infiltration of fat in the pancreas and other organs such as the liver, heart, and striated muscle has been well described in obese individuals and those with insulin resistance [20]. This relation has been well documented in autopsy, CT, and MRI studies [21]. This condition was initially called pancreatic lipomatosis and, more recently, pancreatic steatosis; its clinical implications are still unclear, but it has been shown in some cases to precede the development of type II diabetes [20]. An association with nonalcoholic fatty liver disease has been demonstrated, mostly in women, particularly related to the presence of intralobular pancreatic fat [22]. Given this association, the term *nonalcoholic fatty pancreas disease* has been proposed, suggesting a common pathophysiology related to insulin resistance and the metabolic syndrome. The exact clinical consequences of fatty infiltration of the pancreas are not known.

The diagnosis of pancreatic steatosis should be suspected in patients with markedly hyperechoic pancreatic parenchyma compared with the liver, but less prominent changes also can be found in normal patients. Some authors recommend additional pancreatic images (CT or MRI) to establish this diagnosis in these unclear cases [23].

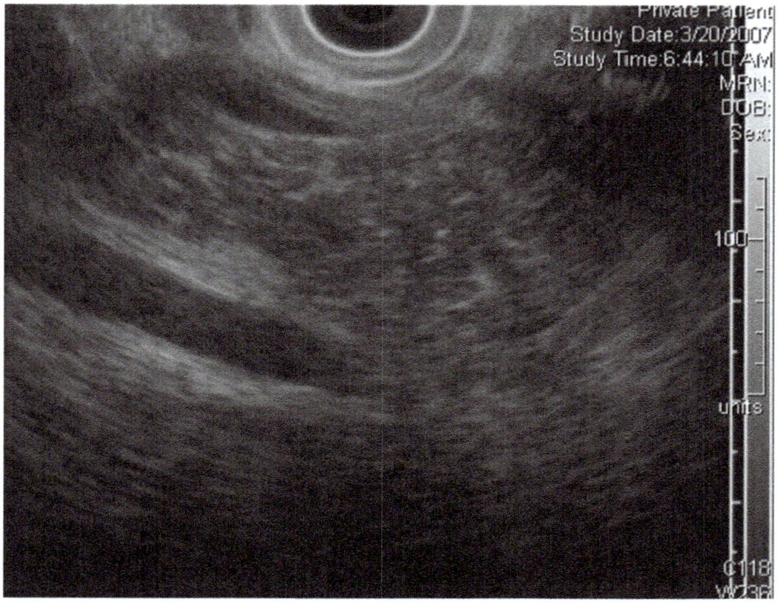

Fig. 6.19 Pancreatic head. Is this chronic pancreatitis?

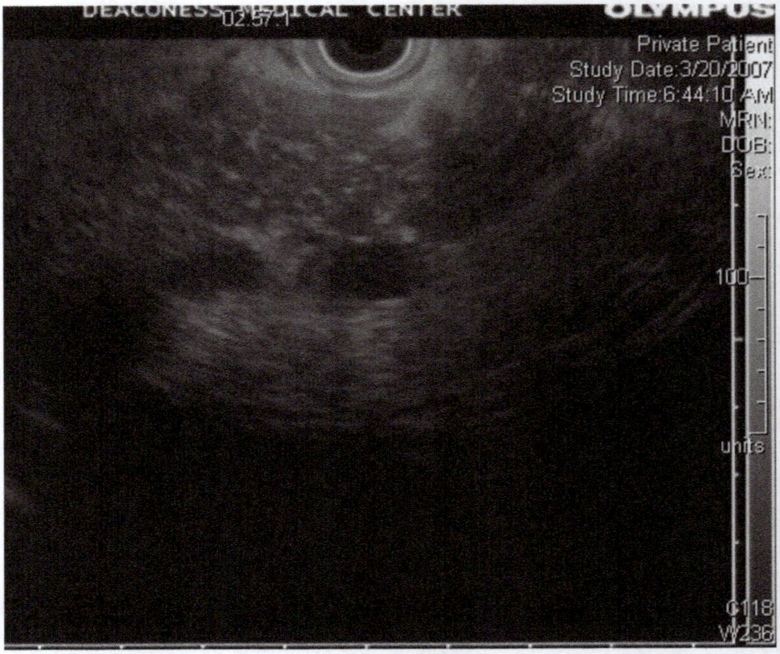

Fig. 6.20 Pancreatic body. This is not "stranding" but septation by fat

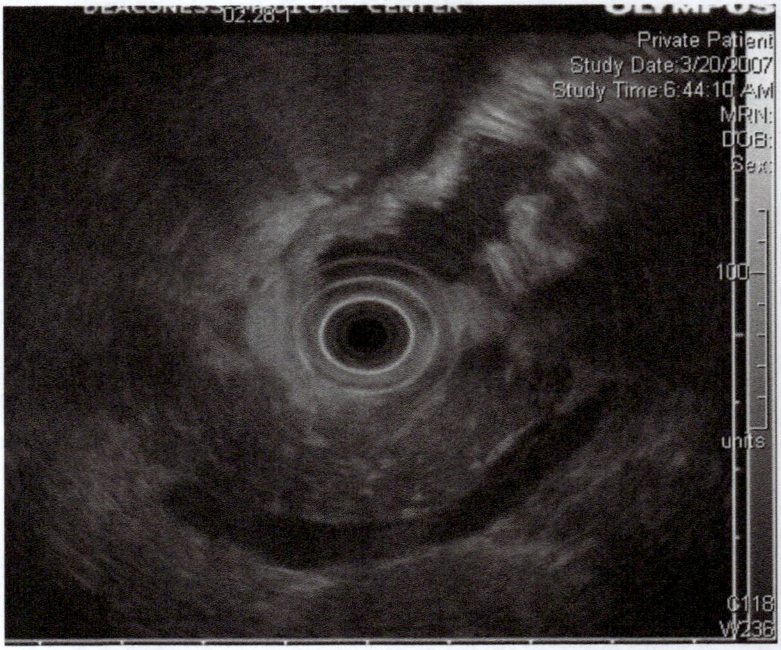

Fig. 6.21 Fatty infiltration of the pancreas, giving it a marbled or lobulated appearance

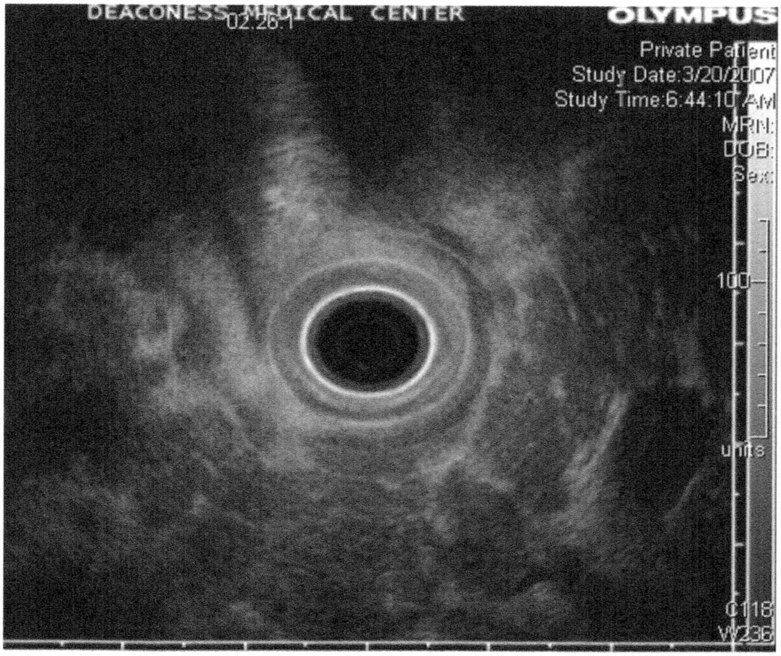

Fig. 6.22 Lobulated appearance of the pancreas seen at a higher frequency

6.2.5 Perivascular Fat Mimicking a Dilated Main Pancreatic Duct

This is a 64-year-old patient who had CT for the evaluation of lower abdominal pain. The CT was interpreted as showing a focally dilated main pancreatic duct, and the patient was referred for EUS evaluation. EUS showed a degree of fatty infiltration of the pancreas but was otherwise unremarkable. Reanalysis of the CT scan shows that fat between the splenic artery and the pancreas was erroneously interpreted as the pancreatic duct. The pancreatic duct, as seen on the labeled CT, Fig. 6.26 takes off into another direction.

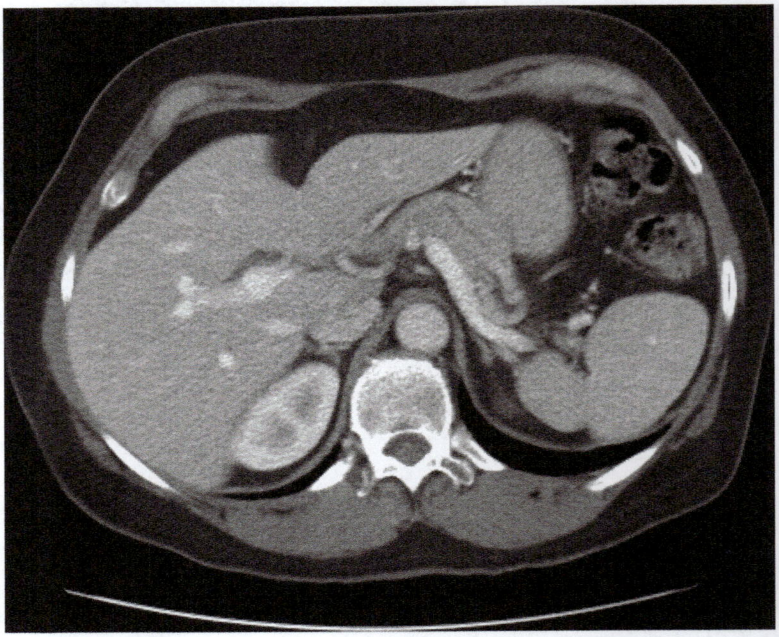

Fig. 6.23 This computed tomography scan shows what initially appeared to be focal dilation of the main pancreatic duct in the body of the pancreas

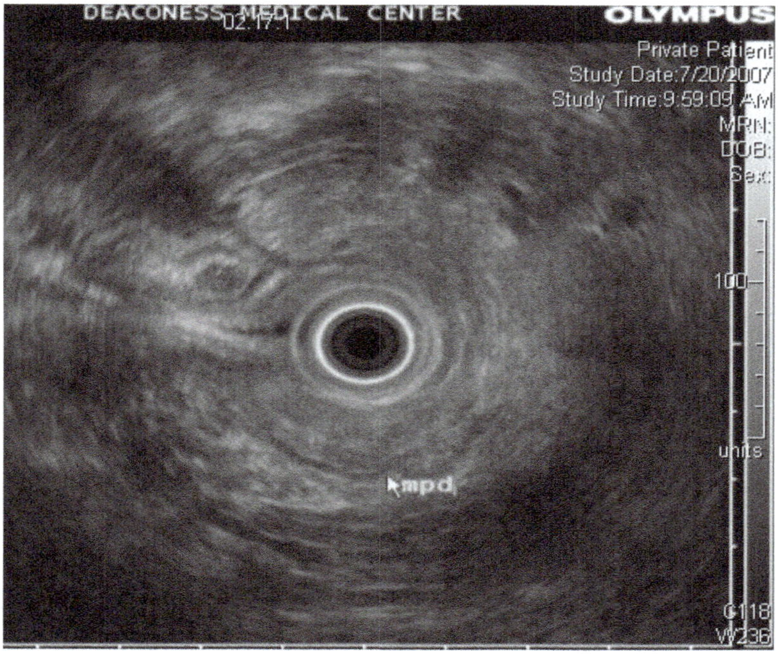

Fig. 6.24 This endoscopic ultrasound image shows some fatty infiltration of the pancreas but is otherwise unremarkable. The main pancreatic duct appears normal

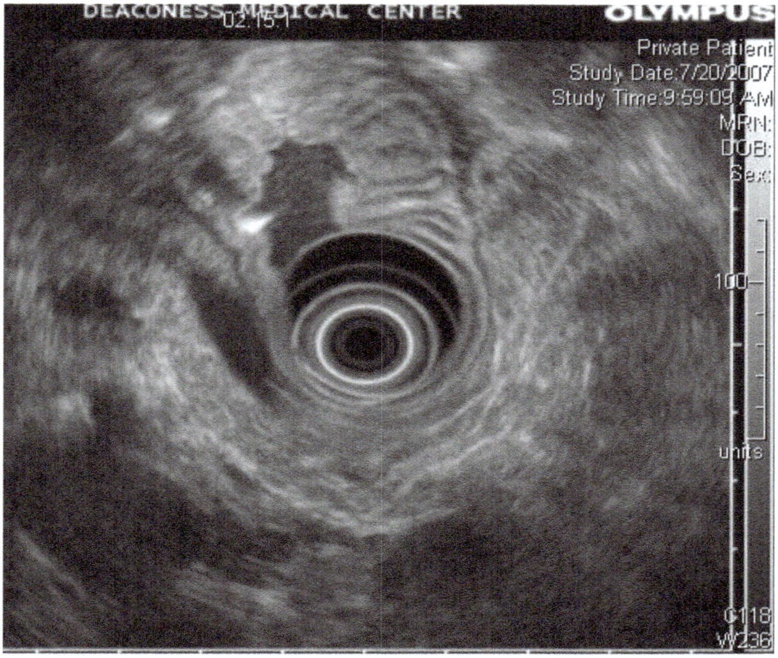

Fig. 6.25 Another view shows no evidence of a dilated main pancreatic duct

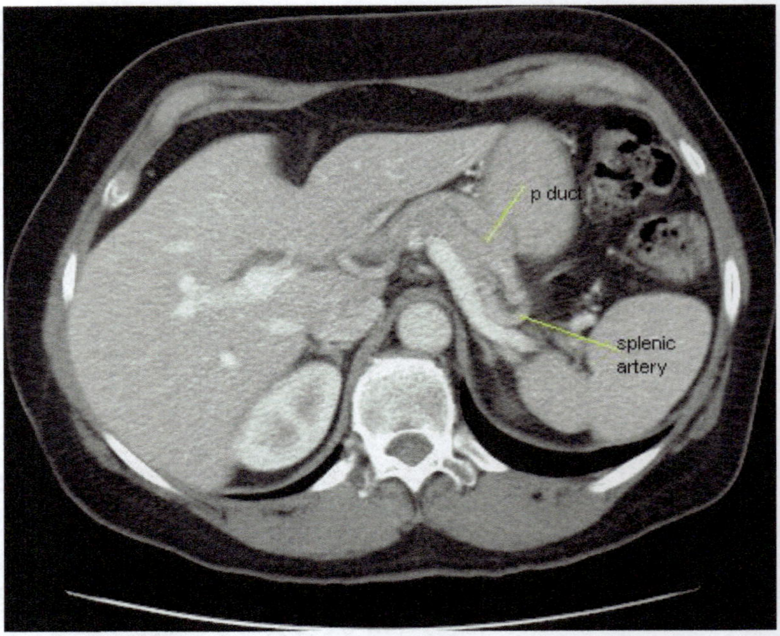

Fig. 6.26 The computed tomography scan was reinterpreted in view of these findings: the dark structure hugging the splenic artery is perivascular fat

6.2.6 Vanishing Pancreatic Mass

This is an 88-year-old woman with a history of esophageal spasms and a Zenker's diverticulum who presented to the emergency department with acute onset of epigastric pain. She was discharged from the emergency department after the pain had significantly improved. Laboratory tests were unremarkable; amylase and lipase levels were apparently not checked at the time. Three months later she returned and had a bilirubin level of 12 mg/dl. An ERCP showed a fairly long stricture in the distal common bile duct. A pancreatic head neoplasm was suspected, although CT of the abdomen was unremarkable except for bile duct dilation. EUS performed at the time showed an ill-defined hypoechoic mass suspicious for tumor, but the fine-needle aspiration (FNA) biopsies were negative. Two months later the patient presented for a follow-up EUS. The jaundice did not recur after removal of the biliary stent. Her CA 19–9 level had decreased from 78 to 42 U/mL, making it likely that the elevation was related to the cholestasis. In place of the previously noted hypodense pseudotumor, small cysts/cystic spaces were now seen. Repeat FNA again was negative. In retrospect it seems that the patient had an unrecognized attack of acute pancreatitis with an inflammatory pseudomass that resolved into small pseudocysts.

Clinical presentation and imaging findings of pancreatic cancer and inflammatory masses of the pancreas, frequently due to chronic pancreatitis, can be similar and their differential diagnosis can be challenging. Both entities can cause pancreatic duct and biliary duct dilation, fluid collection, and lymphadenopathy [24]. Pancreatic cancer can occur in patients with underlying chronic pancreatitis, and these tumors can also be associated with peritumoral inflammatory changes. A variable proportion of patients referred for presumed pancreatic cancer are found to have inflammatory masses of focal pancreatitis [25].

Additional EUS-based techniques such as elastography and contrast enhancement are emerging techniques that may provide better accuracy than standard EUS in the evaluation of solid pancreatic lesions. These techniques are expected to minimize unnecessary FNA and improve diagnostic efficiency, although further research is still necessary to define their clinical roles [26, 27].

An aggressive workup, including FNA, of all suspicious lesions is recommended by some experts, given the morbidity and mortality of pancreatic resections of up to 30 % and 5 %, respectively, although better surgical results are obtained in large referral centers. On the other hand, arguments to not undergo preoperative biopsy in patients with potentially resectable masses and good operability include the fact that FNA/biopsies can be falsely negative in up to 10 % of cases and surgical delays are likely to allow the cancer to progress to more advanced stages that are no longer curable.

One of the concerns with FNA is the risk of tumoral seeding at the needle tract. This is not an issue with masses at the head of the pancreas, for which EUS-guided FNA is performed via a transduodenal approach because the duodenum is removed with the Whipple operation. A few reports of track seeding have been reported in patients undergoing transgastric FNA/biopsies of lesions at the body and tail of the pancreas [28, 29]; this risk seems to be very low given the scarcity of reports, but we recommend that it be discussed as part of the informed consent.

It is clear that FNA is appropriate in patients with large masses that appear to be unresectable so that a histologic diagnosis and the need for palliative therapy can be established. FNA is also appropriate in cases where the diagnosis is not clear based on history and imaging findings; as demonstrated in this case, inflammatory masses can have a presentation that is difficult to distinguish from pancreatic cancer.

Fig. 6.27 Ill-defined hypoechoic area with bile duct compression and jaundice. Is this a pancreatic tumor?

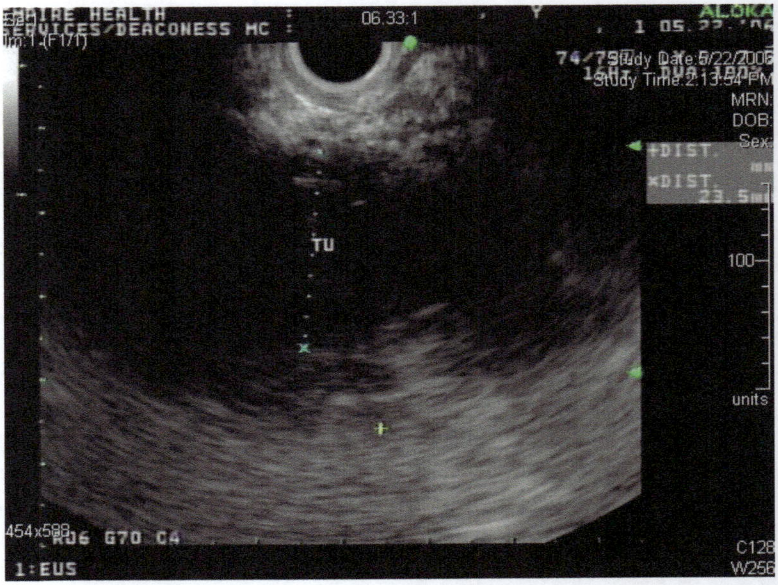

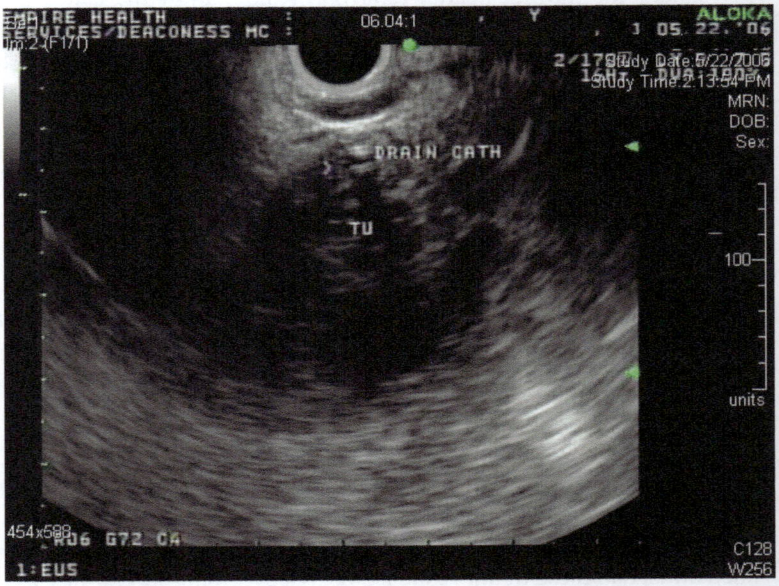

Fig. 6.28 Ill-defined hypodense area in the pancreatic head with a biliary stent

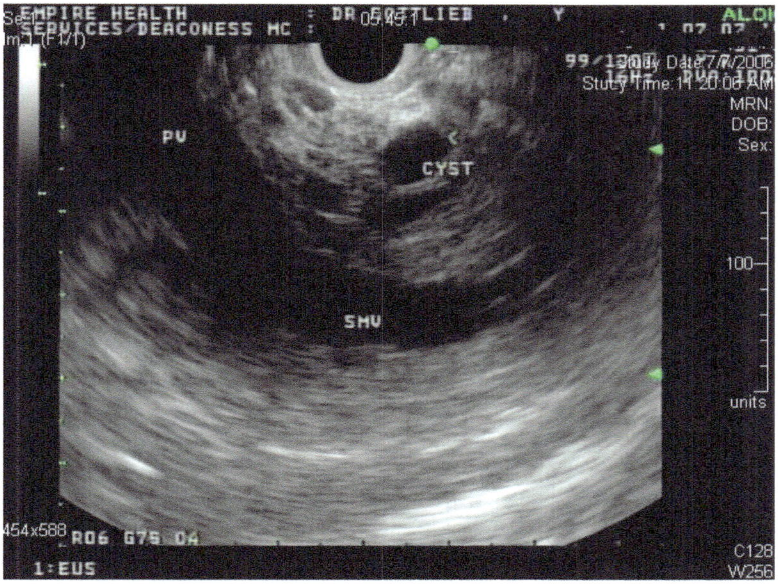

Fig. 6.29 Pseudomass followed by cyst in the same location in the head of the pancreas

6.2.7 Pancreatic Cancer

6.2.7.1 Stage IV Pancreatic Cancer with Extensive Collaterals

This is a 76-year-old patient with a large pancreatic mass with pulmonary metastases. CT showed ascites and extensive venous collaterals surrounding the pancreatic head. A percutaneous CT-guided biopsy was contemplated, but because of the venous collaterals in the biopsy path the patient was referred for EUS-guided FNA instead. Figures 6.31 and 6.32 show the corresponding EUS, which indicates a rather diffuse mass and two vessels next to it, both with a portal venous system spectral Doppler profile. One of them is the portal vein, and the other is a rather large collateral. Five passes were made into the mass, avoiding adjacent vessels.

This case demonstrates one of the most common scenarios seen in the practice of EUS: a patient with obstructive jaundice secondary to advanced adenocarcinoma of the pancreatic head. It is obvious that these patients are not candidates for surgical resection, and the goal of therapy is to provide palliative care. While biliary stents provide acceptable palliation of biliary obstruction, a tissue diagnosis is necessary to proceed with palliative chemotherapy and radiation, which helps to minimize abdominal pain and improve quality of life.

EUS has become the method of choice to obtain histologic diagnosis in this situation, where ERCP brushings are frequently falsely negative, and the same applies to percutaneous biopsies. EUS also provides the option to perform celiac plexus block/neurolysis to better control abdominal pain.

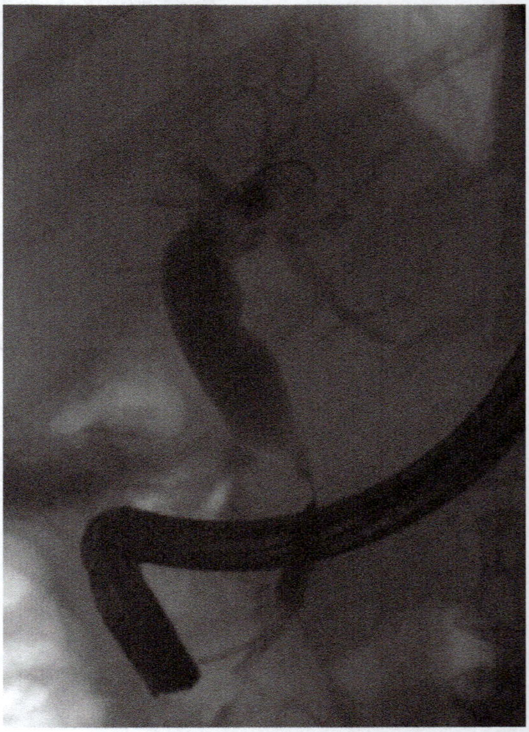

Fig. 6.30 Bile duct stricture secondary to a pancreatic head mass

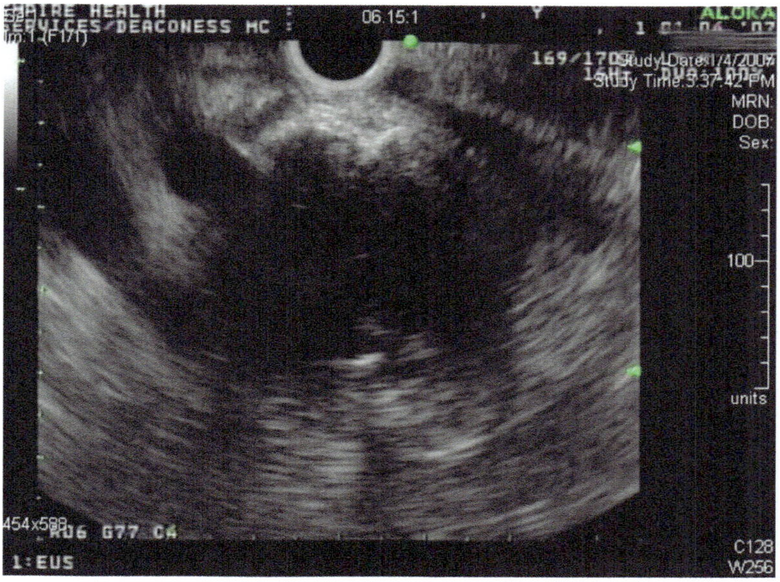

Fig. 6.31 This mass is fairly ill defined at its borders and appears to be diffusely infiltrative

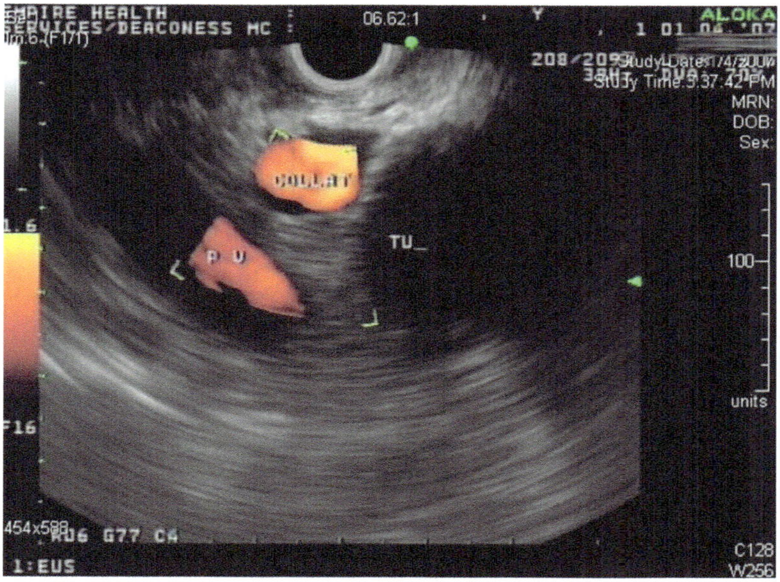

Fig. 6.32 Power Doppler shows the portal vein and a large collateral

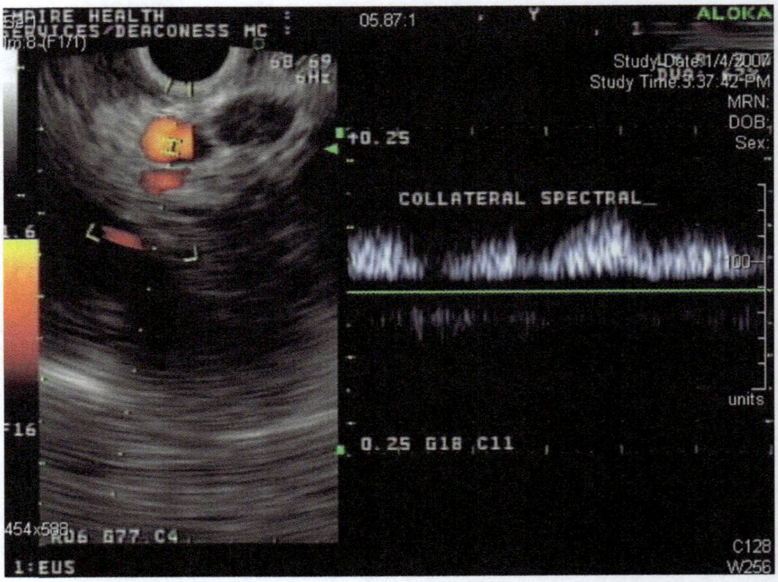

Fig. 6.33 Spectral Doppler confirms that this vessel belongs to the portal venous system

6.2.8 T2 Adenocarcinoma of the Pancreas

This is a 90-year-old patient with a 2.2-cm mass in the head of the pancreas and obstructive jaundice. The gallbladder is massively distended. Note the attachment of the tumor to the portal vein but no signs of invasion. EUS-guided FNA biopsies were performed and a Wallstent was placed the following day.

A palliative approach is also recommended in this 90-year-old patient. In this case a surgical resection would be feasible in expert hands, even with some limited involvement of the portal vein; however, a decision was made to avoid surgery because of the patient's advanced age and existing comorbidities. EUS provided cytological diagnosis and tumor staging; once diagnosis of tissue malignancy was confirmed the patient underwent ERCP with placement of a self-expandable, uncovered metal stent.

It is important to remember than uncovered biliary metal stents are not removable and they are only approved for malignant indications. Fully covered metal biliary stents that can be removed are now available and have been used safely for benign biliary disease; unfortunately they are associated with more frequent complications, particularly migration, compared with uncovered metal stents in the management of distal malignant biliary obstruction [30]. Therefore, we recommend that the evaluation of patients be started with EUS and include histologic confirmation to establish a clear diagnosis before ERCP and stent placement.

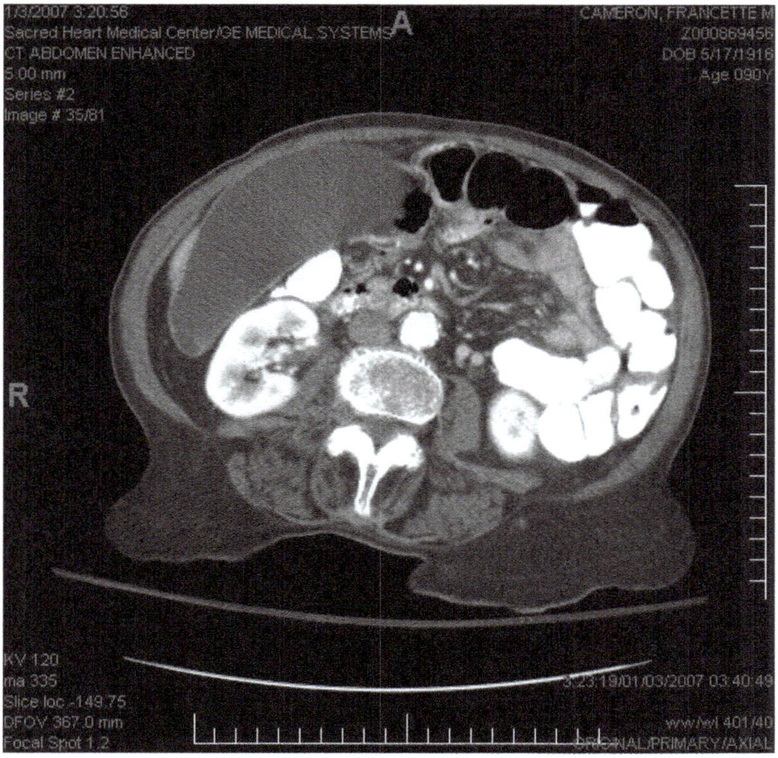

Fig. 6.34 Distended gallbladder in biliary obstruction

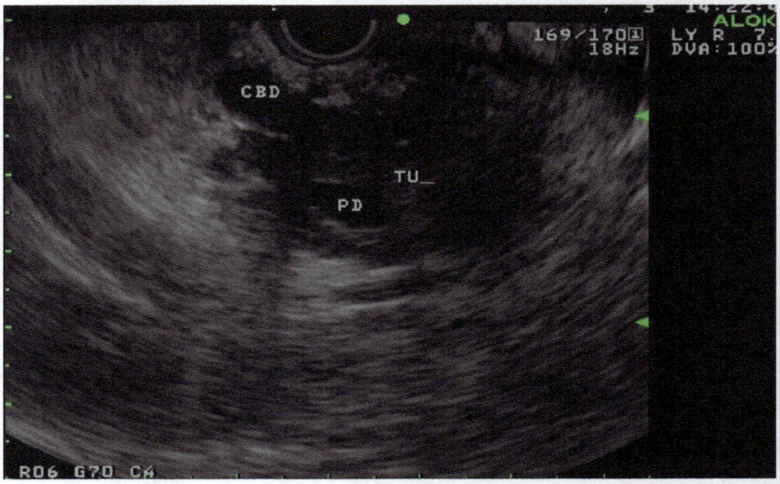

Fig. 6.35 Pancreatic mass on endoscopic ultrasound

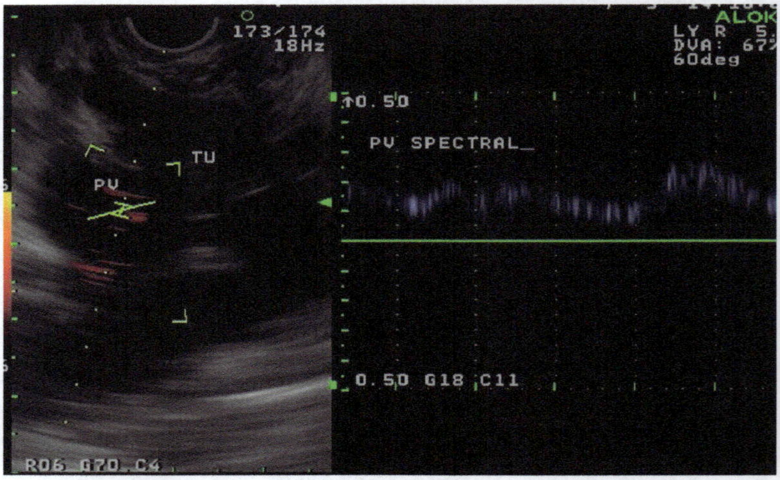

Fig. 6.36 Doppler study showing a portal vein pancreatic mass

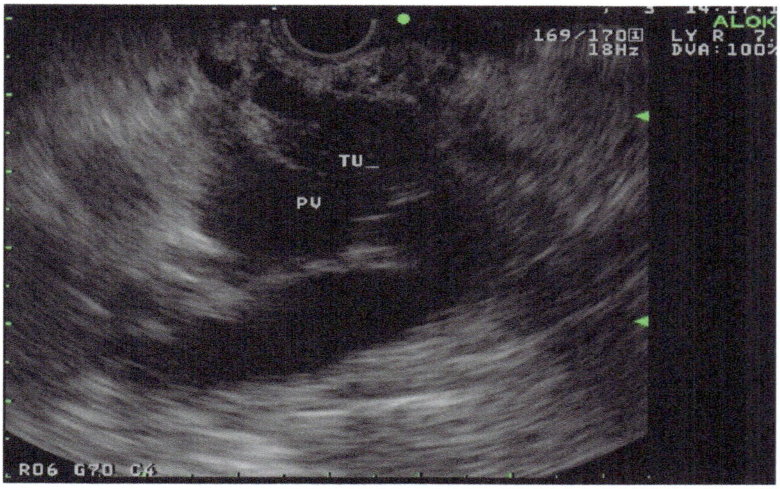

Fig. 6.37 The mass as it relates to the portal vein

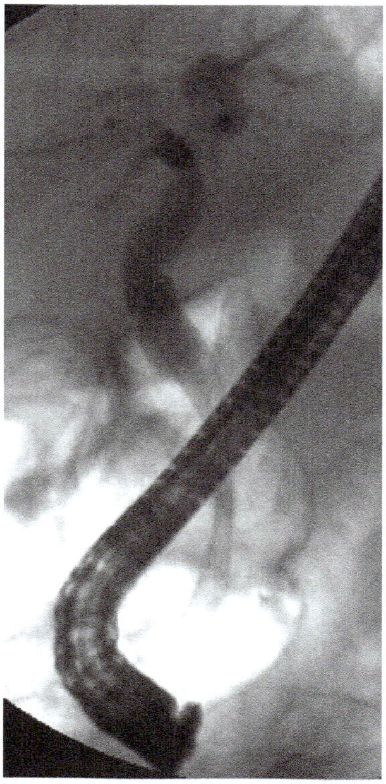

Fig. 6.38 A Wallstent bridging the biliary stricture

6.2.9 Pancreatic Tail Mass

This is a 75-year-old man who has not been feeling well for approximately 2 months; he is complaining of epigastric pain and a 15-lb weight loss. CT of the abdomen showed a large pancreatic tail mass (6 cm in diameter), which had led to splenic vein thrombosis with gastric collaterals, retroperitoneal invasion, and an apparent adrenal metastasis. Corresponding EUS and CT images are shown in Figs. 6.39 and 6.40, respectively. This case highlights that pancreatic tail cancers can grow to a large size before becoming symptomatic. They also are more likely to have metastasized to the liver by the time they are discovered. This tumor also illustrates an infiltrating growth pattern with tumor pseudopodia that may reflect a more aggressive tumor biology. EUS-guided FNA biopsies were positive for adenocarcinoma.

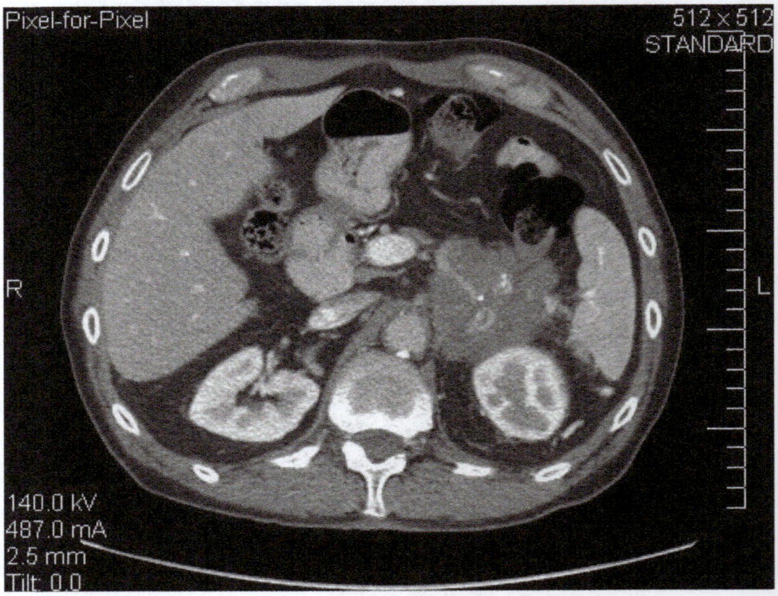

Fig. 6.39 A 6-cm-diameter mass in the pancreatic tail infiltrating into the retroperitoneum

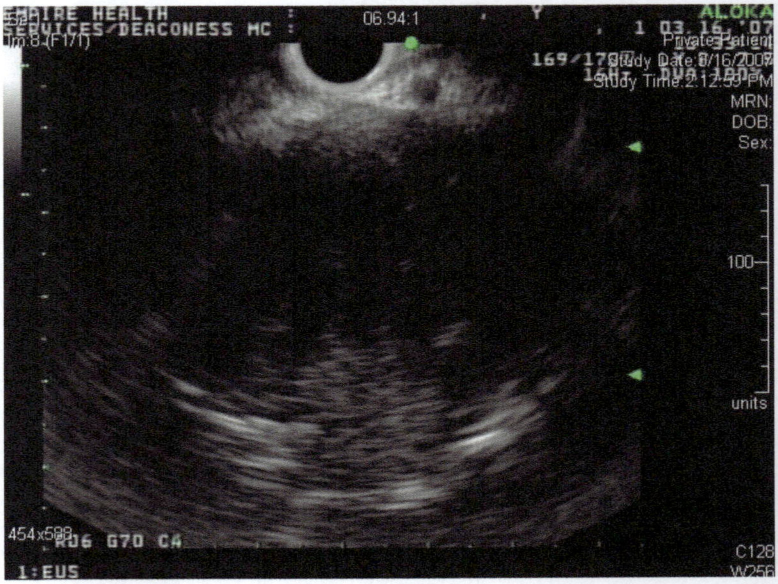

Fig. 6.40 Endoscopic ultrasound appearance of the pancreatic mass. Very large masses sometimes fill the entire field of view. Care must be taken to see the forest in spite of all the trees

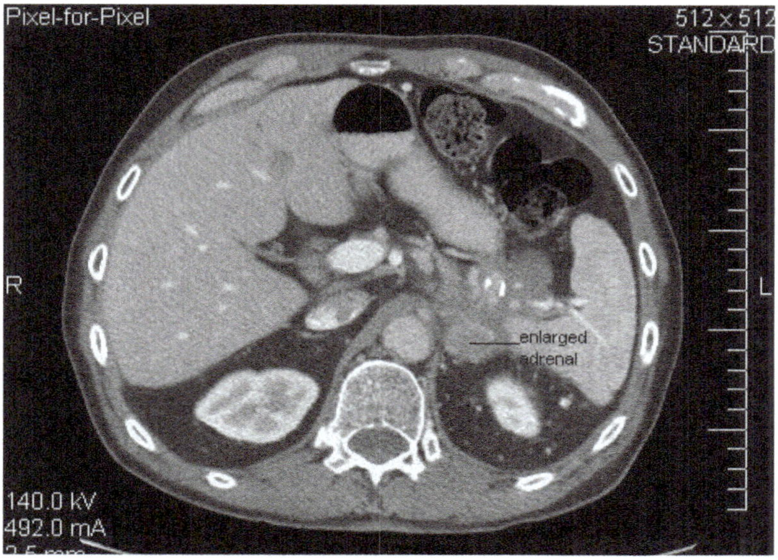

Fig. 6.41 A different level of the computed tomography shows an enhancing mass in the region of the adrenal

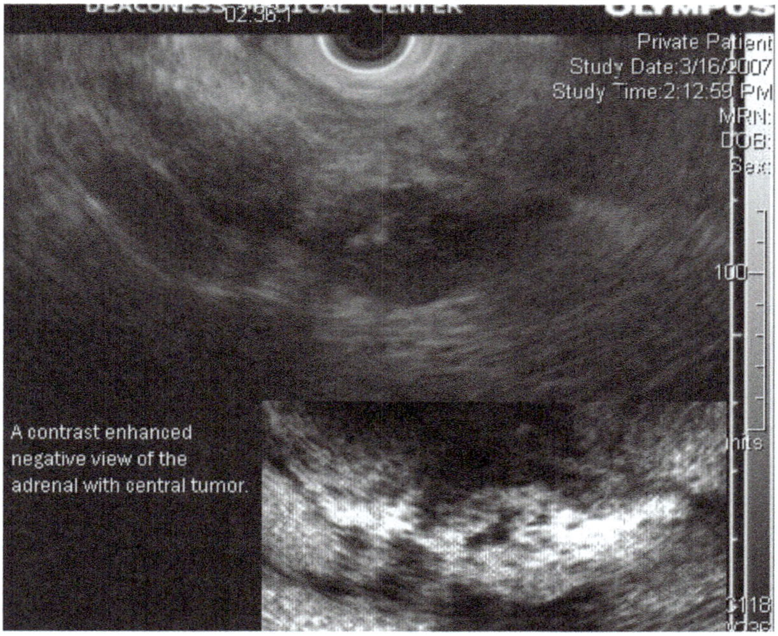

Fig. 6.42 The left adrenal is shown with a central tumor. The inset shows a contrast-enhanced negative image of it

6.2.10 Calcifications in a Hypoechoic Pancreas Tumor

Hypoechoic masses, especially in patients with underlying chronic pancreatitis, may be benign or malignant and may represent inflammation, neoplasia, or relative sparing from the chronic pancreatitis in that location. In patients with an otherwise normal pancreas, calcifications in a hypoechoic mass do not indicate benign disease, as this case demonstrates. In the majority of cases pancreatic calcifications are seen in chronic pancreatitis. However, they occur infrequently in pancreatic adenocarcinomas without pre-existing chronic pancreatitis.

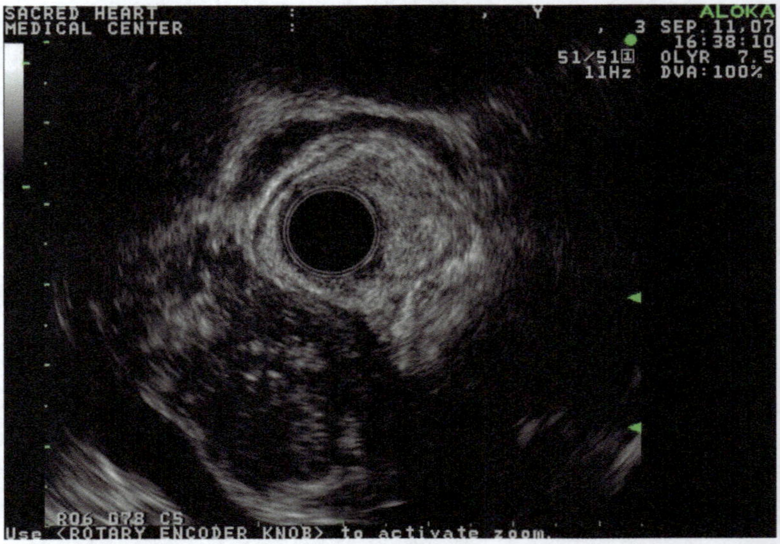

Fig. 6.43 Isolated pancreatic calcifications in a hypoechoic pancreas mass do not establish a diagnosis of benign disease (radial endoscopic ultrasound using a GF-UE160 echoendoscope)

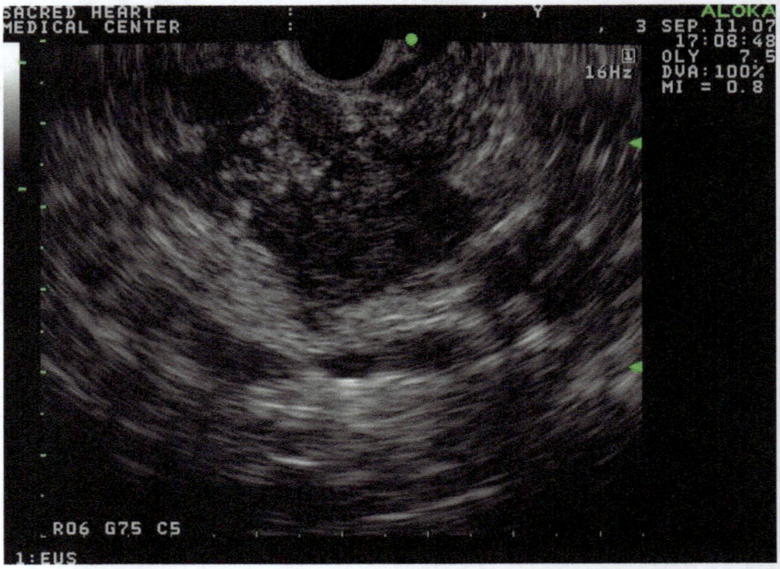

Fig. 6.44 The linear endoscopic ultrasound echoendoscope reveals a different aspect of the same tumor shown in Fig. 6.43 (carcinoma proven by biopsy). Note the fluffy calcifications in the tumor mass

6.2.11 Chronic Pancreatitis and Pancreatic Cancer

This patient had presented elsewhere a year earlier with a pancreatic pseudocyst that resolved. Over the past 6 months he had lost approximately 40 lb of weight and eventually was not able to eat but had no jaundice. CT showed chronic calcific pancreatitis with a dilated and irregular pancreatic duct, gastric outlet obstruction, a dilated bile duct, and a mass in the pancreatic head. EUS showed a relatively small (2.8 cm) tumor in the head of the pancreas close to the duodenum that had infiltrated into the duodenum, causing gastric outlet obstruction symptoms. While this tumor could have originated from the duodenum and grown into the pancreas, it was felt that most imaging was consistent with a pancreatic head primary tumor.

There is a well-known relationship between long-standing severe chronic pancreatitis and pancreatic cancer; the standardized incidence ratio of pancreatic cancer in chronic pancreatitis is 14–18. This association is further increased by cigarette smoking. The mechanisms involved are likely related to the progressive accumulation of genetic mutations caused by pancreatitis-induced DNA damage and incomplete repair in an inflammatory environment [31]. Pre-existing imaging abnormalities make the diagnosis of a newly developing pancreatic cancer more difficult, as discussed earlier. Even FNA cytology may not be diagnostic because of background inflammatory changes.

Duodenal infiltration, as demonstrated in this case, affects prognosis but does not affect resectability since the duodenum is removed with a Whipple operation. Obstruction of the gastric outlet secondary to tumoral obstruction was traditionally managed surgically, providing a gastroenteric bypass as well as a bilioenteric bypass; however, current endoscopic stenting techniques can provide satisfactory palliative results, shorter hospitalization, and a faster return to oral intake [32].

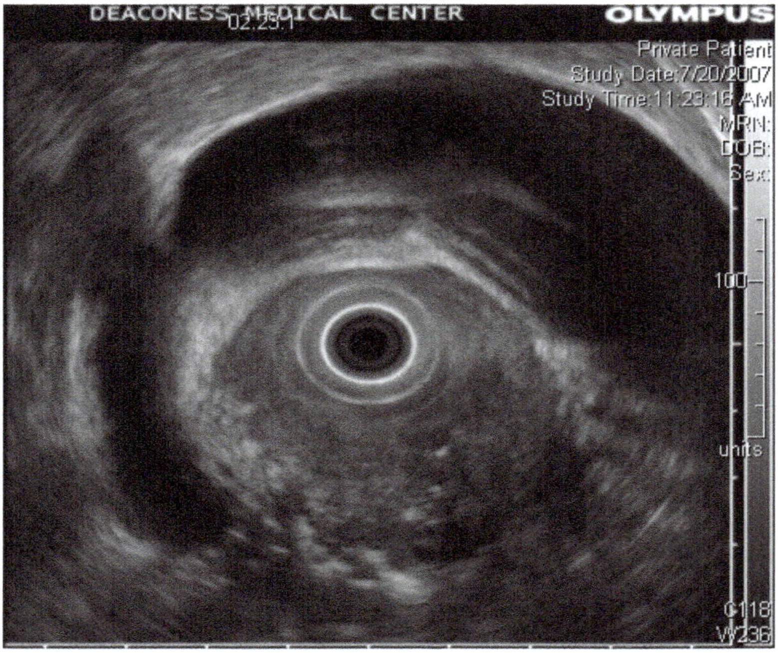

Fig. 6.45 This radial endoscopic ultrasound image demonstrates a dilated bile duct and gallbladder as well as circumferential invasion of the duodenum by tumor

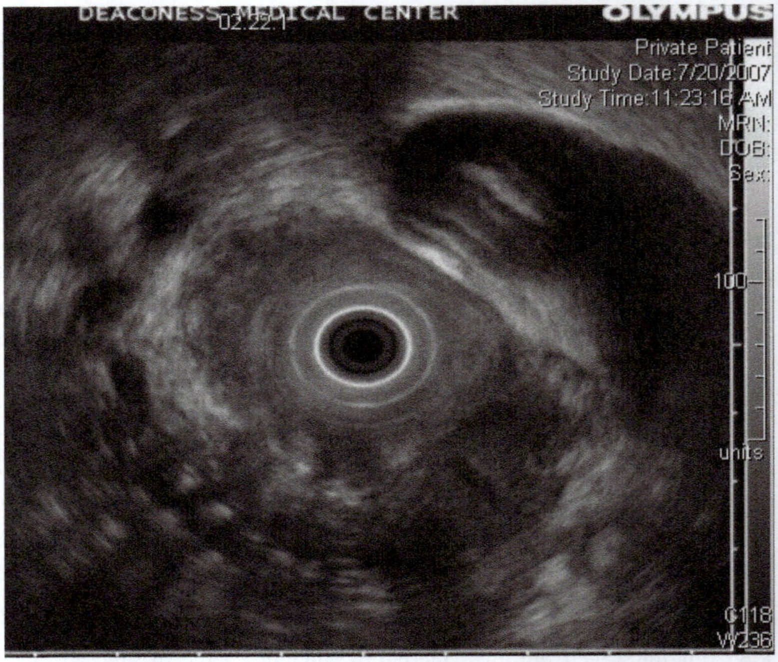

Fig. 6.46 This image shows calcifications in the pancreas head, a hypoechoic tumor close to the duodenum, and duodenal invasion

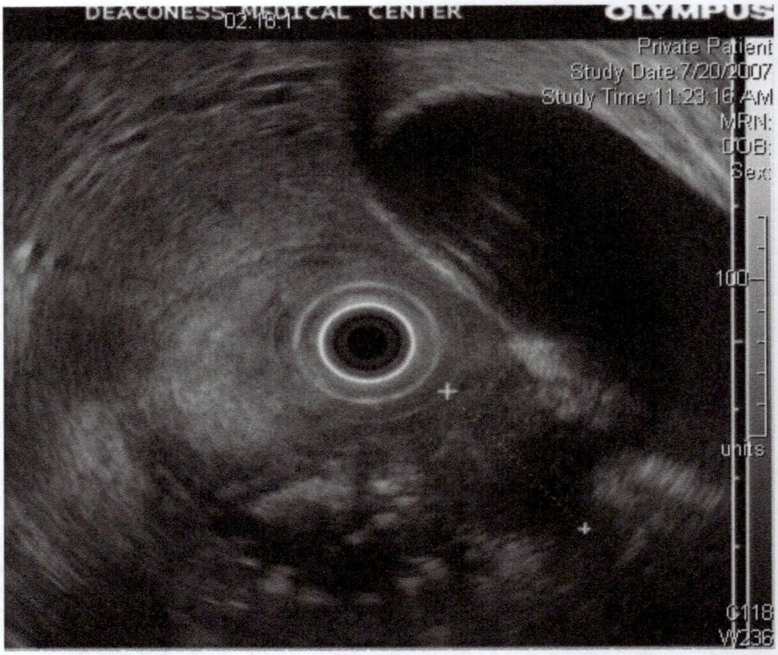

Fig. 6.47 This image focuses on the hypoechoic tumor in the pancreas. It measures 2.8 cm in diameter

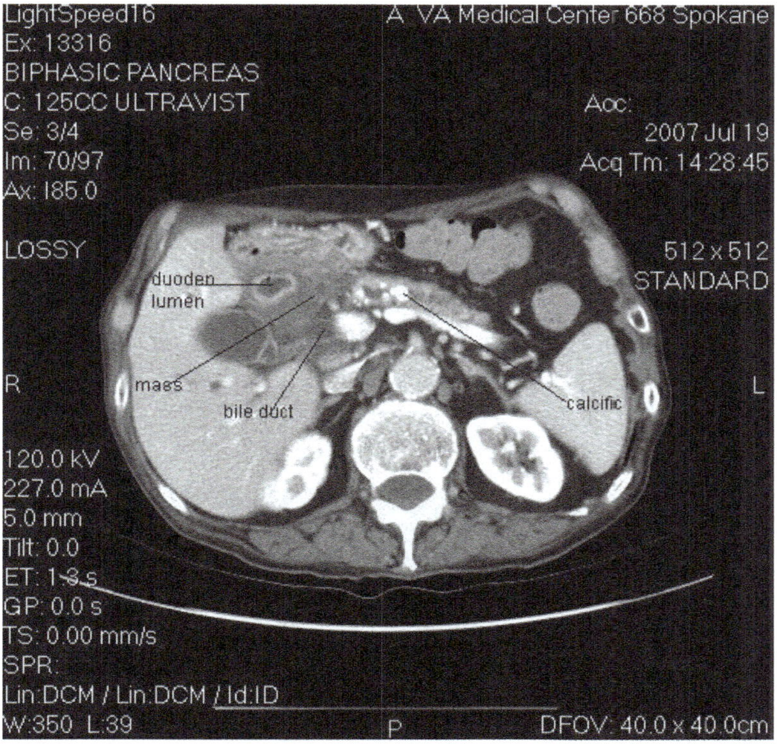

Fig. 6.48 This computed tomography scan shows severe chronic calcific pancreatitis and the periduodenal mass

6.2.12 Small Pancreatic Cancer

This is a 69-year-old asymptomatic man who underwent CT for other reasons and was found to have a small pancreatic body mass (1.3 cm). In this particular case the small pancreatic cancer was hypodense on CT and associated with upstream dilation of the pancreatic duct.

Upstream dilation of the pancreatic duct in this case made the cancer easily recognizable. As we have seen elsewhere, this is often not the case, and one must search for more subtle signs of a mass effect. For example, a visible pancreatic duct in the body and tail of the pancreas can be a sign of a problem if the pancreatic duct in the head area is not visualized well. Tumors that are less than 1.5–2 cm in size have a distinctly better prognosis than those that are larger. For example, in one study from Japan the 5-year survival rate and the median length of survival in patients with tumor diameters of 15 mm or less were 75 % and 62 months, respectively [33]. However, regional lymph nodes should be careful evaluation using EUS, even in patients with a small tumors, to rule out metastatic disease because it is a major prognostic factor [33].

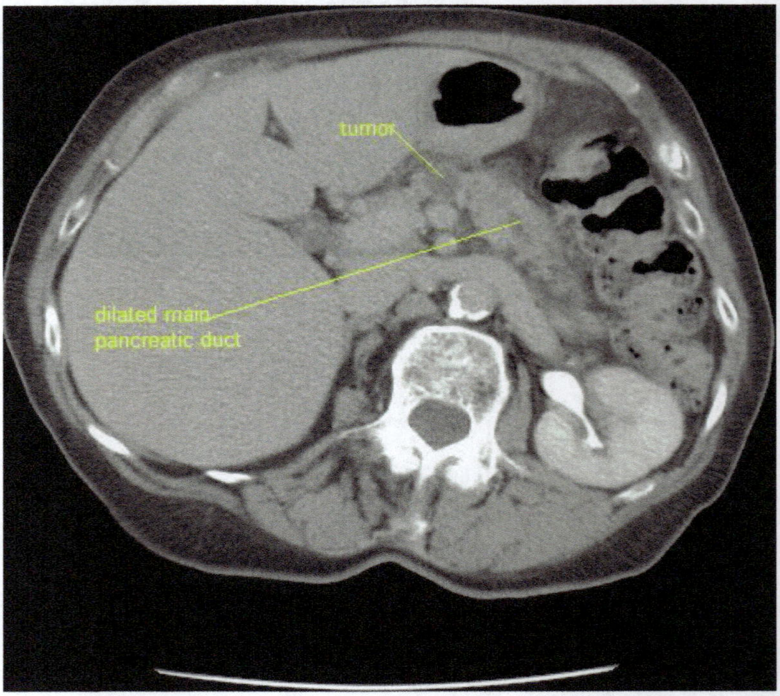

Fig. 6.49 This is a 1.3-cm-diameter mass in the pancreatic body that is obstructing the upstream pancreatic duct

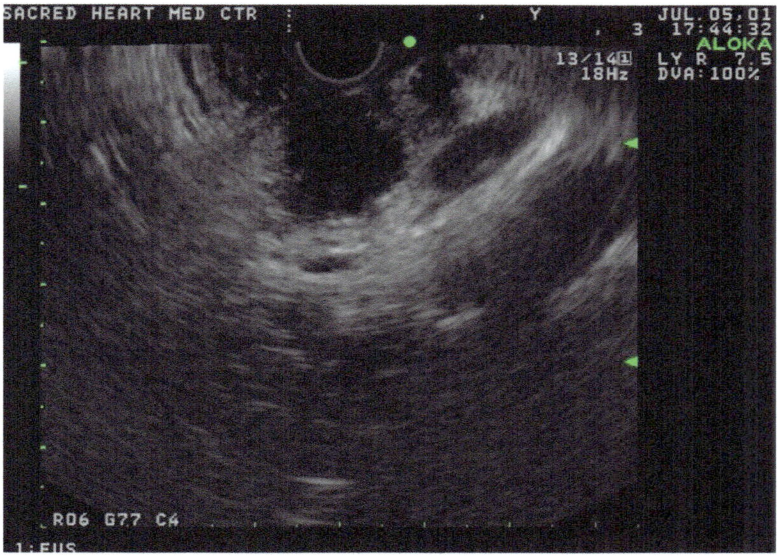

Fig. 6.50 This is the mass seen with the linear array endoscopic ultrasound instrument before fine-needle aspiration biopsy

6.2.13 Isodense Pancreatic Cancer

On contrast-enhanced CT pancreatic cancers are generally hypodense compared to normal pancreas. Up to 10 % of pancreatic cancers may, however, appear isodense. This can pose diagnostic difficulties. This is a 71-year-old patient with weight loss and nonspecific abdominal pain. The initial CT was unremarkable but the patient continued to have complaints. MRI clearly shows a mass lesion suspicious for pancreatic cancer. On a subsequent EUS a 2.2-cm, hypoechoic pancreatic mass was found and biopsied. Cytology was positive for adenocarcinoma. A triangular periportal lymph node that was suspicious because of its size (2.0 cm) also was biopsied but was negative for metastatic disease. To complicate matters, the patient was found to have a small mass in the liver on transabdominal ultrasound, which preoperative percutaneous biopsy showed to be only fibrosis. He had a Whipple pancreaticoduodenectomy. Fortunately, the liver mass was biopsied intraoperatively again and showed hepatocellular carcinoma. The hepatoma was the ablated with radiofrequency energy.

The diagnosis of pancreatic cancer at early stages is of great importance given that the disease can be curable with surgical resection of small tumors. Multidetector CT is faster than helical CT, allowing better timing of the images during the arterial phase and thinner sections. Unfortunately, the diagnosis of small pancreatic cancers can be challenging even with multidetector CT; tumors may appear isodense to normal, particularly on delayed contrast phases (portal or venous), and secondary signs such as ductal dilatation or distortion of the pancreatic contour are minimal. As discussed earlier, the presence of chronic pancreatitis may also affect the diagnostic accuracy of imaging signs of cancer.

EUS is considered the most sensitive test for the detection of pancreatic tumors, particularly those smaller than 2 cm, with reported sensitivity between 91 and 100 %. The specificity of EUS alone is limited, but EUS-guided FNA is able to provide a final diagnosis with high specificity.

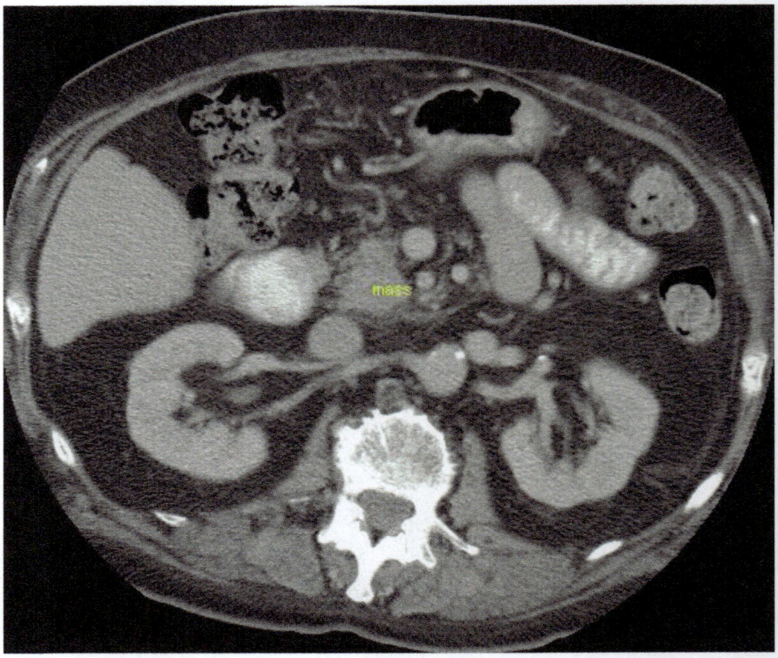

Fig. 6.51 This is a pancreatic mass that is isodense to the normal pancreas and was difficult to discern

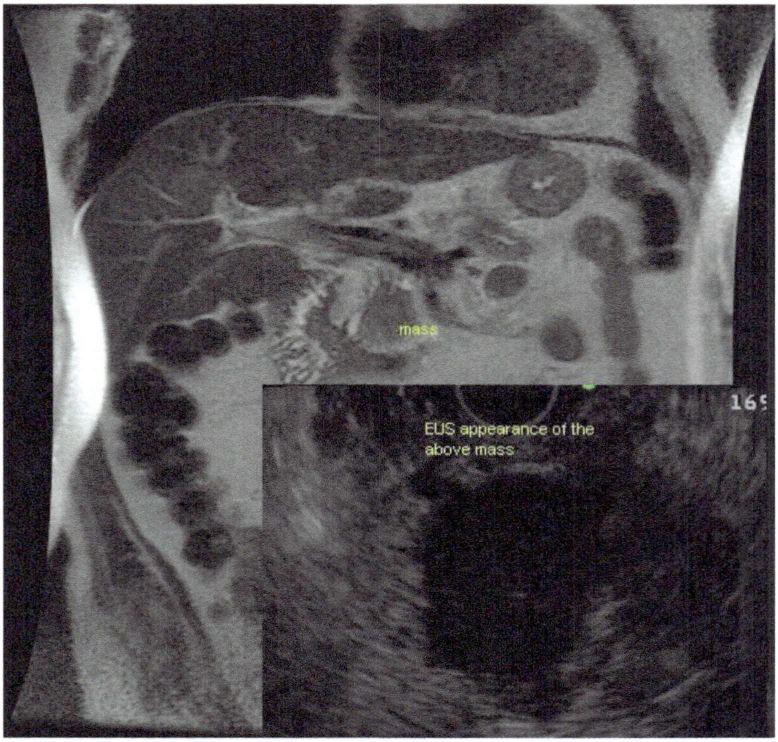

Fig. 6.52 Endoscopic ultrasound with magnetic resonance imaging overlay of the pancreatic head tumor

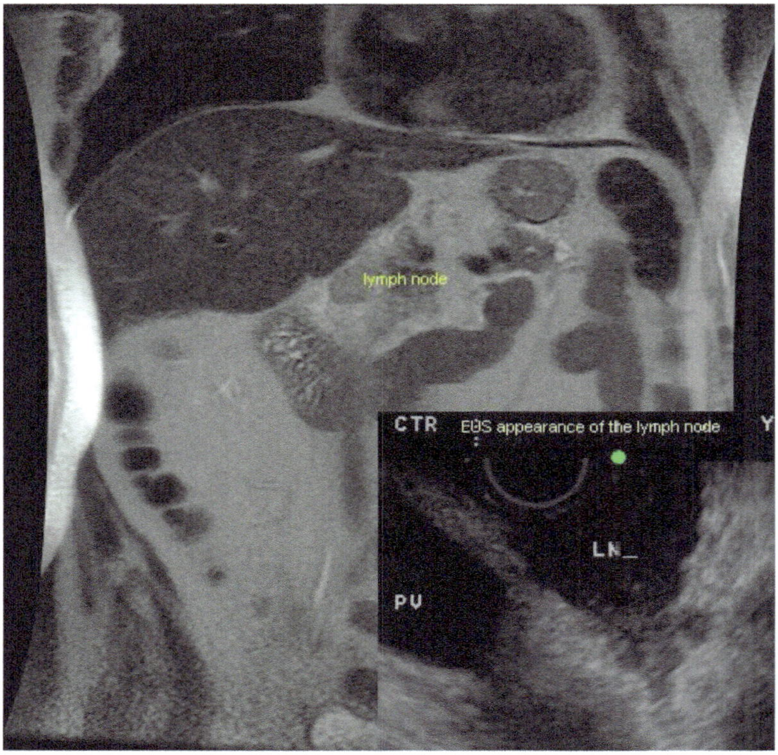

Fig. 6.53 Endoscopic ultrasound with magnetic resonance imaging overlay of the periportal lymph node

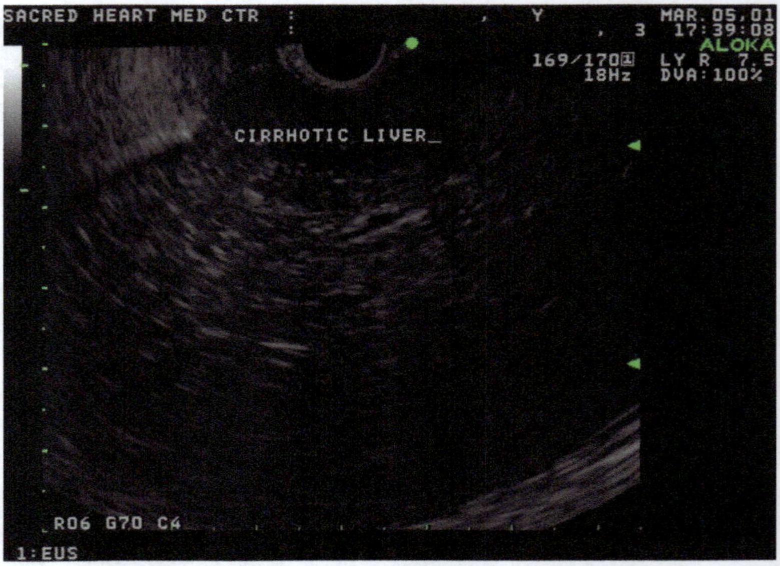

Fig. 6.54 Increased echogenicity of the liver, consistent with fibrosis/cirrhosis

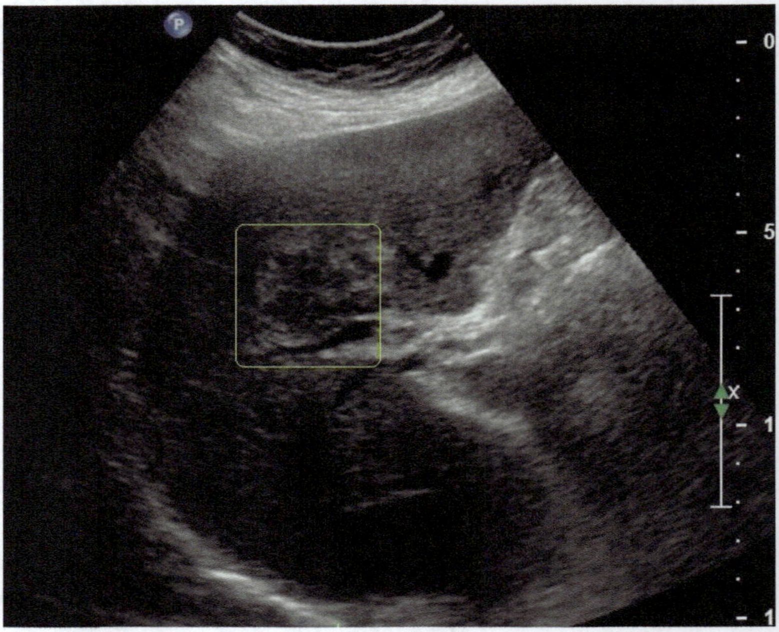

Fig. 6.55 A small, round lesion in the liver was seen on transabdominal ultrasound. Biopsies showed fibrosis only

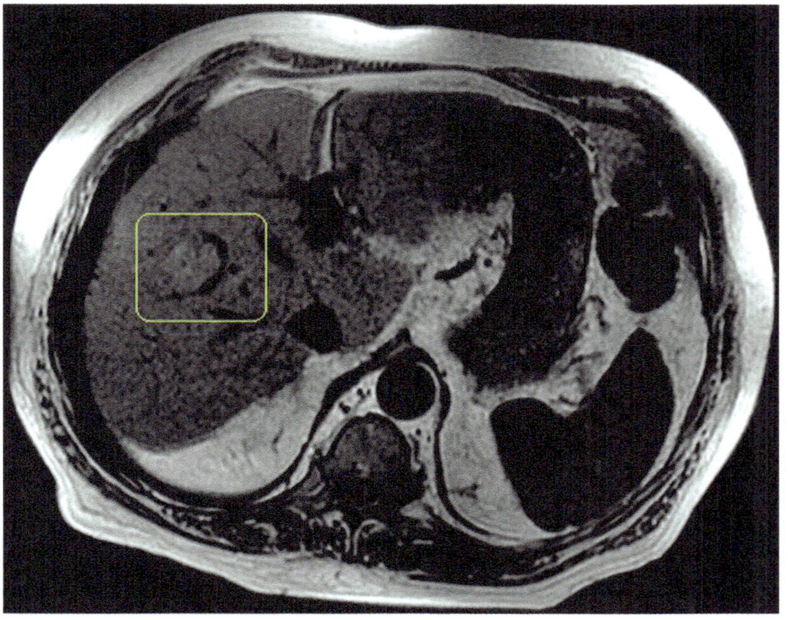

Fig. 6.56 The liver lesion can also be identified retrospectively on the magnetic resonance image. The lesion was biopsied intraoperatively again, revealing hepatoma

6.2.14 Large Pancreatic Head in Relation to Body

This is a 72-year-old patient with a history of prostate cancer who was initially found to have mildly abnormal liver tests. CT was performed 1 year before and again shortly before this EUS. A year ago the pancreatic head measured 2.8 cm; currently it is at least 3.2 cm. Compared with the pancreatic tail the head is indeed large. Moreover, the main pancreatic duct in the body/tail region is dilated, whereas in the head it is difficult to identify. The most recent CT scan was interpreted as showing possible fatty infiltration of the head of the pancreas but, fortunately, an EUS was recommended. EUS shows a hypoechoic mass that was aggressively biopsied (seven passes), showing cells that were read as suspicious for neoplasia. Soon after the patient developed obstructive jaundice consistent with a neoplasm.

It has been suggested that EUS is losing ground as the best imaging modality for the detection of pancreatic cancer to CT and MRI. There are reports that illustrate that this is not the case; EUS has been found to be more sensitive than standard cross-sectional imaging studies for small lesions (<2 cm in diameter) [34]. This case also illustrates that subtle signs of possible pancreatic cancer should trigger EUS evaluation: a dilated main pancreatic duct is always ominous.

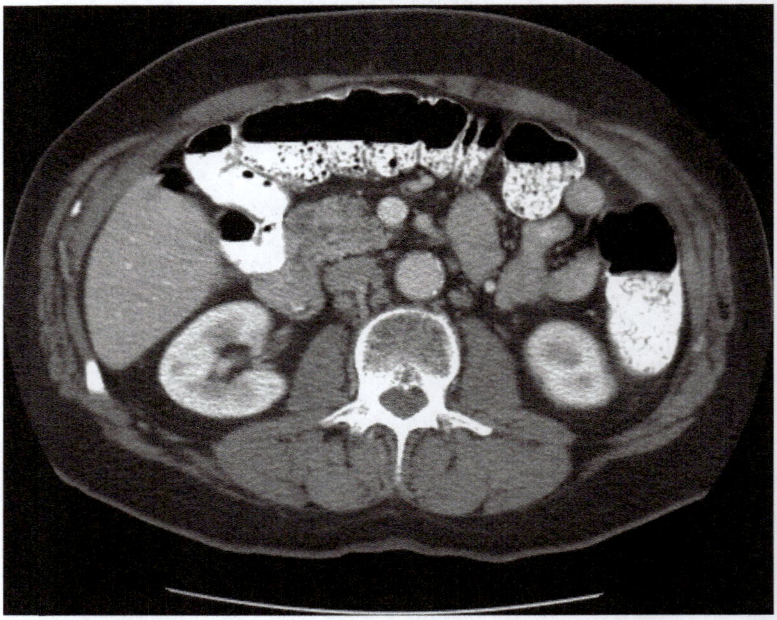

Fig. 6.57 This computed tomography scan shows the dimensions of the head of the pancreas 1 year before this presentation

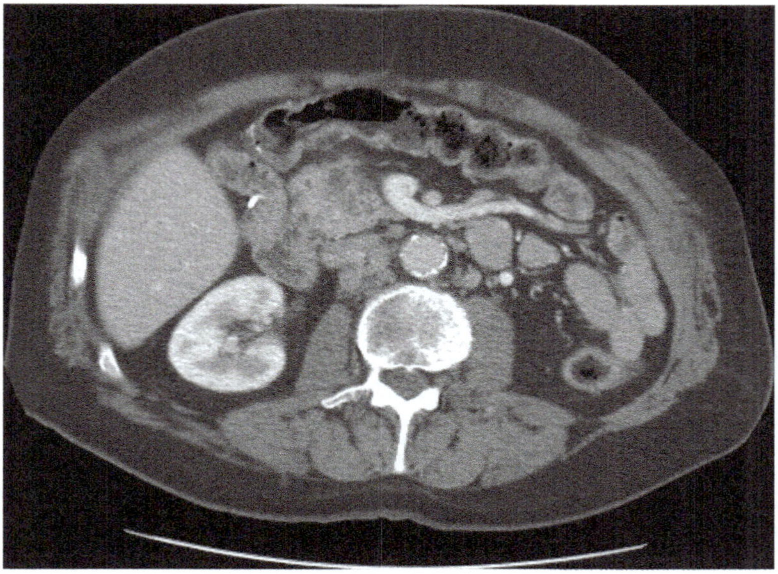

Fig. 6.58 The currently computed tomography scan shows an increased size of the pancreas head, which also appears inhomogeneous. There is no well-defined mass

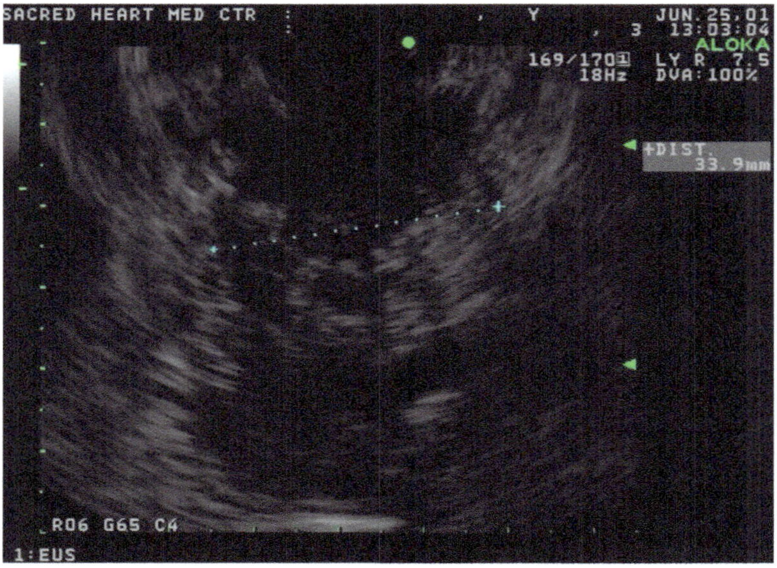

Fig. 6.59 A 3.2-cm mass is seen on this linear array endoscopic ultrasound image

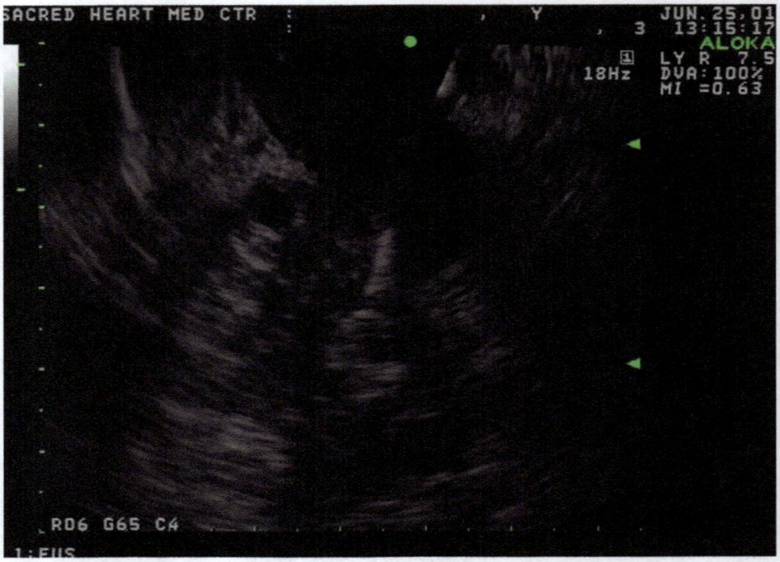

Fig. 6.60 A fine needle passes into the mass during aspiration cytology. Despite seven such passes only few suspicious appearing cells were present in the sample

6.2.15 Gardner's Syndrome and Pancreatic Cancer

This is a 65-year-old woman with Gardner's syndrome after colectomy who received a Whipple pancreaticoduodenectomy for an ampullary neoplasm approximately 10 years ago. Three months before her EUS evaluation she underwent abdominal CT, which incidentally showed a small hypodense area measuring 10.3 mm in diameter in the tail region of the pancreas. To document the stability of this small – and probably inconsequential – lesion, follow-up CT was arranged 3 months later and revealed substantial growth: the lesion now measured 22.2 mm in diameter. On a volume basis this corresponds to a doubling time of only 26 days, indicating a rapidly growing tumor. EUS-guided FNA biopsies revealed adenocarcinoma.

Gardner's syndrome is a variant of familial adenomatous polyposis (FAP) and is characterized by gastrointestinal polyps, multiple osteomas, and skin and soft tissue tumors (desmoid tumors). There is an increased risk of other malignancies, especially ampullary carcinomas. Patients with FAP or Gardner's syndrome also seem to be at increased risk for pancreatic neoplasms, and increased vigilance is necessary [35].

Reports of malignancies of the pancreas in association with FAP/Gardner's syndrome involve a variety of cell lines. Exocrine, endocrine, and stromal pancreatic tissues have all been reported as sites for malignancies in association with FAP/Gardner's syndrome. Individuals with FAP/Gardner's syndrome may have a 100- to 200-fold increased risk of developing periampullary carcinoma when compared with the general population [36]. The incidence of ampullary tumors is increased 200- to 300-fold among patients with hereditary polyposis syndromes, such as FAP, and hereditary nonpolyposis colorectal cancer [37, 38]. However, the risk of pancreatic adenocarcinoma in FAP/Gardner's syndrome has been reported to be increased more than fourfold compared with the general population (relative risk, 4.46; 95 % confidence interval, 1 2–11.4); however, the absolute lifetime risk is still low at about 2 % [39]. FAP is caused by mutations in the *5q21* gene locus, but most pancreatic carcinomas are associated with other mutations such as *K-ras* (12p12), *17p*, *18q* (*DCC* locus), and *p53* (17p13). Whether there is a true linkage or association by coincidence is unclear. However, pancreatic adenocarcinoma has been described in a variety cancer susceptibility syndromes associated with germline mutations in the *p16*, *BRCA1*, *BRCA2*, and *APC* genes [35]. Needless to say, more reports and studies are considered necessary to support linkage and/or association.

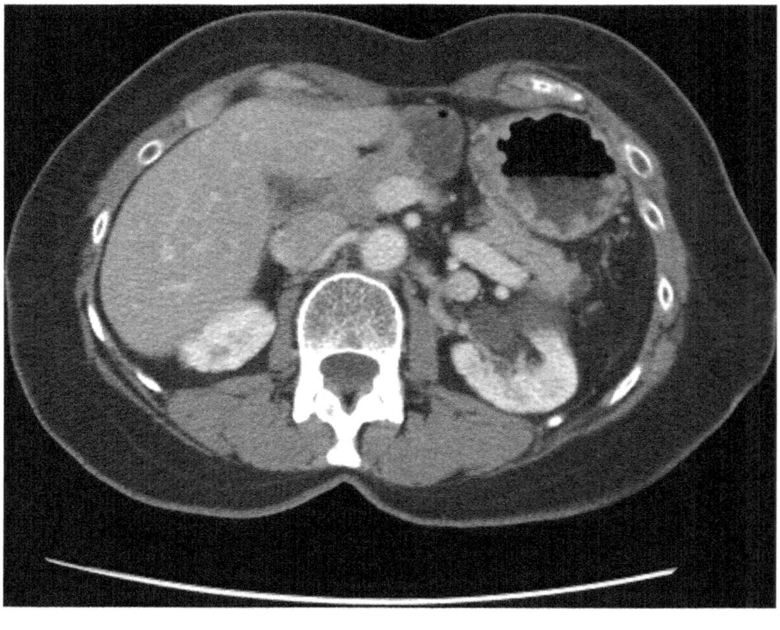

Fig. 6.61 This computed tomography scan shows a 10-mm-diameter hypodense pancreatic tail lesion

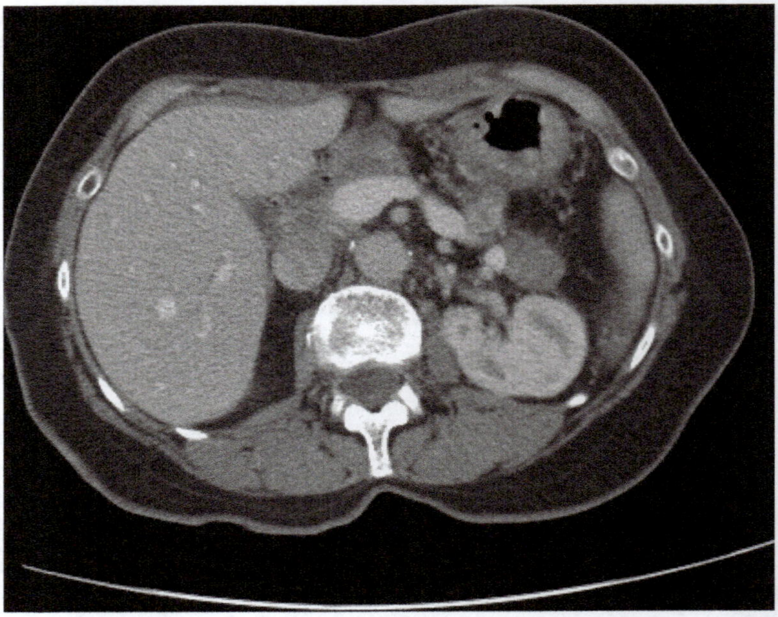

Fig. 6.62 A follow-up computed tomography scan 3 months later (88 days) shows that the lesion has increased from 10.3 to 22.2 mm, corresponding to a doubling time of only 26 days

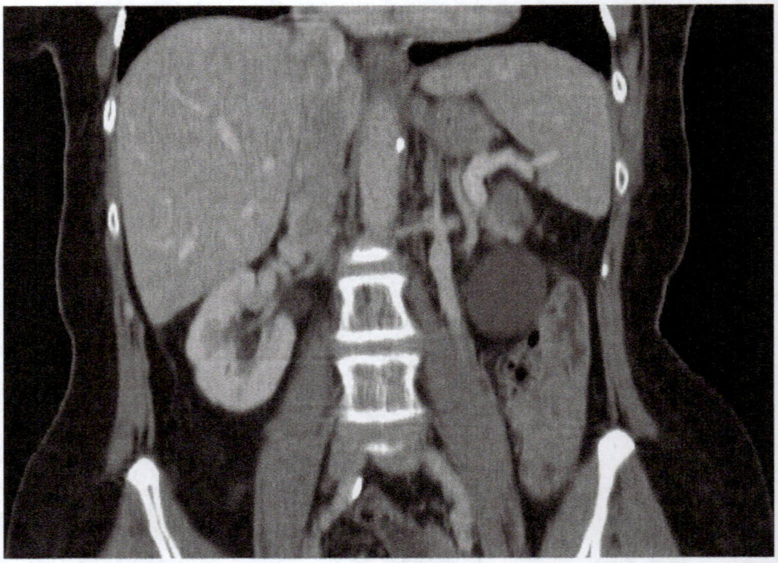

Fig. 6.63 This is a coronal reconstruction of the same pancreatic tail mass

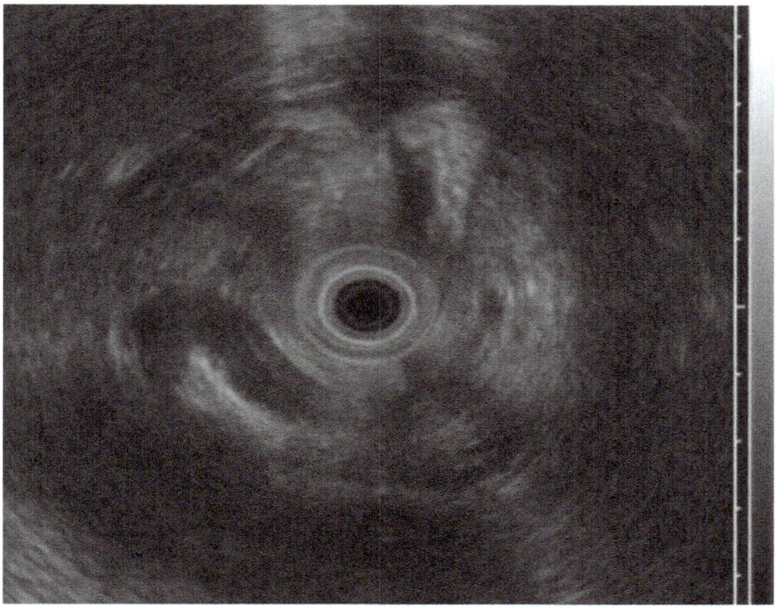

Fig. 6.64 This is a radial endoscopic ultrasound representation of the pancreatic tail mass

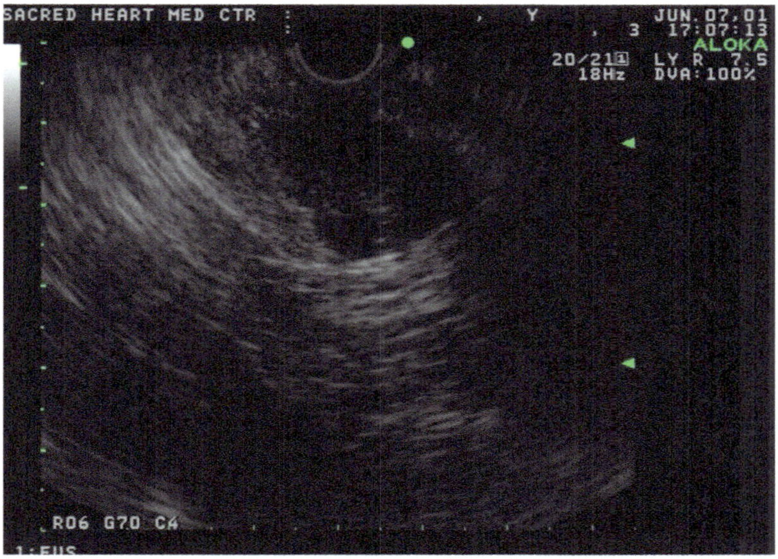

Fig. 6.65 This is a linear endoscopic ultrasound representation of the same pancreatic tail mass before biopsy

6.2.16 Missed Pancreatic Cancer

This is a 69-year-old woman who initially presented with epigastric pain and was found to have mildly elevated pancreatic and liver enzymes. CT showed a dilated bile duct and pancreatic duct but no mass lesion. ERCP with sphincterotomy was performed but no referral for EUS was made, and she improved. Ultimately it was thought that she had dysfunction of the sphincter of Oddi. A year later she returned with increasing abdominal pain, and repeat CT showed a mass in the head of the pancreas. EUS then was requested and showed a 4.4-cm mass wrapping around the superior mesenteric vein. Biopsies confirmed adenocarcinoma.

Both EUS and CT can miss pancreatic cancers. In one study the time interval between abnormalities seen on CT and the clinical diagnosis of pancreatic cancer was investigated, and the authors concluded that CT findings definite or suspicious for pancreatic cancer were present in 50 % of the scans obtained 2–6 and 6–18 months before the diagnosis of pancreatic cancer in those patients who had prior CT scans with an original reading that did not suggest pancreatic cancer [40]. The authors conclude that "an alternating regimen of CT with endoscopic sonography or MRI may prove beneficial by exploiting the strengths of each technique."

An analysis of EUS studies in which a diagnosis of pancreatic adenocarcinoma was missed by experts revealed factors that may increase the likelihood of false-negative EUS evaluation, including chronic pancreatitis, diffusely infiltrative adenocarcinoma, prominent dorsal/ventral split appearance, and acute pancreatitis within the last 4 weeks. If done within 3 months, repeat EUS was able to detect tumors that were initially missed [41].

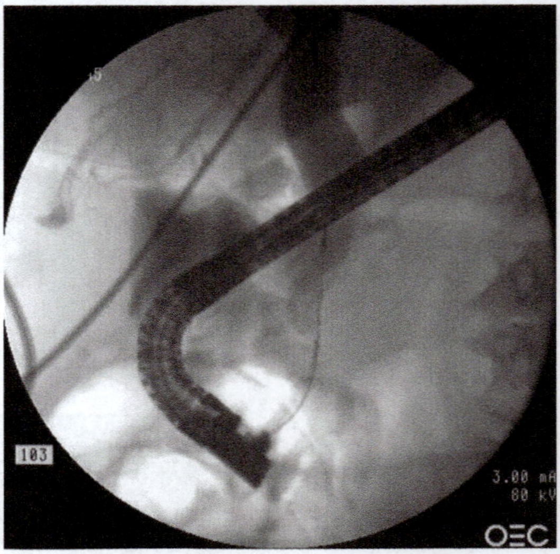

Fig. 6.66 This endoscopic retrograde cholangiopancreatography shows mild dilation of the bile duct ascribed to dysfunction of the sphincter of Oddi 12 months earlier

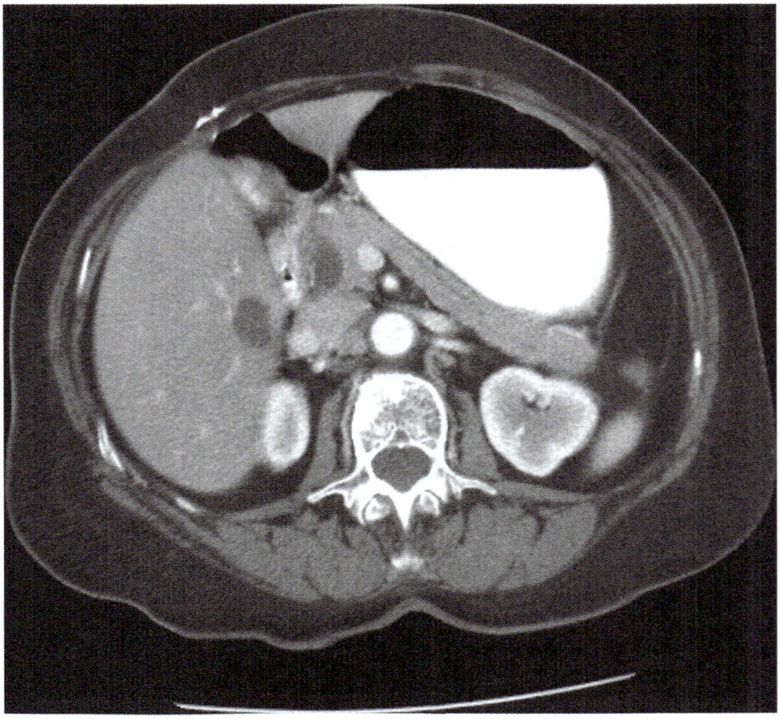

Fig. 6.67 This computed tomography scan shows the dilated common bile duct 12 months before the current presentation

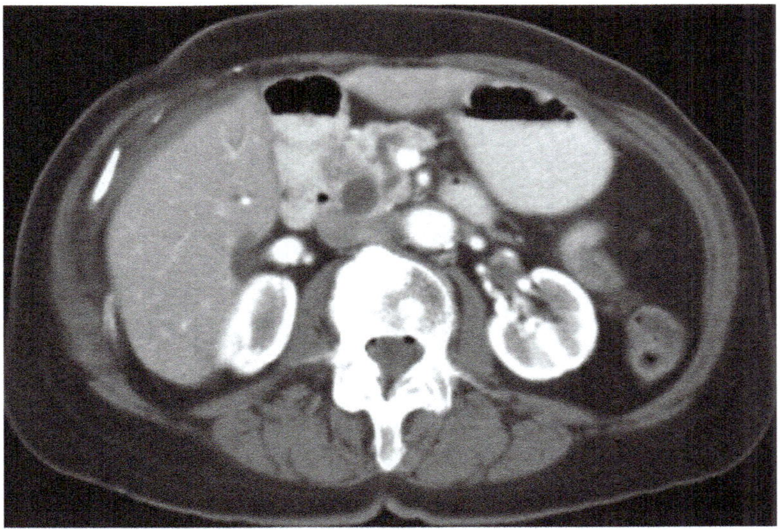

Fig. 6.68 In comparison, the dilated bile duct as seen by the current computed tomography

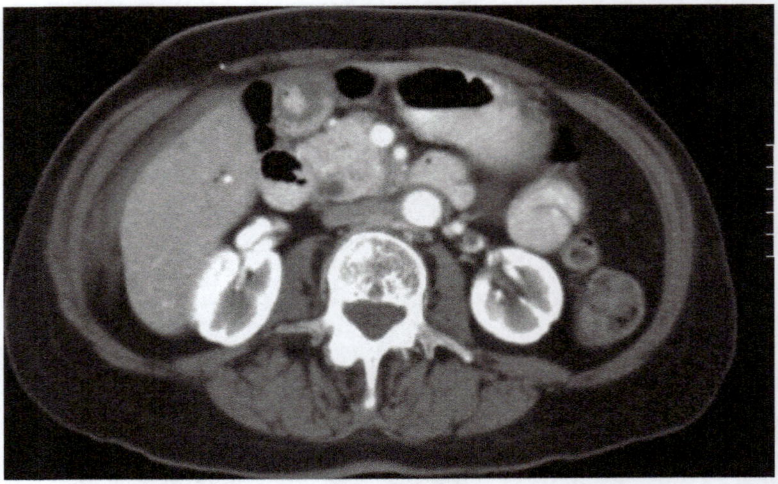

Fig. 6.69 An enhancing mass lesion in the head of the pancreas appears to be present

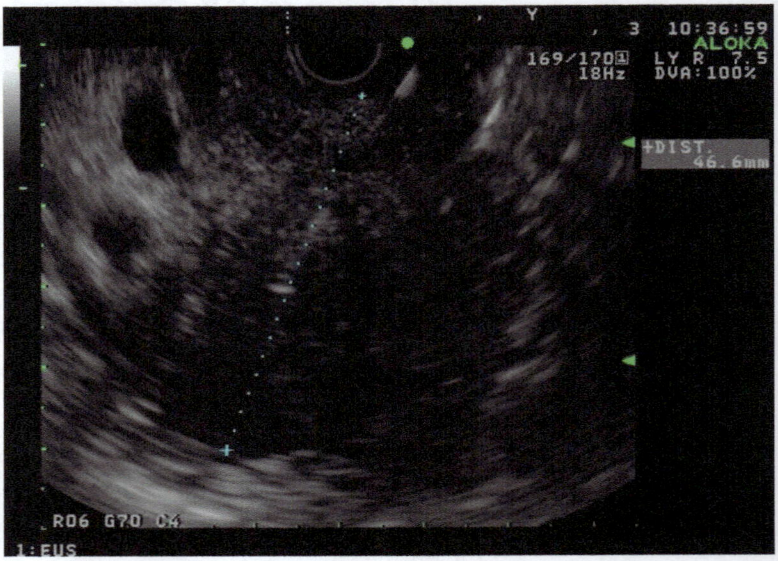

Fig. 6.70 On endoscopic ultrasound a large hypoechoic mass is seen in the head of the pancreas

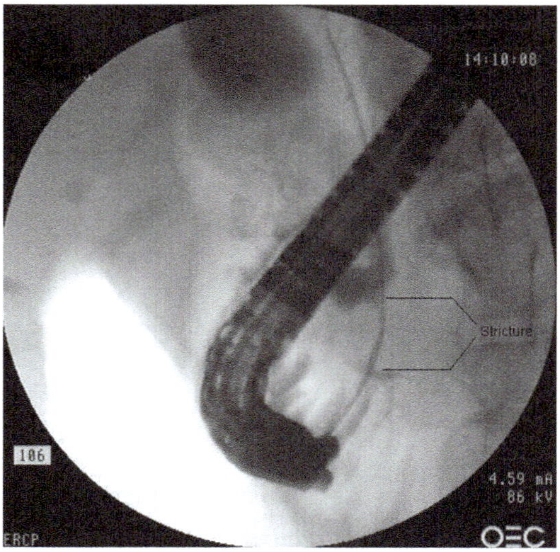

Fig. 6.71 In the interim the patient had developed jaundice. This image from a recent endoscopic retrograde cholangiopancreatography shows a distal common bile duct stricture with typical tumor shelf and upstream dilation of the bile duct

6.2.17 Ovarian Cancer Metastatic to the Pancreas?

This is a 54-year-old patient who developed mid-epigastric discomfort. CT was obtained when she complained of increasing abdominal girth. It showed ascites and a complex cystic ovarian mass as well as a pancreatic body mass but no biliary dilation. The cancer antigen 125 levels were 668 U/ml, but the CA 19–9 levels were even higher (1,277 U/ml). Cytology of the ascites was positive for adenocarcinoma. EUS was requested to obtain an FNA biopsy of the pancreatic mass to rule out a possible pancreatic primary tumor. The mass in the body of the pancreas (shown in Figs. 6.73 and 6.75) was biopsied and a routine exam of the pancreas head conducted. This surprisingly showed extensive collaterals surrounding a nearby second hypoechoic mass. The finding of multiple pancreatic tumors itself would suggest that the pancreas lesions were metastatic. However, immunohistochemistry of the pancreatic FNA strongly supported a pancreatic primary tumor. Cancer antigen 125 levels can be elevated in cancers other than ovarian carcinoma, for example, in pancreatic adenocarcinomas. On the basis of these results the patient's surgery for debulking of the initially suspected ovarian primary tumor was canceled and she was referred for chemotherapy instead.

Metastatic tumors of the pancreas are relatively uncommon and generally asymptomatic; these lesions are usually identified on surveillance imaging. This diagnosis should be strongly considered in cases with atypical imaging findings including the absence of ductal dilation, hypervascularity, size of the lesion >5 cm, intravenous tumor thrombus, and intralesional ducts or cysts [42]. Most of these metastases are found as solitary pancreatic lesions, in contrast to the multifocal involvement of other organs [43].

Renal and lung cancers are the most common primary tumors that metastasize to the pancreas [44]. Renal cancer metastases are hypervascular compared with primary adenocarcinoma or lung metastases. Other tumors that can metastasize to the pancreas include colorectal cancer, breast cancer, melanoma, soft-tissue sarcoma, and, rarely, ovarian cancer [43]. Cystic-appearing lesions have been reported in patients with metastatic colon cancer, melanoma, and ovarian cancer [43].

EUS-guided FNA plays an important role in establishing the diagnosis of metastatic cancer in the pancreas. Immunohistochemistry techniques and cytologic morphology are important in determining the type of primary tumor.

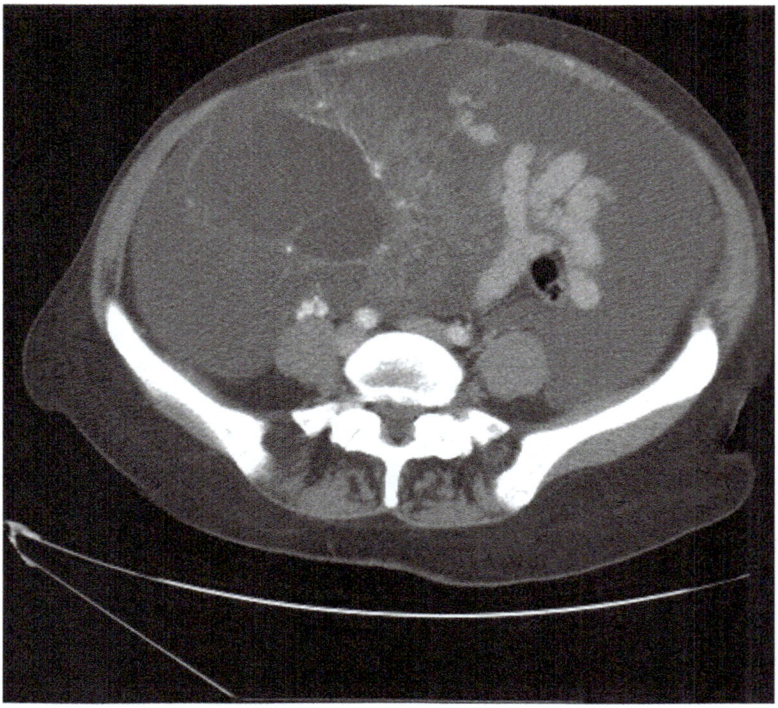

Fig. 6.72 A complex, multicystic pelvic mass surrounded by ascites

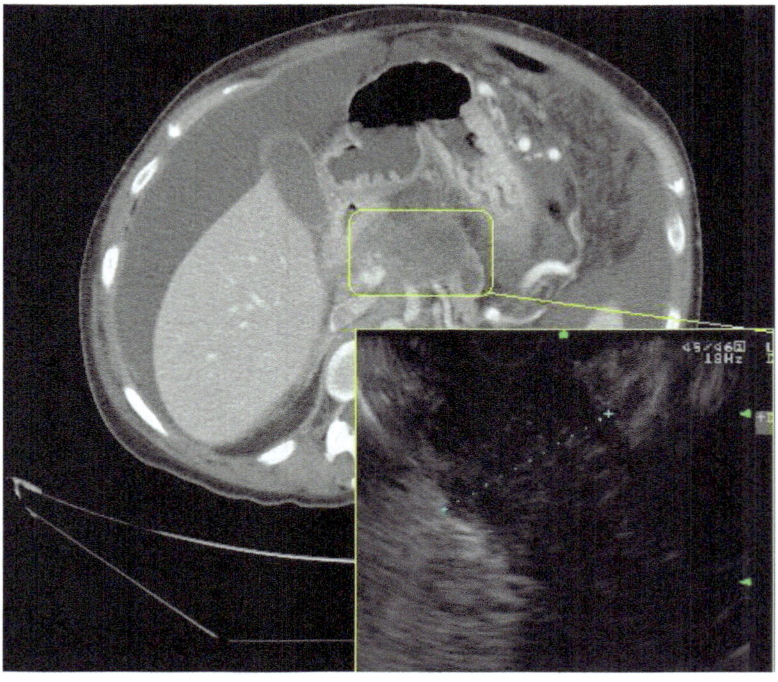

Fig. 6.73 Appearance of the pancreatic body mass on computed tomography and endoscopic ultrasound

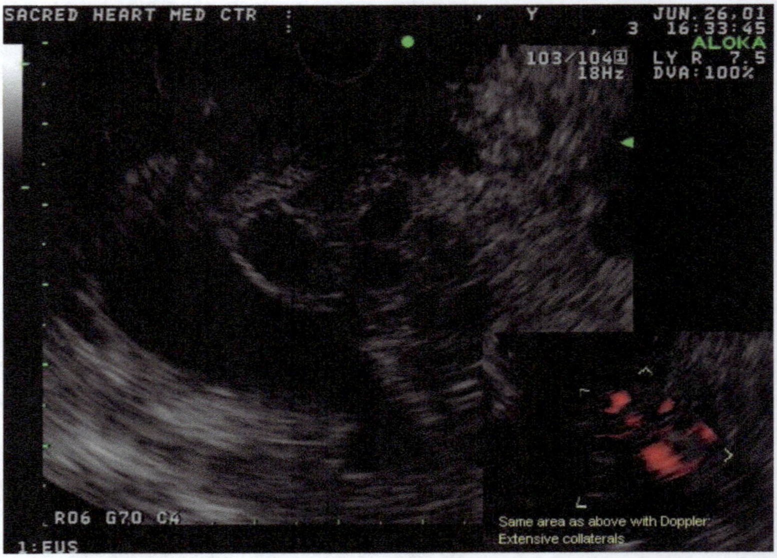

Fig. 6.74 This image shows extensive collaterals caught mostly in cross section

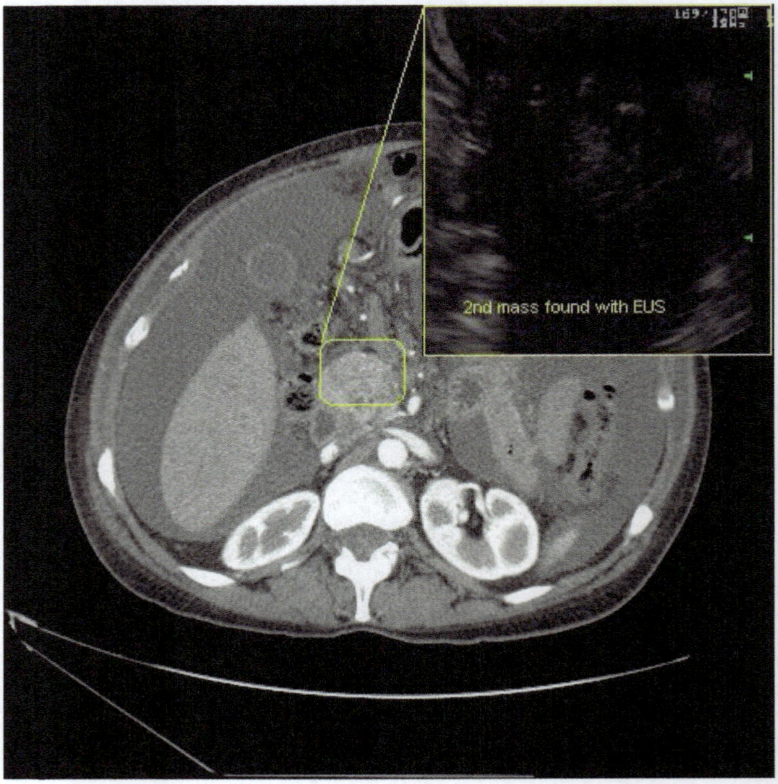

Fig. 6.75 A second hypoechoic tumor, this time in the head, is easily visible with endoscopic ultrasound but seen only retrospectively on computed tomography

6.2.18 Characteristic Appearance of a Wallstent on EUS

This is a 59-year-old man who presented with obstructive jaundice and was found to have a pancreatic mass. Unfortunately, several liver metastases were already present. CT was also interesting because it showed almost complete atrophy of the pancreatic body and tail from obstruction of the main pancreatic duct. A self-expandable metal stent was placed across the bile duct stricture before obtaining a tissue diagnosis. EUS-guided biopsies were performed after stent placement to confirm the diagnosis. The characteristic appearance of the lattice of the Wallstent in cross section is shown.

Evaluation of patients using EUS before performing ERCP has been recommended by the American Society of Gastrointestinal Endoscopy [45] to better evaluate the nature of underlying disease (benign vs. malignant), determine the extent and invasion to adjacent structures (staging), and guide stent selection of plastic versus self-expandable metal stents (SEMSs) [46]. Biliary stents can make the EUS evaluation of the mass and adjacent anatomic structures challenging because of their acoustic shadow; inflammatory reaction around the stent may have a negative effect on the yield of FNA [47]. However, in a recent study the presence of a biliary stent did not effect the diagnostic yield of EUS-guided FNA performed by expert endosonographers. The authors recommended a combination of maneuvers to overcome the reverberation effect induced by SEMSs, including [46]:

- Tracing the SEMS from the hilum to the papilla and targeting the area where the reverberation is minimal, which is expected to correspond to the site of tumor.
- A pull-through maneuver from the second portion of duodenum, torquing the endoscope to deflect the acoustic shadowing to reveal the mass.
- Flushing the duodenal lumen with water and aspirating air.

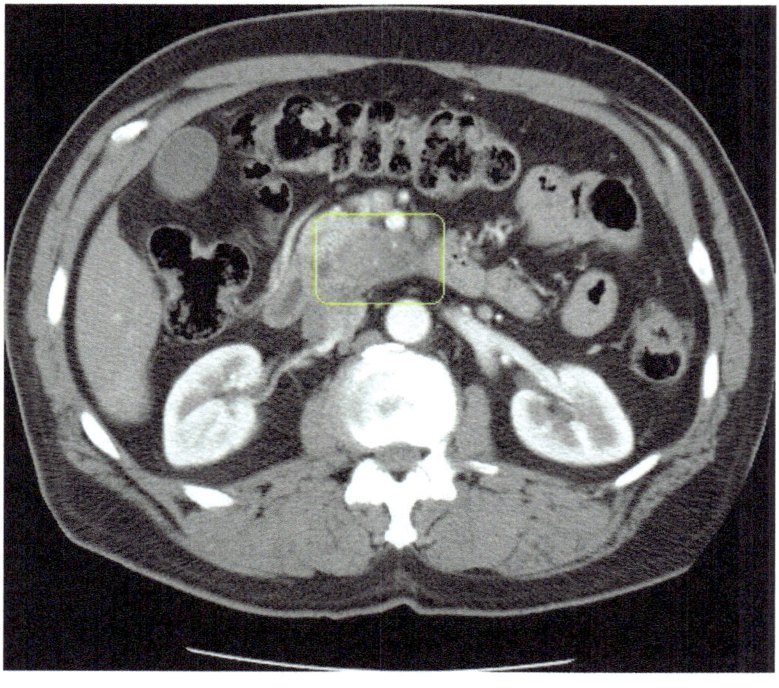

Fig. 6.76 Pancreatic mass on computed tomography

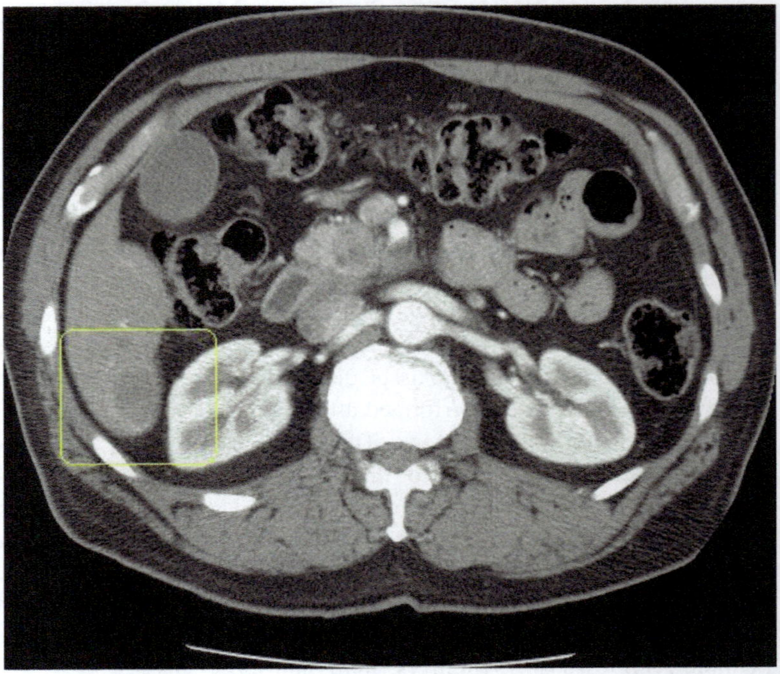

Fig. 6.77 One of several liver metastases from pancreatic adenocarcinoma

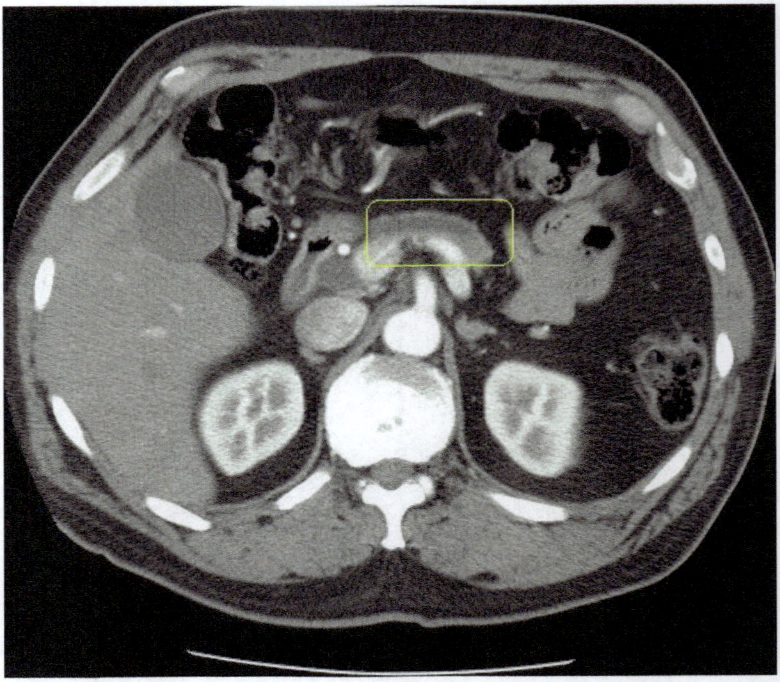

Fig. 6.78 Advanced atrophy of the pancreatic body and tail secondary to an obstructing pancreatic mass

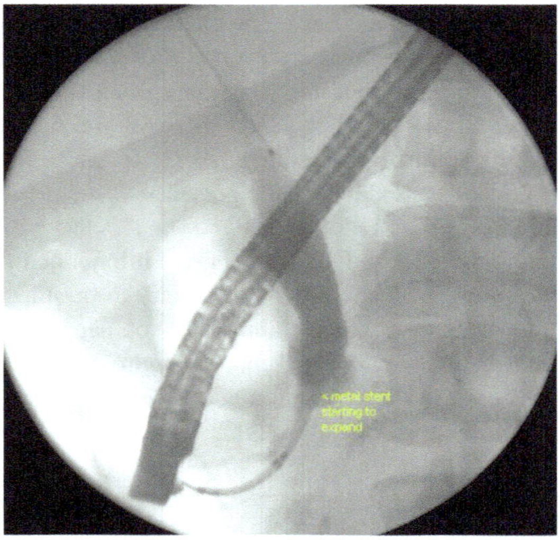

Fig. 6.79 A biliary metal stent in the beginning stages of deployment

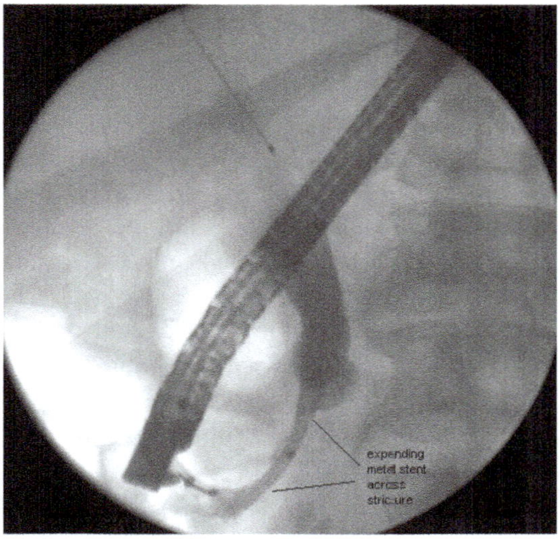

Fig. 6.80 A biliary metal stent fully deployed in pancreatic adenocarcinoma

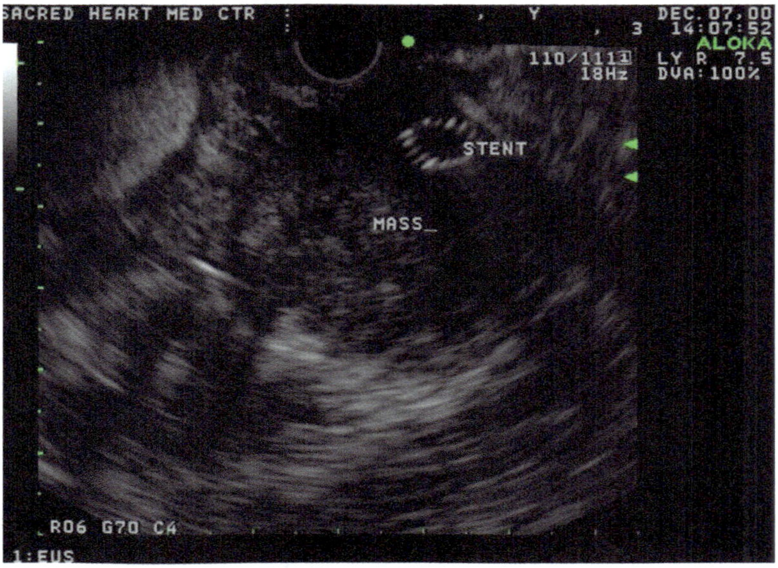

Fig. 6.81 Cross-sectional appearance of the biliary metal stent with endoscopic ultrasound

6.2.19 FNA Biopsies Through a Wallstent

This case indicates that insertion of a metal stent into the bile duct before definitive tissue diagnosis can be problematic. A frail 87-year-old woman had a mass in the head of the pancreas, which led to obstructive jaundice that was palliated with a SEMS placed in the bile duct. The mass was biopsied later using EUS-guided FNA; unfortunately, the cytology was signed out as only "suspicious for malignancy." A CT-guided core biopsy then was performed and returned nondiagnostic material. The medical oncologists convinced us to go back once more, at which time we performed biopsies through an (uncovered) SEMS (as shown in Figs. 6.82 and 6.83), finally confirming the diagnosis.

As discussed before the presence of the metal creates serious streak artifacts that deteriorate imaging by both EUS and CT. Additional endoscopic maneuvers may be necessary to optimize the endosonographic approach to pancreatic masses in patients with biliary endoprosthesis. In this case we demonstrated that FNA can be successfully performed through a SEMS.

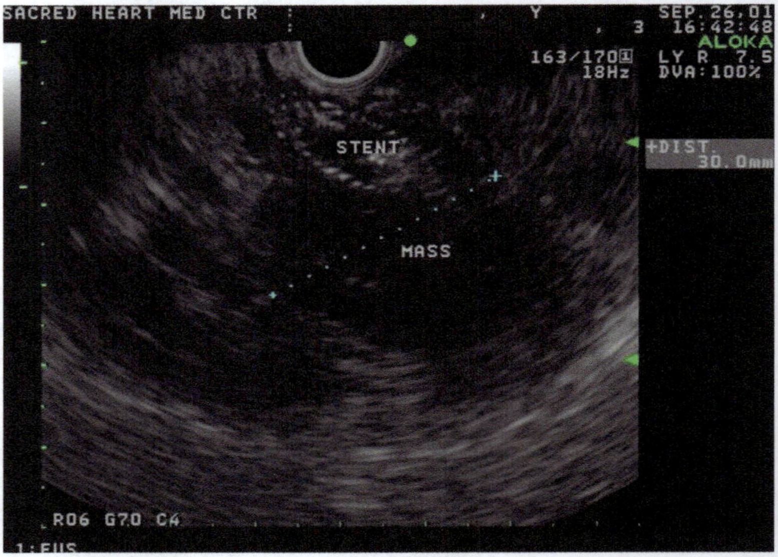

Fig. 6.82 This Wallstent in the common bile duct blocks the path of the needle used for fine-needle aspiration

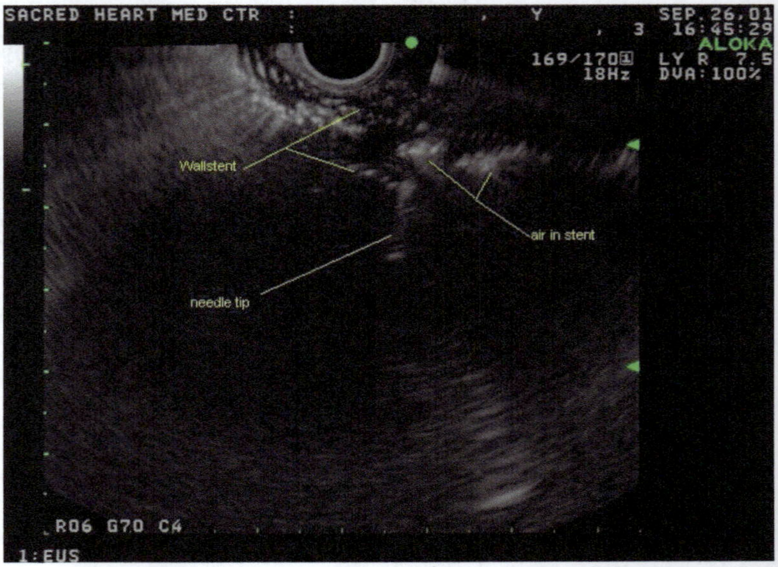

Fig. 6.83 Fortunately, biopsies through an uncovered Wallstent are not particularly difficult

6.2.20 Neuroendocrine Tumors

6.2.20.1 Simultaneous Metastatic Carcinoid and Symptomatic Insulinoma

This is a 75-year-old patient who 3 years earlier presented with unrelenting diarrhea. CT showed multiple liver lesions. Biopsies were consistent with metastatic carcinoid based on characteristic findings on immunohistochemistry. A primary tumor was not apparent. The patient did well with octreotide and the lesions stabilized or may have regressed somewhat. The patient recently exhibited increasingly bizarre behavior: furniture in her home, where she lives by herself, was found to be rearranged in peculiar ways. She had spells of profound weakness and was admitted to the hospital with pneumonia. There she was observed to have seizures. A blood glucose level was repeatedly very low: at one time it was 4 mg/dl (range, 65–99 mg/dl). C-peptide and insulin levels were high. A repeat CT was obtained in Fig. 6.84. The carcinoid tumor lesions were again seen in the liver, but the CT was otherwise read as not showing any other suspicious lesions. An octreotide scan was negative for lesions other than those present in the liver. EUS was requested and showed a 1.7×1.0-cm, hypoechoic, well-circumscribed lesion consistent with a neuroendocrine tumor in the body of the pancreas. It was aspirated for cytology, which confirmed a neuroendocrine tumor. Armed with these findings, the EUS examiner went back to the CT scan, and it was now possible – in retrospect – to identify the lesion. This case illustrates a key point: EUS is an interrogation technique. It helps answer specific questions. When a finding is confusing or its relevance not immediately apparent, the area in question can be "interrogated" from different perspectives and angles. This is not possible with CT.

Approximately 5 % of pancreatic tumors are neuroendocrine in origin All these lesions produce hormones/peptides to some degree, but only some release enough to cause systemic manifestations; these are called functional neuroendocrine tumors.

EUS is an excellent tool with which to identify neuroendocrine tumors of the pancreas that have not previously been seen by other imaging techniques, confirm the disease by obtaining tissue diagnosis, and detect regional lymph node metastases. EUS has been shown to have a high sensitivity (75–94 %) in the detection of pancreatic gastrinomas and insulinomas [48]. It is important to remember that approximately 50 % of gastrinomas are located in the pancreas, while the rest tend to be at the duodenal wall.

The majority of these lesions are solid and well circumscribed on EUS, CT, or MRI, but they can appear cystic, as discussed in the following case. Neuroendocrine tumors can ocassionally cause biliary obstruction in patients with local desmoplastic effect, typically associated to production of serotonin, and in cases with very large tumor that compresses the bile duct [42].

Neuroendocrine tumors can present as single or multiple lesions, and a complete examination of the pancreas is important to rule out synchronous lesions. Tumor size is considered the best predictor of aggressive behavior [49].

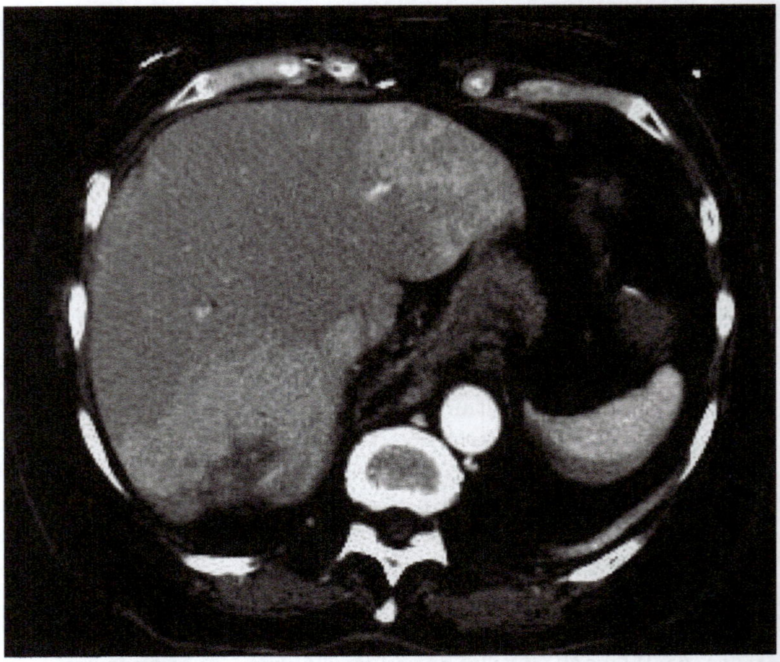

Fig. 6.84 Computed tomography scan shows large liver masses representing metastatic carcinoid

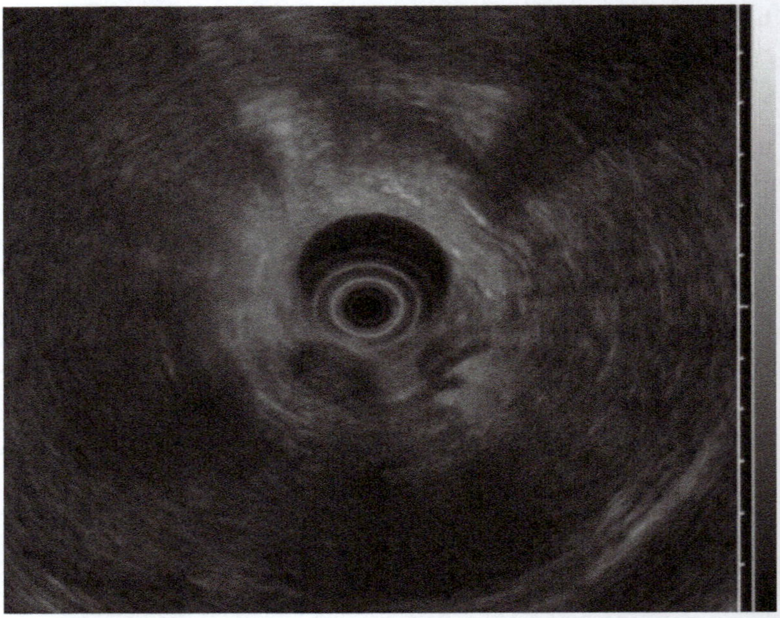

Fig. 6.85 Endoscopic ultrasound shows a hypoechoic mass in the body of the pancreas

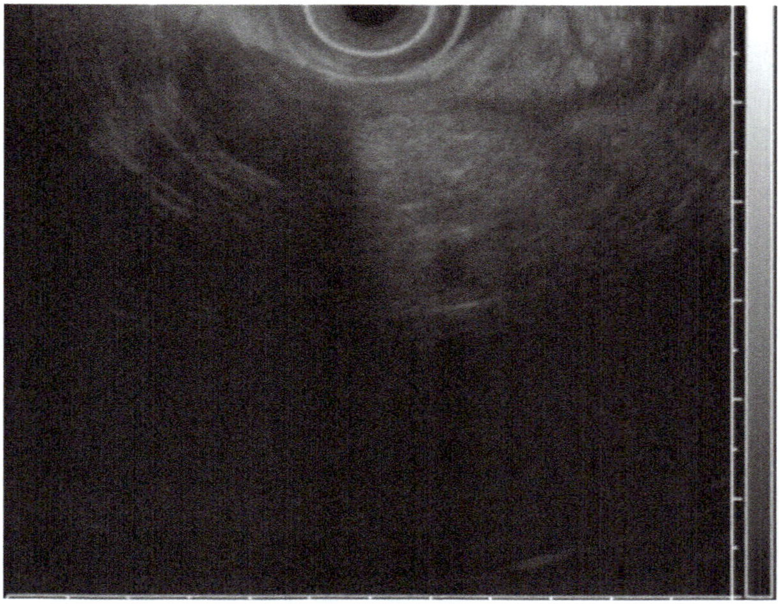

Fig. 6.86 A close-up of the lesion with the radial endoscopic ultrasound scope

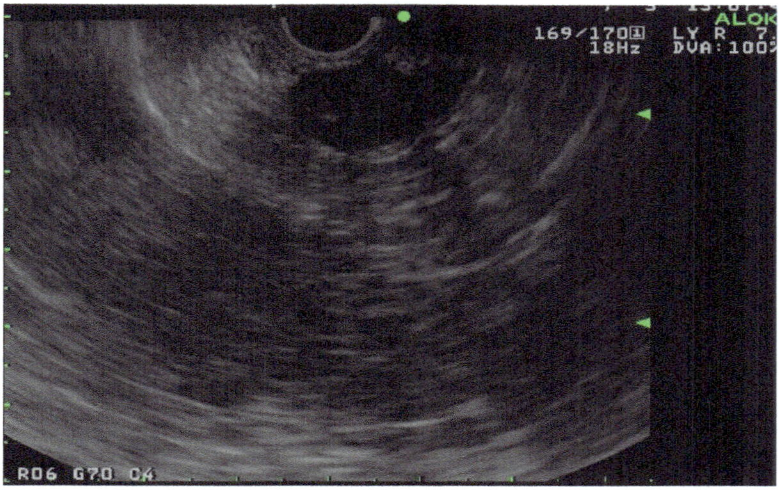

Fig. 6.87 The presumed insulinoma as seen with the linear array echoinstrument

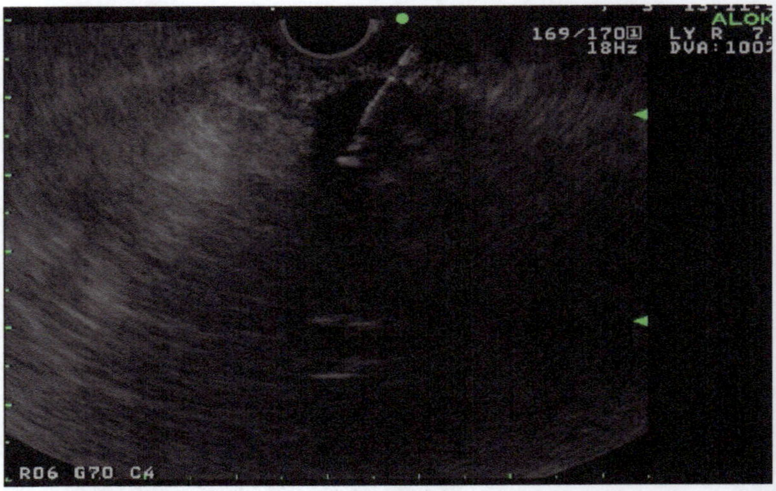

Fig. 6.88 Biopsy of the presumed insulinoma

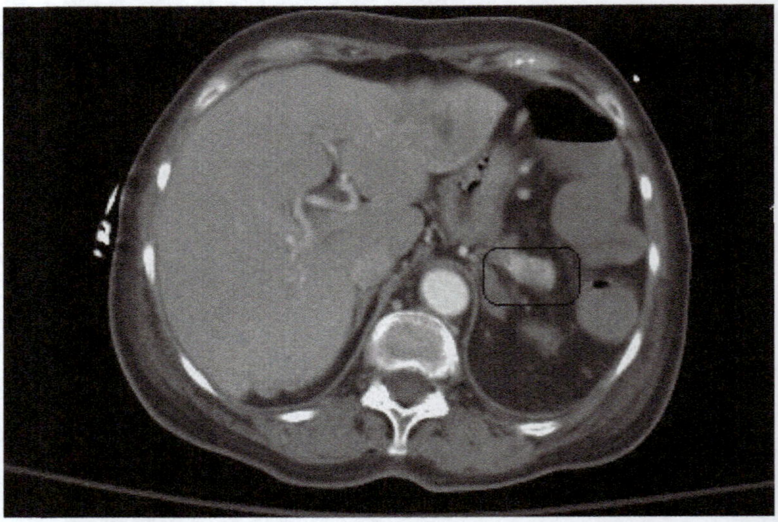

Fig. 6.89 The insulinoma seen in retrospect on the computed tomography scan

6.2.20.2 Cystic Neuroendocrine Tumors of the Pancreas

Cystic neuroendocrine tumors of the pancreas are uncommon. In a recent series from Indiana University, only 13 patients were diagnosed over a 7-year period [50].

This is a 51-year-old patient with a known stable-appearing pancreatic tail lesion that has not changed in size for more than 1 year. EUS evaluation was requested. A mixed solid-cystic structure in the pancreatic tail was found. FNA cytology of the solid wall showed synaptophysin-positive epithelioid cells consistent with a neuroendocrine tumor. Another mixed solid-cystic neuroendocrine tumor can be seen on the DAVE Project website http://daveproject.org/ViewFilms.cfm?Film_id=58.

A cystic component can be found in a subgroup of pancreatic tumors, including ductal adenocarcinoma, acinar cell carcinoma, and up to 5–10 % of pancreatic neuroendocrine tumors [51, 52]. They are expected to have malignant potential similar to solid counterparts [53]. Possible mechanisms postulated to be related to the development of the cystic component include the development of intratumoral hemorrhage and necrosis. The diagnosis of pancreatic cystic neuroendocrine tumors may be challenging if no solid component is identified. Fluid carcinoembryonic antigen (CEA) levels are low in these tumors compared with mucinous pancreatic cystic neoplasms [52].

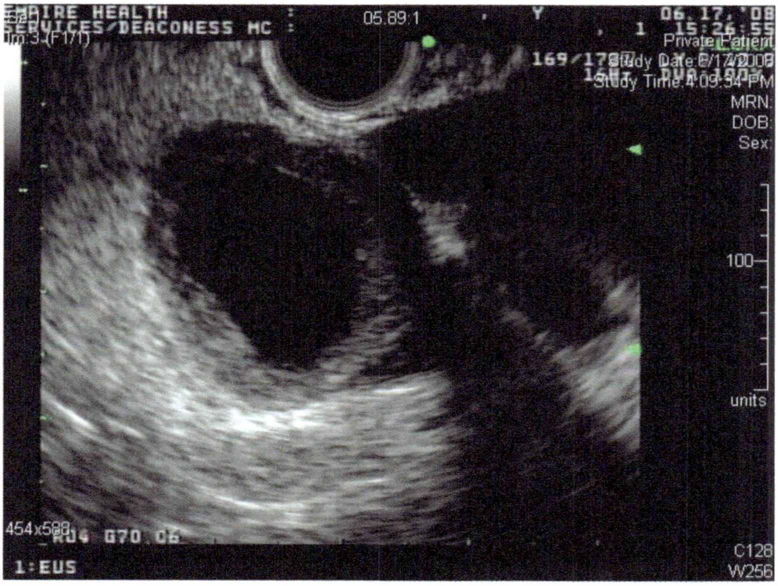

Fig. 6.90 This is an unusual solid-cystic tumor of the pancreas consisting of a thick-walled rim and an anechoic interior

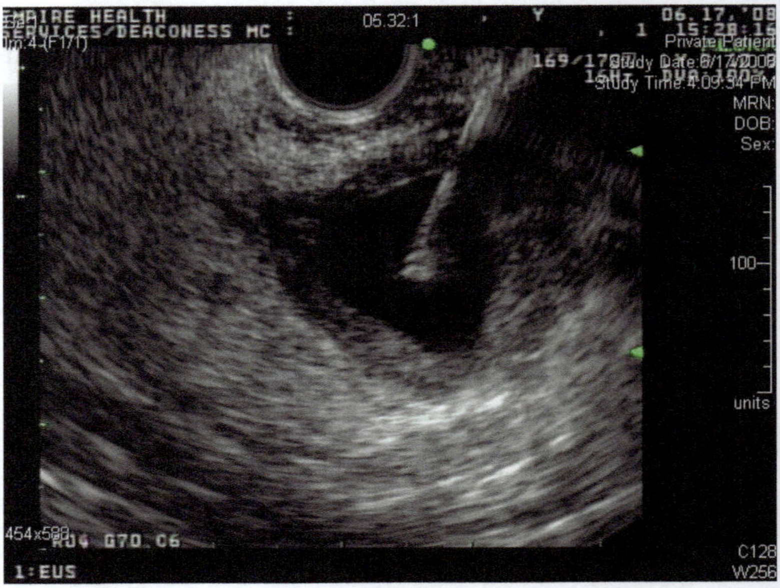

Fig. 6.91 Fine-needle aspiration cytology of the cyst wall was performed after clear fluid had been aspirated from the center. Cytology revealed a low-grade neuroendocrine tumor

6.2.21 Primary Pancreatic Lymphoma

This is an 80-year-old man who presented with shortness of breath. He has a history of chronic lymphocytic leukemia in remission. A chest radiography showed a right lower lobe infiltrate and a pleural effusion. A CT angiogram was done to rule out pulmonary embolism; none was present but the study showed a large, infiltrating mass in the pancreatic tail. CA 19–9 levels were within normal limits. The subsequent EUS showed a lobulated or almost septated mass with a small cystic component deemed to be atypical for a pancreatic adenocarcinoma. A differential diagnosis of neuroendocrine tumor was entertained. EUS-guided FNA of the mass surprisingly revealed a high-grade B-cell lymphoma.

Primary pancreatic lymphoma is a rare form of extranodal lymphoma of the gastrointestinal tract that accounts for approximately 0.5 % of all pancreatic masses [54]. Diffuse, large B-cell lymphoma accounts for approximately 80 % of cases of primary pancreatic lymphoma; other variants include follicular lymphoma, small lymphocytic lymphoma, and T-cell lymphoma [55].

Although imaging can suggest features that are not typical of ordinary adenocarcinoma, the diagnosis requires biopsy. Standard treatment of primary pancreatic lymphoma with chemotherapy and/or radiotherapy achieves a 3-year disease-free survival rate of 44 % [55, 56].

Because the presentation can mimic that of pancreatic adenocarcinoma, EUS-guided FNA plays an important role, providing tissue that can establish this diagnosis. Immunohistochemistry staining and flow cytometry are key for cytologic diagnosis.

Several features are suggestive of lymphoma in patients with pancreatic mass, such as lack of obstructive jaundice [56, 57], dilation of the bile duct or pancreatic duct despite involvement of the head of the pancreas, lack of invasion of surrounding vascular structures, calcifications within the tumor, elevated levels of lactate dehydrogenase and β2 microglobulin, and lack of elevated levels of CA19–9 [58].

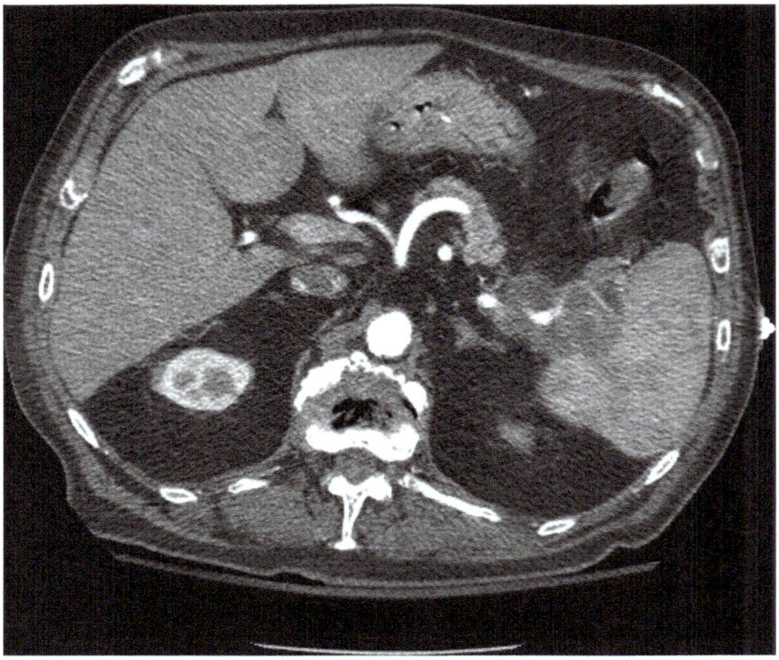

Fig. 6.92 A pancreatic tail tumor as seen on computed tomography

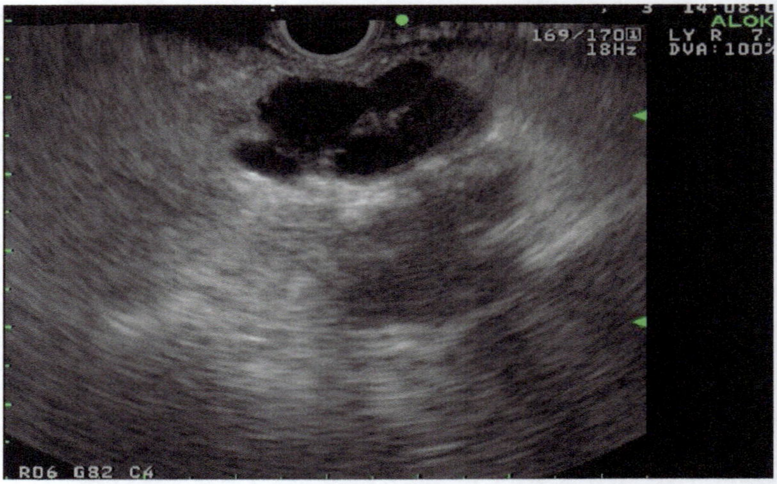

Fig. 6.93 EUS of the pancreatic tail tumor shows a mixed solid-cystic mass with sub-components

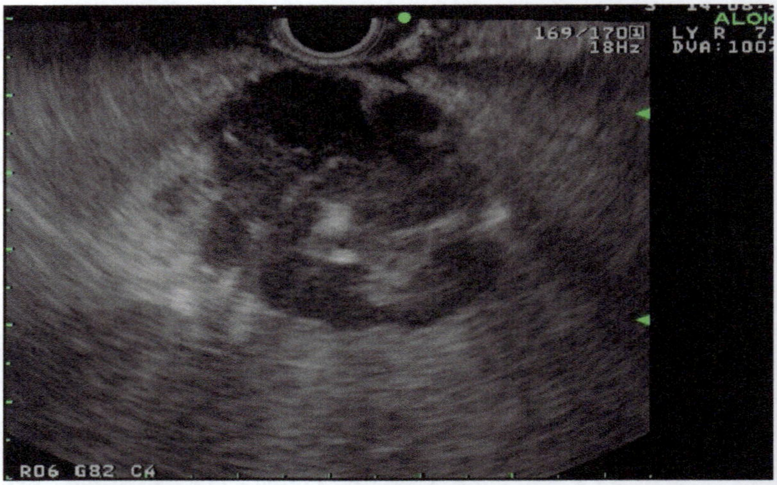

Fig. 6.94 This endoscopic ultrasound image of the pancreatic tail mass shows the septation or subcomponents

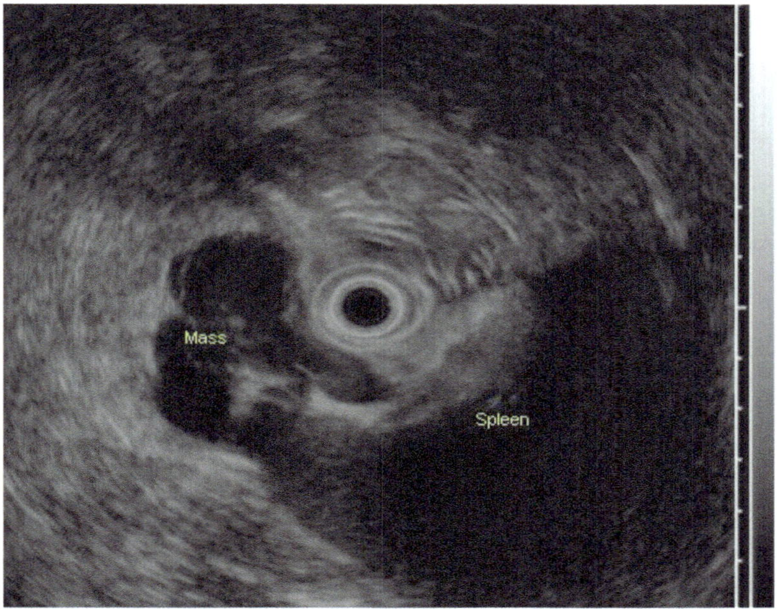

Fig. 6.95 The pancreatic tail mass with its relationship to the spleen as seen on radial endoscopic ultrasound

6.2.22 Mycosis Fungoides Infiltrating the Pancreas

This is a 52-year-old patient who was diagnosed 5 years ago with a cutaneous T-cell lymphoma (mycosis fungoides) that had a waxing and waning course. Overall he did very well with local radiation treatment. He came to see us when he developed abdominal pain, jaundice, and a mass in the head of the pancreas. EUS showed a "peculiar, hypoechoic, infiltrative ill-defined expansion of the entire pancreatic head." A differential diagnosis between pancreatic lymphoma and autoimmune pancreatitis was offered. Indeed, FNA biopsies revealed neoplastic cells consistent with T-cell lymphoma. A biliary stent was placed and the patient received systemic chemotherapy.

Secondary involvement by non-Hodgkin's lymphoma is more common than primary pancreatic lymphoma. A set of four criteria, known as Behrns' diagnostic criteria, have been developed to distinguish secondary involvement [59, 60]. These criteria include:

- Mass located within the pancreas
- Lymphadenopathy confined to the peripancreatic region
- No hepatic or splenic involvement
- Normal white cell count

Cutaneous T-cell lymphoma usually has an indolent course; visceral metastasis is a late event, and symptomatic pancreatic involvement is exceedingly rare.

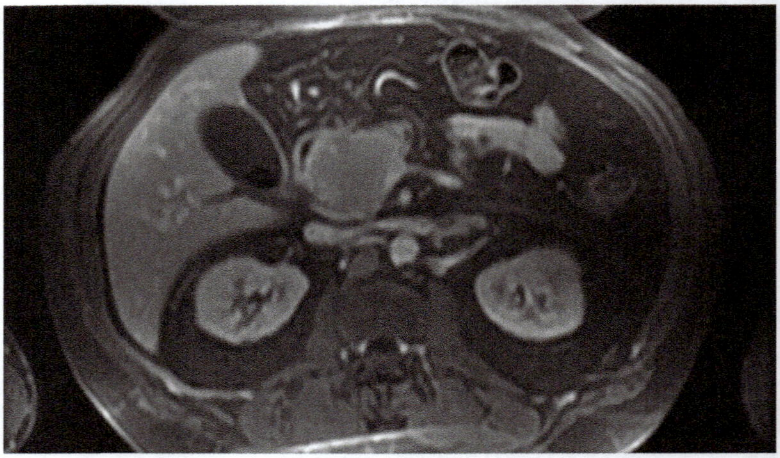

Fig. 6.96 This magnetic resonance image shows a large mass in the pancreatic head. It is difficult or impossible to discern normal parenchyma from abnormal

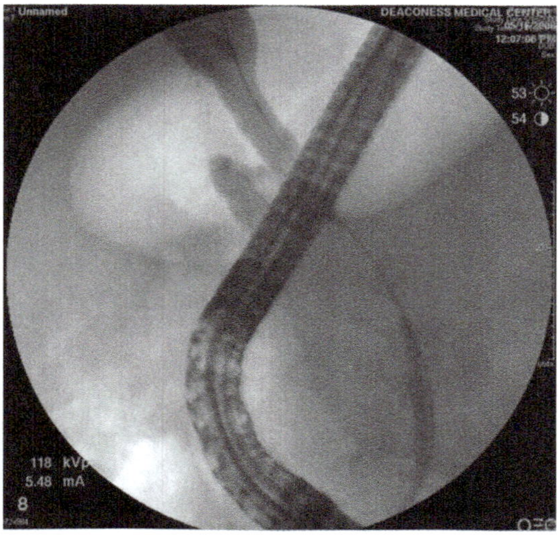

Fig. 6.97 This endoscopic retrograde cholangiopancreatography image shows a long stricture in the common bile duct

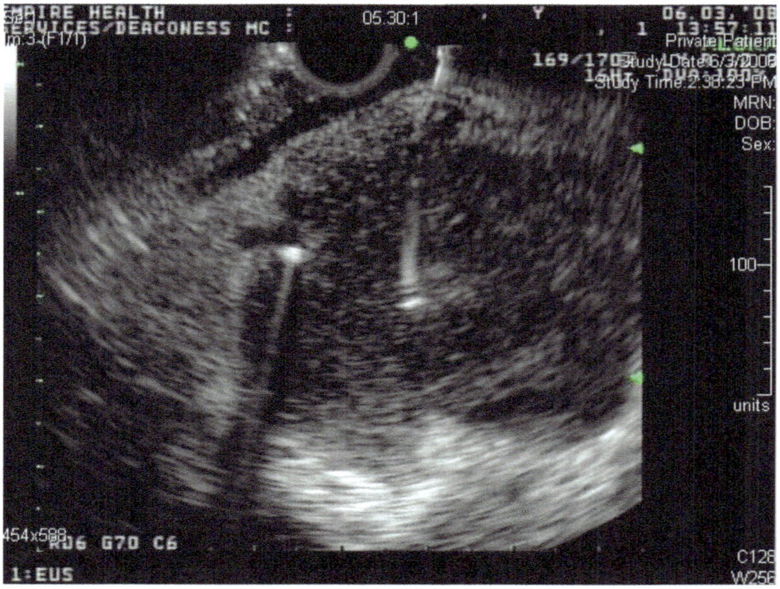

Fig. 6.98 Endoscopic ultrasound showed a process that seemed to involve the entire head of the pancreas, making it look hypoechoic throughout. A needle is seen entering the mass during fine-needle aspiration

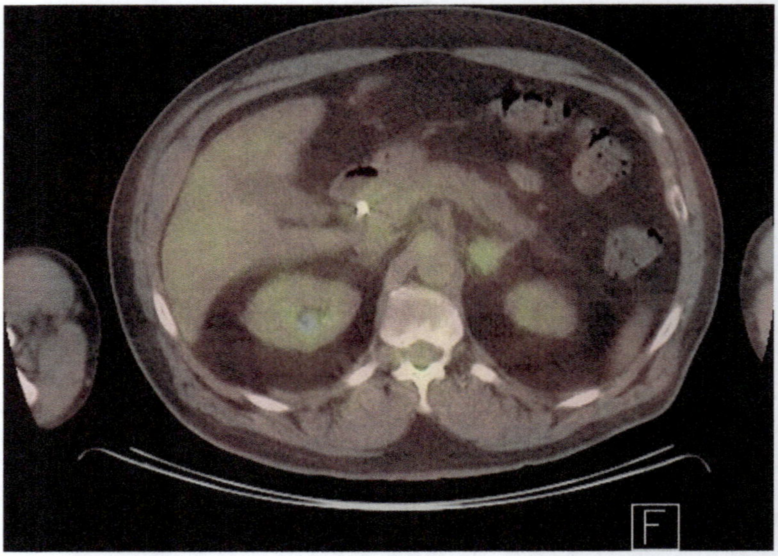

Fig. 6.99 This positron emission tomography–computed tomography scan shows a stent in place in the bile duct but no increased activity in the head of the pancreas

6.2.23 Pancreatic Cysts

6.2.23.1 Pancreatic Cyst with Complex Vessel Relationships

Pancreatic cysts are frequently aspirated during EUS. The safety of this procedure is outstanding in experienced hands. However, there are circumstances when it may be better not to biopsy or aspirate. This is a 74-year-old patient with end-stage primary biliary cirrhosis currently undergoing evaluation for liver transplant. Small cysts in the pancreatic body were seen on abdominal CT performed as a routine part of the evaluation before the transplant. EUS shows that the largest of four cysts measures only 8 mm. The cyst is on a needle trajectory that includes the renal artery and vein. The splenic artery is also close. Even if this were a mucinous cystic neoplasm it would not preclude the performance of a liver transplant if otherwise indicated.

Small cysts are sometimes difficult to penetrate and a certain amount of overshooting may occur. This is no problem only if the parenchyma is behind the cyst. The needle is just carefully withdrawn into the cyst lumen and the aspiration performed. In this case we felt that the risk of lacerating the renal artery, although small, would outweigh the possible benefit of the FNA. The transplant center requested further workup by ERCP, which demonstrated filling defects consisting of mucoid material in the main pancreatic duct (mucicarmine stain was positive). This is characteristic for mucinous pancreatic duct ectasia or intraductal papillary neoplasm.

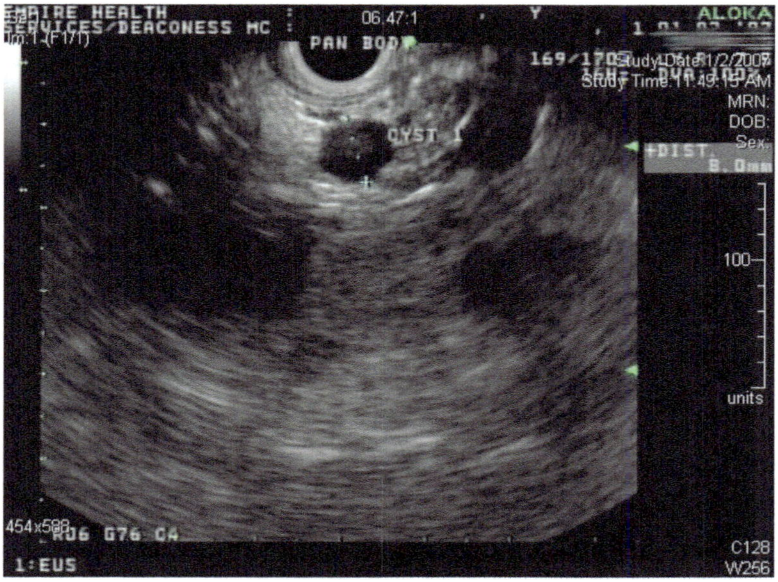

Fig. 6.100 Small cyst in the pancreatic body

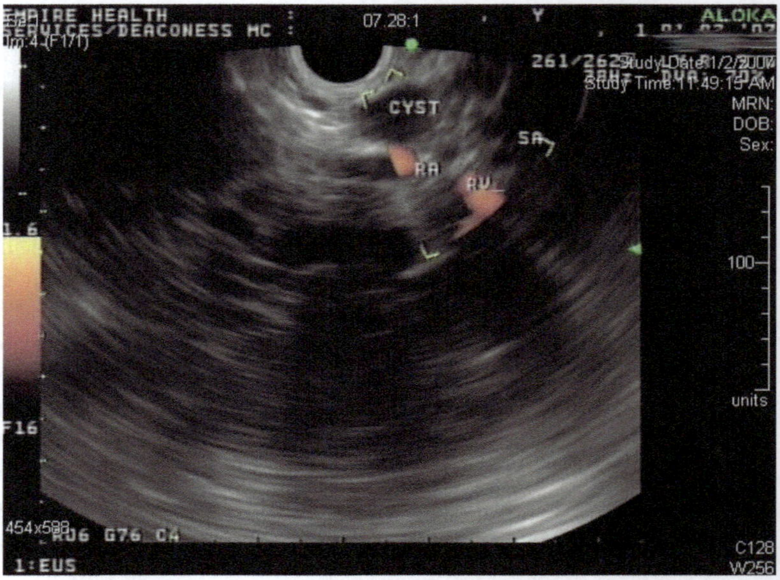

Fig. 6.101 Doppler study of vessels surrounding the pancreatic cyst

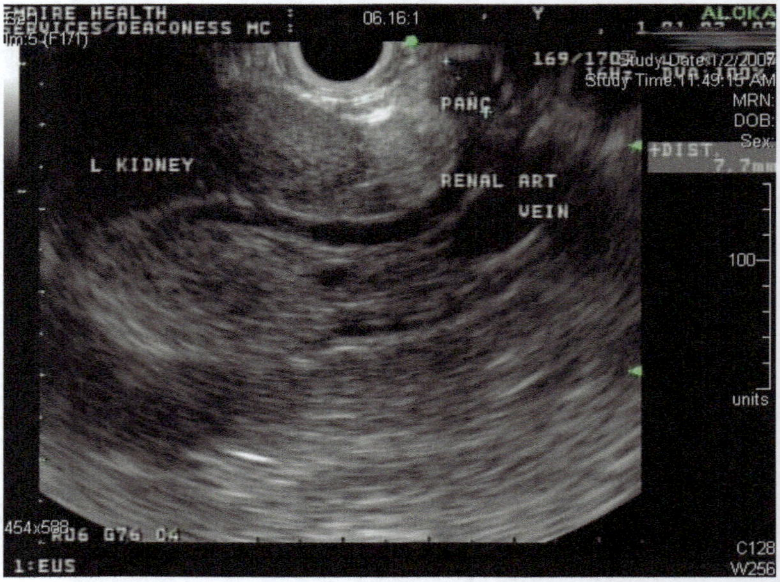

Fig. 6.102 Renal artery and renal vein in the biopsy trajectory

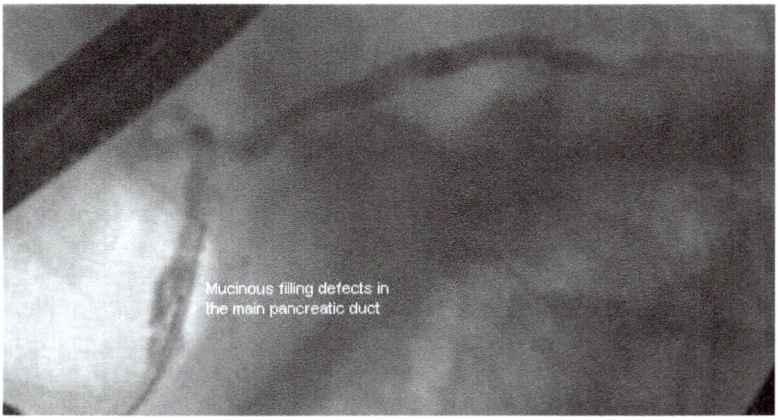

Fig. 6.103 This endoscopic retrograde cholangiopancreatography image shows subtle filling defects consisting of mucoid material in the main pancreatic duct close to the head

6.2.23.2 Pancreatic Cyst with a Small Polypoid Structure Inside

This is a 76-year-old patient with a cystic lesion in the head of the pancreas that was slowly increasing in size. EUS evaluation was requested and the images clearly show the superior resolution of this method compared to CT. There is a small polypoid structure in one of the cyst components, a finding clearly not consistent with a serous cystadenoma (SCA) despite the fact that the cyst aspirate was water-clear. The patient was referred for surgery.

Pancreatic cysts are frequently found incidentally during abdominal imaging studies; one of the largest series reported a prevalence of pancreatic cysts of 2.4 % (66/2803) detected by MRI done as a preventive examination in patients with a mean age of 51 years. An autopsy series from Japan reported pancreatic cysts in 24.3 % of cases (73/300), with higher prevalence in older individuals; 16 % of these cysts had atypical epithelium and 3 % had carcinoma in situ [61].

The differential diagnosis of cystic lesions of the pancreas is extensive. A didactic review of these lesions can be found online at http://www.radiologyassistant.nl/en/p4ec7bb77267de/pancreas-cystic-lesions.html/.

One of the main concerns with these lesions is the risk of premalignant changes or existing malignancy that can be difficult to demonstrate. This subgroup of cystic lesions includes mucinous cystic neoplasms such as intraductal papillary mucinous neoplasm (IPMN), mucinous cystic neoplasm (MCN), and solid pseudopapillary neoplasm, as well as neuroendocrine tumors and adenocarcinomas with cystic degeneration.

EUS is important in the evaluation of these cystic lesions. The presence of septations with all cyst compartments >10 mm in diameter, solid component of the lesion, mural nodularity, irregular wall thickening, and upstream dilation of the pancreatic duct are key features that suggest malignancy or precancerous behavior [62, 63]. It is important to keep in mind that malignancy cannot be excluded by small size alone.

Central calcification and a microcystic pattern are suggestive of a SCA that has minimal malignant potential. The presence of peripheral calcifications and a macrocystic pattern are suggestive of MCN, which has a greater risk of malignant transformation. Communication with the pancreatic duct can be found in patients with pseudocyst and those with IPMN.

Unfortunately, the presence of these features in pancreatic cystic lesions and their recognition by endosonographers is variable. Therefore, the correlation with final diagnosis based on imaging alone has great variability [64].

As mentioned earlier, EUS also allows FNA of solid components or nodularity in addition to aspiration of the cyst fluid for analysis. Cytologic analysis of fluid should be performed, although it has a low yield because of low cellularity. CEA fluid level is considered important in determining the likelihood of a mucinous cyst with premalignant potential, as demonstrated by Brugge et al. [65] and Cizginer et al. [66].

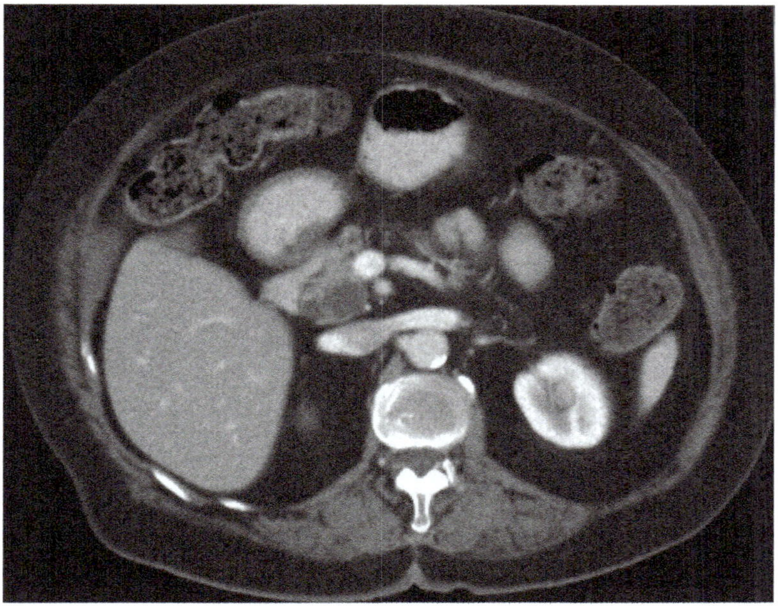

Fig. 6.104 Complex pancreatic cyst on computed tomography

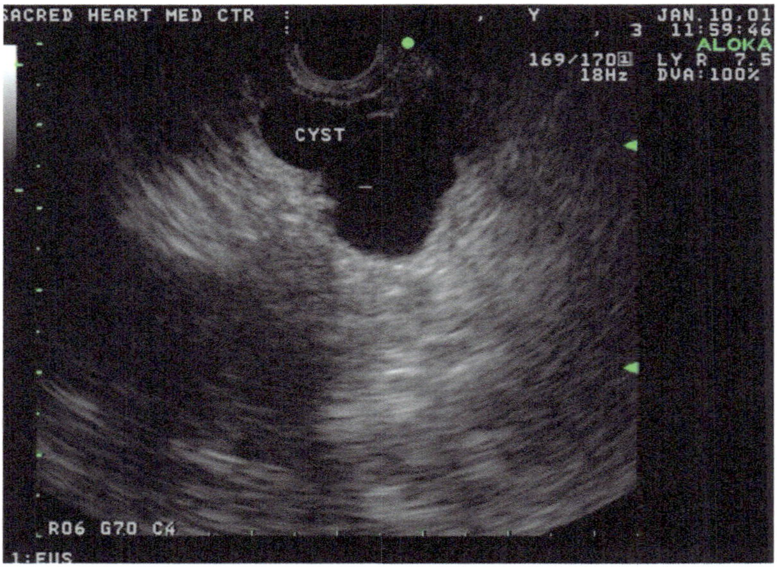

Fig. 6.105 Much better detail is seen on endoscopic ultrasound: there are two cyst components

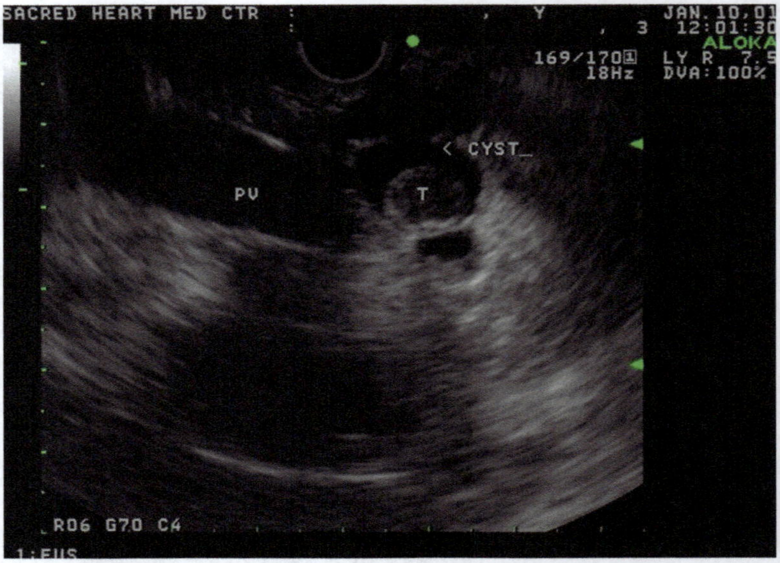

Fig. 6.106 There is a small polypoid structure inside the cyst

6.2.23.3 Pancreatic Pseudocyst

This is a 65-year-old man who is currently asymptomatic but was recently evaluated for symptoms suggestive of kidney stones. Noncontrast CT showed a mass posterior to the head of the pancreas. MRI suggested a cystic nature. EUS evaluation was requested. The FNA aspirate appeared to have water density and was brown, suggesting the presence of decomposed hemoglobin. The overall impression was that of a pseudocyst. However, given the absence of a history suggestive of pancreatitis, the cyst wall with the adherent solid elements was biopsied as well. The fluid chemistry reported amylase content of 42,941 U/l and lipase content of 84,941 U/l. The cytology was negative for neoplastic disease. After aspiration the cyst was almost completely collapsed.

Pseudocysts typically appear on EUS as anechoic lesions with a thick wall and without septations. Debris can be found on dependent areas of the cysts. Features of chronic pancreatitis are frequently found in the pancreatic parenchyma.

New pancreatic cystic lesions in patients with chronic pancreatitis are most likely pseudocysts. However, it is important to keep in mind that IPMNs can trigger pancreatitis; therefore, this diagnosis should be considered in patients who present with pancreatitis and are found to have pancreatic cystic lesions on initial imaging. In doubtful cases FNA can be performed to help establish the difference: typical fluid from pseudocysts is thin and muddy-brown; contains debris, neutrophils, macrophages, histiocytes; and has a high level of amylase (>5,000 U/ml) but not mucin, whereas fluid from IPMNs tends to be more viscous and may contain mucinous columnar cells, mucin, and elevated levels of CEA [67].

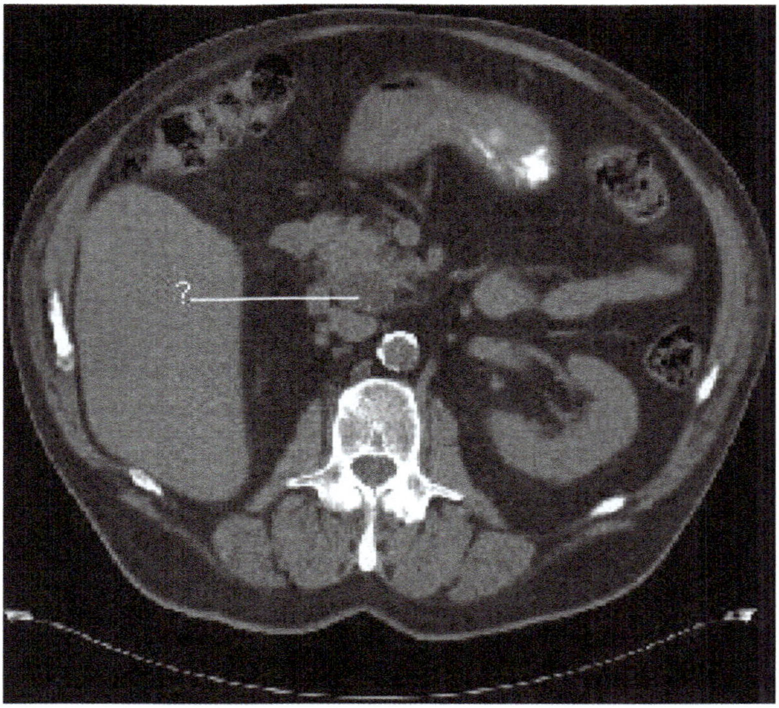

Fig. 6.107 A noncontrast computed tomography scan shows a mass posterior to the head of the pancreas

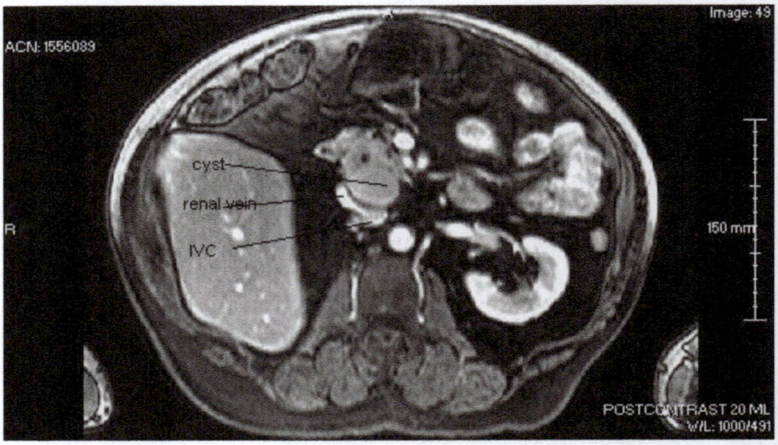

Fig. 6.108 Magnetic resonance imaging shows a cystic-appearing lesion compressing the inferior vena cava and renal vein

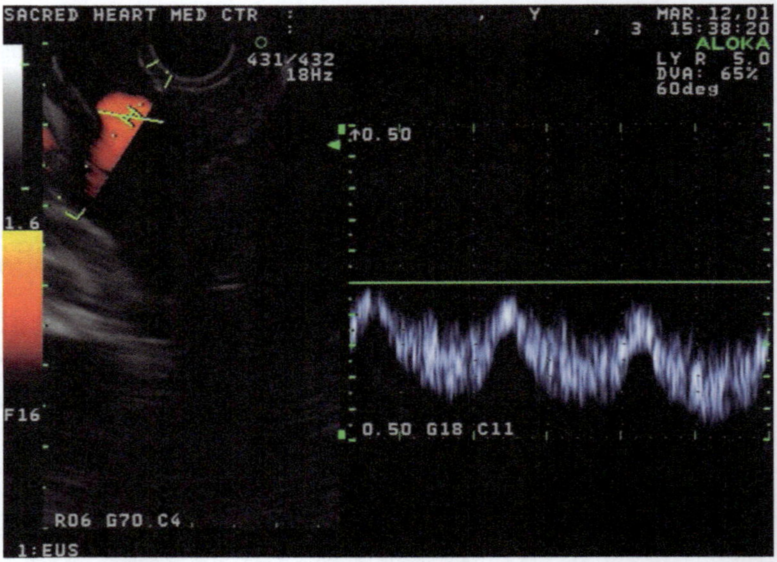

Fig. 6.109 Endoscopic ultrasound with a spectral Doppler signal shows the inferior vena cava being compressed by the cyst

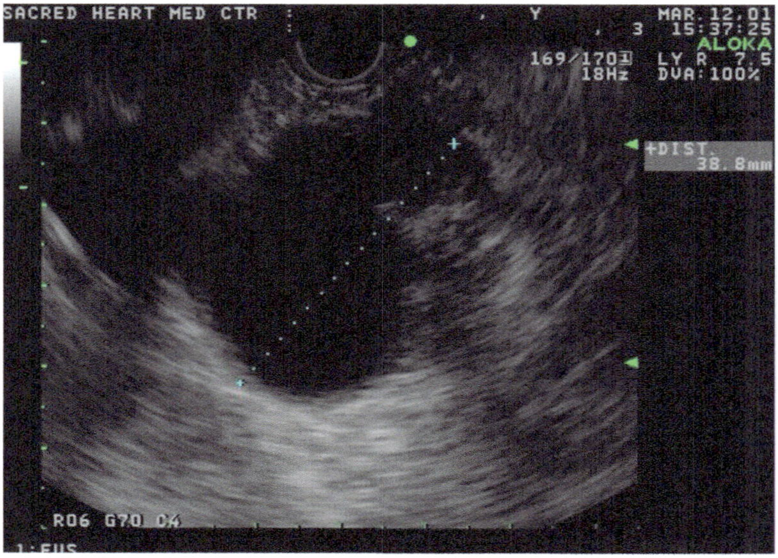

Fig. 6.110 Appearance of the pancreatic cyst on linear array endoscopic ultrasound

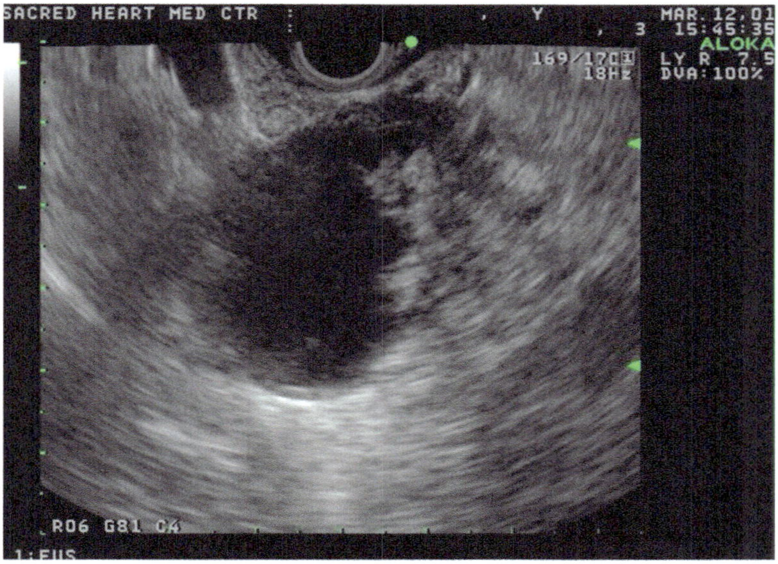

Fig. 6.111 Debris versus neoplastic growth adhering to the cyst wall

6.2.23.4 Mucinous Cystic Neoplasm of the Pancreas

This is a 68-year-old patient who developed acute pancreatitis. A CT scan showed an abnormality in the head of the pancreas, which prompted a, MRI (shown in Fig. 6.113). ERCP showed a dilated main duct in the head of the pancreas with apparent intraductal filling defects, which upon removal appeared rather mucoid. EUS evaluation was requested and shows multiple cysts morphologically consistent with a mucinous cystadenoma (previously called macrocystic adenoma). As expected, the aspirate was extremely mucoid. Surprisingly, the cyst fluid CEA was only 3.9 ng/ml. Overall, the impression was that of a ductal mucin-producing cystic tumor of the pancreas, and a Whipple pancreaticoduodenectomy was recommended.

MCNs (mucinous cystadenoma and mucinous cystadenocarcinoma) comprise approximately a third of pancreatic cystic neoplasms. Pathologically these lesions have ovarian-like stroma and an endoderm-derived, mucin-producing epithelium that secretes glycoproteins including CEA. They are more common in women than men and usually involve the tail or body of the pancreas, without communication with the pancreatic duct. Peripheral (wall) calcifications are highly suspicious for MCNs, but unfortunately only about 25 % of them have this sign. False positives may be due to vascular or ductal calcification [69, 70]. Unlike SCAs, mucinous cystic tumors of the pancreas can be entirely benign, dysplastic, or frankly malignant, and removal is strongly recommended in most cases.

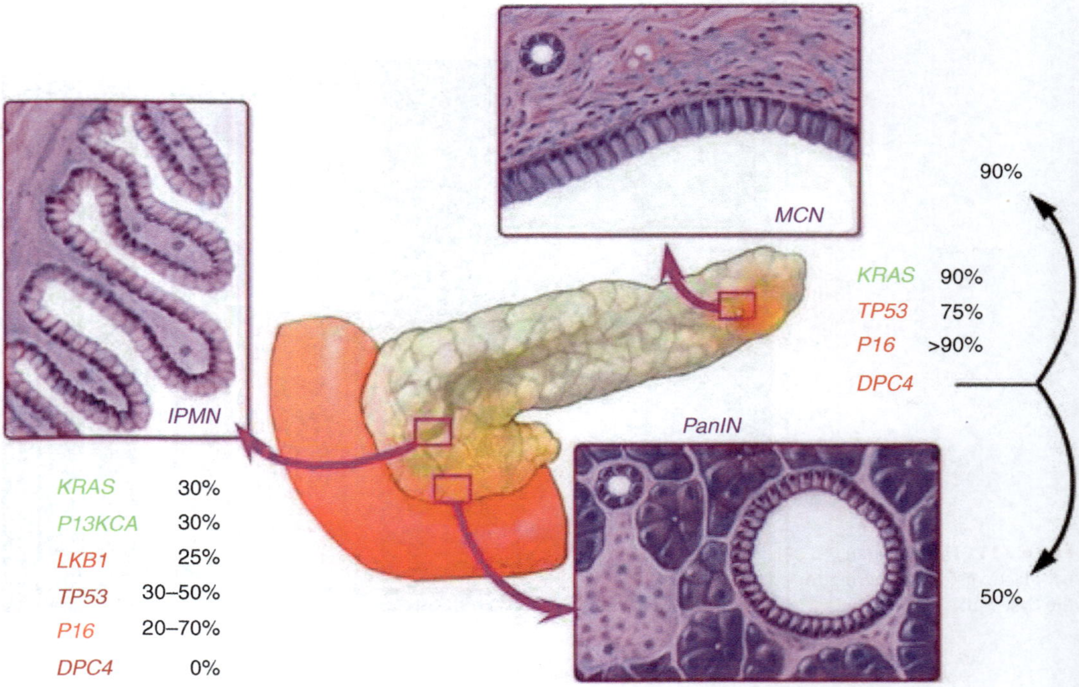

Fig. 6.112 Preinvasive neoplasms of the pancreatic ducts. Pancreatic intraepithelial neoplasia, the most common precursors to pancreatic ductal adenocarcinoma, arise in the terminal ductules and typically progress to invasive disease at the head of the gland. Mucinous cystic neoplasms also develop in the periphery of the gland, though typically in the body and tail, and exhibit a characteristic "ovarian stroma." Intraductal papillary mucinous neoplasms are macroscopic cysts that form in the main or large branch ducts, most commonly in the pancreatic head, and have a genetic profile distinct from the other two classes of precursors (*boxes* indicate completely unique genetic events) (From Hingorani [68])

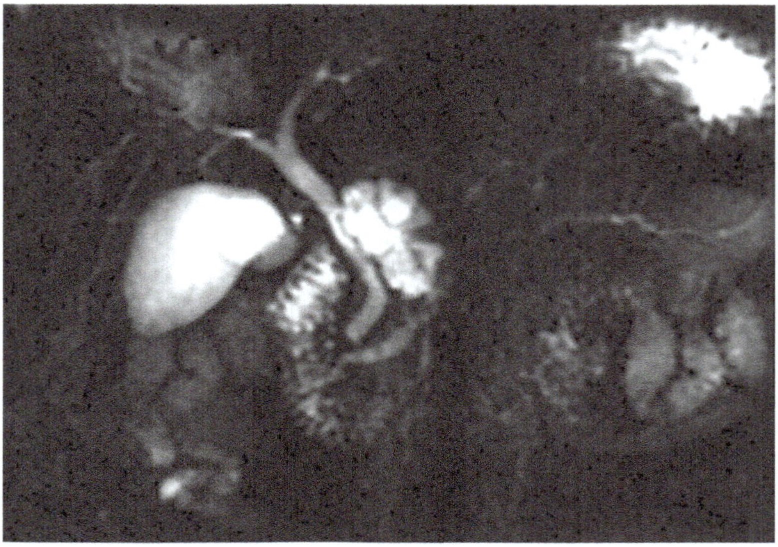

Fig. 6.113 Mucinous cystic neoplasm seen on magnetic resonance cholangiopancreatography

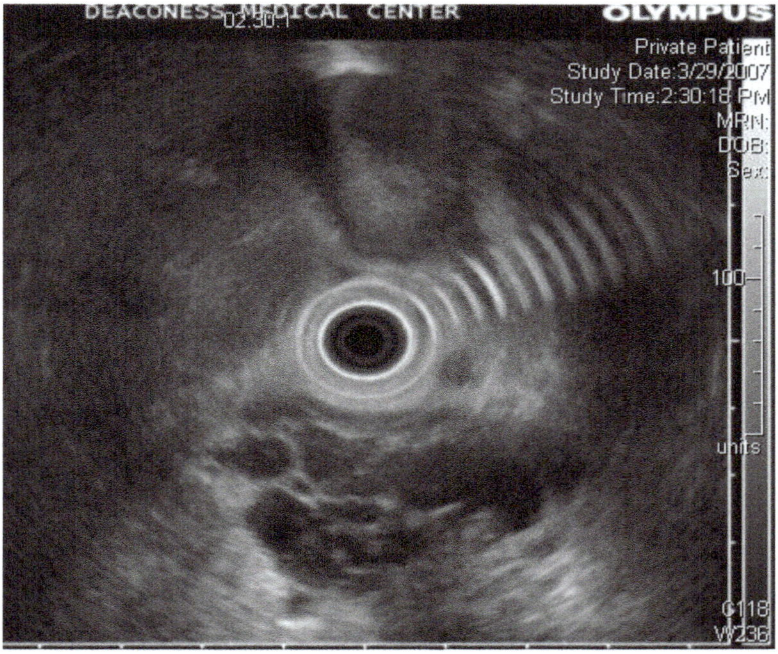

Fig. 6.114 Endoscopic ultrasound shows a macrocystic neoplasm

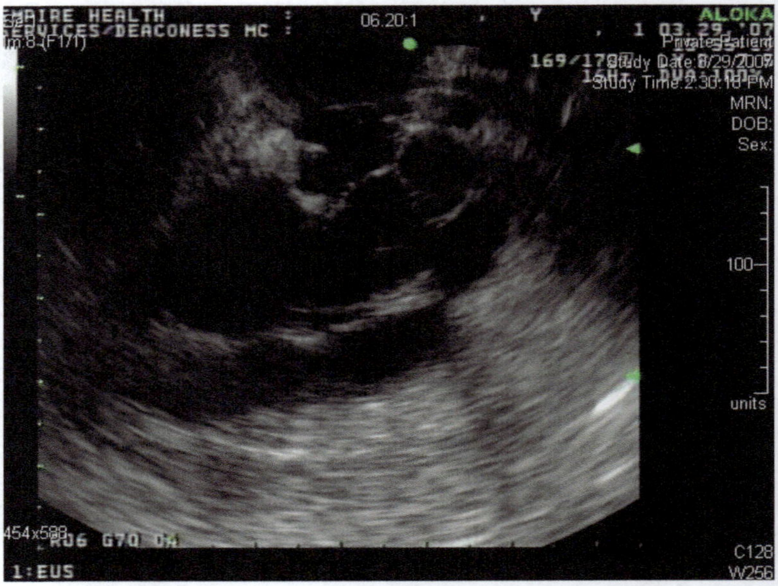

Fig. 6.115 This is an image of the same polycystic mass in the pancreatic head, seen using a linear array echoinstrument

6.2.24 Serous Cystadenoma

This is a 47-year-old woman who complained of back pain. A CT scan showed a cystic mass in the body and tail regions of the pancreas. EUS evaluation and FNA aspiration were requested. EUS showed "several individually simple appearing cysts arranged in a cluster of grapes configuration." FNA aspiration showed clear cyst fluid with low amylase, lipase, and CEA contents. All of this was characteristic of an SCA. Expectant management was recommended but the patient elected to have surgery, hoping that this would improve her back pain. The surgical specimen confirmed the preoperative diagnosis of an SCA.

SCAs are lined by a single layer of cuboidal or flattened cells. These lesions are almost uniformly benign. As mentioned above, central calcification and a microcystic honeycomb pattern on EUS are suggestive of SCAs as opposed to mucinous cystadenomas, which are macrocystic or oligocystic. SCAs can occasionally occur as macrocystic lesions and may not be distinguishable from mucinous cystadenomas by imaging alone. Most do not require surgical intervention, but according to one well-regarded group, tumors larger than 4 cm in size should be removed even if they are asymptomatic [71].

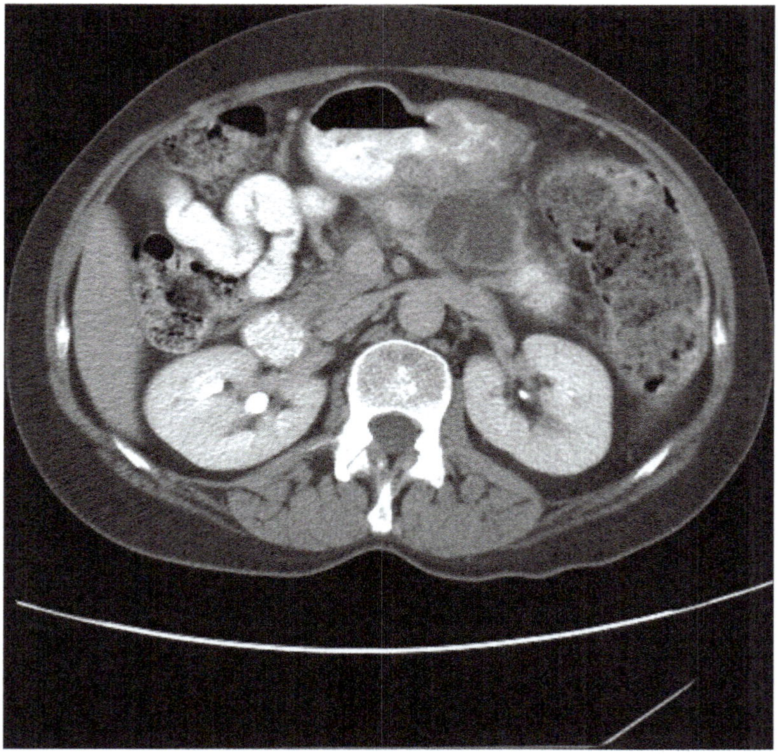

Fig. 6.116 Computed tomography appearance of a serous cystadenoma

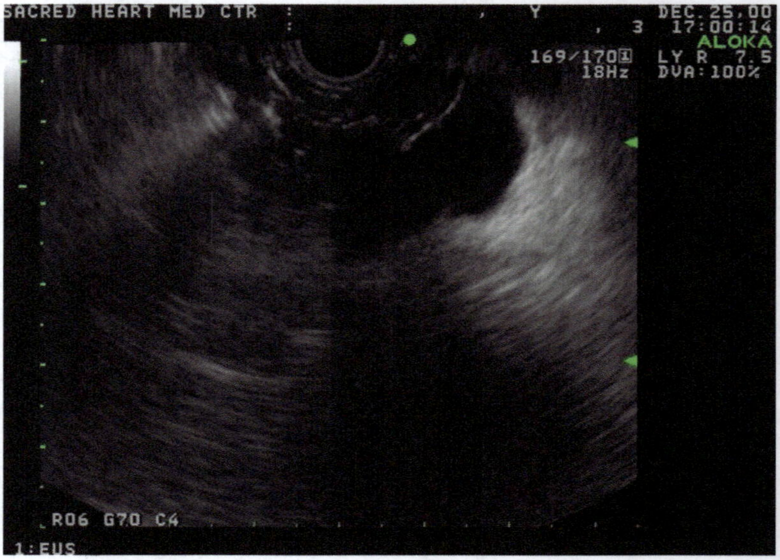

Fig. 6.117 Endoscopic ultrasound appearance of a serous cystadenoma. The cluster of grapes configuration is not apparent on this single image

References

1. Atri M, Nazarnia S, Mehio A, Reinhold C, Bret PM. Hypoechogenic embryologic ventral aspect of the head and uncinate process of the pancreas: in vitro correlation of US with histopathologic findings. Radiology. 1994;190:441–4.
2. Donald JJ, Shorvon PJ, Lees WR. A hypoechoic area within the head of the pancreas – a normal variant. Clin Radiol. 1990;41:337–8.
3. Savides TJ, Gress FG, Zaidi SA, Ikenberry SO, Hawes RH. Detection of embryologic ventral pancreatic parenchyma with endoscopic ultrasound. Gastrointest Endosc. 1996;43:14–9.
4. Rovasio RA. Development and structure of the pancreas. In: Neoptolemos JP, Urrutia R, Abbruzzese JL, Büchler MW, editors. Pancreatic cancer. New York: Springer; 2010; Book doi:10.1007/978-0-387-77498-5, Chapter doi:10.1007/978-0-387-77498-5_2.
5. Prat F, et al. Early EUS of the bile duct before endoscopic sphincterotomy for acute biliary pancreatitis. Gastrointest Endosc. 2001;54:724–9.
6. Stabuc B, et al. Acute biliary pancreatitis: detection of common bile duct stones with endoscopic ultrasound. Eur J Gastroenterol Hepatol. 2008;20:1171–5.
7. Kotwal V, Talukdar R, Levy M, Vege SS. Role of endoscopic ultrasound during hospitalization for acute pancreatitis. World J Gastroenterol. 2010;16: 4888–91.
8. Sugiyama M, Wada N, Atomi Y, Kuroda A, Muto T. Diagnosis of acute pancreatitis: value of endoscopic sonography. AJR Am J Roentgenol. 1995;165: 867–72.
9. Sugiyama M, Atomi Y. Acute biliary pancreatitis: the roles of endoscopic ultrasonography and endoscopic retrograde cholangiopancreatography. Surgery. 1998; 124:14–21.
10. Schmitz-Moormann P, et al. Comparative radiological and morphological study of human pancreas. Pancreatitis like changes in postmortem ductograms and their morphological pattern. Possible implication for ERCP. Gut. 1985;26:406–14.
11. MacCarty RL, Stephens DH, Brown Jr AL, Carlson HC. Retrograde pancreatography in autopsy specimens. Am J Roentgenol Radium Ther Nucl Med. 1975;123:359–66.
12. Luetmer PH, Stephens DH, Ward EM. Chronic pancreatitis: reassessment with current CT. Radiology. 1989;171:353–7.
13. Albashir S, Bronner MP, Parsi MA, Walsh RM, Stevens T. Endoscopic ultrasound, secretin endoscopic pancreatic function test, and histology: correlation in chronic pancreatitis. Am J Gastroenterol. 2010;105:2498–503.
14. Chong AKH, et al. Diagnostic performance of EUS for chronic pancreatitis: a comparison with histopathology. Gastrointest Endosc. 2007;65:808–14.
15. Varadarajulu S, Eltoum I, Tamhane A, Eloubeidi MA. Histopathologic correlates of noncalcific chronic pancreatitis by EUS: a prospective tissue characterization study. Gastrointest Endosc. 2007;66:501–9.
16. Sahai AV, et al. Prospective assessment of the ability of endoscopic ultrasound to diagnose, exclude, or establish the severity of chronic pancreatitis found by endoscopic retrograde cholangiopancreatography. Gastrointest Endosc. 1998;48:18–25.
17. Stevens T, et al. Multicenter comparison of the interobserver agreement of standard EUS scoring and Rosemont classification scoring for diagnosis of chronic pancreatitis. Gastrointest Endosc. 2010;71: 519–26.
18. Wallace MB, et al. The reliability of EUS for the diagnosis of chronic pancreatitis: interobserver agreement among experienced endosonographers. Gastrointest Endosc. 2001;53:294–9.
19. Catalano MF, et al. EUS-based criteria for the diagnosis of chronic pancreatitis: the Rosemont classification. Gastrointest Endosc. 2009;69:1251–61.
20. Van Herpen NA, Schrauwen-Hinderling VB. Lipid accumulation in non-adipose tissue and lipotoxicity. Physiol Behav. 2008;94:231–41.
21. Mathur A, et al. Nonalcoholic fatty pancreas disease. HPB (Oxford). 2007;9:312–8.
22. Van Geenen E-JM, et al. Nonalcoholic fatty liver disease is related to nonalcoholic fatty pancreas disease. Pancreas. 2010;39:1185–90.
23. Ustundag Y, Ceylan G, Hekimoglu K. Pancreatic hyperechogenicity on endoscopic ultrasound examination. World J Gastroenterol. 2011;17:2061–2.
24. Wolfson D, et al. Management of pancreatic masses. Pancreas. 2005;31:203–17.
25. Smith CD, Behrns KE, van Heerden JA, Sarr MG. Radical pancreatoduodenectomy for misdiagnosed pancreatic mass. Br J Surg. 1994;81:585–9.
26. Iglesias-Garcia J, Domínguez-Muñoz JE. Endoscopic ultrasound image enhancement elastography. Gastrointest Endosc Clin N Am. 2012;22:333–48, x–xi.
27. Kitano M, Sakamoto H, Kudo M. Endoscopic ultrasound: contrast enhancement. Gastrointest Endosc Clin N Am. 2012;22:349–58, xi.
28. Ahmed K, Sussman JJ, Wang J, Schmulewitz N. A case of EUS-guided FNA-related pancreatic cancer metastasis to the stomach. Gastrointest Endosc. 2011;74:231–3.
29. Katanuma A, et al. Tumor seeding after endoscopic ultrasound-guided fine-needle aspiration of cancer in the body of the pancreas. Endoscopy. 2012;44(Suppl 2 UCTN):E160–1.
30. Telford JJ, et al. A randomized trial comparing uncovered and partially covered self-expandable metal stents in the palliation of distal malignant biliary obstruction. Gastrointest Endosc. 2010;72:907–14.
31. McKay CJ, Glen P, McMillan DC. Chronic inflammation and pancreatic cancer. Best Pract Res Clin Gastroenterol. 2008;22:65–73.
32. Chandrasegaram MD, et al. Endoscopic stenting versus operative gastrojejunostomy for malignant gastric outlet obstruction. Surg Endosc. 2012;26: 323–9.
33. Shimada K, Sakamoto Y, Sano T, Kosuge T, Hiraoka N. Reappraisal of the clinical significance of tumor

size in patients with pancreatic ductal carcinoma. Pancreas. 2006;33:233–9.
34. Coté GA, Smith J, Sherman S, Kelly K. Technologies for imaging the normal and diseased pancreas. Gastroenterology. 2013;144:1262–71.e1.
35. Elkharwily A, Gottlieb K. The pancreas in familial adenomatous polyposis. JOP. 2008;9:9–18.
36. Pauli RM, Pauli ME, Hall JG. Gardner syndrome and periampullary malignancy. Am J Med Genet. 1980;6:205–19.
37. Quirk DM, Rattner DW, Fernandez-del Castillo C, Warshaw AL, Brugge WR. The use of endoscopic ultrasonography to reduce the cost of treating ampullary tumors. Gastrointest Endosc. 1997;46:334–7.
38. Jagelman DG, DeCosse JJ, Bussey HJ. Upper gastrointestinal cancer in familial adenomatous polyposis. Lancet. 1988;1:1149–51.
39. Giardiello FM, et al. Increased risk of thyroid and pancreatic carcinoma in familial adenomatous polyposis. Gut. 1993;34:1394–6.
40. Gangi S, et al. Time interval between abnormalities seen on CT and the clinical diagnosis of pancreatic cancer: retrospective review of CT scans obtained before diagnosis. AJR Am J Roentgenol. 2004; 182:897–903.
41. Bhutani MS, et al. The No Endosonographic Detection of Tumor (NEST) Study: a case series of pancreatic cancers missed on endoscopic ultrasonography. Endoscopy. 2004;36:385–9.
42. Coakley FV, et al. Pancreatic imaging mimics: part 1, imaging mimics of pancreatic adenocarcinoma. AJR Am J Roentgenol. 2012;199:301–8.
43. Atiq M, et al. Role of endoscopic ultrasonography in evaluation of metastatic lesions to the pancreas: a tertiary cancer center experience. Pancreas. 2012. doi:10.1097/MPA.0b013e31826c276d.
44. Mesa H, et al. Diagnosis of nonprimary pancreatic neoplasms by endoscopic ultrasound-guided fine-needle aspiration. Diagn Cytopathol. 2004;31:313–8.
45. Baron TH, et al. The role of endoscopy in the evaluation and treatment of patients with pancreaticobiliary malignancy. Gastrointest Endosc. 2003;58:643–9.
46. Ranney N, et al. Impact of biliary stents on EUS-guided FNA of pancreatic mass lesions. Gastrointest Endosc. 2012;76:76–83.
47. Fisher JM, Gordon SR, Gardner TB. The impact of prior biliary stenting on the accuracy and complication rate of endoscopic ultrasound fine-needle aspiration for diagnosing pancreatic adenocarcinoma. Pancreas. 2011;40:21–4.
48. Kim MK. Endoscopic ultrasound in gastroenteropancreatic neuroendocrine tumors. Gut Liver. 2012; 6:405–10.
49. Raman SP, Hruban RH, Cameron JL, Wolfgang CL, Fishman EK. Pancreatic imaging mimics: part 2, pancreatic neuroendocrine tumors and their mimics. AJR Am J Roentgenol. 2012;199:309–18.
50. Baker MS et al. Pancreatic cystic neuroendocrine tumors: preoperative diagnosis with endoscopic ultrasound and fine-needle immunocytology. J Gastrointest Surg. 2008;12(3):450–6.
51. Adsay NV. Cystic neoplasia of the pancreas: pathology and biology. J Gastrointest Surg. 2008;12:401–4.
52. Charfi S, et al. Cystic pancreatic endocrine tumors: an endoscopic ultrasound-guided fine-needle aspiration biopsy study with histologic correlation. Cancer. 2009;117:203–10.
53. Singhi AD, et al. Cystic pancreatic neuroendocrine tumors: a clinicopathologic study. Am J Surg Pathol. 2012;36:1666–73.
54. Zucca E, Bertoni F, Roggero E, Cavalli F. The gastric marginal zone B-cell lymphoma of MALT type. Blood. 2000;96:410–9.
55. Li Z, Zhang S, Vasdani N, Castillo E. Clues for diagnosing primary pancreatic lymphoma. Case Rep Gastroenterol. 2012;6:438–45.
56. Battula N, Srinivasan P, Prachalias A, Rela M, Heaton N. Primary pancreatic lymphoma: diagnostic and therapeutic dilemma. Pancreas. 2006;33:192–4.
57. Du X, et al. Primary pancreatic lymphoma: a clinical quandary of diagnosis and treatment. Pancreas. 2011;40:30–6.
58. Merkle EM, Bender GN, Brambs HJ. Imaging findings in pancreatic lymphoma: differential aspects. AJR Am J Roentgenol. 2000;174:671–5.
59. Alexander RE, et al. Primary pancreatic follicle center-derived lymphoma masquerading as carcinoma. Gastroenterol Hepatol (N Y). 2011;7:834–8.
60. Behrns KE, Sarr MG, Strickler JG. Pancreatic lymphoma: is it a surgical disease? Pancreas. 1994;9: 662–7.
61. Kimura W, Nagai H, Kuroda A, Muto T, Esaki Y. Analysis of small cystic lesions of the pancreas. Int J Pancreatol. 1995;18:197–206.
62. Tanaka M, et al. International consensus guidelines for management of intraductal papillary mucinous neoplasms and mucinous cystic neoplasms of the pancreas. Pancreatology. 2006;6:17–32.
63. Sedlack R, et al. Utility of EUS in the evaluation of cystic pancreatic lesions. Gastrointest Endosc. 2002;56:543–7.
64. Ahmad NA, et al. Interobserver agreement among endosonographers for the diagnosis of neoplastic versus non-neoplastic pancreatic cystic lesions. Gastrointest Endosc. 2003;58:59–64.
65. Brugge WR, et al. Diagnosis of pancreatic cystic neoplasms: a report of the cooperative pancreatic cyst study. Gastroenterology. 2004;126:1330–6.
66. Cizginer S, et al. Cyst fluid carcinoembryonic antigen is an accurate diagnostic marker of pancreatic mucinous cysts. Pancreas. 2011;40:1024–8.
67. Jacobson BC, et al. ASGE guideline: the role of endoscopy in the diagnosis and the management of cystic lesions and inflammatory fluid collections of the pancreas. Gastrointest Endosc. 2005;61:363–70.
68. Hingorani SR. A new preclinical paradigm for pancreas cancer. In: Han H, Grippo P, editors. Drug discovery in pancreatic cancer. New York: Springer;

2010. p. 73–93, Book doi:10.1007/978-1-4419-1160-5, Chapter doi:10.1007/978-1-4419-1160-5_4.
69. Reddy RP, et al. Pancreatic mucinous cystic neoplasm defined by ovarian stroma: demographics, clinical features, and prevalence of cancer. Clin Gastroenterol Hepatol. 2004;2:1026–31.
70. Gress F, Gottlieb K, Cummings O, Sherman S, Lehman G. Endoscopic ultrasound characteristics of mucinous cystic neoplasms of the pancreas. Am J Gastroenterol. 2000;95:961–5.
71. Tseng JF, et al. Serous cystadenoma of the pancreas: tumor growth rates and recommendations for treatment. Ann Surg. 2005;242:413–9, discussion 419–21.

Adrenals and Spleen, Peritoneum, and Retroperitoneum

7

Contents

7.1 **General Principles** ... 385
7.1.1 Anatomy and Technique ... 385

7.2 **Cases and Discussions** ... 386
7.2.1 Adrenal Biopsy ... 386
7.2.2 Myelolipoma Inside an Adrenal Adenoma ... 390
7.2.3 Paraganglioma ... 392
7.2.4 Accessory Spleen ... 394
7.2.5 Ascites ... 396
7.2.6 Omentum ... 398
7.2.7 Fluid in the Lesser Sac ... 400
7.2.8 Mesenteric Cysts ... 402
7.2.9 Omental Cake ... 405
7.2.10 Peritoneal Carcinomatosis ... 409
7.2.11 Retroperitoneal Carcinomatosis ... 411

References ... 414

7.1 General Principles

The adrenals, spleen, and peritoneal structures each do not supply enough material for separate chapters of their own; this is the only reason they are combined here. Visualization of the adrenal glands by endoscopic ultrasound (EUS) has been demonstrated for almost two decades; a reliable approach to the left adrenal gland was initially reported by Chang et al. [1] in 1996. More recently, several groups have shown several techniques that allow visualization and fine-needle aspiration (FNA) of the right adrenal gland, as described below.

A careful examination of adrenal glands is frequently requested by referring providers to rule out metastatic disease, evaluate imaging abnormalities or masses, or obtain tissue by FNA.

The spleen can be easily found from the proximal part of the stomach, opposite the liver and above the kidney. The splenic hilum can be found following the splenic vein by clockwise torque and slight withdrawal of the echoendoscope.

7.1.1 Anatomy and Technique

The left adrenal gland can usually be found from the proximal part of the stomach, adjacent to the upper pole of the left kidney, between the kidney and the aorta. Both radial and linear scanning echoendoscopes can be used to visualize it.

The EUS approach to the right adrenal gland is more challenging and has been described from the antrum, duodenal bulb, and descending

K. Gottlieb, G. Marino, *Diagnostic Endosonography*,
DOI 10.1007/978-3-642-39118-7_7, © Springer-Verlag Berlin Heidelberg 2014

duodenum by different authors. Preference of technique depends on local expertise; a scanning frequency of 5 MHz is recommended for better visualization of deep landmark anatomic structures. Examination from the duodenal bulb requires a linear scanning echoendoscope [2]. The endoscope is positioned in the duodenal bulb with a long gastric approach; once the portal vein is visualized, a longitudinal view of inferior vena cava (IVC) can be found by clockwise rotation and elevation of the tip of the endoscope. The IVC can be traced toward the hilum to detect the right adrenal gland. The adjacent upper pole of the right kidney can be found by rotating the endoscope. Uemura et al. [2] reported successful visualization of the right adrenal gland in 87 % of patients (131/150) with this technique.

Visualization of the right adrenal gland from the second portion of the duodenum starts with identification of the right kidney by linear scanning EUS. Slow withdrawal of the endoscope for a few centimeters with counterclockwise torque may provide visualization of the adrenal gland, often behind the IVC. Additional gentle maneuvering can provide a safe window between the inferior margin of the liver and the IVC for detailed examination and FNA [3].

Another approach to visualize the right adrenal gland from the antrum has been described by Dietreich and Kann [4]. The tip of the endoscope is placed in the antrum, in front of the pylorus, and the patient is turned into the right decubitus position. The endoscope is flexed toward the right, leaning behind the angular notch, and is gently retracted to find the landmark structures: the upper pole of the right kidney, IVC, portal vein, and margin of the liver. The right adrenal gland can then be found behind the IVC.

While ascites is a frequent finding on EUS exams, more localized collections, for example, in the lesser sac, are less frequently encountered and may raise unique differential diagnostic possibilities. These collections can easily be aspirated with EUS-FNA, and this could effect the management of patients, particularly if malignant cells are found. The normal omentum is rarely observed during EUS exams, but familiarity with its appearance on ultrasound may avert misinterpretation when it becomes visible. Cases with mesenteric cysts and different forms of peritoneal carcinomatosis conclude this chapter.

Box 7.1: Resources

- NIH State-of-the-Science Conference 2002: Management of the Clinically Inapparent Adrenal Mass (Incidentaloma) http://consensus.nih.gov/2002/2002AdrenalIncidentalomasos021Program.pdf
- "The Incidentally Discovered Adrenal Mass." Review article (full online access provided by the *New England Journal of Medicine*) http://www.nejm.org/doi/full/10.1056/NEJMcp065470
- DAVE Project – Gastroenterology: Ascites – Malignant Ascites EUS FNA: http://daveproject.org/ascites-malignant-ascites-eus-fna/2003-12-05/

7.2 Cases and Discussions

7.2.1 Adrenal Biopsy

This is a 46-year-old woman who presented initially with hematuria. As part of the workup, a computed tomography (CT) scan of the abdomen was performed and showed a pancreatic cystic mass. The patient was referred for EUS evaluation. The EUS showed a solid lesion instead but it was not clear whether it was coming from the pancreas, adrenals (no normal adrenals were seen on EUS), or – least likely –the kidney. A FNA biopsy was performed and the cytology was most consistent with a benign adrenal adenoma. This was an unplanned adrenal biopsy but it obviously helped to reassure the patient and referring physicians.

Adrenal masses, defined as lesions with a diameter of 1 cm or more [5], can be found incidentally on EUS in patients evaluated for another reason. The prevalence of these lesions is markedly increased in older individuals. In these cases the endoscopist must obtain all the information that EUS can provide. Size of the mass, shape, definition of margins, and sonographic pattern are key predictors of malignant disease, as discussed below. Eloubeidi et al. [6] have reported that altered adrenal shape correlates better with probability of malignancy than size or echogenic pattern. A clear understanding of the differential diagnosis and the current approach to these lesions is necessary to optimize the role of EUS and avoid inappropriate manipulation if it is not indicated.

In patients with an adrenal mass and known malignancy (including lung, kidney, breast, gastrointestinal tract, pancreas, and liver tumors) the probability of adrenal metastases increases to approximately 50 % [7]. In these cases the diagnosis cannot be made with imaging alone. Biopsy is also usually necessary when bilateral involvement is present; however, management is not clear in those with unilateral involvement, and surgical resection without biopsy may be considered.

The most common adrenal incidentalomas include adrenocortical adenomas, adrenocortical carcinomas, metastases, myelolipomas, pheochromocytomas, adrenal cysts, ganglioneuromas, and infectious lesions.

- Adrenocortical adenomas typically have a slow growth rate, less than a centimeter per year, reaching a total diameter no larger than 3 cm, and have a well-defined round or oval smooth margin. Nonhypersecreting, benign adrenocortical adenomas are the most common type of adrenal incidentaloma.
- Adrenocortical carcinomas usually have an irregular margin and heterogeneous density because of areas of necrosis, hemorrhage, and calcifications and can grow rapidly, reaching large diameters (>4 cm).
- Metastasis to the adrenal gland frequently occurs as bilateral lesions of variable growth rate and size.
- Myelolipomas are lesions formed by myeloid, erythroid, and adipose tissue. Fat can be identified on imaging studies including EUS, giving them a typical appearance, as shown in the following case 7.2.2.
- Pheocromocytomas also have a round or oval shape but may develop cystic changes and hemorrhage. Their rate of growth is slow but they can reach large diameters (>4 cm) [5].
- Infectious lesions include tuberculosis, fungal infections (such as histoplasmosis, coccidiomycosis, blastomycosis, parasitic infections), cytomegalovirus, and bacterial abscess.

Full access to an excellent review of this topic is available at the *New England Journal of Medicine* website (see Box 7.1). Important questions about the management of this entity are controversial, and there are no comprehensive guidelines. The 2003 National Institutes of Health state-of-the science statement [8] was an attempt to define this problem and its management options, but only limited information regarding the role of EUS was available at that time, and the role of EUS-guided FNA has not been standardized. More recent publications have reported a better yield with EUS-guided biopsy than with CT-guided percutaneous FNA/biopsy, with comparable safety. We recommend that endosonographers establish discussion and communication with endocrinologists and specialized surgeons to develop a clear protocol. Evaluation of hormonal activity by focused history, physical examination, and laboratory testing is the first step in the evaluation of these lesions.

EUS-guided FNA sampling of the left adrenal gland is not difficult, and its safety and effectiveness have been reported multiple times [9]. EUS imaging and FNA of the right adrenal gland is more challenging, but excellent safety and diagnostic results also have been reported by EUS experts [2, 3, 6]. EUS-guided FNA minimizes the length of the needle path, traversing only the wall of the stomach or duodenum and avoiding vascular structures and the pancreas, spleen, liver, and lungs; therefore it is considered a safer technique than CT-guided FNA [2, 6], which can cause pneumothorax, hemorrhage, pancreatitis, needle track seeding, and abscess.

Some important points to remember include the following:

- Most adrenal incidentalomas do not require tissue sampling.
- FNA may be indicated in cases suspicious for malignancy or infectious cause if imaging diagnosis is not sufficient.
- Pheochromocytoma should be ruled out before FNA to avoid a hypertensive crisis.

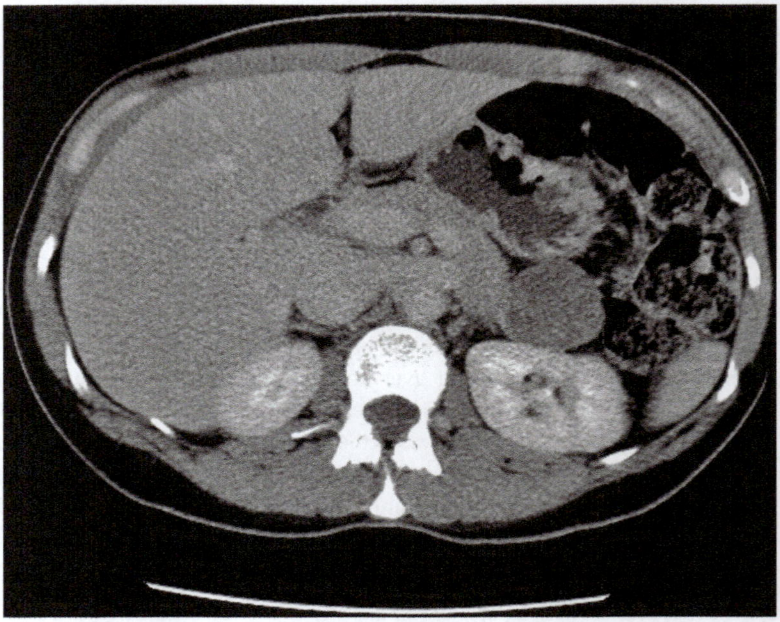

Fig. 7.1 Four-centimeter-diameter mass between the pancreas and kidney on computed tomography

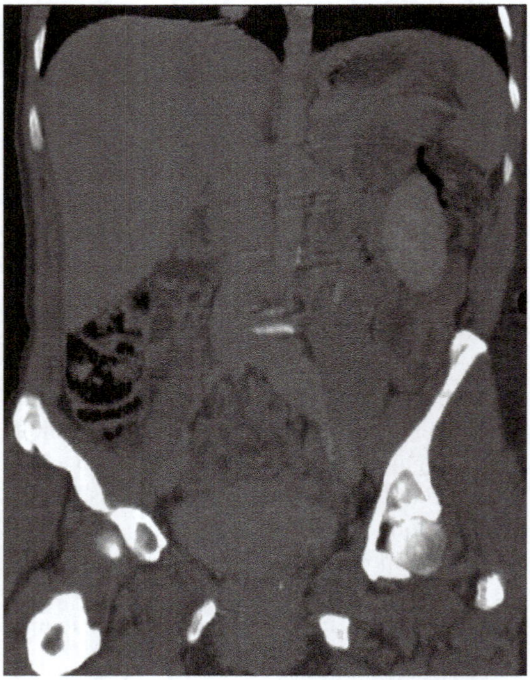

Fig. 7.2 Computed tomography with coronal reconstruction showing a mass between the pancreas and kidney

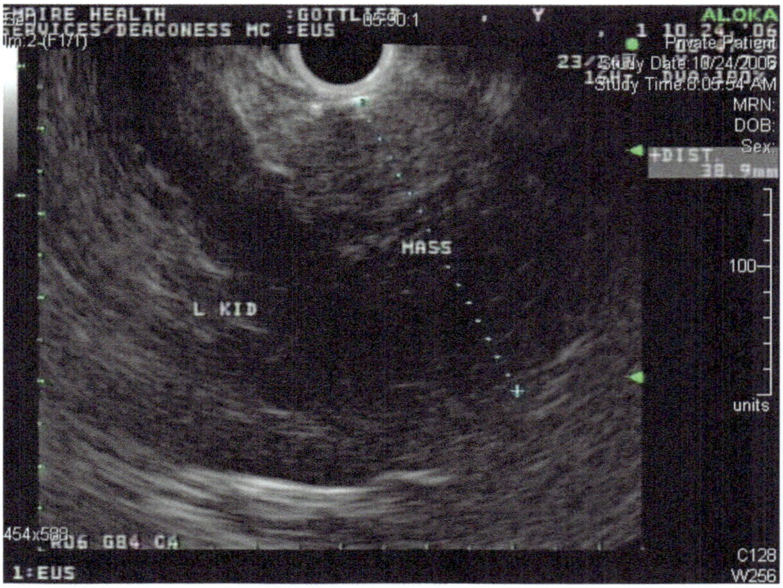

Fig. 7.3 Endoscopic ultrasound appearance of the mass between the left kidney (*L KID*) and pancreas

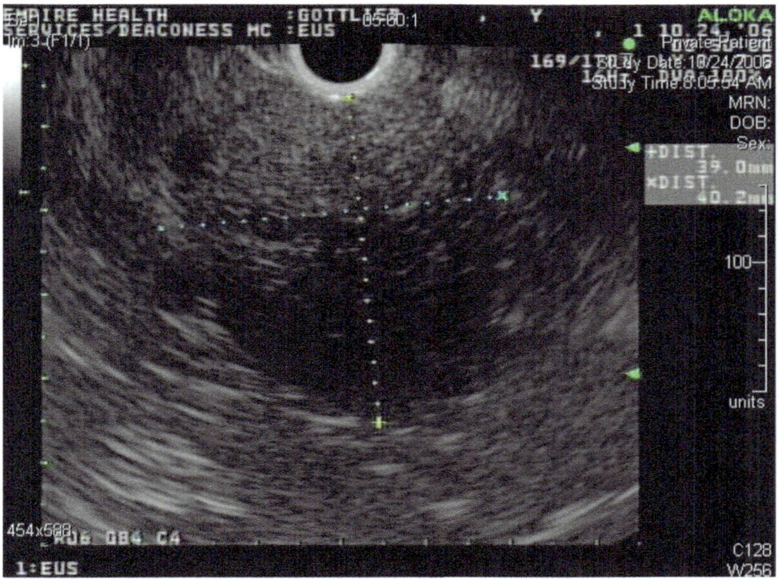

Fig. 7.4 Another view of the 4-cm-diameter adrenal mass

7.2.2 Myelolipoma Inside an Adrenal Adenoma

This is a 66-year-old patient with a known stable adrenal adenoma. She was referred for the evaluation of one episode of acute pancreatitis with unclear etiology. EUS shows the adrenal adenoma, which contains two internal, spherical, echogenic structures consistent with myelolipomas of the adrenal gland. The exam of the pancreas was unremarkable.

Adrenal myelolipoma is a rare benign neoplasm composed of mature adipose tissue and a variable amount of hematopoietic elements. Most lesions are small and asymptomatic, discovered incidentally at autopsy or on imaging studies performed for other reasons. The sonographic appearance varies with the composition of the neoplasm. If the tumor contains predominantly fatty components, it appears uniformly hyperechoic. If the tumor contains a predominance of myeloid cells, it may appear heterogeneous or hypoechoic.

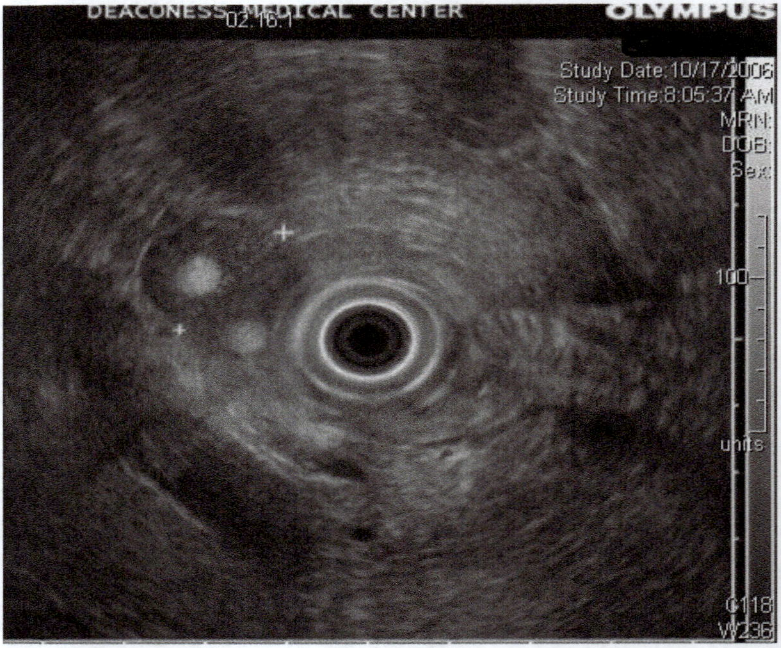

Fig. 7.5 Adrenal myelolipoma

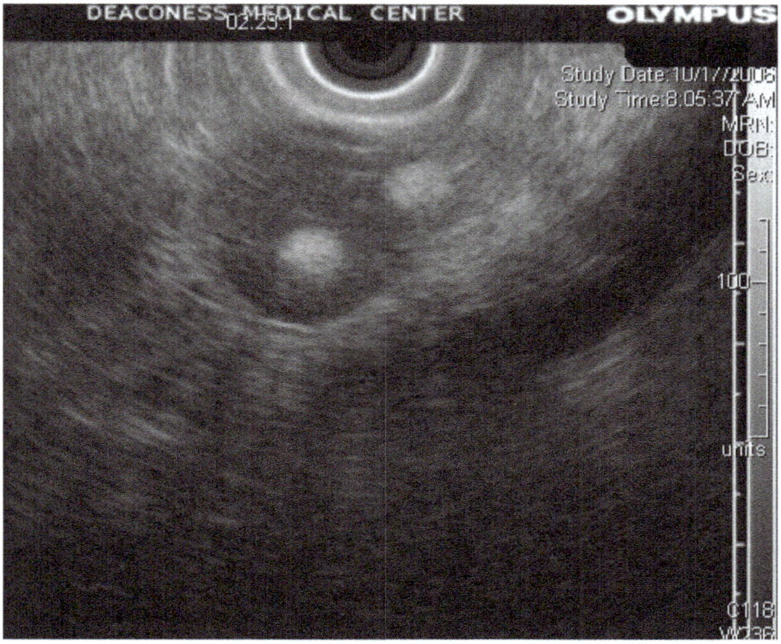

Fig. 7.6 Adrenal myolipoma (close-up)

7.2.3 Paraganglioma

This is a 72-year-old man with well-controlled hypertension who was incidentally found to have a large peripancreatic mass. The CT scan shows inhomogenous enhancement and the EUS shows a hypoechoic, spherical, well-circumscribed tumor separate from the pancreas. The FNA aspirate was unusually bloody, confirming the vascular nature of the neoplasm. A neuroendocrine tumor was suspected. The cytology was nondiagnostic and the tumor was surgically excised. The final histology – confirmed by outside consultation – was consistent with a paraganglioma/pheochromocytoma.

Paraganglia are ganglia that derive from the autonomic nervous system. The parasympathetic paraganglia (carotid body, supracardiac paraganglia) and the sympathetic paraganglia (chromaffin paraganglia, adrenalin system) often are differentiated. The Zuckerkandl organ (organum nervosum Zuckerkandl, para-aortic ganglia) is the most common extra-adrenal site of pheochromocytoma. Tumors of the paraganglia are rare and mostly benign but have a significant risk of recurrence.

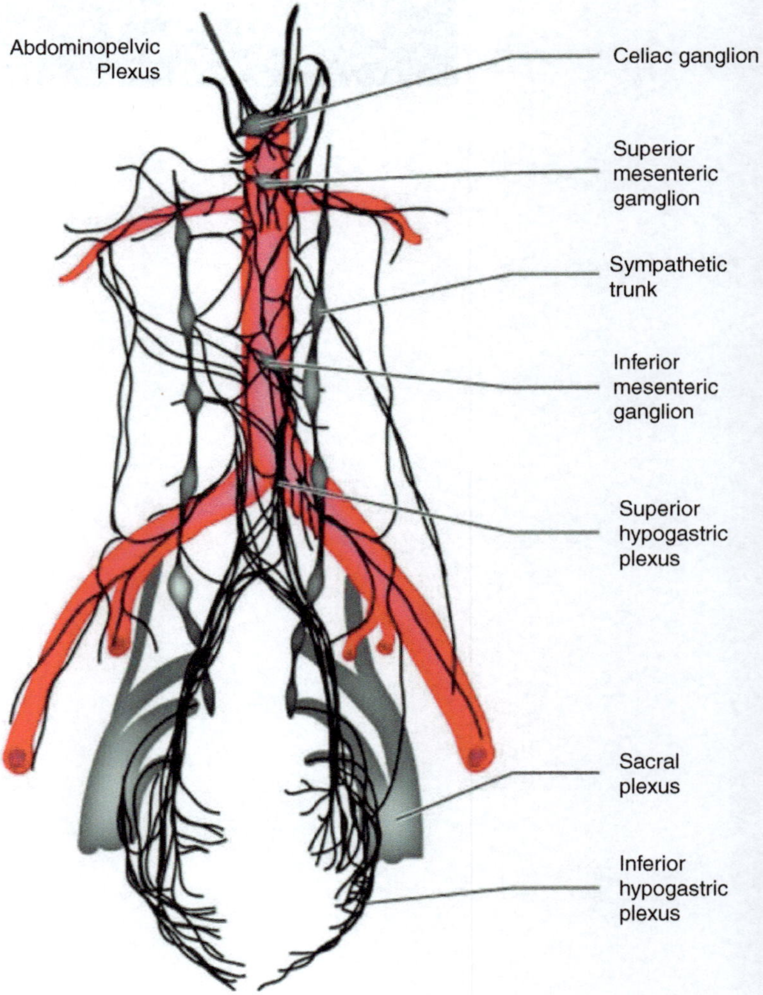

Fig. 7.7 The abdominopelvic autonomic nervous system. The abdominopelvic plexus can be seen as a complex network of fibers wrapped around the anterior and lateral aspects of the abdominal aorta, dividing just below the aorta to course into the endopelvic fascia of the pelvic basin (From Willard and Schuenke [10])

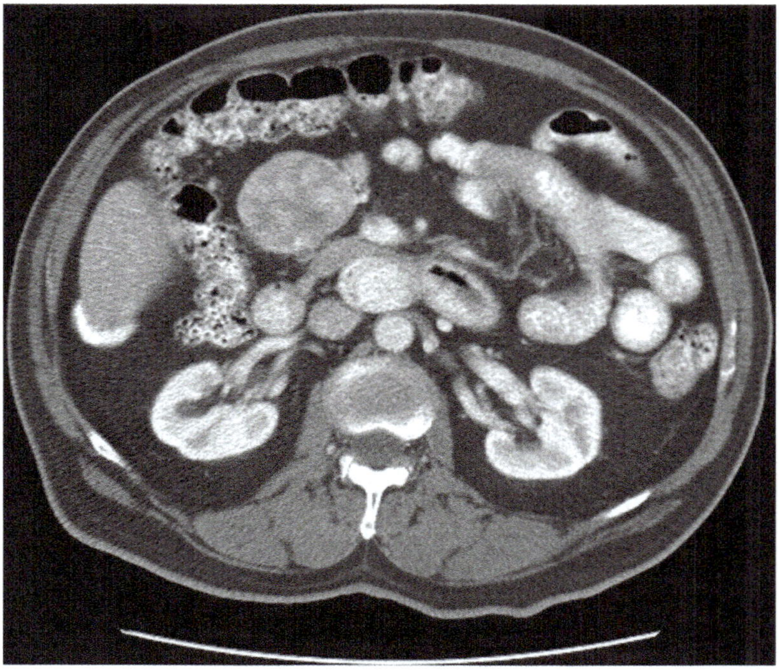

Fig. 7.8 Paraganglioma on computed tomography

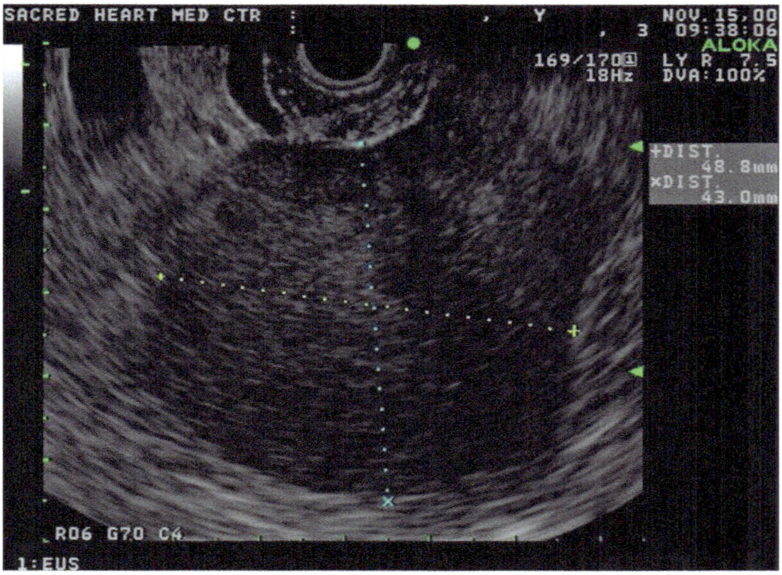

Fig. 7.9 Paraganglioma on endoscopic ultrasound

7.2.4 Accessory Spleen

This is a 57-year-old woman referred to us for the evaluation of a pancreatic cyst. Incidentally noted was the splenule shown both on abdominal CT and radial EUS.

Accessory spleens have been found in 10 % of cases from an autopsy series [11] and in up to 16 % of patients undergoing contrast-enhanced abdominal CT [12], usually as an incidental finding because most of them are asymptomatic. Supernumerary spleens, splenunculi, or splenules are congenital foci of healthy splenic tissue that are separate from the main body of the spleen. They are usually located around the splenic hilum (80 %), tail of the pancreas, greater omentum, and splenic ligaments; they are less commonly found in the bowel mesentery, left ovary and broad ligament, left scrotum and inguinal region, pelvis, and retroperitoneum [13]. Intrapancreatic accessory spleen can mimic pancreatic tumors, particularly neuroendocrine tumors [14]. Typically, accessory spleens appear on CT scans as well-marginated, round masses that are smaller than 2 cm and enhance homogeneously on contrast-enhanced images with an intensity similar to the spleen. When accessory spleens are smaller than 1 cm, their attenuation may be lower than that of the spleen because of partial volume effects [12]. On EUS accessory spleens have a well-defined margin and a homogeneous sonographic pattern but they can be hyperechoic or hypoechoic [13]. ^{99m}Technetium heat-damaged red blood cell scintigraphy combined with single-photon emission CT or superparamagnetic iron oxide–enhanced magnetic resonance imaging can be useful to establish the diagnosis in doubtful cases.

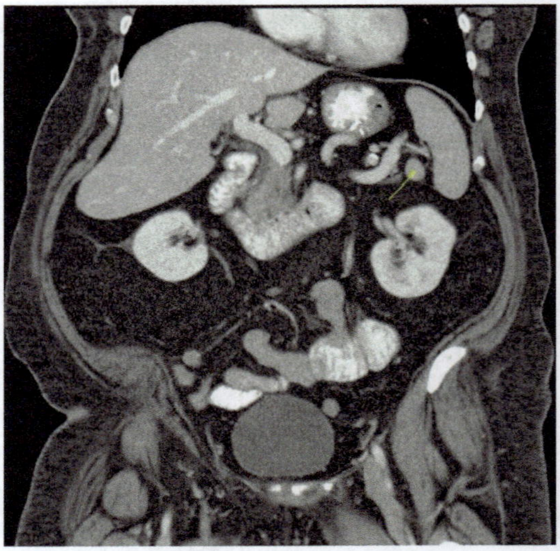

Fig. 7.10 This coronal reconstruction of an abdominal computed tomography scan shows the splenule (accessory spleen) in a typical location (*yellow arrow*)

It is important to recognize accessory spleens because they can be mistaken for enlarged lymph nodes or hypervascular tumors. In unclear cases EUS-guided FNA may establish the diagnosis [15].

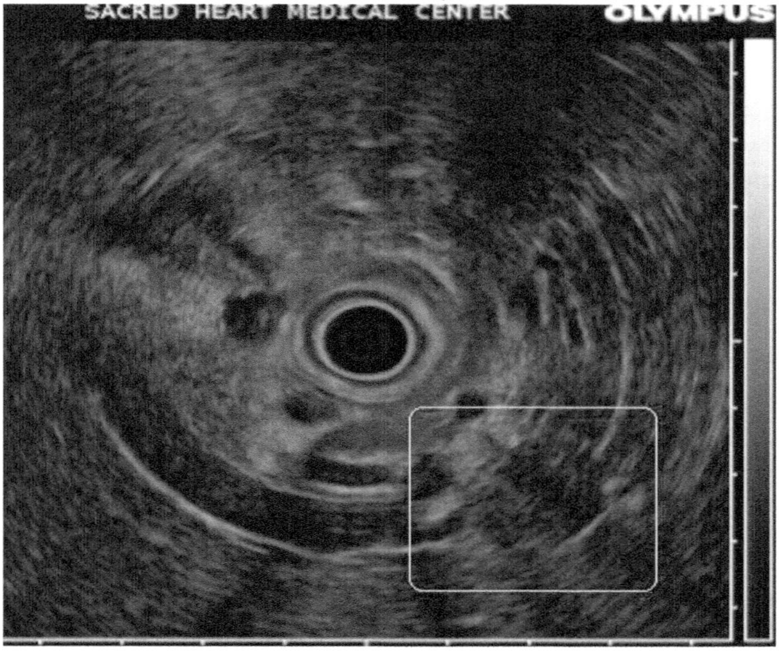

Fig. 7.11 The same splenule as seen on a radial endoscopic ultrasound (within *yellow outline*). Note the prominent splenic vein

7.2.5 Ascites

This is a 42-year-old woman with apparent idiopathic pancreatitis who was referred for EUS evaluation. She has a family history of pancreatic cancer (her mother, a maternal grandmother, and a brother). She may belong to kindred of patients with familial pancreatitis or familial pancreatic cancer. Her daughter, who was16 years old at the time, was evaluated several years ago by the same examiner for a pancreatic tail cyst. The EUS examination is fairly unremarkable except for the presence of ascites surrounding the gallbladder and liver, as seen in these images. EUS is more sensitive than CT and transabdominal ultrasound in the detection of ascites [16, 17]. In this case the ascites is inflammatory in nature. Small amounts of ascites not related to pancreatic necrosis, as well as pleural and pericardial effusions, are frequent in acute pancreatitis, and most resolve spontaneously [18]. In the setting of a malignant-appearing mass lesion, however, aspiration of even small amounts of ascites with EUS guidance will frequently show malignant cells [19].

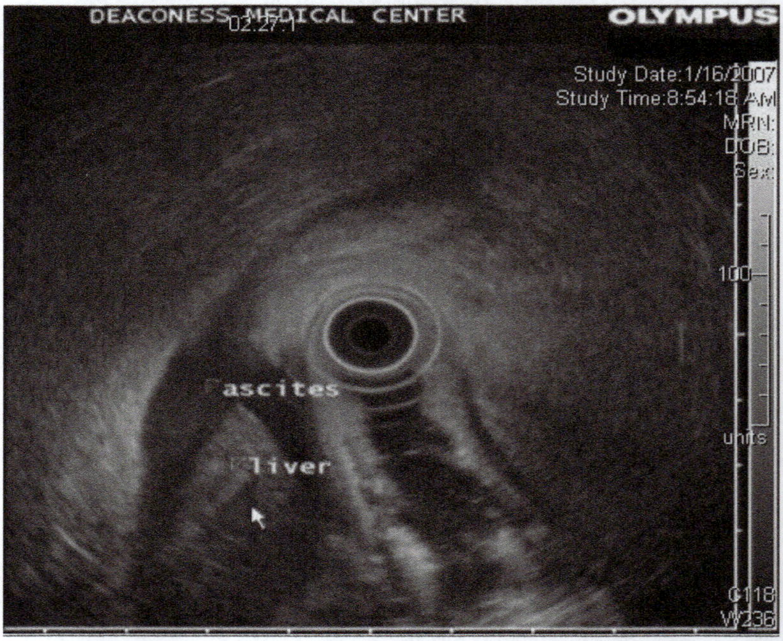

Fig. 7.12 Idiopathic acute pancreatitis. Ascites is surrounding the tip of the left lobe of the liver in the setting of acute pancreatitis

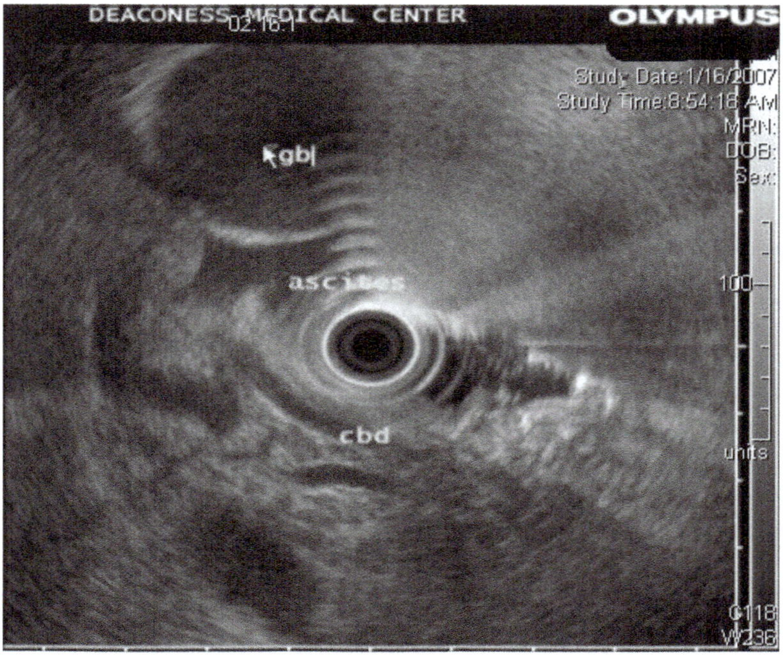

Fig. 7.13 Ascites surrounding the gallbladder (*gb*). *cbd* common bile duct

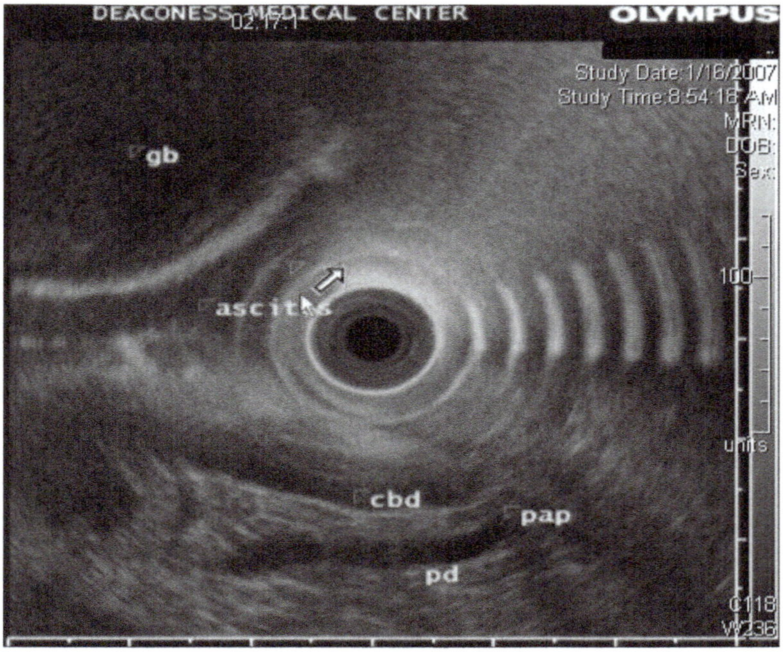

Fig. 7.14 Close-up of ascites surrounding the gallbladder (*gb*) (*arrow*). *cbd* common bile duct, *pd* pancreatic duct, *pap* papilla of vater

7.2.6 Omentum

The normal omentum is rarely identifiable on CT and magnetic resonance imaging; ultrasound visualization of a normal omentum is also rare. This is a 56-year-old liver transplant candidate with significant ascites who was referred for EUS evaluation for other reasons. The EUS images show normal omentum in a lesser sac filled with ascites (posterior to the stomach). Lesser sac hernias make up only about 1–4 % of all internal hernias. The herniated organs may include the small intestine, cecum, proximal colon, transverse colon, omentum, and gallbladder. The entrance of the herniation into the lesser sac is usually through the foramen of Winslow [20].

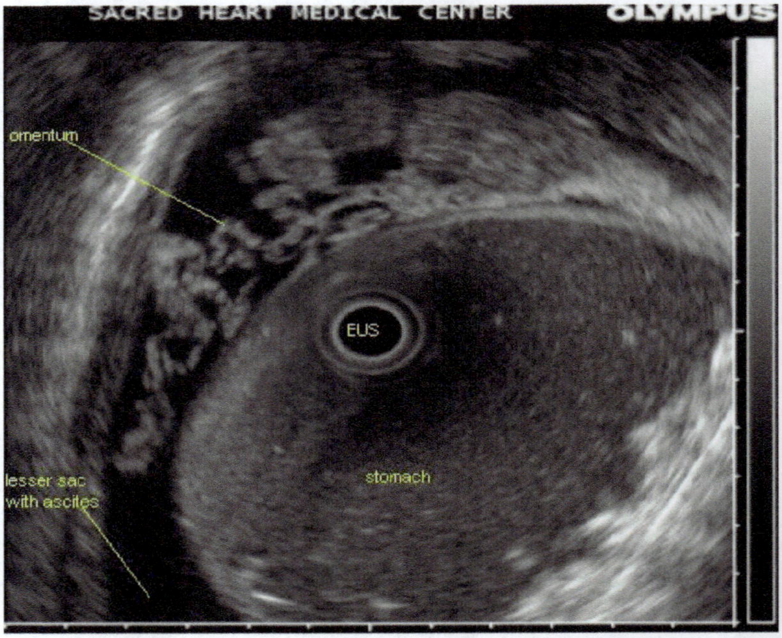

Fig. 7.15 This endoscopic ultrasound (EUS) image shows omentum herniated into the lesser sac in a patient with portal hypertension and ascites

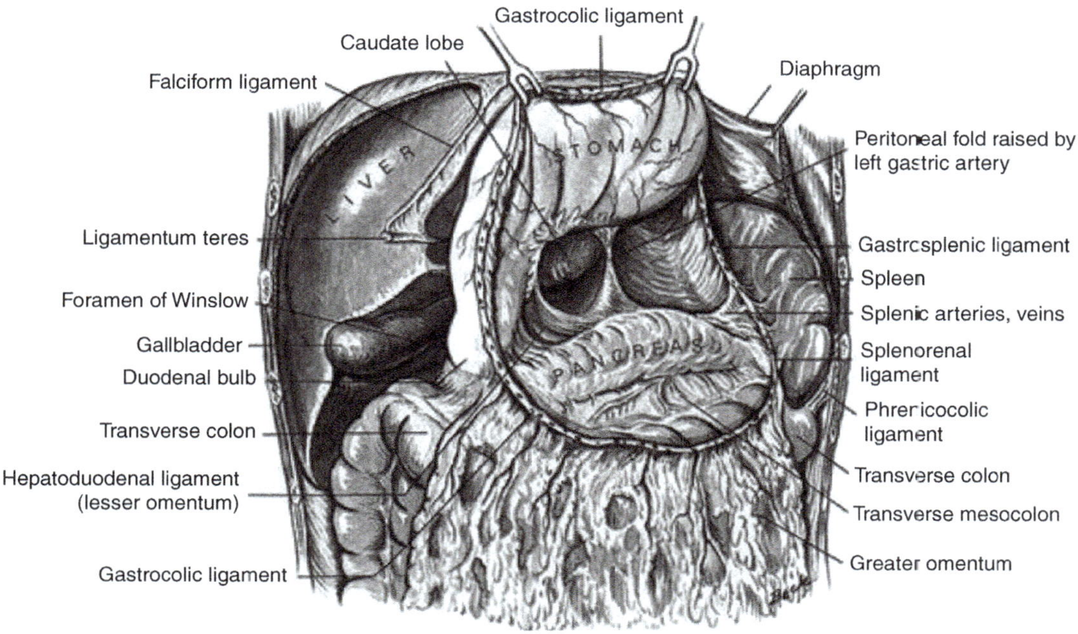

Fig. 7.16 The lesser sac and its relationships shown with the stomach upraised: foramen of Winslow (*arrow*) (From Meyers and Charnsangavej [21])

7.2.7 Fluid in the Lesser Sac

This is a 53-year-old patient with ovarian cancer who developed recurrent disease shortly after debulking surgery and chemotherapy. She then underwent debulking again and hyperthermic intraperitoneal chemotherapy at another institution. Several weeks after discharge she was readmitted with signs of peritonitis and was found to have a perforation of the sigmoid colon. Another 3 months later she was referred to us with what appeared to be a soft-tissue density on CT scan suspicious for recurrent cancer. EUS showed this to be a fluid collection in the lesser sac. Straw-colored fluid was aspirated with EUS guidance. The fluid cytology was positive for adenocarcinoma, and amylase and lipase contents were within normal limits.

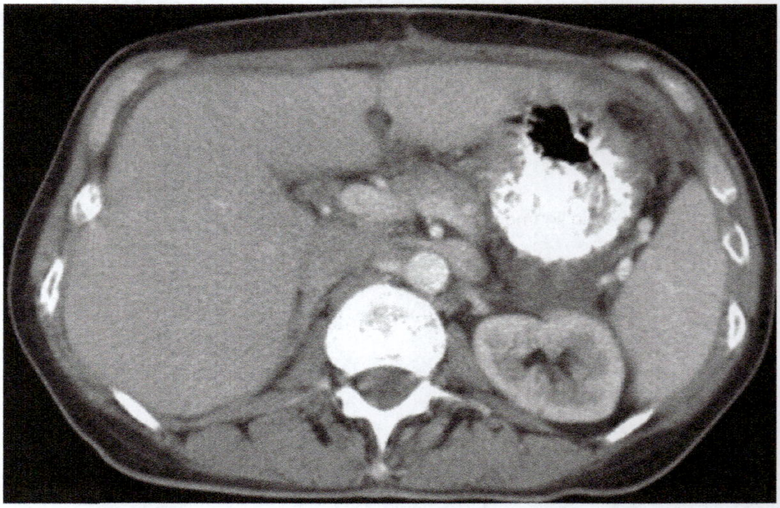

Fig. 7.17 This computed tomography scan was interpreted as showing a soft-tissue mass posterior to the stomach, suspicious for recurrent ovarian cancer

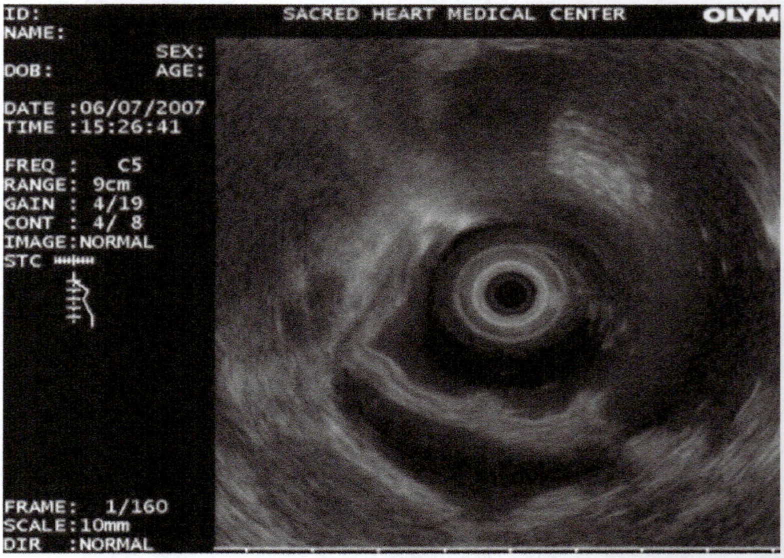

Fig. 7.18 The endoscopic ultrasound shows that the computed tomography abnormality is actually fluid. Aspiration of the ascitic fluid showed malignant cells consistent with adenocarcinoma

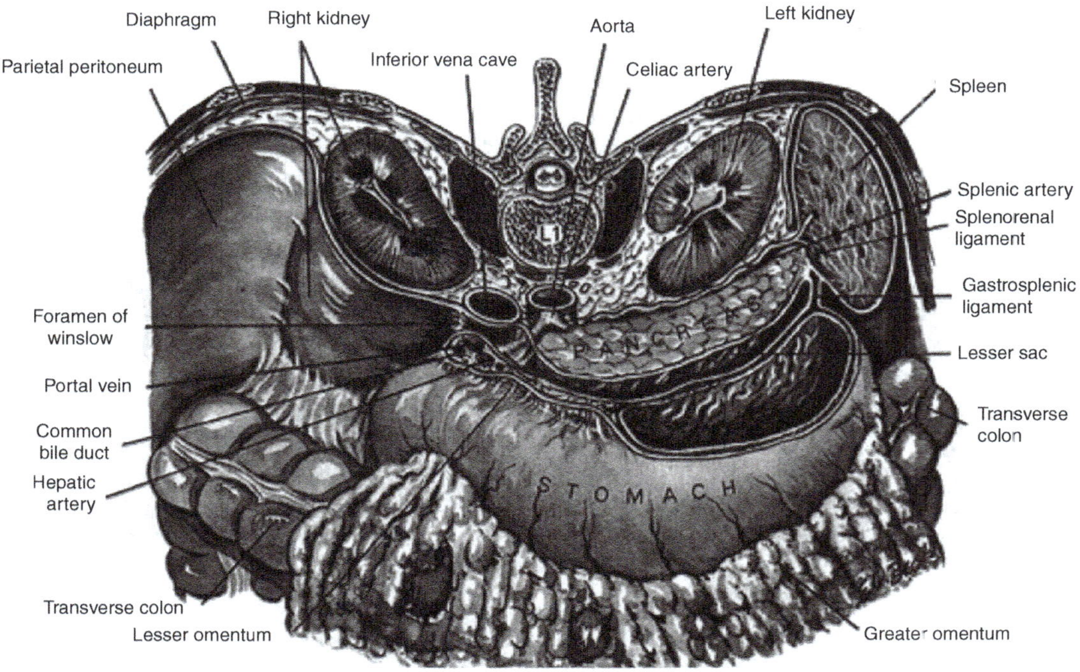

Fig. 7.19 The lesser sac and its relationships. The foramen of Winslow is generally only large enough to admit the introduction of one to two fingers, but in vivo it represents merely a potential communication between the greater and lesser peritoneal cavities (From Meyers and Charnsangavej [21])

7.2.8 Mesenteric Cysts

This is a 68-year-old woman who underwent CT evaluation for nonspecific abdominal pain. She is otherwise fairly healthy and has no weight loss. The CT report suggested the possibility of a retroperitoneal lymphocele, and a lymphangiogram was performed. This study was unremarkable. The patient was then referred for EUS evaluation. The EUS images are characteristic of a mesenteric cyst, which denotes a point of origin or attachment rather than a specific pathologic diagnosis.

Mesenteric and omental cysts are rare: the incidence is about 1 per 140,000 general hospital admissions. Mesenteric cysts can occur anywhere in the mesentery of the gastrointestinal tract, and they may extend from the base of the mesentery into the retroperitoneum. They range in size from incidental small masses to structures that fill the abdomen. The etiology is controversial. These benign cysts can be simple or multiple, unilocular or multilocular, and are typically lined by cuboidal or columnar cells. Ultrasound demonstrates fluid-filled cystic structures with thin internal septi. Internal echoes occur with debris, from hemorrhage, or with infection [22]. Experience with mesenteric and omental cysts is scant. Most of them are benign; however, given the inability to obtain a precise preoperative diagnosis, some authors recommend surgical removal even if they are asymptomatic. Our patient did not want to undergo surgery and her physicians decided to perform serial imaging follow-up.

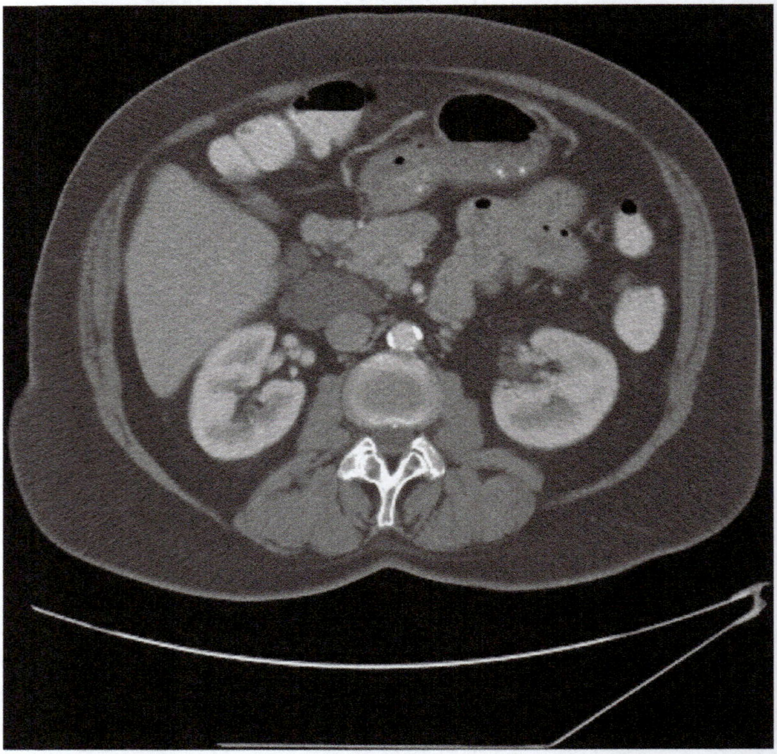

Fig. 7.20 There is a cystic structure adjacent to the inferior vena cava

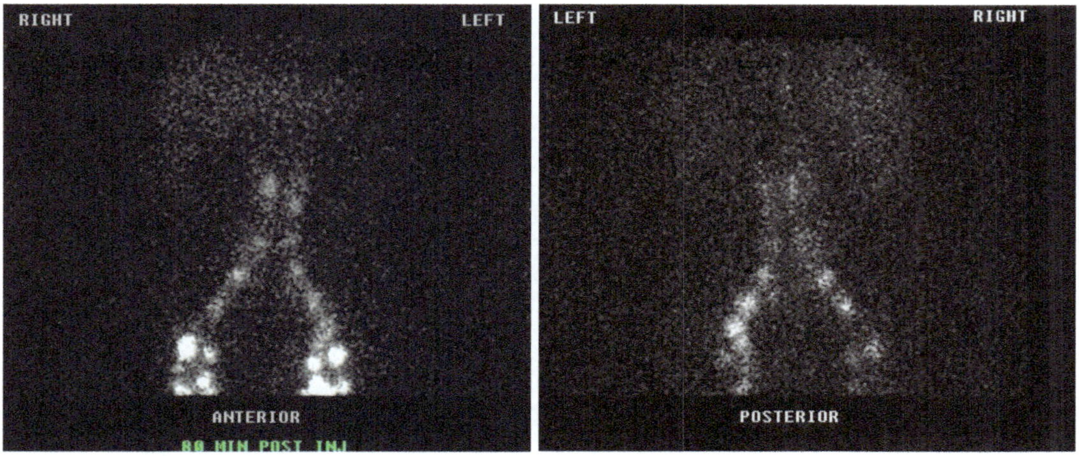

Fig. 7.21 A mesenteric lymphangiogram was unremarkable

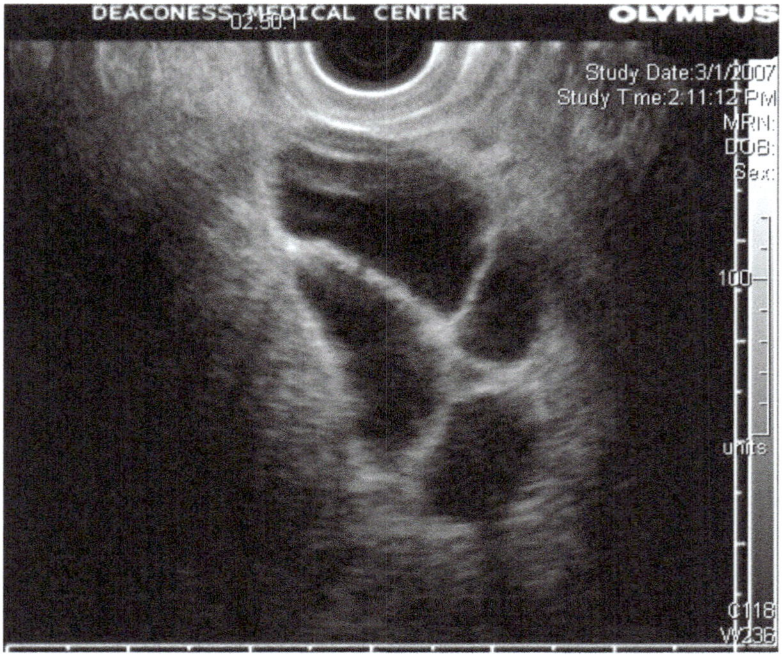

Fig. 7.22 Endoscopic ultrasound appearance of the mesenteric cyst. The septations are not apparent on the computed tomography scan

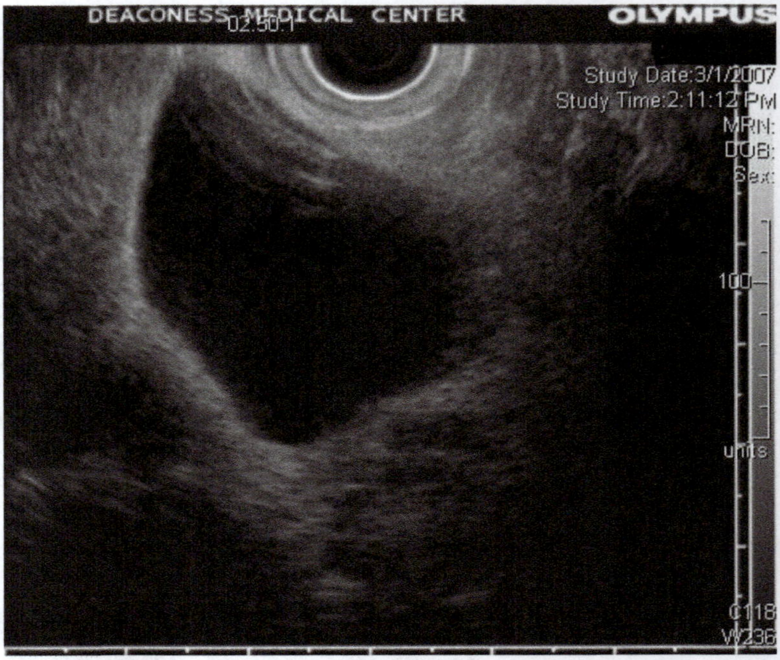

Fig. 7.23 The largest of a group of several mesenteric cysts shows a clear interior without debris and a smooth cyst wall

7.2.9 Omental Cake

Omental metastatic disease, or omental cake, is the infiltration of the omentum by tumor cells and is caused most often by metastatic ovarian cancer and less frequently by metastatic stomach and colon cancer. Benign etiologies, such as tuberculous peritonitis, are rare in developed countries [23]. The descriptive term is particularly appropriate when the thickened omentum is outlined by surrounding ascites, assuming a placental or cake-like aspect.

This is a 60-year-old woman who had vague abdominal pain. A CT scan showed peritoneal carcinomatosis and ascites. Pancreatobiliary EUS was requested to search for a potential primary tumor, which was not apparent on CT. The EUS images of the omental cake were obtained from scanning positions in the distal duodenum. No other pathology was found. A rectal EUS was performed during the same session and revealed a peculiar hypoechoic tumor, potentially originating from the ovary, with brightly echogenic focal areas consistent with fat. (For a review of the ultrasound appearance of adnexal massses we refer the reader to Braun et al. [24].) The ascites cytology showed adenocarcinoma, with immunohistochemistry supporting an origin from the ovary or breast.

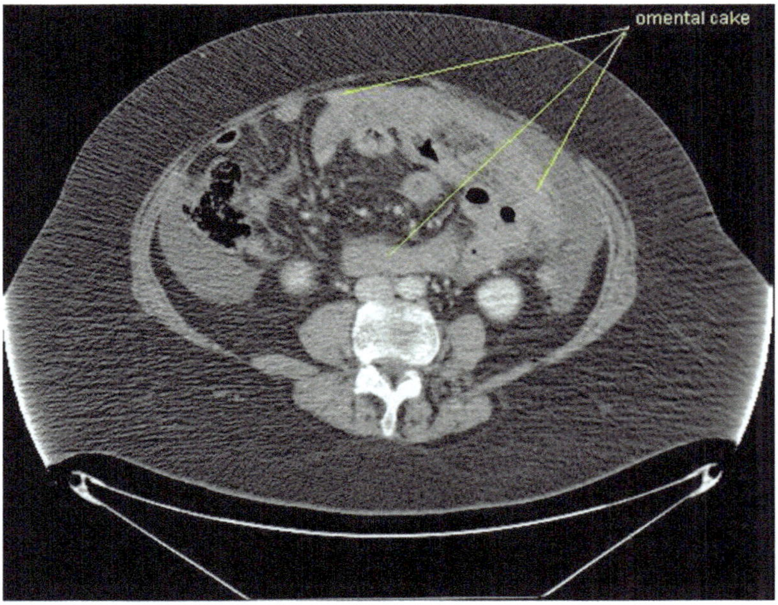

Fig. 7.24 This computed tomography scan shows the omental cake and a moderate amount of ascites

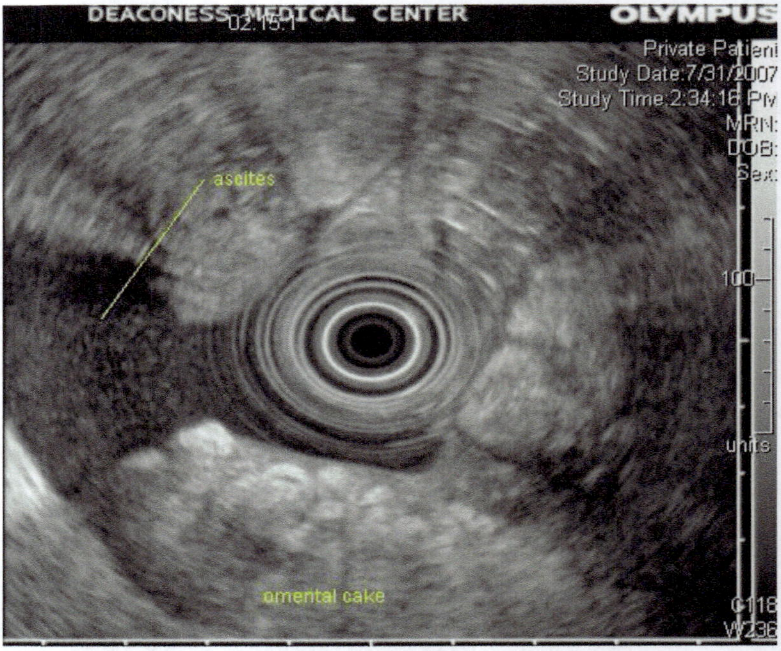

Fig. 7.25 The bright echoes in the lower half of the image represent a conglomerate of omental fat

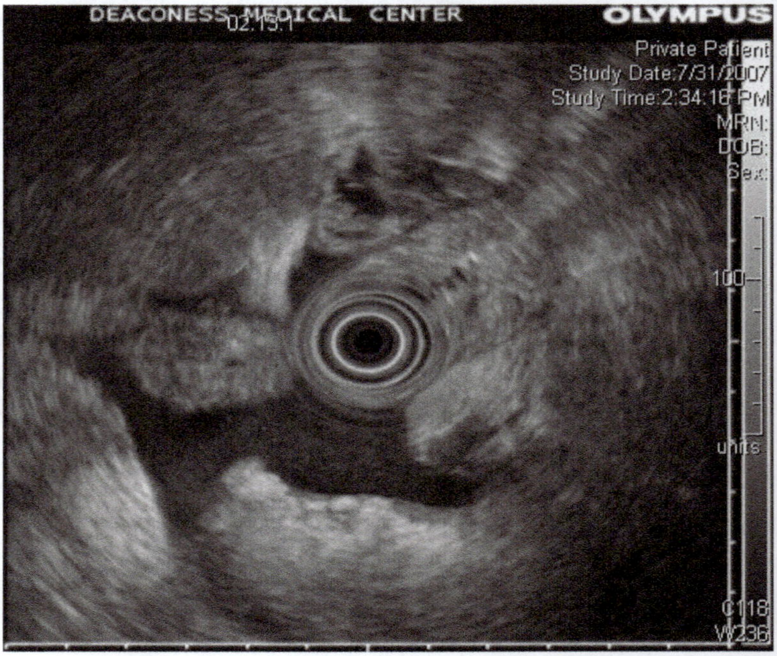

Fig. 7.26 A different aspect of the same omental cake

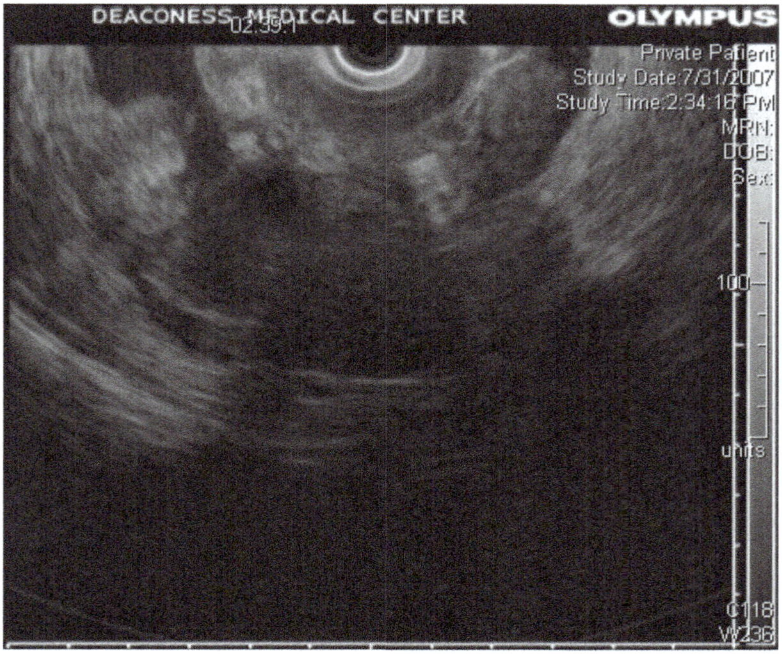

Fig. 7.27 A poorly defined infiltrating hypoechoic mass is seen from the rectosigmoid

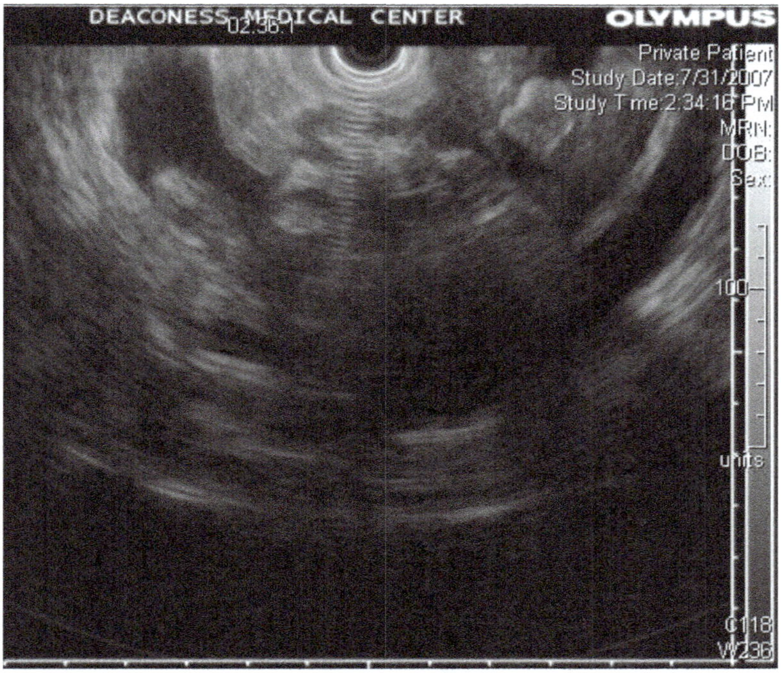

Fig. 7.28 After identification of the mass on transrectal ultrasound, the computed tomography scan was reevaluated. Notice the brighter echoes close to the transducer

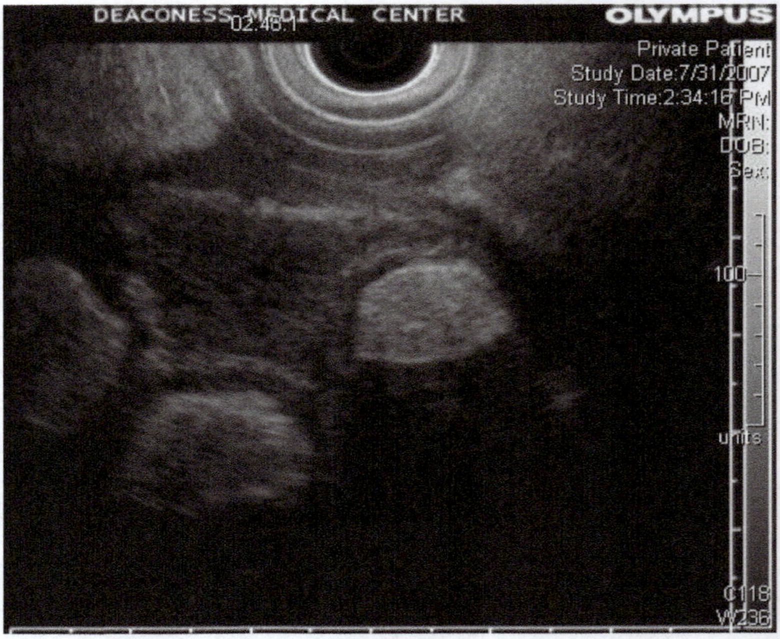

Fig. 7.29 This is a close-up at higher frequency. Peculiar polycyclic, brightly echogenic "plugs" are seen in the otherwise hypoechoic mass

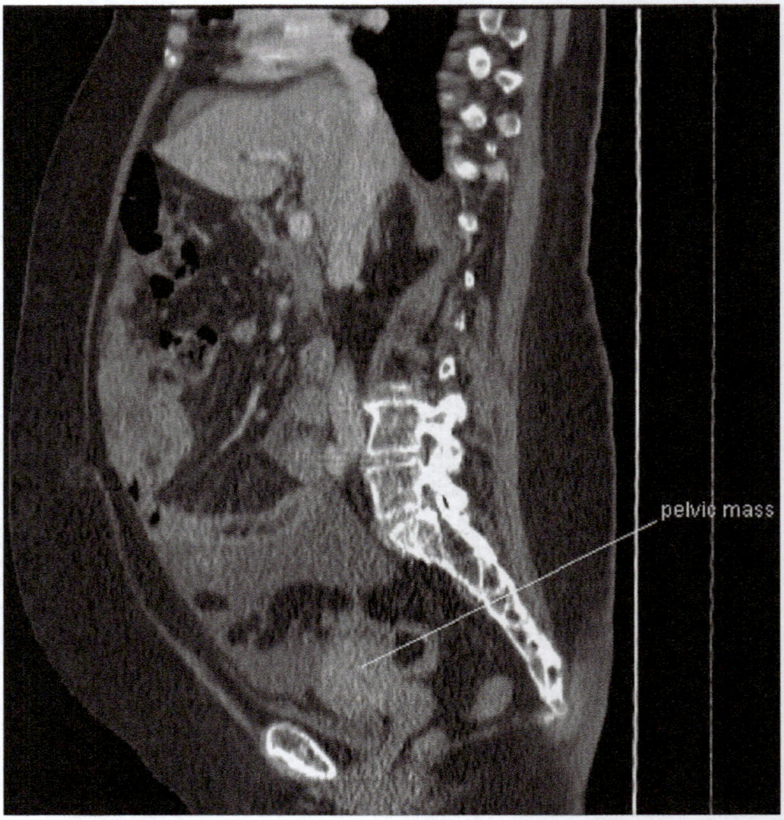

Fig. 7.30 The sagittal computed tomography reconstruction shows the tumor clearly. It is most likely an ovarian cancer

7.2.10 Peritoneal Carcinomatosis

This is a previously healthy 75-year-old male who presented to a local emergency department complaining of some abdominal discomfort but mostly of leg pain. Abnormal liver tests prompted a CT scan of the abdomen, which showed numerous abnormalities. A rather large mass next to the ascending colon (not shown) was suspected to be the primary tumor, but colonoscopy and upper endoscopy were negative. At this point the pancreatic abnormality was subjected to EUS evaluation. FNA biopsies were positive for adenocarcinoma consistent with a pancreatic origin. Any remaining doubts about whether the pancreatic mass was really the primary tumor were dispelled by the results of the carbohydrate antigen 19-9 serum levels: >700,000 ng/ml (normal up to 35 ng/ml). This level was verified by repeat analysis; it is interesting that even higher CA-19-9 levels have been reported in similar circumstances [25]. The leg pain was caused by a popliteal vein clot, and a small pulmonary embolism also was present.

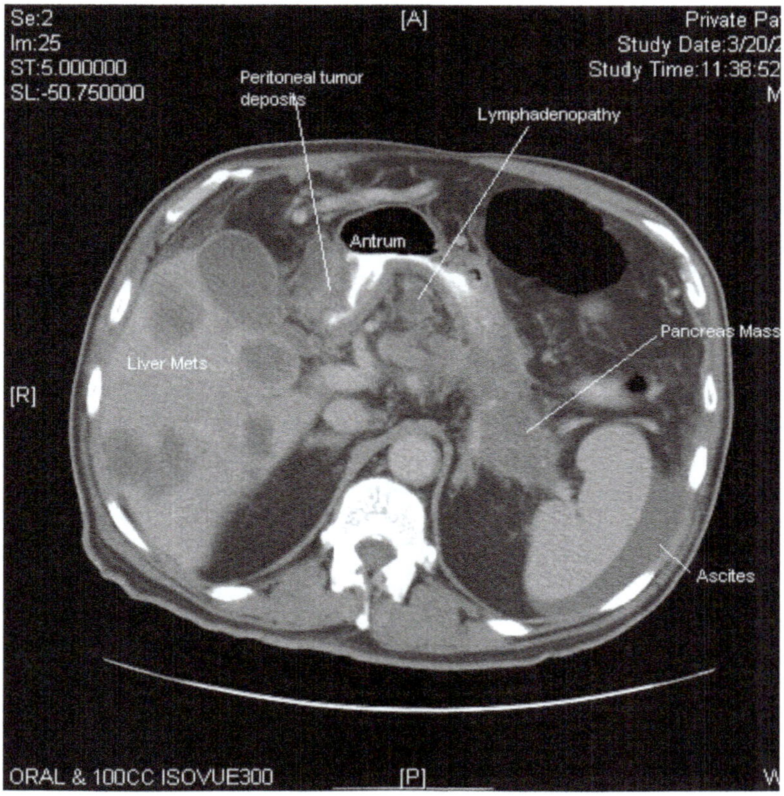

Fig. 7.31 This computed tomography scan shows multiple abnormalities such as liver metastases, a pancreatic mass, carcinomatosis, ascites, and enlarged lymph nodes

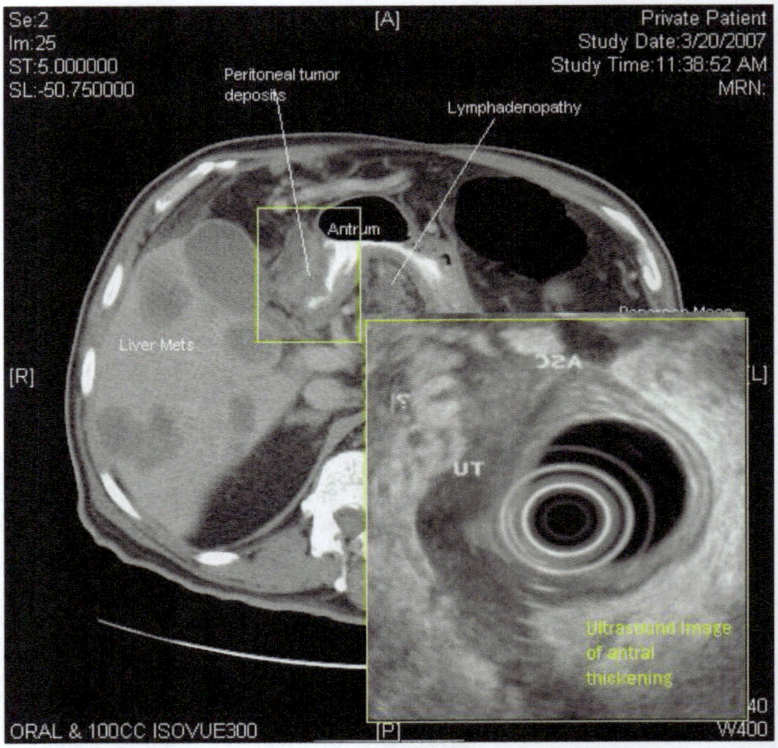

Fig. 7.32 In this computed tomography scan, an endoscopic ultrasound inset shows a close-up of the antral narrowing secondary to peritoneal tumor deposits. The antral wall itself is normal

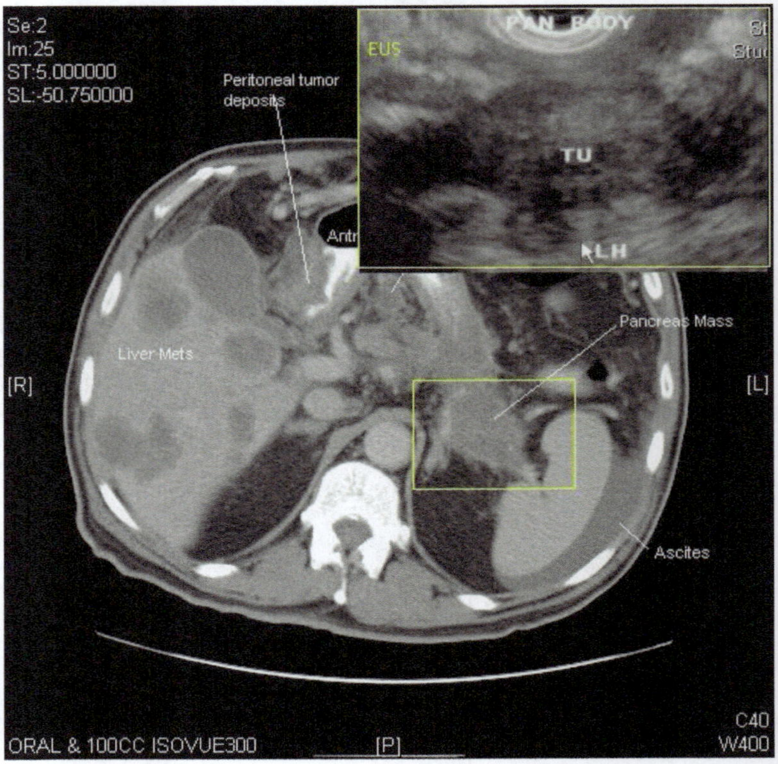

Fig. 7.33 The endoscopic ultrasound (EUS) inset in this computed tomography image shows the cancerous tumor (*tu*) in the pancreatic tail, *LN* lymph node

7.2.11 Retroperitoneal Carcinomatosis

This is a 79-year-old patient who was admitted to the hospital with a 4-week history of nausea and vomiting. She also had noticed a decreased urine output. Her medical history was remarkable for coronary artery disease, diabetes, and a cholecystectomy. Laboratory data revealed evidence of acute renal failure, and therefore only a noncontrast CT scan was obtained (shown).

This was thought to represent retroperitoneal fibrosis. The endoscopic ultrasound shows a diffuse infiltrative process that is fairly unilateral, involves chiefly the right kidney and ureter, and extends toward the retroperitoneal portion of the duodenum, which is narrowed, leading to partial gastric outlet obstruction (see Fig. 7.37). Given the fact that a core biopsy of this tumor could easily be accomplished with CT guidance, we did not pursue EUS-guided FNA. The CT-guided biopsies revealed an undifferentiated carcinoma, with immunohistochemistry not entirely typical but suggestive of renal cell origin.

Current imaging techniques are insufficiently specific to allow for confident differentiation between idiopathic retroperitoneal fibrosis and secondary retroperitoneal fibrosis due to malignancy, infection, or other causes. As a result, open or imaging-guided biopsy remains the mainstay of diagnostic confirmation [26].

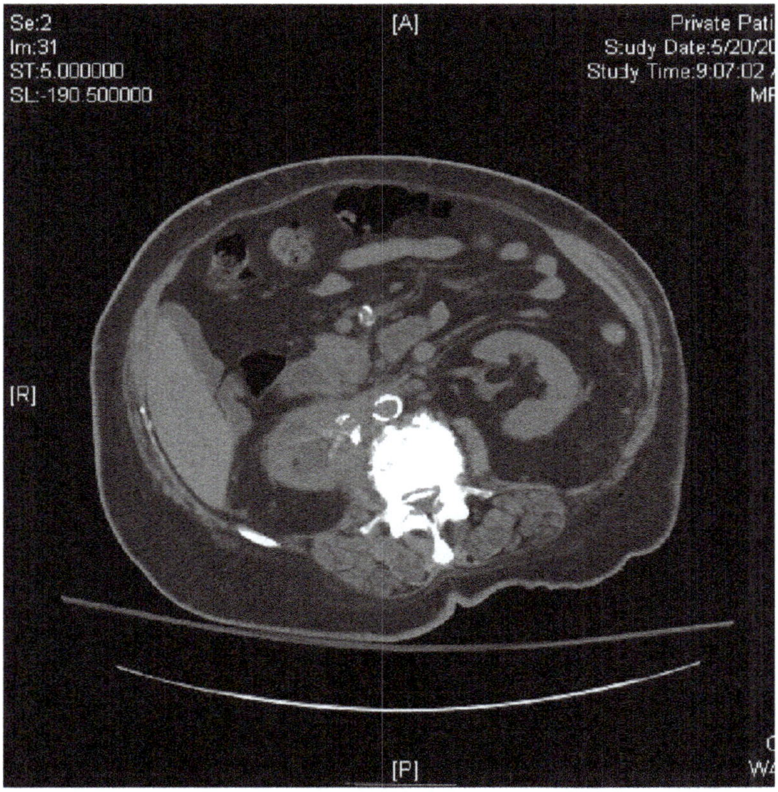

Fig. 7.34 This is a retroperitoneal process involving the right ureter and the duodenum

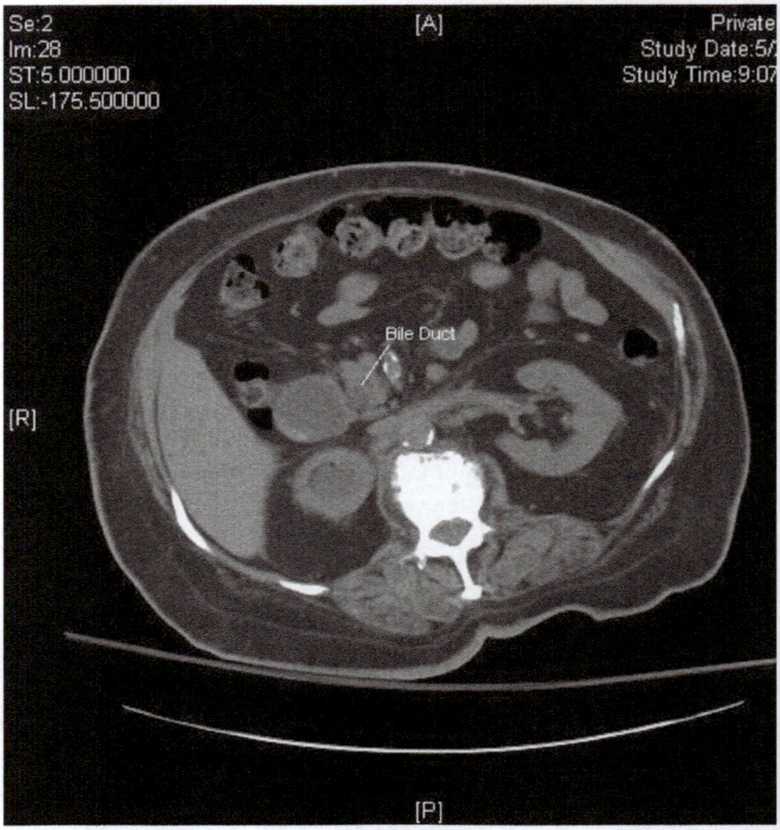

Fig. 7.35 The duodenum is distended, indicating a distal obstruction

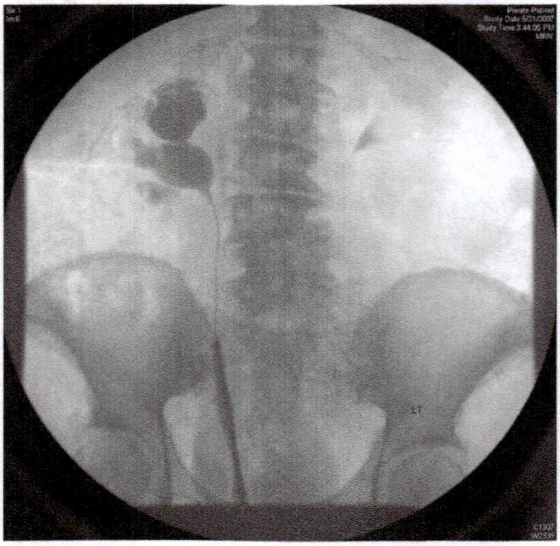

Fig. 7.36 This retrograde urography shows a dilated right renal collecting system and a long ureteral stricture *LT* left

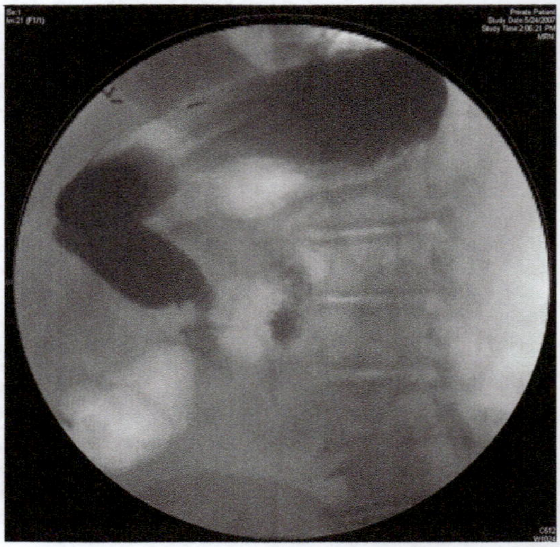

Fig. 7.37 The duodenal narrowing is demonstrated on this upper gastrointestinal barium study

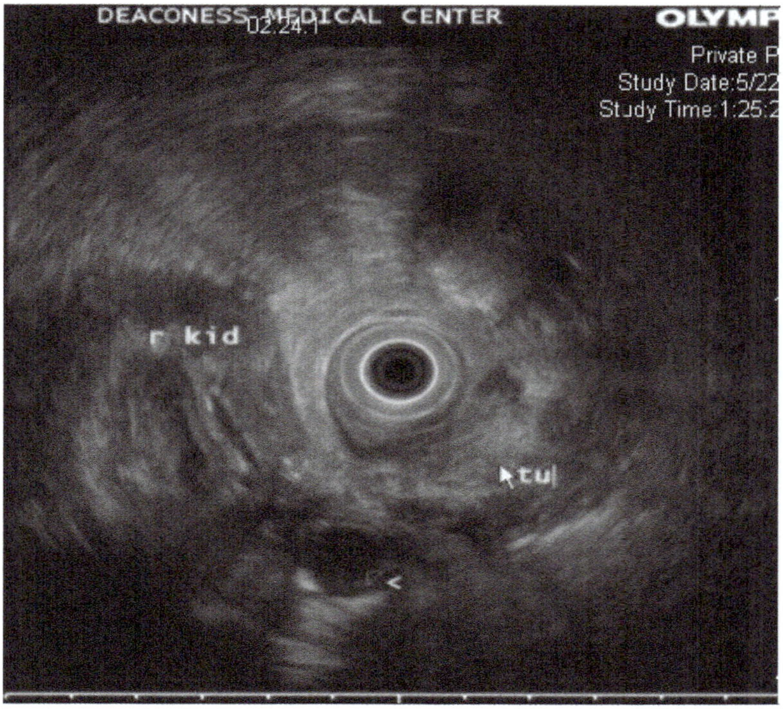

Fig. 7.38 The duodenum (*duo*) is involved by an extensive retroperitoneal process (tu). *R kid* right kidney

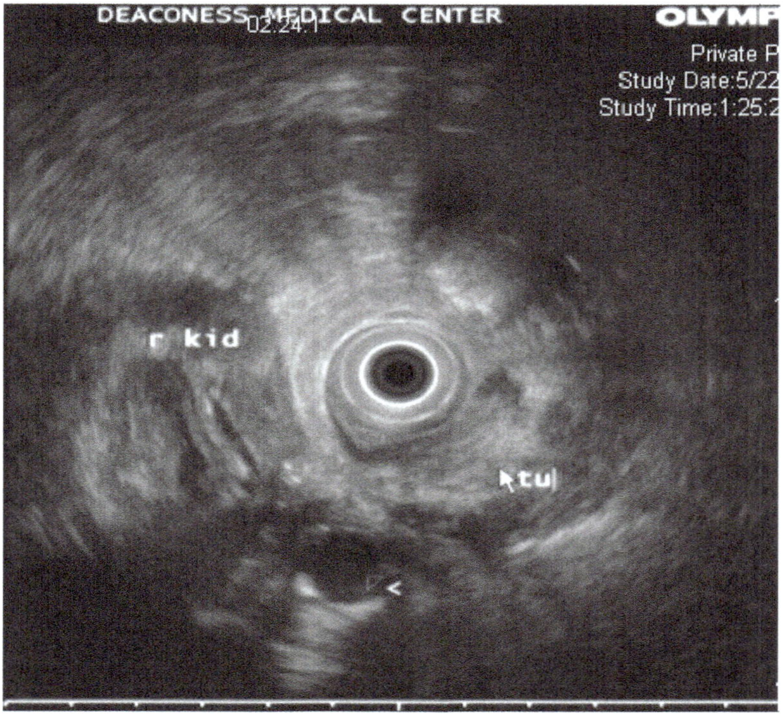

Fig. 7.39 The structure labeled with an *arrowhead* (<) is the renal vein, later confirmed by Doppler, encased by tumor. *R kid* right kidney, *tu* retroperitoneal process

References

1. Chang KJ, Erickson RA, Nguyen P. Endoscopic ultrasound (EUS) and EUS-guided fine-needle aspiration of the left adrenal gland. Gastrointest Endosc. 1996;44(5):568–72.
2. Uemura S, Yasuda I, Kato T, Doi S, Kawaguchi J, Yamauchi T, et al. Preoperative routine evaluation of bilateral adrenal glands by endoscopic ultrasound and fine-needle aspiration in patients with potentially resectable lung cancer. Endoscopy. 2013;45(3):195–201. doi: 10.1055/s-0032-1325988. Epub 2013 Jan 8.
3. Eloubeidi MA, Morgan DE, Cerfolio RJ, Eltoum IA. Transduodenal EUS-guided FNA of the right adrenal gland. Gastrointest Endosc. 2008;67(3):522–7.
4. Dietreich CF, Kann PH. Endoscopic ultrasound imaging of the adrenals. In: Endoscopic ultrasound: an introductory manual and atlas. New York: Thieme; 2011.
5. Young Jr WF. Clinical practice. The incidentally discovered adrenal mass. N Engl J Med. 2007;356(6):601–10.
6. Eloubeidi MA, Black KR, Tamhane A, Eltoum IA, Bryant A, Cerfolio RJ. A large single-center experience of EUS-guided FNA of the left and right adrenal glands: diagnostic utility and impact on patient management. Gastrointest Endosc. 2010;71(4):745–53.
7. Lenert JT, Barnett Jr CC, Kudelka AP, Sellin RV, Gagel RF, Prieto VG, et al. Evaluation and surgical resection of adrenal masses in patients with a history of extra-adrenal malignancy. Surgery. 2001;130(6):1060–7.
8. Grumbach MM, Biller BMK, Braunstein GD, Campbell KK, Carney JA, Godley PA, et al. Management of the clinically inapparent adrenal mass ("incidentaloma"). Ann Intern Med. 2003;138(5):424–9.
9. DeWitt J, Alsatie M, LeBlanc J, McHenry L, Sherman S. Endoscopic ultrasound-guided fine-needle aspiration of left adrenal gland masses. Endoscopy. 2007;39(1):65–71.
10. Willard FH, Schuenke MD. The neuroanatomy of female pelvic pain. In: Pain in women. New York: Springer; 2013. p. 17–58.
11. Halpert B, Gyorkey F. Lesions observed in accessory spleens of 311 patients. Am J Clin Pathol. 1959;32(2):165–8.
12. Mortelé KJ, Mortelé B, Silverman SG. CT features of the accessory spleen. AJR Am J Roentgenol. 2004;183(6):1653–7.
13. Barawi M, Bekal P, Gress F. Accessory spleen: a potential cause of misdiagnosis at EUS. Gastrointest Endosc. 2000;52(6):769–72.
14. Arkadopoulos N, Athanasopoulos P, Stafyla V, Karakatsanis A, Koutoulidis V, Theodosopoulos T, et al. Intrapancreatic accessory spleen issues: diagnostic and therapeutic challenges. JOP. 2009;10(4):400–5.
15. Krishna SG, Heif MM, Sharma SG, Pandey T, Rego RF. Intrapancreatic accessory spleen: investigative dilemmas and role of EUS-guided FNA for diagnostic confirmation. JOP. 2011;12(6):603–6.
16. Lee YT, Ng EKW, Hung LCT, Chung SCS, Ching JYL, Chan WY, et al. Accuracy of endoscopic ultrasonography in diagnosing ascites and predicting peritoneal metastases in gastric cancer patients. Gut. 2005;54(11):1541–5.
17. Nguyen PT, Chang KJ. EUS in the detection of ascites and EUS-guided paracentesis. Gastrointest Endosc. 2001;54(3):336–9.
18. Maringhini A, Ciambra M, Patti R, Randazzo MA, Dardanoni G, Mancuso L, et al. Ascites, pleural, and pericardial effusions in acute pancreatitis. A prospective study of incidence, natural history, and prognostic role. Dig Dis Sci. 1996;41(5):848–52.
19. Wardeh R, Lee JG, Gu M. Endoscopic ultrasound-guided paracentesis of ascitic fluid. Cancer Cytopathol. 2011;119(1):27–36.
20. Yoo E, Kim JH, Kim M-J, Yu J-S, Chung J-J, Yoo H-S, et al. Greater and lesser omenta: normal anatomy and pathologic processes. Radiographics. 2007;27(3):707–20.
21. Meyers MA, Charnsangavej C. Intraperitoneal spread of infections and seeded metastases. In: Meyers' dynamic radiology of the abdomen. New York: Springer; 2011. p. 69–107.
22. Ji H, Ros PR. Tumors of the Mesentery and Omentum. In Radiologic-Pathologic Correlations from Head to Toe, pp. 447–473. Springer Berlin Heidelberg, 2005.
23. Mamlouk MD, van Sonnenberg E, Shankar S, Silverman SG. Omental cakes: unusual aetiologies and CT appearances. Insights Imaging. 2011;2(4):399–408.
24. Brown DL, Dudiak KM, Laing FC. Adnexal masses: US characterization and reporting1. Radiology. 2010;254(2):342–54.
25. Al-Khallaf H, Monaghan PJ, Ourfali A, Elsammak M, Ambrosio C, Sodi R, et al. The highest ever reported level of carbohydrate antigen 19-9: a case report. J Med Cases. 2011;2(2):71–5.
26. Cronin CG, Lohan DG, Blake MA, Roche C, McCarthy P, Murphy JM. Retroperitoneal fibrosis: a review of clinical features and imaging findings. AJR Am J Roentgenol. 2008;191(2):423–31.

Colon, Rectum, and Anus

8

Contents

8.1 **General Principles** 415
8.1.1 Anatomy of the Rectal Wall and Perirectal Structures: Correlation with EUS 415
8.1.1.1 Anal Canal 415
8.1.1.2 Rectum 416
8.1.2 Endoscopic Ultrasound Probes 419
8.1.3 Preparation 419
8.1.4 Endoscopic Ultrasound Examination Technique 419

8.2 **Cases and Discussions** 421
8.2.1 Progression of Rectal Cancer from T2N0 to T3N1 421
8.2.2 T3N1 Rectal Carcinoma: Response to Treatment 425
8.2.2.1 EUS for the Evaluation of Rectal Cancer 427
8.2.3 Colon Cancer Metastatic to Mediastinal Lymph Nodes 428
8.2.4 Large Colon Polyp 431
8.2.5 Large Villous Adenoma with High-Grade Dysplasia 433
8.2.6 Anal Cancer with Extensive Intramural Spread into the Rectum 435
8.2.7 Anorectal Melanoma 438
8.2.8 Diffuse Cavernous Rectal Hemangioma 442
8.2.9 Cystic Lymphangioma of the Colon 445
8.2.10 Coccygeal Chordoma 449

References 452

8.1 General Principles

Endoscopic ultrasound (EUS) allows a detailed examination of the anal canal, rectum, and adjacent pelvic structures and has become an important tool in the evaluation of colorectal and pelvic disorders. A clear understanding of the anatomy, EUS probe options, and appropriate preparation and technique, as explained in this chapter, is necessary for optimal results.

8.1.1 Anatomy of the Rectal Wall and Perirectal Structures: Correlation with EUS

8.1.1.1 Anal Canal

The anal canal extends from the anal verge to the anorectal junction, where the puborectalis encircles the rectum [1]. The dentate line is approximately 2 cm from the anal verge and it is an important landmark to help predict the type of tissue obtained by biopsies and pattern of spread of neoplastic lesions. Anal glands, located mainly at the submucosal space but extending as far as the external anal sphincter, open at the level of the anal crypts above the dentate line. The epithelium appears endosonographically as a faint layer; the submucosa and subcutaneous connective tissue are seen as a well-defined hyperechoic layer. The internal anal sphincter is a caudal extension of the circular inner layer of the muscularis propria of the rectum [1] and can be seen as a hypoechoic circumferential cylinder, approximately 2–4 mm

K. Gottlieb, G. Marino, *Diagnostic Endosonography*,
DOI 10.1007/978-3-642-39118-7_8, © Springer-Verlag Berlin Heidelberg 2014

in thickness, in the superior three fourths of the anal canal. The external anal sphincter surrounds the internal anal sphincter below the puborectalis and is formed by striated muscle, appearing as a hyperechoic ring in contrast to hypoechoic smooth muscle layers. The external sphincter is approximately 7–9 mm in thickness in young patients and becomes thinner with age [2, 3]. The anterior portion of the external sphincter is shorter and slopes downward in women, which can lead to a false-positive diagnosis of anterior sphincter tear or defect if the endoscopist is not aware of this normal variation [4].

8.1.1.2 Rectum

As the probe is advanced proximally from the external sphincter, the puborectalis can be found posteriorly, adjacent to the rectum, appearing as a hyperechoic sling. Additional muscles that form the levator ani have a hyperechoic appearance but are usually not well visualized sonographically.

The rectal wall has a thickness of 2–4 mm. Only the upper third and anterior wall of the middle third of rectum are above the peritoneal reflection and covered by a hyperechoic serosal layer. The posterior peritoneal reflection is approximately 12–15 cm from the anal verge, while the anterior peritoneal reflection is 6–8 cm from the anal verge [1]. The best landmark for the upper border of the rectum is the confluence of the taenia coli at the rectosigmoid junction; however, this confluence cannot be visualized endoscopically; therefore the National Cancer Institute has defined the rectum as the last 12 cm from the anal verge when measured using a rigid proctosigmoidoscope [5]. Three endoluminal curves known as the valves of Houston can be visualized endoscopically. These folds are formed by mucosa and submucosa but not muscularis propria as seen in the partially distended rectum. The middle valve is the most consistently located and is correlated with the anterior peritoneal reflection [1]. The peritoneal reflection is difficult to see sonographically but its limits correlate with the superior margin of bladder in men and superior margin of the uterus and bladder in women [6].

Rectal wall layers seen on sonography include the hyperechoic borderline between the lumen and mucosa, the hypoechoic mucosa, hyperechoic submucosa, hypoechoic muscularis propria, and hyperechoic perirectal fat. The two components of the muscularis propria – circular (internal) and longitudinal (external) – may be identifiable, separated by a thin layer of hyperechoic connective tissue. As mentioned above, only the upper third of the rectum and the anterior wall of the middle third of the rectum as well as the transverse colon and sigmoid are covered by a serosal layer that appears hyperechoic. Retroperitoneal portions of the colon, that is, ascending and descending, are covered by adventitia. The ileocecal valve also has a five-layer pattern but the wall is thickened at that level.

Landmark structures for anatomic reference around the rectum are the prostate, seminal vesicles, and bladder in men and the vagina, uterus, and bladder in women. Flexible endoscopes allow advancement to the distal sigmoid and evaluation of iliac vessels and possible adjacent lymphadenopathy. Pericolonic organs including the liver, pancreas, kidneys, spleen, vascular structures, ovaries (sometimes), and lymph nodes can also be visualized during colonic EUS.

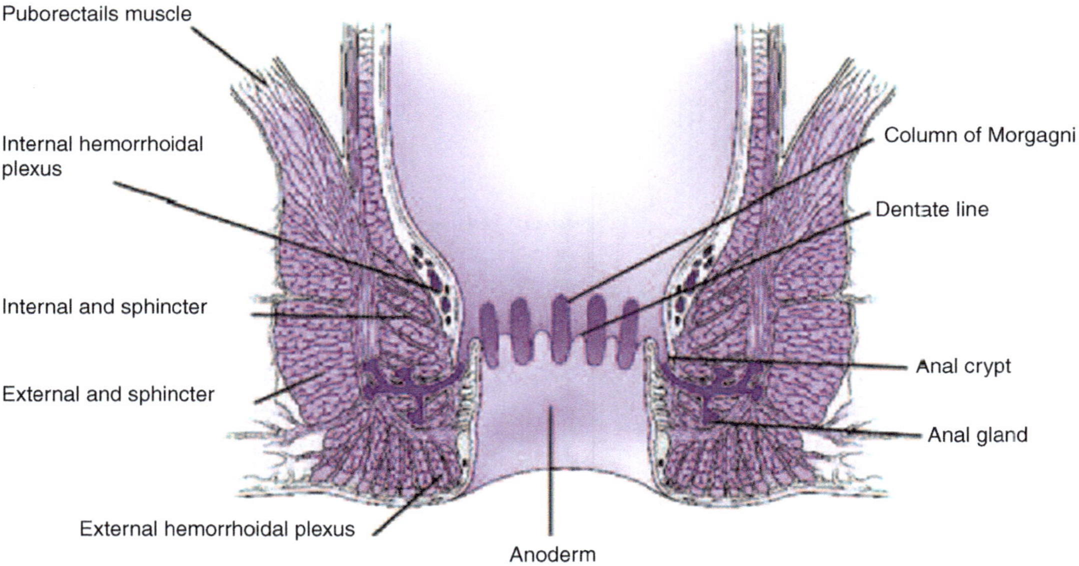

Fig. 8.1 Anatomy of the anal region (From Ehrenpreis [7])

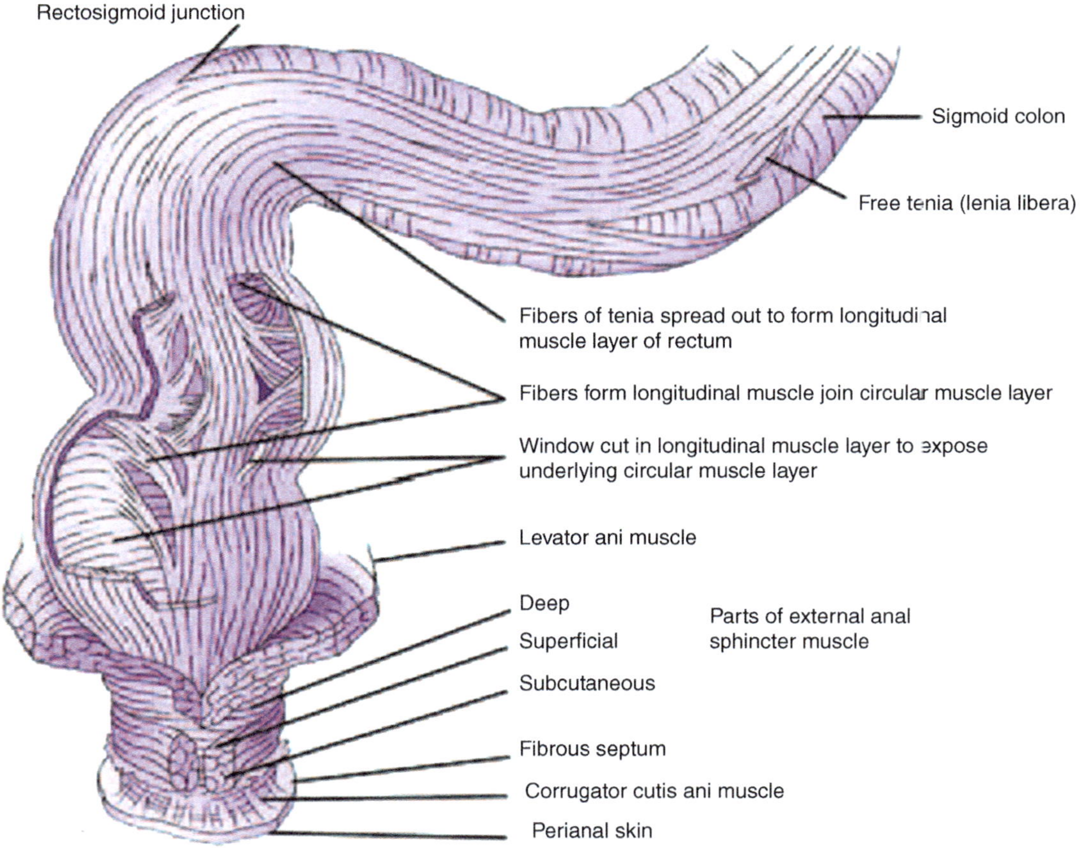

Fig. 8.2 Rectal muscle anatomy (From Ehrenpreis [7])

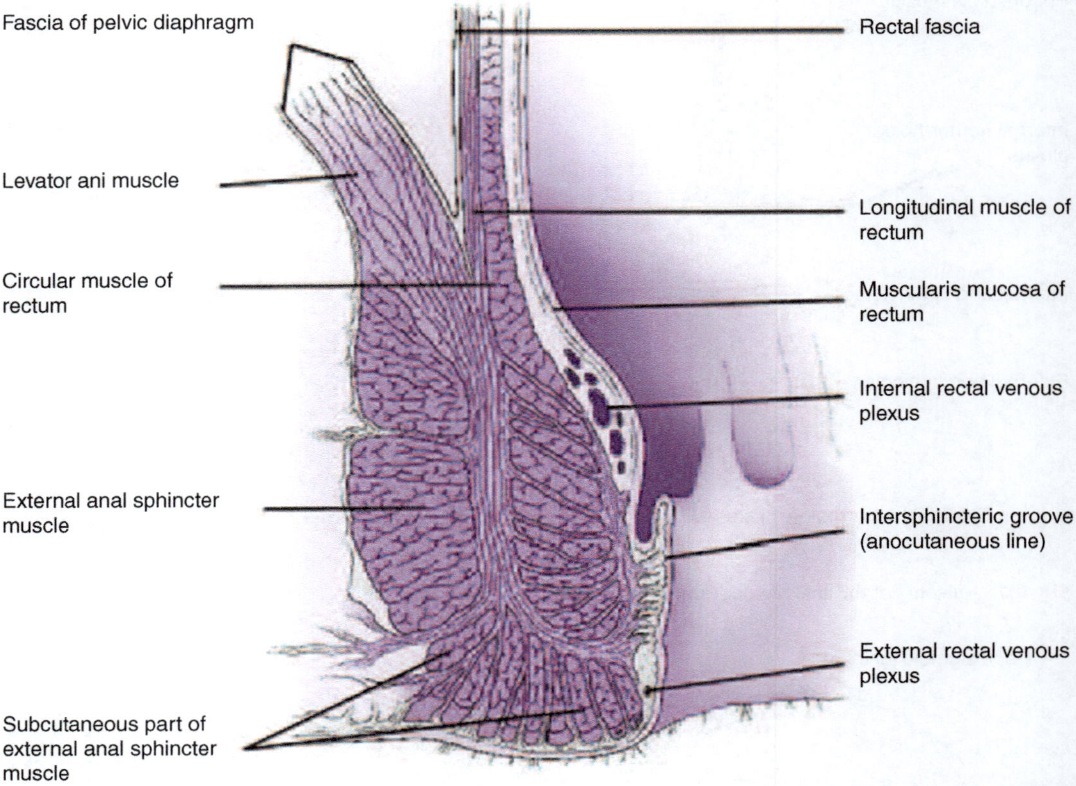

Fig. 8.3 Anal muscle anatomy (From Ehrenpreis [7])

8.1.2 Endoscopic Ultrasound Probes

EUS examination can be performed with rigid probes as well as flexible radial scanning or linear scanning video-endoscopes. Colorectal surgeons and radiologists are more comfortable using rigid probes, but flexible endoscopes are now widely available to gastroenterologists who are trained to use them. Forward-viewing endoscopes allow advancement through the entire colon. Flexible video-endoscopes allow direct optical visualization and confirmation of appropriate scanning or a fine-needle aspiration (FNA) target, avoiding false readings from residual stool. The endoscope can be maneuvered to advance above partially obstructing lesions, and the distance of lesions to the dentate line can be measured [8].

Miniprobe catheters that can be passed through regular endoscope channels also are available. These have a higher scanning frequency (12–20 MHz) and allow detailed evaluation of superficial lesions, particularly those limited to mucosa or submucosa [9].

8.1.3 Preparation

The rectum can be prepared for endoscopy using enemas; two enemas 1 h before the procedure have been reported as appropriate for EUS evaluation of rectal cancer [10]. However, poor preparation and small amounts of stool can interfere with appropriate interpretation, in which case additional enemas may be necessary or, as an alternative, patients can undergo standard colonoscopy preparation [11]. Ideally, patients should avoid urinating before anorectal EUS; this helps to improve bladder visualization. Conscious sedation is not necessary for anorectal EUS unless patients have painful anorectal pathology or painful rectal cancer.

8.1.4 Endoscopic Ultrasound Examination Technique

Endoscopic examination is usually performed first to localize the lesion, evaluate any anatomic distortion to ensure that the echoendoscope can be passed in patients with rectal masses, and evaluate the adequacy of the preparation. If proctosigmoidoscopy is performed it is ideal to minimize air insufflation, and all air should be removed during withdrawal.

To evaluate rectal or colonic lesions the endoscope is advanced and water instilled until the target lesion is covered with water to optimize acoustic coupling; this may require turning the patient so the lesion is placed in the dependent position. Scanning should be performed with the endoscope as parallel to the wall as possible to minimize tangential imaging with magnification of wall thickness. EUS balloons can help examine areas that are not well covered with water; however, caution should be taken not to compress the lesion with the balloon, which might distort staging or measurements.

Evaluation of perirectal lymph nodes requires complete removal of air and careful scanning around the distal sigmoid/rectum, which can be better achieved starting proximally from a point where iliac vessels have been visualized and slowly withdrawing the probe toward the anal canal. An appropriate focal distance should be maintained between the probe and the surface of the rectum or lesion to provide optimal sonographic images.

Adjacent anatomic structures, including the prostate, seminal vesicles, bladder in men and the vagina, uterus, and bladder in women, should be easily recognized. A consistent position of adjacent anatomic landmarks such as prostate or uterus at the top or bottom of the EUS screen allows systematic interpretation and defines the location of the lesions being evaluated. For complete staging in patients with rectal cancer, it is necessary to inspect the iliac vessels, which are usually found between 20 and 25 cm from the anus, and look for perivascular lymph nodes.

Forward-viewing optics are ideal for deeper insertion of echoendoscopes into the colon under direct visualization of the lumen; this is helpful to avoid diverticular perforation or forceful passage. Standard side-viewing echoinstruments, however, also have been used by experienced examiners [12]. The intubation technique is similar to standard colonoscopy but the larger distal end of the endoscope requires more careful manipulation, and it may be more difficult to advance through sharply angulated segments. Bhutani and Nadella [13] have reported no difficulties performing a complete EUS evaluation of up to 45 cm from the anus using radial or linear scanning, oblique view endoscopes. Detailed sonographic visualization of target lesions is better performed during withdrawal of the echoendoscope after water infusion or using the balloon for acoustic coupling.

Examination of the anal canal and sphincters using radial scanning probes without balloon insufflation is usually preferred, although linear scanning instruments have been reported to provide better evaluation of perianal fistulae. Air bubbles can be visualized as hyperechoic tracks or beads at fistulous tracks, and the application of gentle pressure during linear scanning may allow documentation of the air bubbles moving within the track [2]. Greater symmetry of the anterior part of the external sphincter has been achieved during endosonography of the anal canal in the prone position [14].

Box 8.1: Resources for the Colon, Rectum, and Anus

- American Joint Committee on Cancer *Cancer Staging Manual*, 7th edition http://www.springer.com/medicine/surgery/book/978-0-387-88440-0
- National Comprehensive Cancer Network*, Clinical Practice Guidelines in Oncology: Rectal and Colonic Carcinoma (2012):
  http://www.nccn.org/index.asp
  http://www.nccn.org/professionals/physician_gls/pdf/rectal.pdf
  http://www.nccn.org/professionals/physician_gls/pdf/colon.pdf
- Dave Project – Gastroenterology: EUS for staging of rectal cancer
  http://daveproject.org/eus-for-staging-of-rectal-cancer/2009-11-09/
- Medical University of South Carolina, Digestive Disease Center: EUS Atlas
  http://www.ddc.musc.edu/professional/education/atlases/EUSatlas/index.cfm

*Registration to the NCCN website is a free service; it is necessary to view these clinical practice guidelines.

Box 8.2: Good Reviews About Anal Cancer

- Anal cancer: ESMO Clinical Recommendations for diagnosis, treatment, and follow-up (*Ann Oncol* 2009) http://annonc.oxfordjournals.org/content/20/suppl_4/iv57.long
- National Comprehensive Cancer Network*, Clinical Practice Guidelines in Oncology: Anal Carcinoma (2013) http://www.nccn.org/professionals/physician_gls/pdf/anal.pdf

*Registration to the NCCN website is a free service; it is necessary to view these clinical practice guidelines.

8.2 Cases and Discussions

8.2.1 Progression of Rectal Cancer from T2N0 to T3N1

Cancer of the rectum, when localized, is a highly treatable and often curable disease. Surgery is the primary treatment and results in cure in approximately 45 % of all patients. The prognosis of rectal cancer is clearly related to the degree of penetration of the tumor through the bowel wall and the presence or absence of nodal involvement. EUS is an accurate method of evaluating tumor stage and the status of the perirectal nodes (detailed discussion in Sect. 8.2.2.1). Accurate staging can influence therapy by helping to determine which patients are candidates for local excision rather than more extensive surgery and for preoperative chemotherapy and radiation therapy to maximize the likelihood of resection with clear margins.

This is a 53-year-old man who was diagnosed with rectal cancer. EUS staging revealed this to be a T2N0 lesion. Unfortunately, he refused standard treatment – despite the urgings of his physicians – and chose alternative treatments instead, which consisted, at least in part, of tea enemas. These were not effective. Four months later he had restaging EUS, which was performed to encourage him to change his mind about treatment. Indeed, the cancer had advanced to a T3N1 stage. Eventually he was convinced to have radiation and chemotherapy.

The histologic T stage of rectal tumors can be estimated sonographically by the deepest layer of visible invasion. The accuracy of EUS evaluation of T stage in the range 69–94 % has been reported [15–17]. Access to the TNM (tumor, node, metastasis) staging system is available online at: http://goo.gl/00RNs.

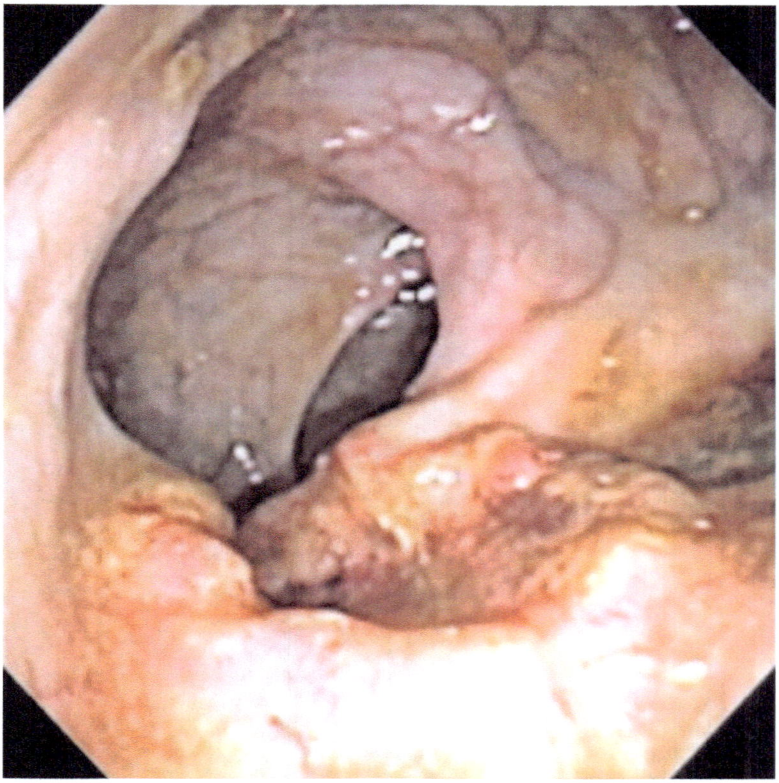

Fig. 8.4 Endoscopic image of a malignant rectal ulcer

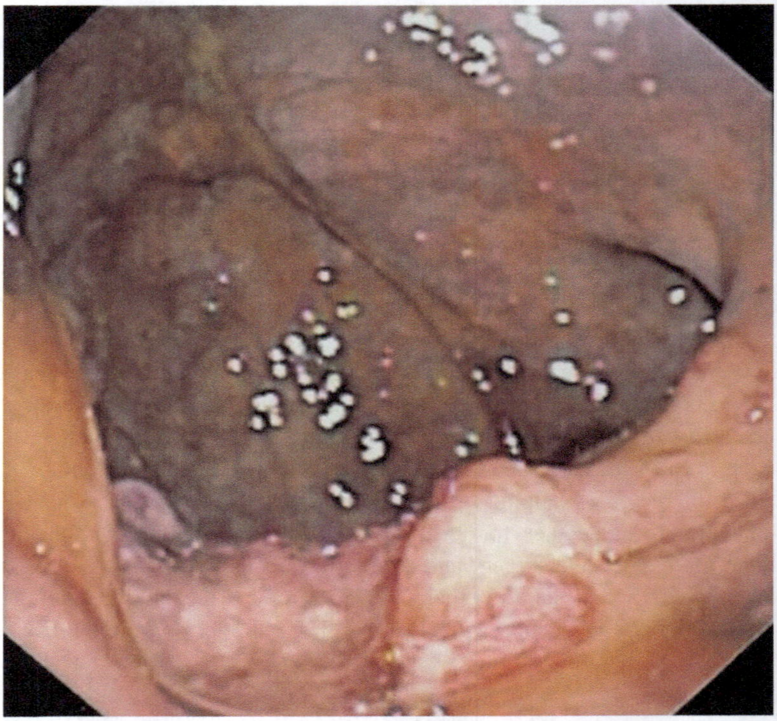

Fig. 8.5 In June, after 4 months of tea enemas, progression of the rectal cancer is seen on endoscopy

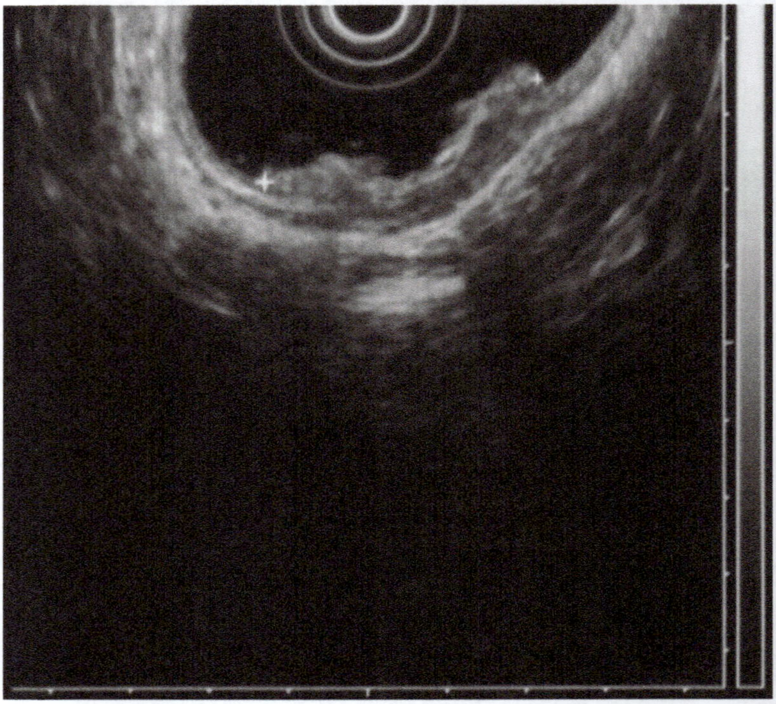

Fig. 8.6 Rectal carcinoma on endoscopic ultrasound (stage uT2N0 at initial presentation)

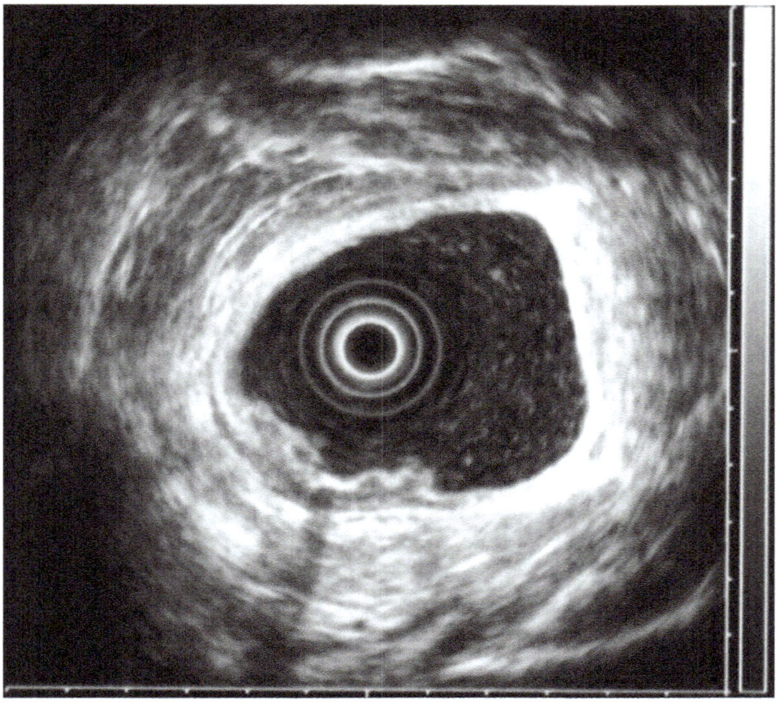

Fig. 8.7 Another view of the stage uT2N0 rectal cancer

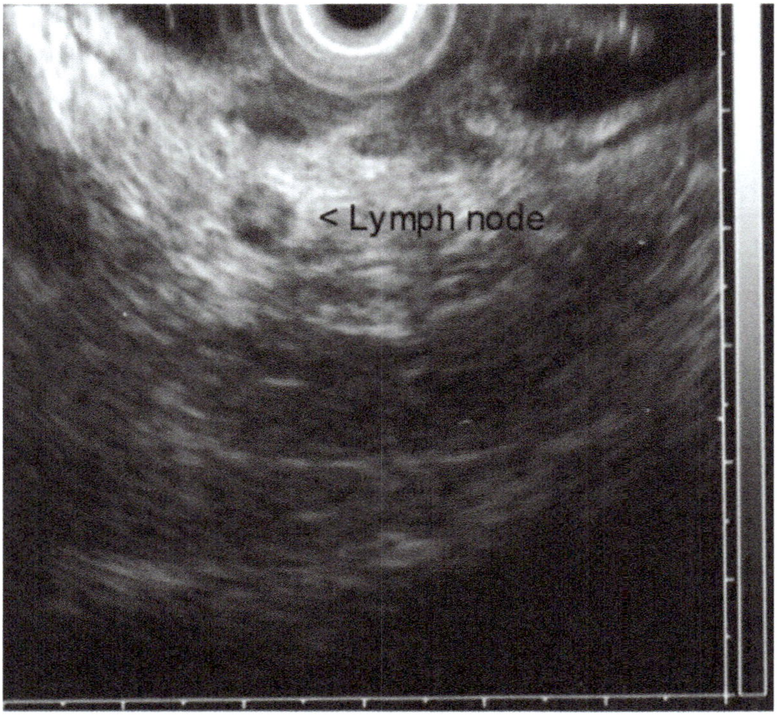

Fig. 8.8 Four months after initial presentation, the rectal cancer has progressed. Malignant lymphadenopathy is now present

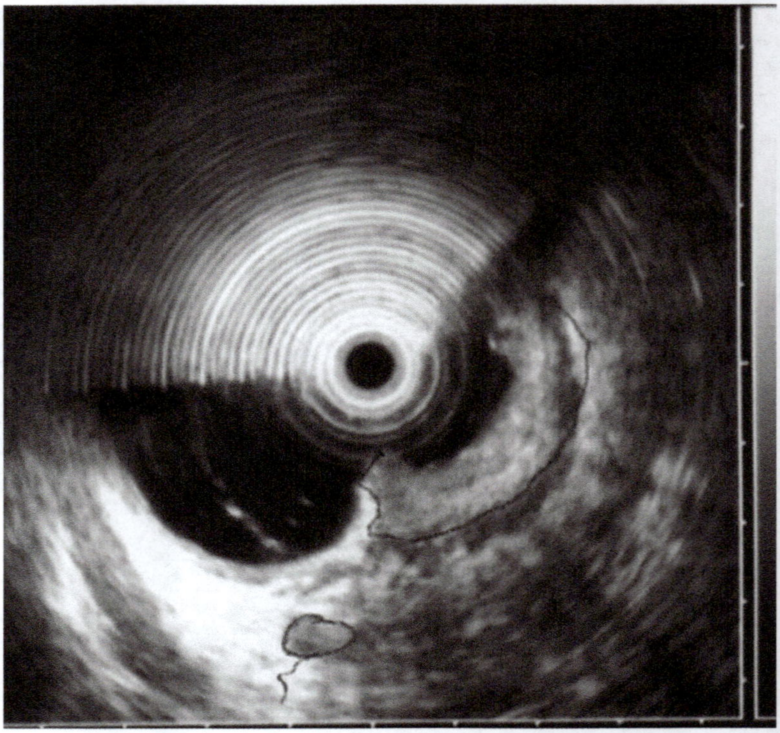

Fig. 8.9 The cancer is now stage T3N1. The tumor penetrates through the muscularis propria (uT3N1)

8.2.2 T3N1 Rectal Carcinoma: Response to Treatment

This is a 45-year-old woman with a large, 80 % circumferential rectal tumor associated with lymphadenopathy. She underwent preoperative radiation and chemotherapy, which resulted in the resolution of the previously noted lymphadenopathy and complete disappearance of viable-appearing tumor in the rectum on surface endoscopy. Instead of a tumor a large confluent ulcer is present. Repeat EUS shows a reduction in the size of the hypoechoic mass. It is impossible to tell whether this represents residual tumor, scarring, inflammation, or all three.

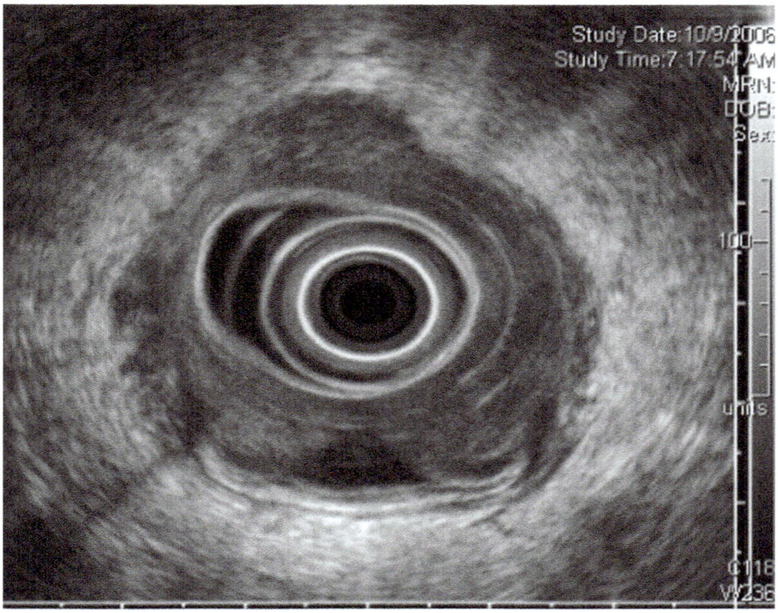

Fig. 8.10 Bulky T3 rectal cancer

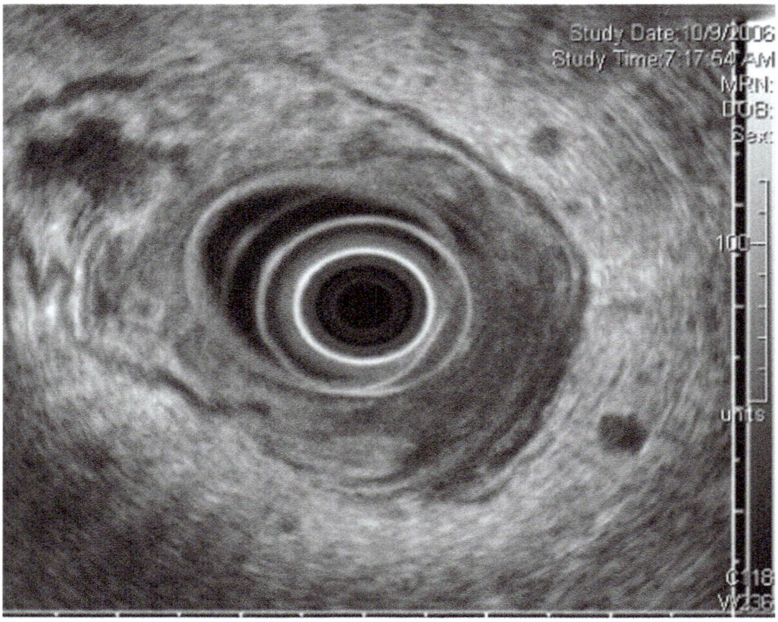

Fig. 8.11 Two small, malignant-appearing lymph nodes adjacent to a rectal cancer

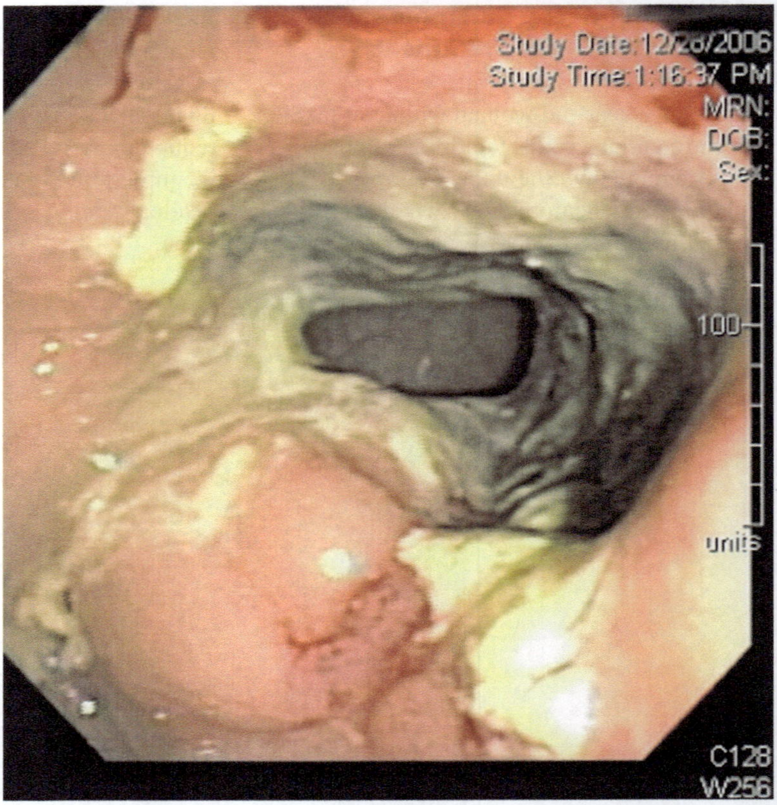

Fig. 8.12 Surface endoscopy view of rectal cancer after chemotherapy; ulceration after treatment is seen

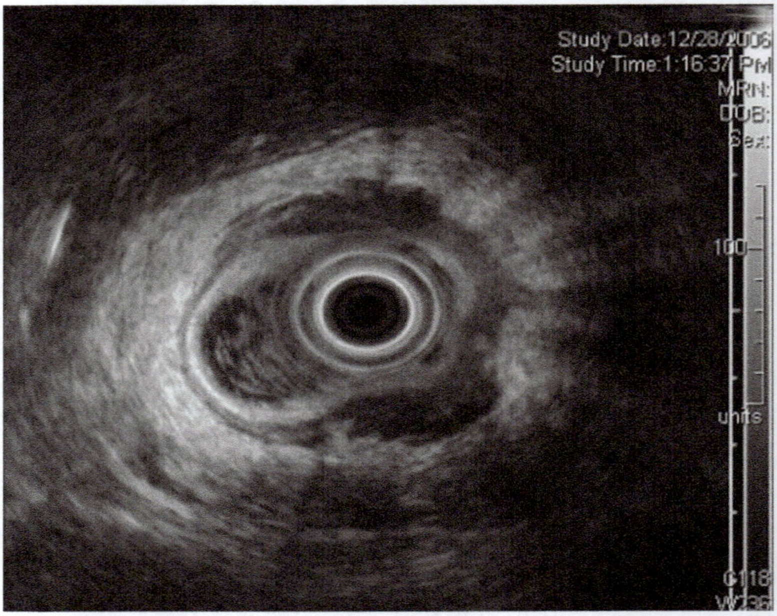

Fig. 8.13 Rectal ultrasound after neoadjuvant chemotherapy and radiation

8.2.2.1 EUS for the Evaluation of Rectal Cancer

Appropriate staging of rectal cancer is necessary to plan the best therapeutic approach, for example, the type of surgery, candidacy for anal preserving surgery, and neoadjuvant chemotherapy and radiation to prevent local recurrence. The risk of local recurrence after surgery without neoadjuvant therapy is approximately 25 %, mostly during the first 2 years [18]. A relative risk reduction of approximately 50 % of local recurrence has been associated with neoadjuvant chemoradiation in selected patients with stage II and III tumors [19]; EUS is one of the most accurate modalities in the assessment of the extent of local tumors [20]. Evaluation of sphincter involvement is also provided by EUS and is important in patients with distal tumors. Other imaging modalities such as computed tomography (CT) and magnetic resonance imaging (MRI) have been used for this purpose. CT provides information regarding distant metastasis but has limited capacity to distinguish mural layers and local depth of invasion. MRI with dedicated coils has an accuracy similar to that of EUS, and it may have an advantage for more advanced lesions [21].

Features that may cause artifacts, including poor preparation, presence of air within tumor ulcerations, previous biopsy or electrocautery defects, previous surgery or radiation, and tangential imaging, should be considered.

EUS can be helpful to evaluate for signs of deep wall invasion, which will determine potential minimally invasive resectability [10], in cases with suspected but unconfirmed malignancy.

Hildebrandt et al. proposed a modification of the TNM system based on EUS findings, adding the prefix *u*, indicating the use of ultrasonographic criteria, as opposed to the prefix *p*, which is used for pathologic postoperative stage. Of course, distant metastases cannot be evaluated by EUS, and therefore only T and M are included in staging [22].

Early stage rectal tumors (uT1: confined to submucosa) without evidence of regional metastasis to lymph nodes are ideal candidates for local excision, transanal surgical resection, or transanal endoscopic microsurgery [23] and are associated with less morbidity than radical surgery [24]. Local recurrence for T1 adenocarcinomas is relatively low: 9.8 % at 5 years.

uT1 and uT2 lesions are usually appropriate for surgery without neoadjuvant chemoradiation. uT3 tumors extend to the serosa or perirectal fat, and uT4 lesions invade adjacent organs including the prostate, seminal vesicles, vagina, uterus, or bladder. T3 and T4 lesions are considered locally advanced and are usually treated with neoadjuvant chemoradiation, which can reduce the risk of local recurrence and provide better patient tolerance [25].

Deep invasion of the wall beyond muscularis propria or evidence of regional lymph node metastasis is associated with a higher local recurrence (up to 40 %) [26]. Preoperative chemoradiation for T3 or N1 tumors has been shown to decrease the relative risk of postoperative local recurrence to approximately 50 % compared with those that did not receive neoadjuvant therapy [19].

Early extension through the muscularis propria (T3) may be difficult to differentiate from adjacent inflammatory or desmoplastic reactions (histologically T2) using ultrasound because these pseudotumorous changes are also hypoechoic and indistinguishable from true neoplasm. This problem can lead to overstaging in up to 18 % [15, 27] and understaging in up to 13 % of tumors [15].

Whether T staging is more difficult after polypectomy because of inflammatory changes is debatable; changes after polypectomy are not expected to cause sonographic changes beyond the rectal wall, and demonstration of disease at this level is considered accurate in diagnosing tumor extension [28]. Overall accuracy of T staging by EUS has been reported between 72 and 92 % [29].

The risk of lymph node metastasis correlates with the depth of invasion; it has been reported in 6–11 % of T1, 10–35 % of T2, and 25–65 % of T3 and T4 tumors [30, 31]. Sonographic criteria for nodal staging of rectal cancer are limited. The typical criteria for suspicion of metastatic lymph nodes developed in the staging of esophageal cancer by EUS include size greater than 1 cm, round shape, and hypoechoic sonographic pattern without hyperechoic core. Unfortunately, these criteria have limited sensitivity and specificity in rectal cancer. The accuracy of diagnosis by ultrasound without FNA has been reported between 64 and 85 % [15, 16, 29], leading to overstaging in up to 25 % and understaging in 11 %. Normal perirectal lymph nodes are usually less than 3 mm in diameter and not visible by EUS; however, up to 78 % of lymph nodes ≤ 5 mm in diameter identified by EUS have been found to have metastatic invasion [32]. Enlargement of lymph nodes > 5 mm is not sufficient to diagnose malignant invasion; metastatic lymph nodes overlap in size with peritumoral inflammatory nodes.

Staging can be improved by performing FNA to confirm nodal or distant metastases [33]. FNA of nonjuxtatumoral lymph nodes has been shown to change therapy in 19 % of patients, particularly in those with early T stage disease. Accuracy of EUS with FNA for nodal staging was 92 % in a study by Shami et al. [29].

One study found that EUS-guided FNA of solid lesions of the lower gastrointestinal tract, including lymph nodes, had a low risk of infections and complications [34]; these authors did not consider EUS-guided FNA a standard indication for antibiotic prophylaxis.

MRI with endorectal coils visualizes the rectal wall very well; however, this technique may be challenging because of difficulty inserting the coil in patients with a stenosing tumor, poor visualization of lesions high in the rectum, and poor resolution of structures surrounding the rectum. MRI with pelvic phased-array coil is noninvasive and allows the entire pelvis to be visualized but has lower resolution of the rectal wall. Some authors have found that MRI is more accurate in the staging of locally advanced tumors [21, 35], whereas EUS can quite accurately stage T1 and T2 tumors. Accuracy of nodal staging by MRI has been reported between 59 and 95 %, similar to that of EUS without FNA. Therefore, MRI and endorectal ultrasound are considered complementary methods in the preoperative staging of rectal cancer [35], and EUS offers the possibility of FNA/histologic diagnosis in patients with suspected imaging.

EUS can also detect recurrent cancer at or near the anastomosis line, which is frequently not detectable by colonoscopy, carcinoembryonic antigen level, digital exam, or other imaging techniques [36]. Many of these lesions arise extraluminally and are not detectable with standard videoendoscopy until they are at an advanced stage. Prospective studies have shown that EUS is superior to CT for detection of recurrent rectal cancer [37, 38]; CT images are frequently distorted by surgical changes, metal clips, or radiation. Lesions smaller than 2 cm diameter may not be accurately detected by CT [2]. Recurrent cancer has been described on EUS as a hypoechoic mass involving a portion of the rectal wall, typically at or just above the site of resection anastomosis [25]. EUS-guided biopsy may be necessary to establish the final diagnosis because similar findings may be due to surgical scarring or radiation. EUS in combination with FNA of suspicious lesions has been shown to have an accuracy of at least 92 % in the detection of early recurrence, leading to curative resection [38, 39]. Surveillance with EUS every 6 months for 2 years after low anterior resection or transanal excision has been recommended by some experts [40]. This aggressive approach is more likely to benefit those with a high risk of recurrence, such as patients with more advanced tumors at diagnosis or those undergoing local excision [2].

8.2.3 Colon Cancer Metastatic to Mediastinal Lymph Nodes

The liver, lungs, bones, peritoneum, and lymph nodes are metastatic sites of colon cancer. Mediastinal lymph nodes are rarely affected. This is a 69-year-old patent who had a transverse colectomy for colon cancer 18 months earlier, the final pathologic stage of which was T3N2. Recent follow-up positron emission tomography showed activity in the right hilar and subcarinal lymph nodes. EUS could not demonstrate the right hilar mass. However, the relatively small subcarinal lymph nodes were aspirated under EUS guidance and found to be positive for metastatic adenocarcinoma, most consistent with a colonic primary tumor.

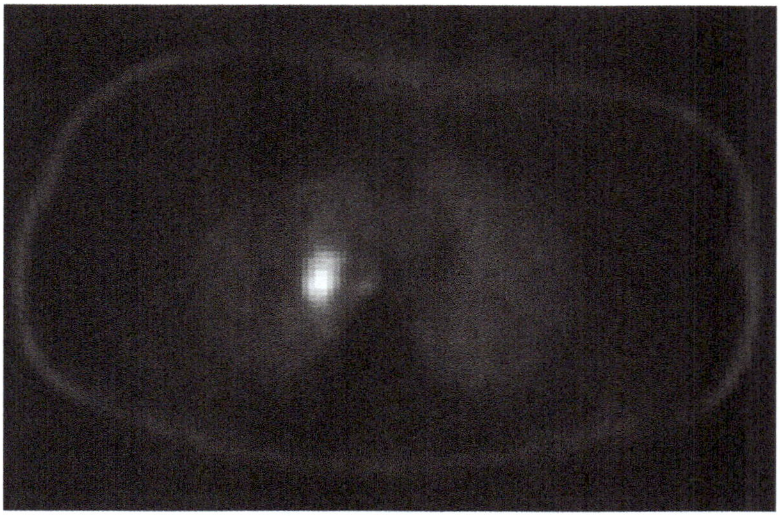

Fig. 8.14 This positron emission tomography scan shows activity in the right hilar area

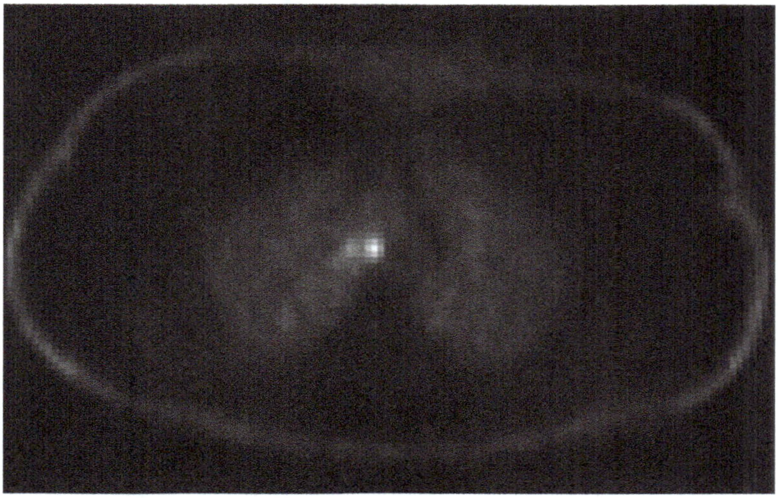

Fig. 8.15 This positron emission tomography scan shows additional smaller and less intense hot spots in a subcarinal location

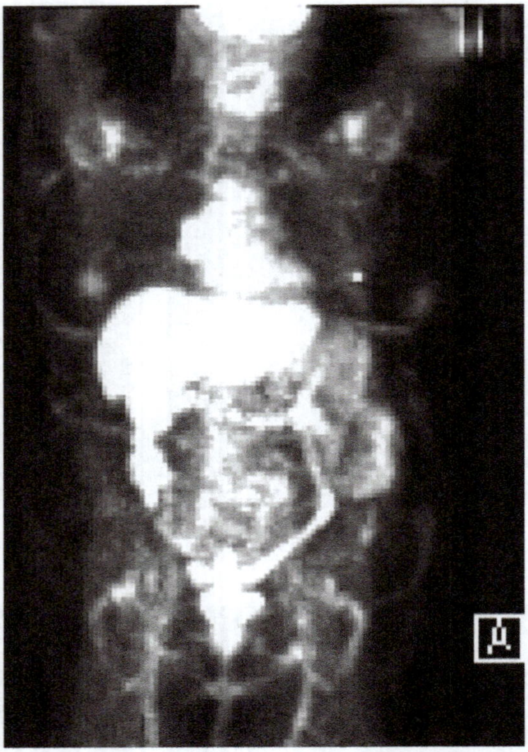

Fig. 8.16 This positron emission tomography scan shows diffuse nonspecific activity throughout the colon. A right hilar hot spot can also be appreciated

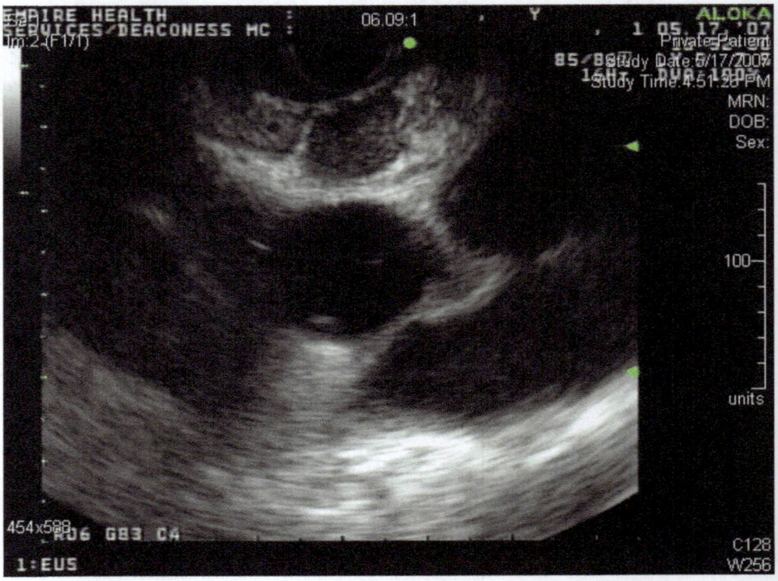

Fig. 8.17 Endoscopic ultrasound appearance of the mildly enlarged subcarinal lymph nodes before fine-needle aspiration biopsy

8.2.4 Large Colon Polyp

This is an 83-year-old patient with rectal bleeding. Colonoscopy showed a 4-cm-diameter mobile polypoid mass located at the rectosigmoid junction. Biopsies revealed high-grade dysplasia, probably reflecting sampling error. An endorectal ultrasound was performed, revealing a large polypoid tumor with a short stalk and no evidence of invasion that was suspicious foci or lymphadenopathy. Given the patient's age, we recommended a snare polypectomy as a reasonable choice and that further management would depend on the extent of stalk invasion (if any).

A significant proportion of large villous adenomas may contain invasive carcinoma; induration and ulceration raise the endoscopic suspicion, but up to 10 % of villous adenomas without these signs and even with negative biopsies can still harbor invasive carcinoma [42]. It is important to determine the likelihood of invasive carcinoma to avoid incomplete endoscopic excision and evaluate the appropriateness of surgical local excision techniques. EUS can demonstrate the presence of invasion into the submucosa [43] or muscularis propria and regional lymph nodes when assisted by FNA. EUS diagnosis of T1 adenocarcinoma versus high-grade dysplasia/in situ carcinoma can be challenging; some experts have reported that hyperechoic foci within homogeneously hyperechoic adenomatous lesions are concerning for focal carcinoma [44–46]. A meta-analysis revealed that 81 % of rectal villous adenomas with focal invasive carcinoma missed by biopsy were accurately diagnosed as malignant by endorectal ultrasound [47]. The authors of that study calculated that performing EUS can reduce the rate of false-negative misdiagnosis in rectal adenomas from 24 to 5 %.

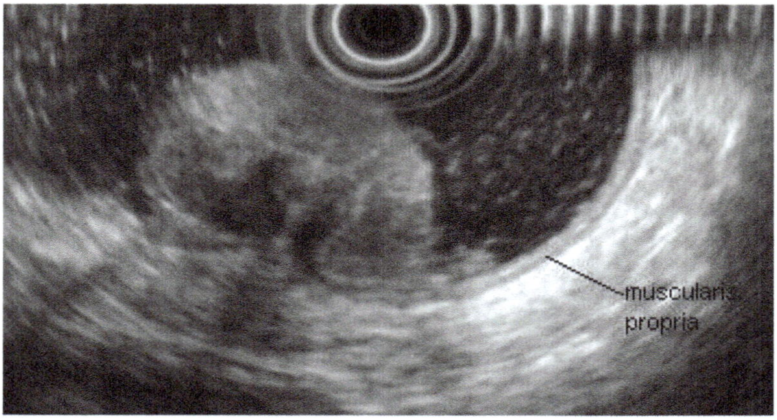

Fig. 8.18 This radial endoscopic ultrasound image shows a 4-cm-diameter polyp at the rectosigmoid junction

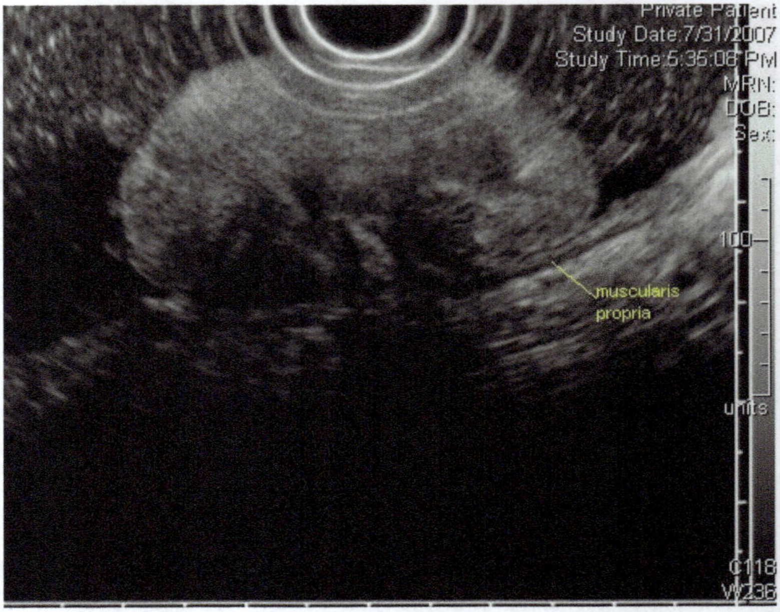

Fig. 8.19 A higher frequency exam of the same polyp also shows an intact muscularis propria

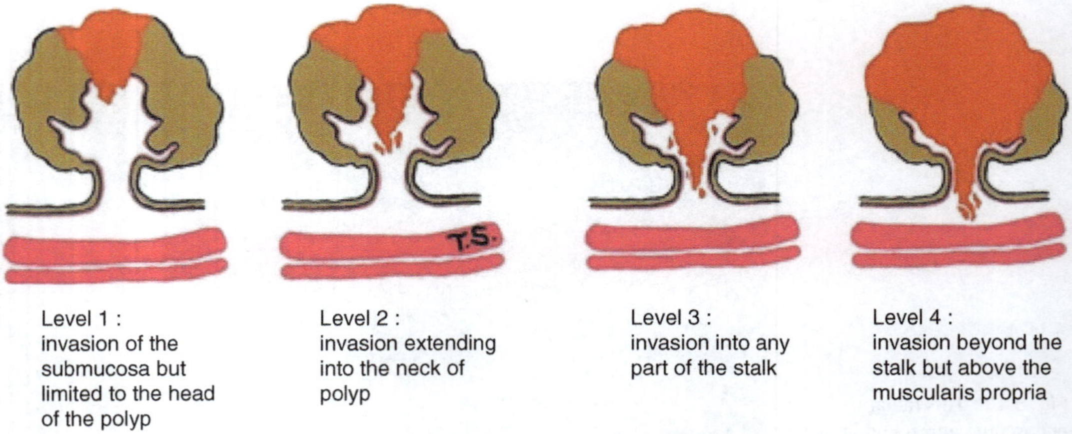

Fig. 8.20 Haggitt levels of invasion in polypoid carcinomas. Haggitt level 4 (in resected polyps) correlates with lymph node metastases and residual disease (From Quirke et al. [41])

8.2.5 Large Villous Adenoma with High-Grade Dysplasia

This is a 66-year-old patient with morbid obesity, sleep apnea, and pulmonary hypertension. He presented with rectal bleeding and was found to have a 50 % circumferential villous-appearing lesion in the rectum. Forceps biopsies confirmed villous adenoma. EUS showed no evidence of invasion into the muscularis. Also note that the mucosa is isoechoic compared with the surrounding areas (except for the muscularis propria, which is the dark layer). Given the features described, the signed EUS report cautioned that a transrectal excision would be difficult or impossible. However, in view of the multiple comorbidities, excision was attempted. The resection was, not surprisingly, incomplete. High-grade dysplasia was found in the resected tumor and the patient subsequently had radiation and chemotherapy before a possible attempt at complete surgical resection.

Adenomatous polyps appear sonographically as lesions arising from the first two layers (interface and mucosa). Larger polyps can have heterogeneous echogenicity, and this feature does not correlate with the presence of carcinoma. Invasive features including involvement of the muscularis propria or transmural involvement preclude endoscopic resection and raise concern about lymphatic metastases. The presence of lymph nodes larger than 1 cm has a high correlation with malignant invasion [48].

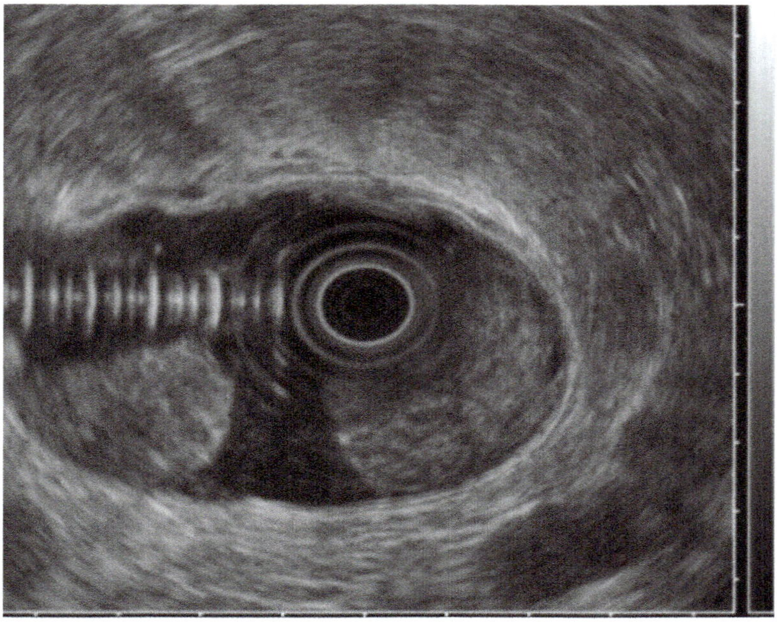

Fig. 8.21 Partial view of a large villous adenoma in the rectum

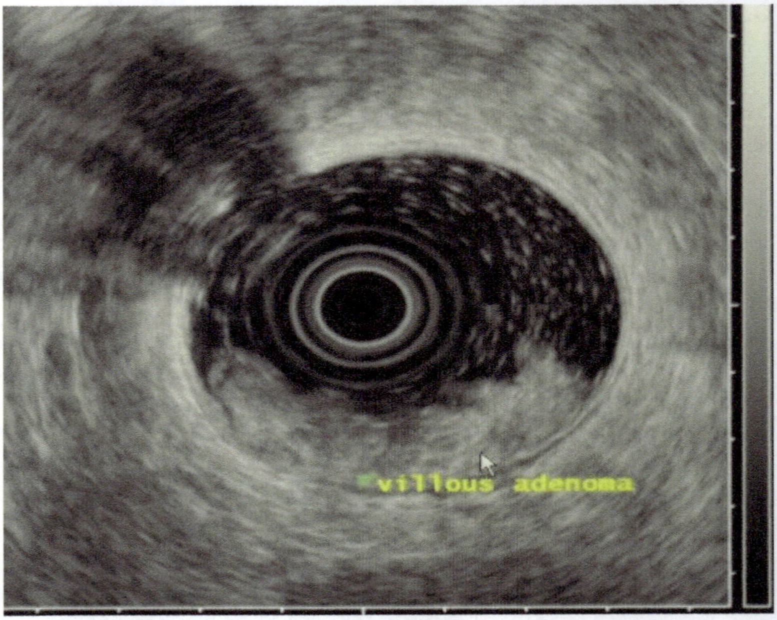

Fig. 8.22 Different aspect of the same villous adenoma shown in Fig. 8.21

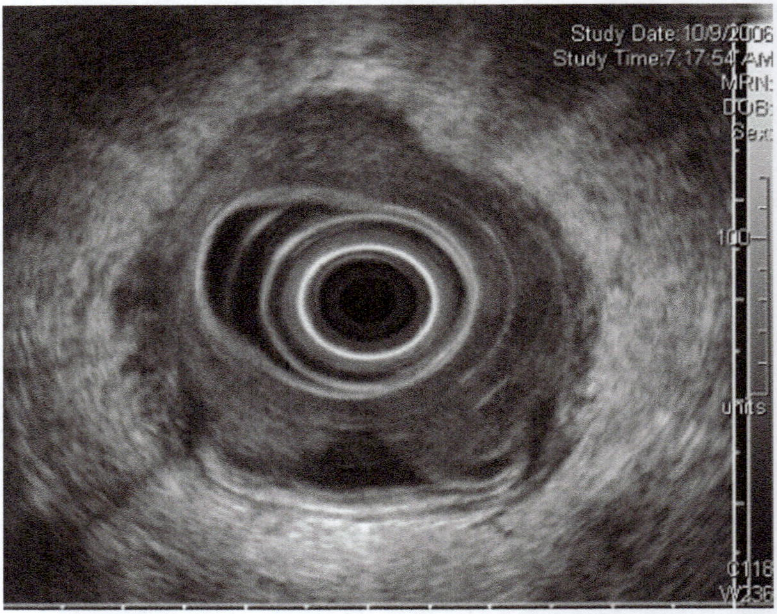

Fig. 8.23 Rectal cancer in a different patient in comparison to (hypoechoic) T3 rectal cancer

8.2.6 Anal Cancer with Extensive Intramural Spread into the Rectum

Anal cancer is a disease that is in part related to infection by the human papillomavirus (HPV). Treatment was revolutionized in the 1970s when chemoradiation was found to cure patients with anal cancer without requiring an abdominoperineal resection (Nigro protocol; for resources see Box 8.1). The staging of anal cancer is heavily influenced by the size of the tumor, and accurate measurements are best obtained with EUS.

This is a 58-year-old woman who noticed a mass in her rectum when she introduced the tip of a hemorrhoid cream applicator. Colonoscopy showed a large submucosal mass in the posterior wall of the lower rectum, which appeared to be partially infiltrating upward through the otherwise largely intact rectal mucosa. Biopsies were diagnostic of squamous cell carcinoma. A 4.7 × 3.6 cm submucosal mass was seen on rectal ultrasound and was connected to the muscularis propria with one small adjacent lymph node. This was identified as intramural spread from a much smaller superficial lesion in the anal canal; during digital rectal examination this was correlated with an indurated cleft-like abnormality in the sphincter. This type of intramural growth pattern is rare.

The differential diagnosis of masses in the rectum and anal canal involves benign and malignant conditions. Malignancies include adenocarcinoma, epidermoid carcinoma, basal cell carcinoma, and other more unusual tumors such as anaplastic sarcoma, lymphoma, undifferentiated cylindrical cellular carcinoma, and metastatic cancer (e.g., breast) [49]. Nonmalignant masses to be considered in the differential diagnosis include Crohn's proctocolitis, rectal prolapse, rectal endometriosis, and colitis cystica profunda.

Colitis cystica profunda typically presents as single or multiple polypoid masses with an irregular surface; these cause thickening of the colonic or rectal wall and histologically consist of mucus-filled cysts. On EUS these cysts vary in size and are found at the level of the mucosa and submucosal layers but do not involve the muscularis propria [50].

The rectosigmoid is the most common site of extrapelvic endometriosis, which appears as subepithelial masses. These lesions appear hypoechoic or heterogeneous because of the presence of cystic areas and have a crescent shape; they involve the muscularis propria, serosa, and occasionally the submucosa or adjacent structures including the rectovaginal septum or uterine wall [51]. EUS is highly accurate in establishing this diagnosis in patients with known pelvic endometriosis. Since the lesions extend beyond the rectal wall, a malignancy cannot be excluded and surgical exploration is generally recommended. A solitary rectal ulcer, ulcerative colitis, and cytomegalovirus colitis can cause severe ulcerations, sometimes with an irregular border that may have a malignant endoscopic appearance.

In patients with inconclusive endoscopic and histopathologic evaluations, EUS may play a diagnostic role, as demonstrated in the case above, that is absolutely necessary to define an appropriate therapeutic plan.

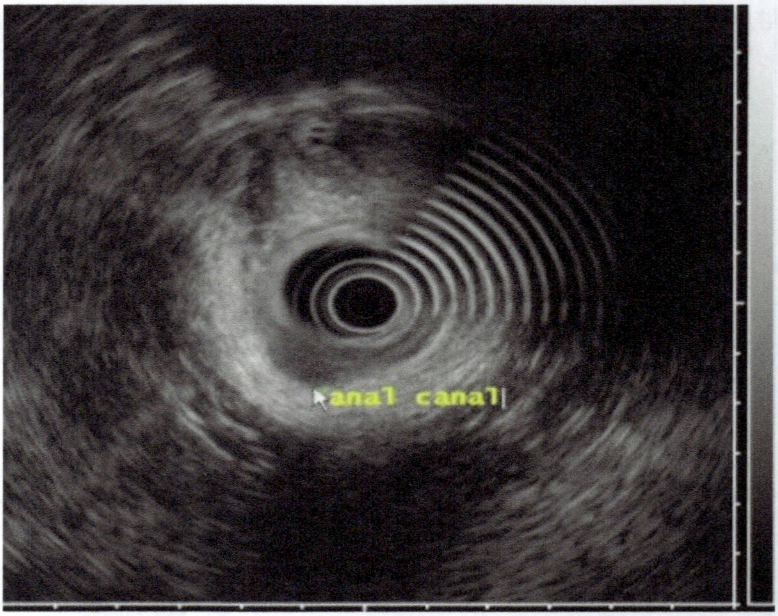

Fig. 8.24 The point of origin of the anal cancer (*arrow*)

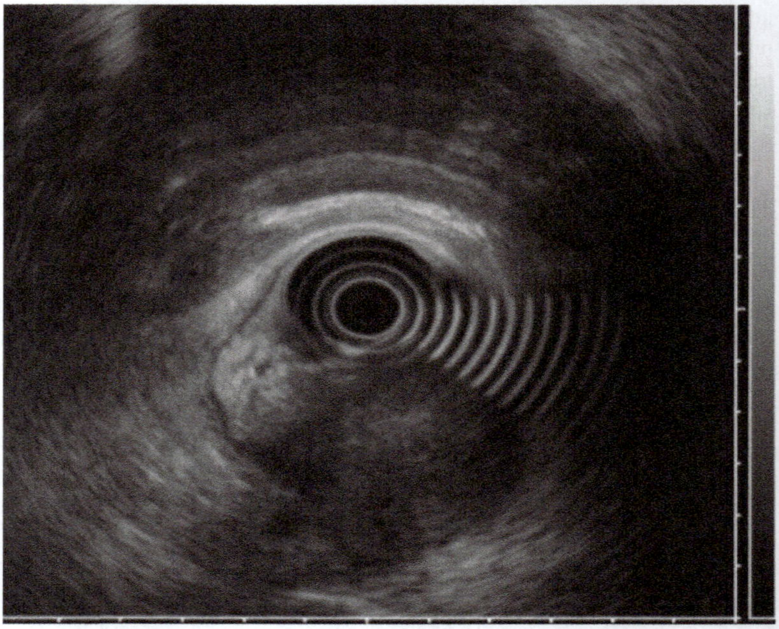

Fig. 8.25 This radial endoscopic ultrasound image shows a large submucosal mass in the lower rectum, connecting to the muscularis propria. Biopsy proved this was a squamous cell carcinoma

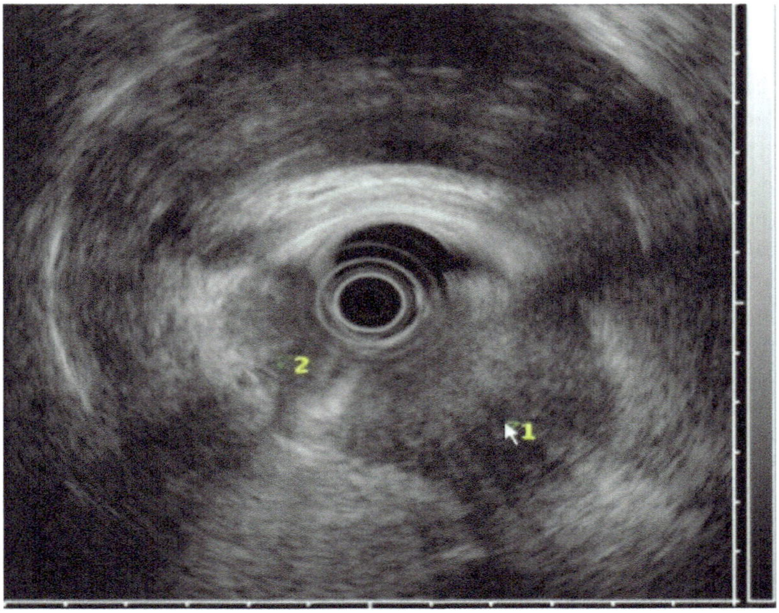

Fig. 8.26 A second smaller lesion (*2*) is seen next to the bulky primary deposit (*1*)

The incidence of anal canal carcinoma has increased, particularly in the younger male population. A tenfold increase in 20- to 49-year-old men was reported in New York between 1979 and 1985 [52]. HPV has been found in 88 % of patients with anal cancer [53]; HPV type 16 is more common in patients with high-grade anal intraepithelial neoplasia, whereas other types of HPV are more often found in patients with low-grade intraepithelial neoplasia [54]. It seems clear that immunosuppression from HIV infection increases the likelihood of HPV infection and subsequent anal intraepithelial neoplasia [54]. Initial symptoms, including bleeding and pain, are frequently attributed inappropriately to other disorders such as hemorrhoids, delaying evaluation.

Simultaneous treatment with external beam radiation and chemotherapy with 5-fluorouracil and mitomycin has been the standard approach for most patients since the development of the Nigro protocol in 1974 [55]. The prognosis of anal cancer correlates well with the size of the tumor and lymph node involvement [54]. Therefore, current anal cancer tumor staging by the American Joint Committee on Cancer is based on tumor size and not depth or layer of penetration. The TNM staging system is available online at http://goo.gl/Qahiu. Staging recommended by the National Comprehensive Cancer Network includes digital examination, inguinal lymph node evaluation, chest imaging, anoscopy, and abdominal/pelvic CT or MRI but not EUS [56].

Early T1N0 (<2 cm) lesions without sphincter involvement (limited to submucosal involvement) are amenable to local surgical excision. EUS may play a significant role in these cases and has been shown to provide accurate information about size, depth of invasion, and assessment of sphincter invasion. A study comparing transanal EUS and MRI in the staging of anal cancer demonstrated a high level of concordance between these studies and suggested that EUS may be better for the evaluation of smaller tumors [57].

EUS should also be considered as a staging technique in patients with contraindications to MRI such as metal implants or claustrophobia [58]. EUS also allows FNA to be performed for the evaluation of possible deep or lymph node recurrence.

8.2.7 Anorectal Melanoma

This is a 60-year-old patient who presented with a "hemorrhoid problem." Several adenomatous-appearing polyps were removed during colonoscopy. A peculiar-appearing deeply ulcerated lesion in the lowermost portion of the rectum extending into the anal canal was seen as well. Histology showed malignant melanoma. Primary anorectal melanoma (ARM) is a rare disorder and the optimal treatment is controversial. In this patient no lymphadenopathy was seen immediately adjacent to the tumor.

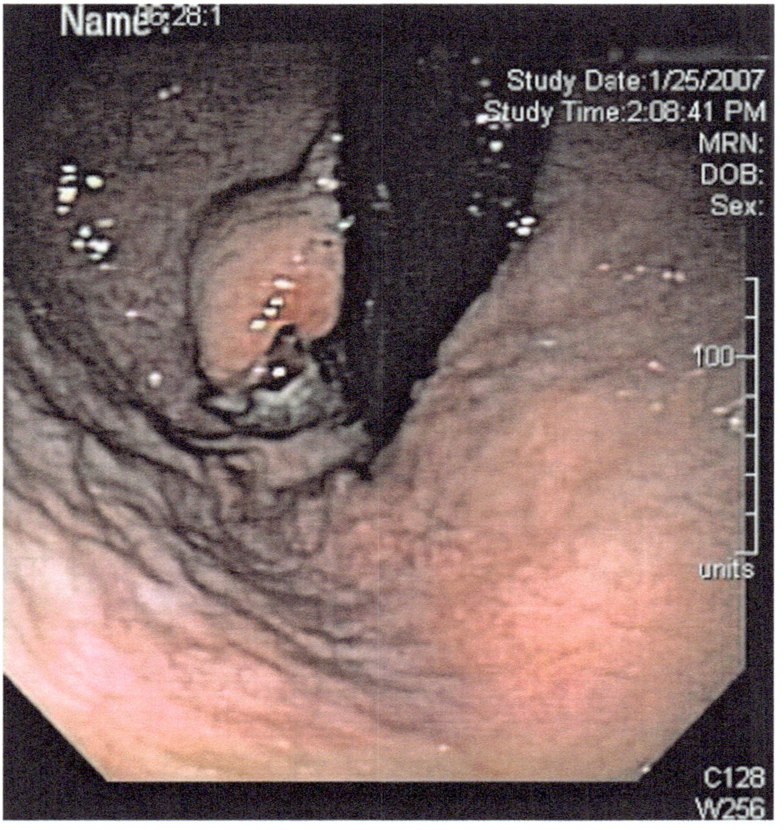

Fig. 8.27 Anorectal melanoma during retroflexion

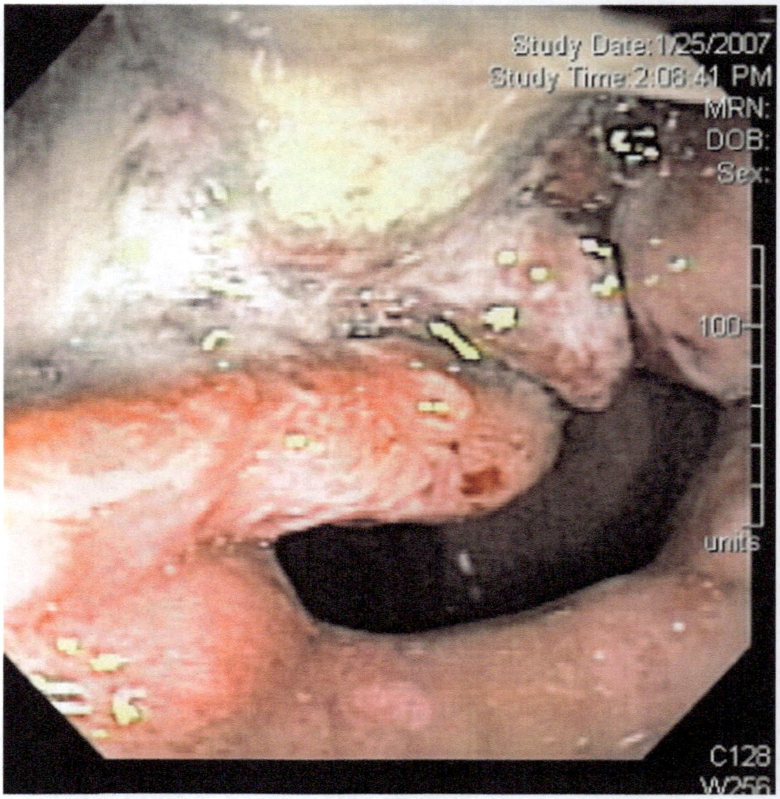

Fig. 8.28 Ulcerated melanoma as seen upon withdrawal from the anal canal

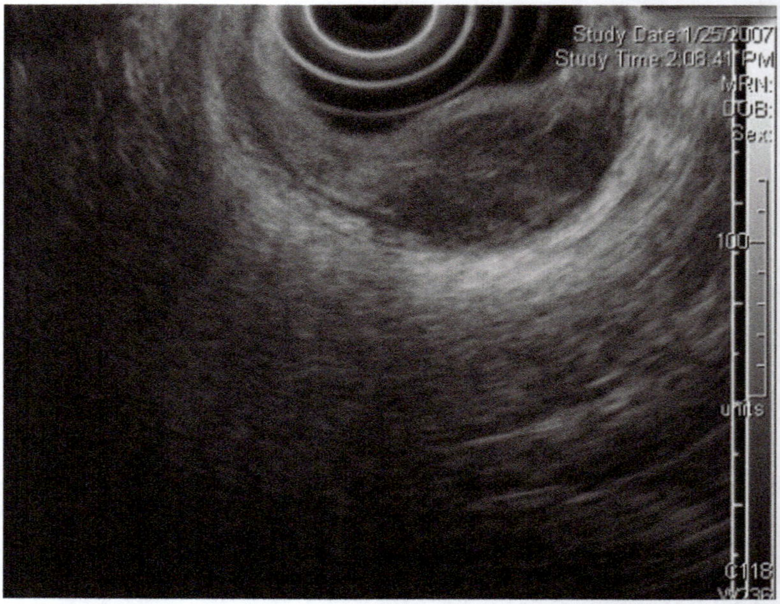

Fig. 8.29 Endoscopic ultrasound image of the anorectal melanoma

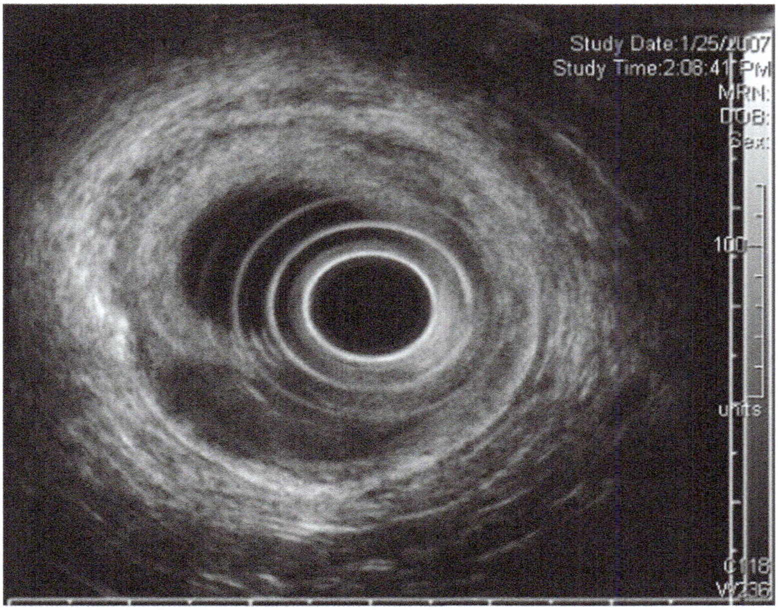

Fig. 8.30 Another endoscopic ultrasound view of the same anorectal melanoma demonstrates invasion through the muscularis propria

ARM is an aggressive condition, usually asymptomatic in its early stages, and associated with nonspecific symptoms as it grows. These symptoms include tenesmus, pruritus, hematochezia, pain, and change in bowel habit. Symptoms typically persist 4–6 months before diagnosis [59], and approximately half of cases are initially misdiagnosed [60]. ARM represents between 1 and 2 % of malignancies of the lower gastrointestinal tract [61]. The ideal management of this disease is not well known because of its uncommon nature and lack of high-quality clinical trials. Perhaps the availability of diagnostic studies such as positron emission tomography–CT, MRI, or EUS with FNA may offer information to better stratify and treat this condition. An average thickness of 7 mm has been reported for ARM [49]. As a reference, a tumor thickness of 4 mm or greater is associated with more aggressive disease in cutaneous melanoma; however, reporting of this value for ARM has not been consistent, and additional studies are required to assess its prognostic value. It is most commonly located at the anal canal or at the dentate line, with less than 10 % of cases have a purely rectal location [49]. Given its tendency to metastasize to bone, chest, liver, and brain, it is recommended that CT of the head, chest, abdomen, and pelvis be obtained as an initial approach to evaluate for distant metastases. Unfortunately, most patients present with metastatic disease, and the 5-year survival has been less than 18 % in most series [62]. It is hoped that the recent introduction of ipilimumab will improve this statistic for patients who are positive for HLA-A*020 [63].

EUS and MRI are capable of providing local tumor staging information for ARM, as for other rectal tumors [64]; however, their application and influence in decision making for this indication has not been well defined. Nodal involvement correlates with outcome; however, groin dissection to evaluate for metastatic lymphadenopathy is a morbid operation and should not be used indiscriminately. The effect of diagnostic techniques including sentinel node biopsy or EUS-guided FNA is not known. Despite all this, it seems clear that EUS is capable of providing evaluation of sphincter involvement, which can change the surgical decision between wide local excision and abdominoperineal resection.

8.2.8 Diffuse Cavernous Rectal Hemangioma

A 29-year-old woman presented with recurring hematochezia and required transfusions during her second and third trimesters of pregnancy. Previous examinations by other endoscopists had shown oozing varicosities in the distal rectum. CT of the abdomen and pelvis revealed diffuse thickening of the rectum and distal sigmoid and multiple wall calcifications at that level. Her rectal bleeding worsened, requiring 1–2 units of red blood cells a day by the 35th week of gestation. Early cesarean delivery was performed, immediately after which bleeding improved significantly.

Anorectal EUS with Doppler revealed pulsatile arterial flow and a sponge-like mass with vascular channels surrounding the rectum, consistent with the diagnosis of diffuse cavernous rectal hemangioma. An MRI demonstrated the classic findings of this entity, including bright signal intensity on T2-weighted images and intermediate signal intensity on T1-weighted images. Blood vessels are signal voided on T1- and T2-weighted images but thrombosed vessels have an intense signal.

Cavernous hemangiomas of the sigmoid colon and rectum are uncommon vascular malformations usually found in young adults with a long history of episodic and painless rectal bleeding. Alternatively, they may present with massive life-threatening hemorrhage [65]. They are usually considered benign hamartomas arising from the submucosal vascular plexus and are clearly differentiated from telangiectasias and angiodysplasias. Large rectal cavernous hemangiomas can infiltrate the entire pelvis and behave aggressively. Colonic hemangiomas are divided into capillary and cavernous types: the former tend to be small and asymptomatic, whereas the latter, which are more frequently encountered, is either discrete and circumscribed or diffuse and expansive (Gentry classification) [66]. Large, tortuous vascular channels with turbulent, sluggish blood flow predispose to the formation of phleboliths. In fact, the clustering of such phleboliths in an unusual location in a young individual with rectal bleeding is suggestive of a cavernous hemangioma of the colon or rectum, although phleboliths are absent or difficult to see in half of cases. Interestingly, our patient had CT for other reasons 2 years before the current presentation and no calcifications were seen. One could speculate that the repeated stop-and-go bleeding during pregnancy together with the repeated activation of local hemostatic mechanisms led to the rapid formation of these calcifications. This diagnosis is often missed, even with repeated colonoscopic examinations, and patients frequently are subjected to hemorrhoidectomies that are of no benefit. CT is useful for the evaluation of rectal hemangiomas [67], but if phleboliths are not present the diagnosis cannot be made with confidence or may be missed altogether. Characteristic MRI findings have been described [68] and consist of rectal wall thickening with high signal intensity on T2-weighted images and abnormal perirectal fat with serpiginous structures. Phleboliths are difficult to see on MRI. Most patients with recurrent rectal bleeding from cavernous rectal hemangiomas are young and otherwise healthy, and few physicians proceed rapidly to pelvic CT or MRI, particularly not during pregnancy. In nonpregnant patients with severe, recurrent bleeding, contrast CT of the abdomen and pelvis is obtained as a next step after a nondiagnostic colonoscopy. Even if the cause is not immediately clear, CT findings may still narrow the selection of further imaging studies, such as angiography (if a vascular fistula is suspected) or MRI (if a space-occupying lesion is found). If locally available, rectal EUS performed with a flexible Doppler-capable instrument may be the diagnostic test of choice because it avoids exposure to radiation or a magnetic field and cost run-ups for lesions that appear inflammatory or neoplastic [69]. No sedation is required, and a high-resolution Doppler evaluation of flow is possible. In addition, biopsies can be obtained with transrectal ultrasound–guided FNA if needed. In patients with diffuse cavernous rectal hemangioma who consider or elect surgery, MRI may give the most information for surgical planning, allowing an individualized surgical approach with the goal of anal sphincter preservation.

Many primary care physicians are not familiar with this rare entity, and it is worth pointing out that not all bright-red blood per rectum is related to benign hemorrhoids. In pregnancy, endorectal ultrasonography may be the imaging modality of choice in perplexing cases.

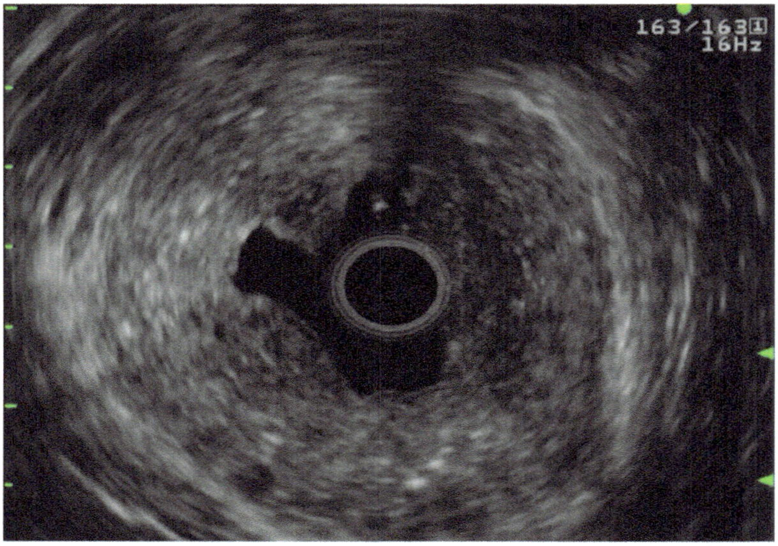

Fig. 8.31 This image, obtained with the GF-UE160 electronic radial echoinstrument, shows the sponge-like nature of the cavernous rectal hemangioma. The vascular channels are much more delicate than the magnetic resonance images suggest

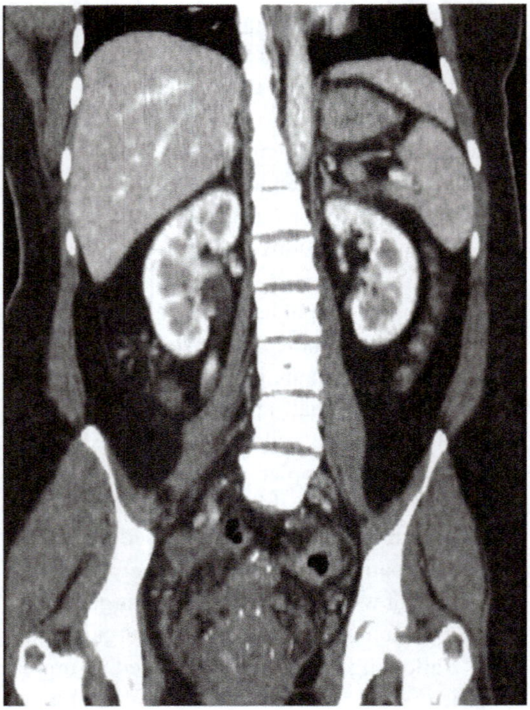

Fig. 8.32 This coronal reconstruction of an abdominopelvic computed tomography scan shows thickening of the rectal wall and scattered perirectal calcifications

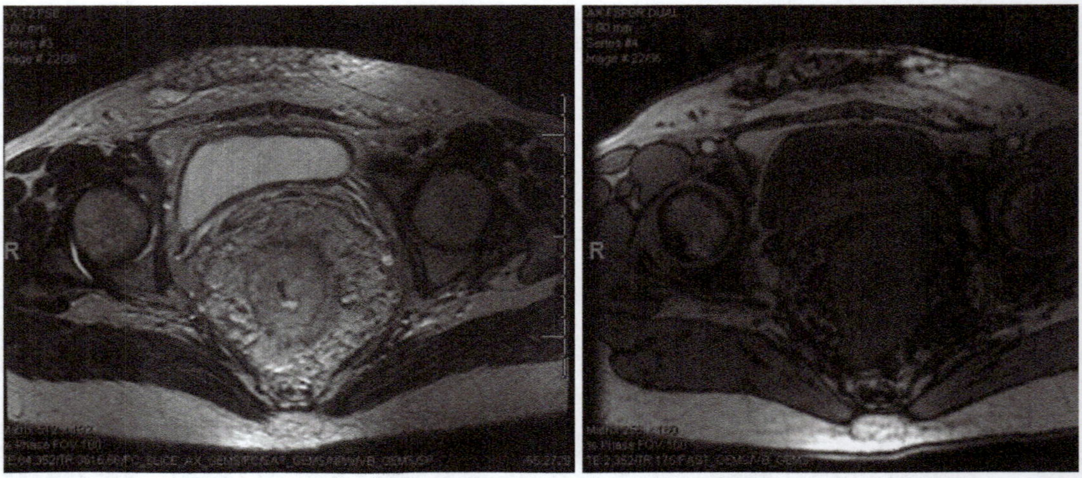

Fig. 8.33 T2-weighted (*left*) and fast spoiled gradient echo (also known as T1 contrast-enhanced fast field echo) (*right*) magnetic resonance images of the rectal cavernous hemangioma at the same level

8.2.9 Cystic Lymphangioma of the Colon

This is a 58-year-old woman from El Salvador who had been evaluated for right upper quadrant pain 5 years before this presentation. A septated liver cyst was found and drained radiologically. There were many white cells but no growth on routine and acid-fast bacilli cultures, and cytology showed no neoplastic cells. The exact nature of the cyst remained undetermined. Follow-up ultrasound, performed because she was again complaining of abdominal pain, showed that the liver cyst had not returned. A colonoscopy showed a submucosal cystic-appearing lesion in the transverse colon, which later was evaluated by EUS and showed the characteristic features of a cystic lymphangioma. The EUS images clearly show that the cyst arises from the submucosa and is surrounded by muscularis propria.

A standard radial scanning ultrasound gastroscope (GF-UM160; Olympus Optical Co, Ltd., Tokyo, Japan) was used in this case, obtaining a field of view that was sufficient to show the entire aspect of this large lesion. Advancement of this instrument through the colon is difficult but possible. Ultrasound catheter miniprobes can be advanced through the working channel of standard colonoscopies and are convenient, but they are not available to all endosonographers [70]. These miniprobes allow better resolution at the expense of penetration depth.

Lymphatic cysts (cystic lymphangiomata and lymphangiomatous, lymphangiectatic, or chylous cysts) of the abdomen are rare. They can occur in the mesentery, omentum, retroperitoneum, and, very rarely, the wall of the stomach, duodenum, or intestine.

Cystic lymphangiomas and benign multicystic peritoneal mesotheliomas have a similar if not identical appearance on imaging studies [12]. Fortunately, both are benign lesions and are differentiated based on their histological appearance. They are characterized by anechoic cysts separated by thin walls on EUS. These two lesions can be indistinguishable unless, as in this case, the layer of origin can be shown. A lesion originating from the bowel wall is, by definition, not a peritoneal lesion. This is one of a handful of cases of colonic cystic lymphangiomas that have been evaluated by EUS.

Other entities to consider in the differential diagnosis include gastrointestinal wall duplication cysts, pancreatic pseudocysts in the bowel wall, and cystic tumors that metastasize to the serosa. Pancreatic pseudocysts and metastatic tumors can be suspected based on the history and additional imaging findings. Duplication cysts commonly present on the mesenteric side of the gut, especially the ileum [12].

Colitis cystica profunda can also present with cystic subepithelial lesions that can involve submucosa and mucosa layers but usually not the muscularis propria. This entity should be considered in the differential diagnosis.

Pneumatosis cystoides coli can have a similar endoscopic appearance, with polypoid round or oval lesions covered by normal mucosa. In this entity the lesions are filled with air, which can be appreciated on CT ; EUS will not show cystic lesions but a shadow due to the presence of air in the submucosa.

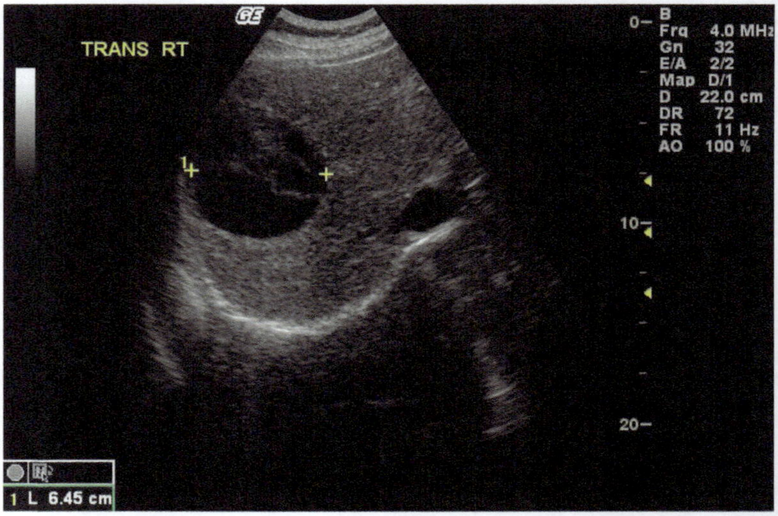

Fig. 8.34 This liver cyst of unknown etiology was aspirated 5 years earlier and did not recur

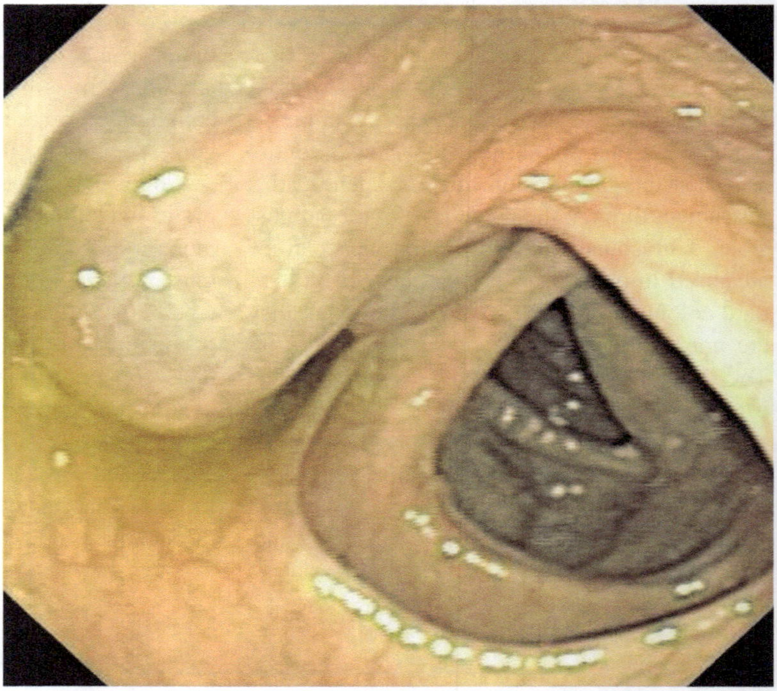

Fig. 8.35 The cystic lymphangioma as it appears during colonoscopy (transverse colon)

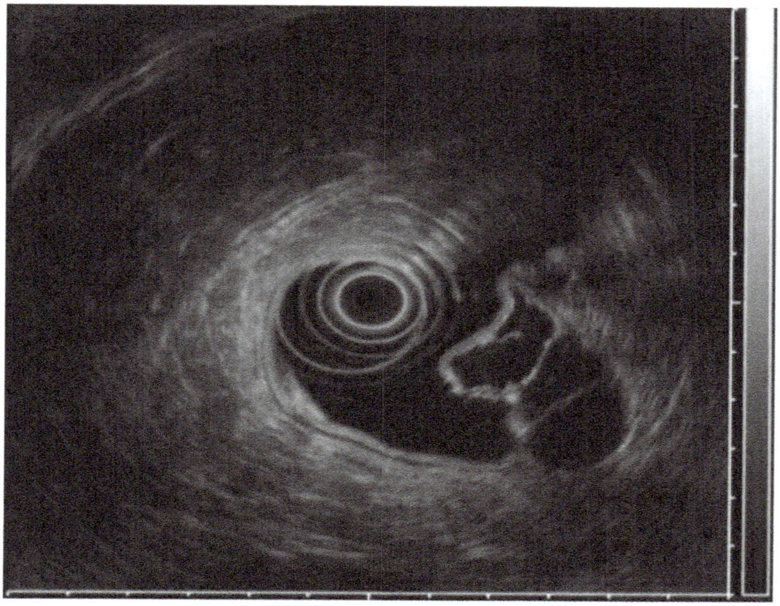

Fig. 8.36 The colonic lymphangioma scanned with the GF-UM130 gastro-videoscope, a difficult instrument to do colonoscopy with

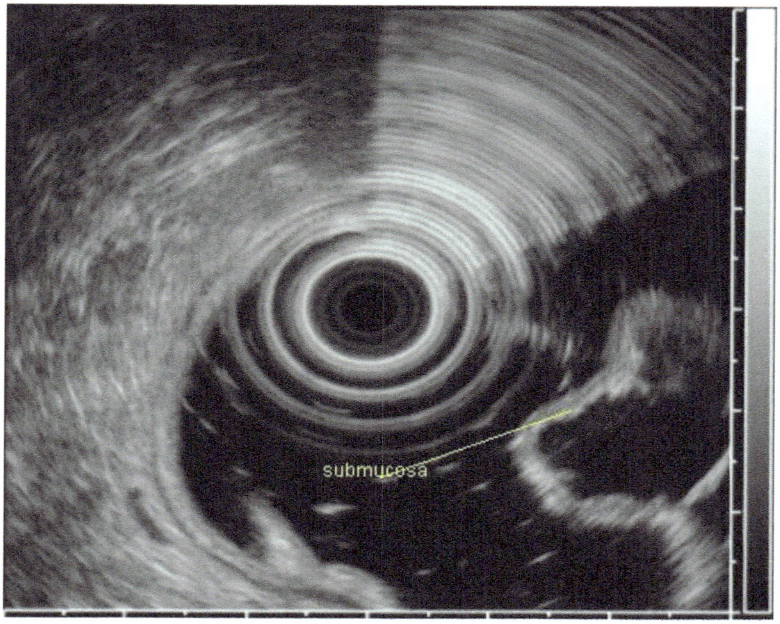

Fig. 8.37 This endoscopic ultrasound image shows a close-up of the mucosal layer (*bright to dark*) and submucosa (*bright*), demonstrating that the cyst originates from the submucosa

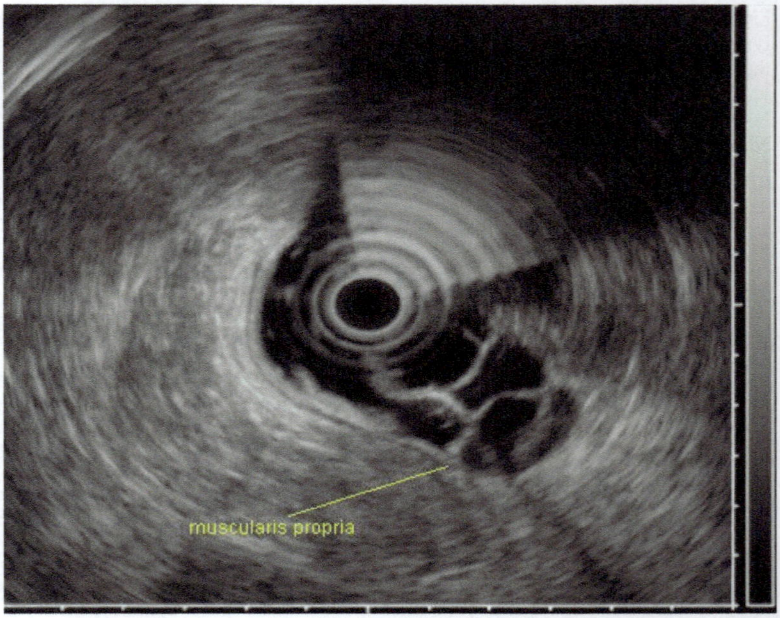

Fig. 8.38 This endoscopic ultrasound image of the cystic lymphangioma shows the course of the muscularis propria surrounding the cyst

8.2.10 Coccygeal Chordoma

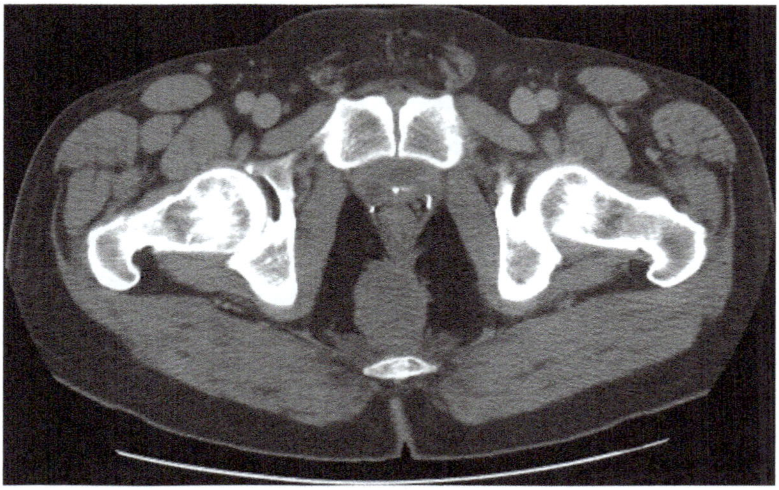

Fig. 8.39 CT reveals a retrorectal mass

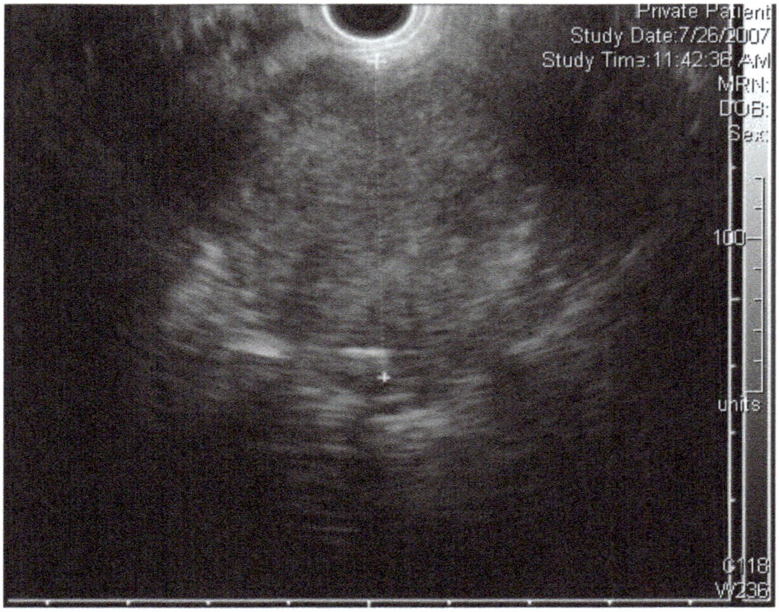

Fig. 8.40 This radial endoscopic ultrasound image shows a 5-cm-diameter mass that is fairly echogenic

This is a 55-year-old patient who developed pelvic pain. CT showed a 5-cm-diameter retrorectal mass. Six years earlier the patient had a radical prostatectomy. His prostate-specific antigen levels remained undetectable. He was referred for EUS-guided transrectal FNA biopsies. Cytology revealed a chordoma, which was confirmed by immunohistochemistry and outside consultation. Chordomas are rare tumors (less than 1 % of central nervous system tumors; 300 cases per year in the USA) thought to arise from ectopic remnants of the notochord. Notochord remnants are usually present as the nucleus pulposus of the intervertebral disks. Extradural remnants are most often located in the sacrococcygeal region. Although not usually metastatic, these tumors behave aggressively locally and have a high tendency to recur locally after surgery.

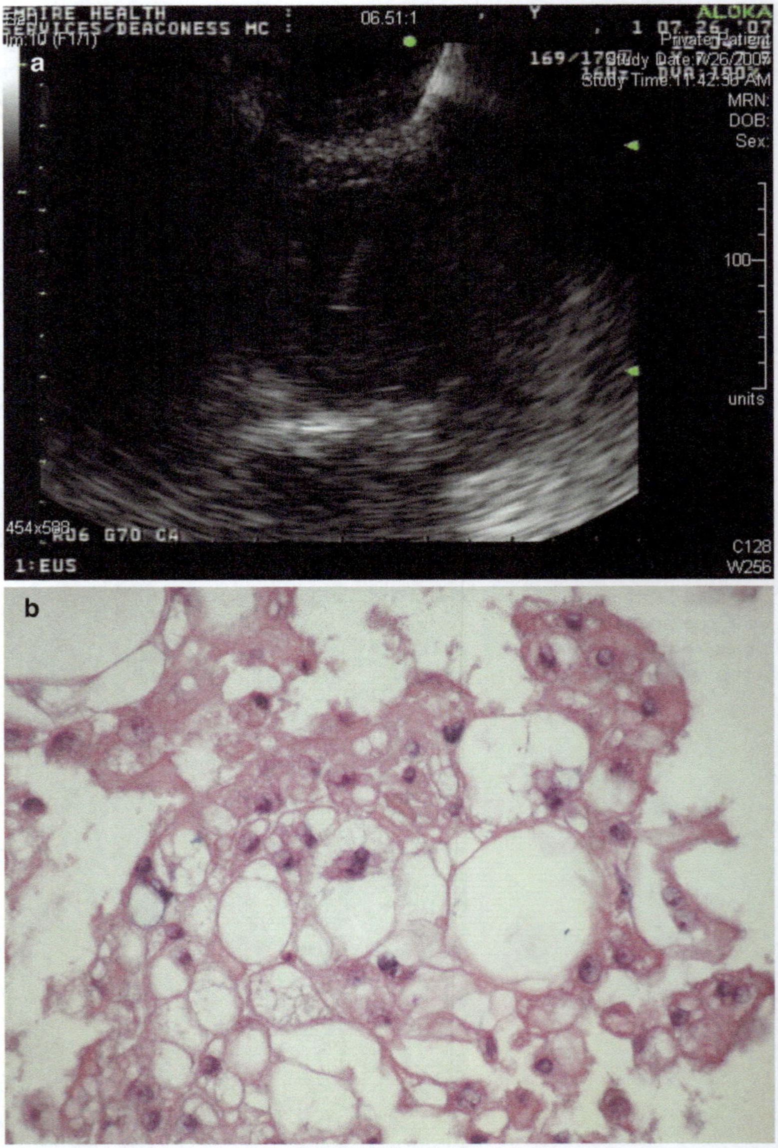

Fig. 8.41 (**a**) Endoscopic ultrasound–guided fine-needle aspiration revealed the characteristic physaliphorous cells of a chordoma. (**b**) A high-resolution image of the histology of the presacral chordoma (Image courtesy of Dr. Karl Anders)

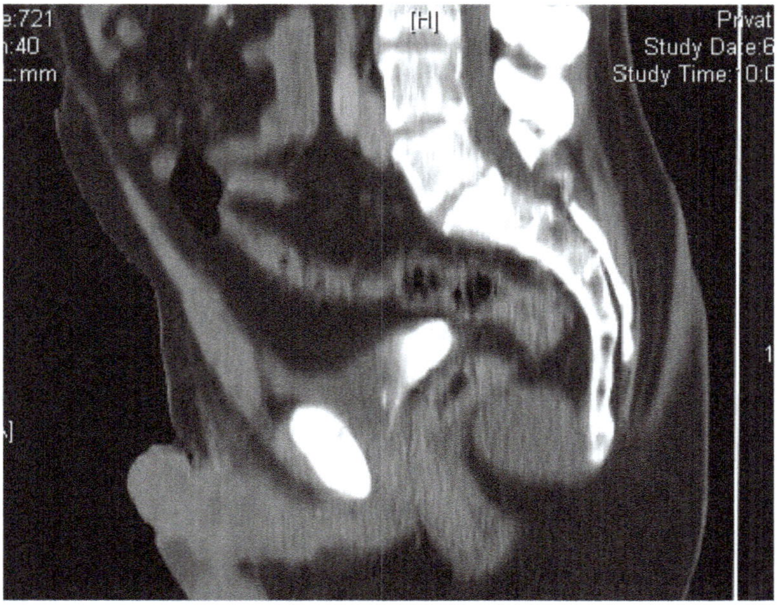

Fig. 8.42 This reconstructed computed tomography scan shows the relationship of the chordoma to the coccyx

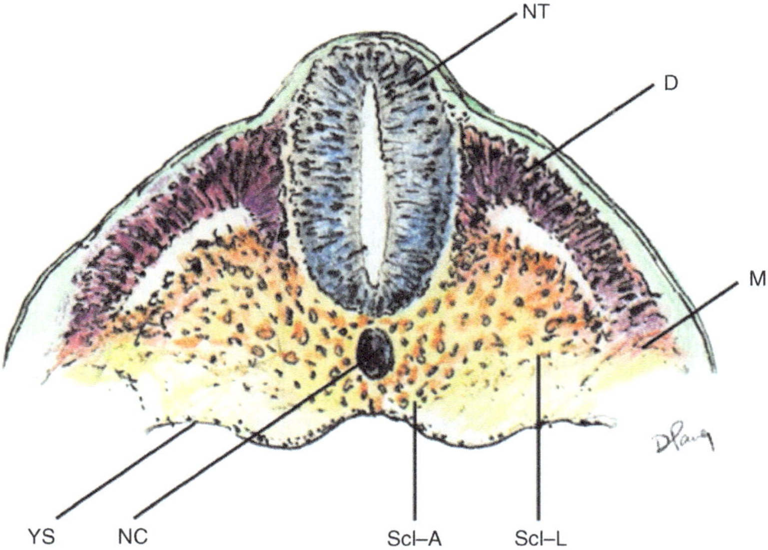

Fig. 8.43 Coronal section of a chick embryo after dorsoventral differentiation of somites, showing axial or perichordal sclerotome (*Scl-A*) surrounding the notochord (*NC*) and lateral sclerotome (*Scl-L*) on both sides of the neural tube (*NT*). *D* dermatome, *M* myotome, *YS* yolk sac membrane (From Pang and Thompson [71])

References

1. Dujovny N, Quiros RM, Saclarides TJ. Anorectal anatomy and embryology. Surg Oncol Clin N Am. 2004;13(2):277–93.
2. Schwartz DA, Harewood GC, Wiersema MJ. EUS for rectal disease. Gastrointest Endosc. 2002;56(1):100–9.
3. Nielsen MB, Hauge C, Rasmussen OO, Sørensen M, Pedersen JF, Christiansen J. Anal sphincter size measured by endosonography in healthy volunteers. Effect of age, sex, and parity. Acta Radiol. 1992;33(5):453–6.
4. Sultan AH, Kamm MA, Hudson CN, Nicholls JR, Bartram CI. Endosonography of the anal sphincters: normal anatomy and comparison with manometry. Clin Radiol. 1994;49(6):368–74.
5. Nelson H, Petrelli N, Carlin A, Couture J, Fleshman J, Guillem J, et al. Guidelines 2000 for colon and rectal cancer surgery. J Natl Cancer Inst. 2001;93(8):583–96.
6. Deutsch J. Chapter 7: Normal rectal endoscopic ultrasound anatomy. In: Buthani MS, Deutsch JC, editors. Digital human anatomy and endoscopic ultrasonography. Hamilton: BC Decker, Inc.; 2005.
7. Ehrenpreis ED. Chapter 1: General information. In: Ehrenpreis ED, et al., editors. Anal and rectal diseases. New York: Springer; 2012. doi:10.1007/978-1-4614-1102-4_1.
8. Savides TJ, Hawes RH. Chapter 28: Endoscopic ultrasound staging of rectal cancer. In: Van Dam J, Sivak MV, editors. Gastrointestinal endosonography. Philadelphia: WB Saunders; 1999.
9. Yoshida M, Tsukamoto Y, Niwa Y, Goto H, Hase S, Hayakawa T, et al. Endoscopic assessment of invasion of colorectal tumors with a new high-frequency ultrasound probe. Gastrointest Endosc. 1995;41(6):587–92.
10. Savides TJ, Master SS. EUS in rectal cancer. Gastrointest Endosc. 2002;56(4 Suppl):S12–8.
11. Chak A. Chapter 2: The radial scanning echoendoscope. In: Gastrointestinal endosonography. Philadelphia: WB Saunders; 1999.
12. Gottlieb K, Elkharwily A. Endoscopic ultrasound evaluation of a cystic lymphangioma of the colon. J Ultrasound Med. 2007;26(12):1803–4.
13. Bhutani MS, Nadella P. Utility of an upper echoendoscope for endoscopic ultrasonography of malignant and benign conditions of the sigmoid/left colon and the rectum. Am J Gastroenterol. 2001;96(12):3318–22.
14. Frudinger A, Bartram CI, Halligan S, Kamm M. Examination techniques for endosonography of the anal canal. Abdom Imaging. 1998;23(3):301–3.
15. Garcia-Aguilar J, Pollack J, Lee S-H, Hernandez de Anda E, Mellgren A, Wong WD, et al. Accuracy of endorectal ultrasonography in preoperative staging of rectal tumors. Dis Colon Rectum. 2002;45(1):10–5.
16. Herzog U, von Flüe M, Tondelli P, Schuppisser JP. How accurate is endorectal ultrasound in the preoperative staging of rectal cancer? Dis Colon Rectum. 1993;36(2):127–34.
17. Kulig J, Richter P, Gurda-Duda A, Gach T, Klek S. The role and value of endorectal ultrasonography in diagnosing T1 rectal tumors. Ultrasound Med Biol. 2006;32(4):469–72.
18. Rau B, Hünerbein M, Barth C, Wust P, Haensch W, Riess H, et al. Accuracy of endorectal ultrasound after preoperative radiochemotherapy in locally advanced rectal cancer. Surg Endosc. 1999;13(10):980–4.
19. Fleming FJ, Påhlman L, Monson JRT. Neoadjuvant therapy in rectal cancer. Dis Colon Rectum. 2011;54(7):901–12.
20. Bipat S, Glas AS, Slors FJM, Zwinderman AH, Bossuyt PMM, Stoker J. Rectal cancer: local staging and assessment of lymph node involvement with endoluminal US, CT, and MR imaging – a meta-analysis. Radiology. 2004;232(3):773–83.
21. Beets-Tan RGH. MRI in rectal cancer: the T stage and circumferential resection margin. Colorectal Dis. 2003;5(5):392–5.
22. Hildebrandt U, Feifel G. Preoperative staging of rectal cancer by intrarectal ultrasound. Dis Colon Rectum. 1985;28(1):42–6.
23. Tsai BM, Finne CO, Nordenstam JF, Christoforidis D, Madoff RD, Mellgren A. Transanal endoscopic microsurgery resection of rectal tumors: outcomes and recommendations. Dis Colon Rectum. 2010;53(1):16–23.
24. Langer C, Liersch T, Markus P, Süss M, Ghadimi M, Füzesi L, et al. Transanal endoscopic microsurgery (TEM) for minimally invasive resection of rectal adenomas and "Low-risk" carcinomas (uT1, G1–2). Z Gastroenterol. 2002;40(2):67–72.
25. Krajewski KM, Kane RA. Ultrasound staging of rectal cancer. Semin Ultrasound CT MR. 2008;29(6):427–32.
26. McCall JL, Cox MR, Wattchow DA. Analysis of local recurrence rates after surgery alone for rectal cancer. Int J Colorectal Dis. 1995;10(3):126–32.
27. Sauer R, Becker H, Hohenberger W, Rödel C, Wittekind C, Fietkau R, et al. Preoperative versus postoperative chemoradiotherapy for rectal cancer. N Engl J Med. 2004;351(17):1731–40.
28. Kruskal JB, Sentovich SM, Kane RA. Staging of rectal cancer after polypectomy: usefulness of endorectal US. Radiology. 1999;211(1):31–5.
29. Shami VM, Parmar KS, Waxman I. Clinical impact of endoscopic ultrasound and endoscopic ultrasound-guided fine-needle aspiration in the management of rectal carcinoma. Dis Colon Rectum. 2004;47(1):59–65.
30. Hu KS, Harrison LB. Adjuvant therapy for resectable rectal adenocarcinoma. Semin Surg Oncol. 2000;19(4):336–49.
31. Kim HJ, Wong WD. Role of endorectal ultrasound in the conservative management of rectal cancers. Semin Surg Oncol. 2000;19(4):358–66.
32. Herrera L, Villarreal JR. Incidence of metastases from rectal adenocarcinoma in small lymph nodes detected by a clearing technique. Dis Colon Rectum. 1992;35(8):783–8.
33. Knight CS, Eloubeidi MA, Crowe R, Jhala NC, Jhala DN, Chhieng DC, et al. Utility of endoscopic ultrasound-guided fine-needle aspiration in the diagnosis and staging of colorectal carcinoma. Diagn

Cytopathol. [Internet]. 19 Sep 2011. http://www.ncbi.nlm.nih.gov/pubmed/21932358. Cited 20 June 2012.
34. Levy MJ, Norton ID, Clain JE, Enders FB, Gleeson F, Limburg PJ, et al. Prospective study of bacteremia and complications With EUS FNA of rectal and perirectal lesions. Clin Gastroenterol Hepatol. 2007;5(6):684–9.
35. Halefoglu A-M, Yildirim S, Avlanmis O, Sakiz D, Baykan A. Endorectal ultrasonography versus phased-array magnetic resonance imaging for preoperative staging of rectal cancer. World J Gastroenterol. 2008;14(22):3504–10.
36. Mellgren A, Sirivongs P, Rothenberger DA, Madoff RD, García-Aguilar J. Is local excision adequate therapy for early rectal cancer? Dis Colon Rectum. 2000;43(8):1064–71; discussion 1071–4.
37. Novell F, Pascual S, Viella P, Trias M. Endorectal ultrasonography in the follow-up of rectal cancer. Is it a better way to detect early local recurrence? Int J Colorectal Dis. 1997;12(2):78–81.
38. Löhnert M, Dohrmann P, Stoffregen C, Hamelmann H. Value of endorectal sonography in the follow-up of patients treated surgically for rectum carcinoma. Zentralbl Chir. 1991;116(7):461–4.
39. Hünerbein M, Totkas S, Moesta KT, Ulmer C, Handke T, Schlag PM. The role of transrectal ultrasound-guided biopsy in the postoperative follow-up of patients with rectal cancer. Surgery. 2001;129(2):164–9.
40. Siddiqui AA, Fayiga Y, Huerta S. The role of endoscopic ultrasound in the evaluation of rectal cancer. Int Semin Surg Oncol. 2006;3:36.
41. Quirke P, Risio M, Lambert R, Karsa L, Vieth M. Quality assurance in pathology in colorectal cancer screening and diagnosis – European recommendations. Virchows Arch. 2011;458(1):1–19. doi:10.1007/s00428-010-0977-6.
42. Nivatvongs S, Nicholson JD, Rothenberger DA, Balcos EG, Christenson CE, Nemer FD, et al. Villous adenomas of the rectum: the accuracy of clinical assessment. Surgery. 1980;87(5):549–51.
43. Starck M, Bohe M, Simanaitis M, Valentin L. Rectal endosonography can distinguish benign rectal lesions from invasive early rectal cancers. Colorectal Dis. 2003;5(3):246–50.
44. Kuntz C, Glaser F, Buhr HJ, Herfarth C. Endorectal ultrasound in diagnosis and therapy planning of broad-base rectal adenomas. Chirurg. 1993;64(4):290–4.
45. Glaser F, Schlag P, Herfarth C. Endorectal ultrasonography for the assessment of invasion of rectal tumours and lymph node involvement. Br J Surg. 1990;77(8):883–7.
46. Derksen EJ, Cuesta MA, Meijer S. Intraluminal ultrasound of rectal tumours: a prerequisite in decision making. Surg Oncol. 1992;1(3):193–8.
47. Worrell S, Horvath K, Blakemore T, Flum D. Endorectal ultrasound detection of focal carcinoma within rectal adenomas. Am J Surg. 2004;187(5):625–9; discussion 629.
48. Dancygier H, Lightdale CJ, Stevens PD. Chapter 2: Endoscopic ultrasonography of the upper gastrointestinal tract and colon. In: Dancygier H, Lightdale CJ, editors. Endosonography in gastroenterology. Stuttgart/New York: Thieme; 1999.
49. Meguerditchian A-N, Meterissian SH, Dunn KB. Anorectal melanoma: diagnosis and treatment. Dis Colon Rectum. 2011;54(5):638–44.
50. Petritsch W, Hinterleitner TA, Aichbichler B, Denk H, Hammer HF, Krejs GJ. Endosonography in colitis cystica profunda and solitary rectal ulcer syndrome. Gastrointest Endosc. 1996;44(6):746–51.
51. Pishvaian AC, Ahlawat SK, Garvin D, Haddad NG. Role of EUS and EUS-guided FNA in the diagnosis of symptomatic rectosigmoid endometriosis. Gastrointest Endosc. 2006;63(2):331–5.
52. Biggar RJ, Burnett W, Mikl J, Nasca P. Cancer among New York men at risk of acquired immunodeficiency syndrome. Int J Cancer. 1989;43(6):979–85.
53. Frisch M, Glimelius B, van den Brule AJ, Wohlfahrt J, Meijer CJ, Walboomers JM, et al. Sexually transmitted infection as a cause of anal cancer. N Engl J Med. 1997;337(19):1350–8.
54. Ryan DP, Compton CC, Mayer RJ. Carcinoma of the anal canal. N Engl J Med. 2000;342(11):792–800.
55. Nigro ND, Vaitkevicius VK, Considine Jr B. Combined therapy for cancer of the anal canal: a preliminary report. Dis Colon Rectum. 1974;17(3):354–6.
56. NCCN Clinical Practice Guidelines in Oncology (NCCN Guidelines®) Anal Carcinoma [Internet]. 2012. http://www.nccn.org/professionals/physician_gls/pdf/anal.pdf
57. Otto SD, Lee L, Buhr HJ, Frericks B, Höcht S, Kroesen AJ. Staging anal cancer: prospective comparison of transanal endoscopic ultrasound and magnetic resonance imaging. J Gastrointest Surg. 2009;13(7):1292–8.
58. Tarantino D, Bernstein MA. Endoanal ultrasound in the staging and management of squamous-cell carcinoma of the anal canal: potential implications of a new ultrasound staging system. Dis Colon Rectum. 2002;45(1):16–22.
59. Pessaux P, Pocard M, Elias D, Duvillard P, Avril M-F, Zimmerman P, et al. Surgical management of primary anorectal melanoma. Br J Surg. 2004;91(9):1183–7.
60. Zhang S, Gao F, Wan D. Effect of misdiagnosis on the prognosis of anorectal malignant melanoma. J Cancer Res Clin Oncol. 2010;136(9):1401–5.
61. Yap LB, Neary P. A comparison of wide local excision with abdominoperineal resection in anorectal melanoma. Melanoma Res. 2004;14(2):147–50.
62. Bullard KM, Tuttle TM, Rothenberger DA, Madoff RD, Baxter NN, Finne CO, et al. Surgical therapy for anorectal melanoma. J Am Coll Surg. 2003;196(2):206–11.
63. Hodi FS, O'Day SJ, McDermott DF, Weber RW, Sosman JA, Haanen JB, et al. Improved survival with ipilimumab in patients with metastatic melanoma. N Engl J Med. 2010;363(8):711–23.
64. Sashiyama H, Takayama W, Miyazaki S-I, Makino H, Matsushita K, Shimada H, et al. The diagnostic value of endoscopic ultrasonography and magnetic resonance imaging for anorectal malignant melanoma: report of a case. Surg Today. 2003;33(3):209–13.

65. Gottlieb K, Coff P, Preiksaitis H, Juviler A, Fern P. Massive hemorrhage in pregnancy caused by a diffuse cavernous hemangioma of the rectum – EUS as imaging modality of choice. Medscape J Med. 2008;10(9):206.
66. Gentry RW, Dockerty MB, Glagett OT. Vascular malformations and vascular tumors of the gastrointestinal tract. Surg Gynecol Obstet. 1949;88(4):281–323.
67. Hsu RM, Horton KM, Fishman EK. Diffuse cavernous hemangiomatosis of the colon: findings on three-dimensional CT colonography. AJR Am J Roentgenol. 2002;179(4):1042–4.
68. Djouhri H, Arrivé L, Bouras T, Martin B, Monnier-Cholley L, Tubiana JM. MR imaging of diffuse cavernous hemangioma of the rectosigmoid colon. AJR Am J Roentgenol. 1998;171(2):413–7.
69. Gottlieb K. Doppler-endosonography with the GF-UE 160 electronic radial echoendoscope – current use and future potential. J Gastrointestin Liver Dis. 2007;16(4):455–61.
70. Irisawa A, Bhutani MS. Cystic lymphangioma of the colon: endosonographic diagnosis with through-the-scope catheter miniprobe and determination of further management. Report of a case. Dis Colon Rectum. 2001;44(7):1040–2.
71. Pang D, Thompson DNP. Embryology and bony malformations of the craniovertebral junction. Childs Nerv Syst. 2011;27(4):523–64.

Index

A
Abdomen
  anatomy
    prostate, 34
    seminal vesicles, 35–36
    uterus, 39
    vagina, 37–38
  Doppler endosonography, upper abdomen
    celiac artery variants, 49–51
    celiac ganglia, 52–53
    celiac vessels and superior mesenteric artery, 47–48
    hepatic veins, 42
    pelvis, 54
    portal vein, 43–44
    splenic vein and splenic artery, 45–46
Abdominopelvic autonomic nervous system, 392
Accessory spleens, 394–395
Adrenal biopsy, 386–389
Adrenal incidentalomas, 387
Adrenal masses, 386–389
Adrenal myelolipoma, 390–391
Adrenocortical adenomas, 387
Adrenocortical carcinomas, 387
Ampullary carcinoma, 211–212
Anal cancer
  EUS *vs.* MRI, 438
  HPV infection, 438
  incidence of, 438
  point of origin, 436
  prognosis of, 438
  staging of, 435
Ann Arbor staging system, 159
Anorectal melanoma (ARM), 438
  EUS, 440–441
  during retroflexion, 439
  symptoms, 442
  tumor thickness, 442
  ulcerated melanoma, 438, 440
Aortic aneurysms, 74–75
Aortic dissections, 76–77
ARR GoldMiner®, 58
Artifacts
  computed tomography
    limitations of, 14–15
    streak artifacts on, 12–13
  contrast resolution, in EUS, 8–11
  generic categories, of ultrasound imaging, 8
  partial volume, 18–21
  reverberation, 16–17
Ascites, 396–397
Ascitic fluid aspiration, 400
Azygos veins
  anatomy, 31–32
  Doppler endosonography, 40–41
  pulmonary emboli, 78–79
  right heart strain, 82

B
Behrns' diagnostic criteria, 364
Bile ducts
  arterial vessel crossing, dilation caused by, 268–269
  choledochocele *vs.* bile duct web, 292–293
  common hepatic ductma, defect in, 290–291
  EUS
    extrapancreatic portion, 302
    intrapancreatic segment, 303
  extrinsic compression by metastatic melanoma, 287–289
  isolated bile duct dilation, 265–267
  liver tests, 265
  malignant bile duct stricture, 280–283
  narcotic, 275–276
  online resources, 235, 236
  PSC, 277–279
  stones, 270–274
  type II choledochal cyst, 284–286
  villous lesions, 294–295
Biliary metal stent, 351, 353
BioText literature search engine, 55

C
Cancer molecular pathology, 66
Carcinosarcoma, of esophagus
  barium esophagogram, 125
  cystic degeneration, 127
  exophytic nature, 128
  polypoid nature, 126
  sausage-shaped tumor, in CT scan, 126
  tumor pseudopodia, 128

K. Gottlieb, G. Marino, *Diagnostic Endosonography*,
DOI 10.1007/978-3-642-39118-7, © Springer-Verlag Berlin Heidelberg 2014

Celiac ganglion, 52–53
Celiac vessels, 47–48
Centrally located primary lung lesions, 109–112
Cholangiocarcinoma, 16, 193
Cholecystitis, 12, 237–239
Choledochocele *vs.* bile duct web, 292–293
Coccygeal chordoma, 449–451
Cognitive biases
  confirmation bias, 3–4
  defense strategies, 2–3
  field-dependence bias, 5–7
  framing in imaging, 3–4
  image perception research, 5
Colon cancer, 428–430
Colonic hemangiomas, 442–443
Comet tail artifact, 16
Computed tomography (CT)
  accessory spleens, 394
  bile duct stent, 243
  bone metastases, 158
  bronchial carcinoid, 90
  bronchial cysts, 94
  celiac ganglion, 52–53
  choledochal cyst, 284, 285
  chordoma-coccyx relationship, 451
  coronal reconstruction, 111
  cystic duct stone, 237
  dilated bile duct, 301, 302, 344, 345
  esophageal duplication cyst, 135
  esophageal leiomyomas, 137–139
  focally dilated main pancreatic duct, 314
  gastric cancer, 152, 154, 184
  hemangiomas, 251, 252
  Hodgkin's lymphoma, 88
  hypodense pancreatic tail lesion, 341–342
  insulinoma, 355, 358
  intraluminal tissue and gallbladder stone, 240, 241
  mediastinal pseudocysts, 98
  metastatic carcinoid, 355, 356
  non-Hodgkin's lymphoma, 218
  omental cake, 405
  pancreatic calcifications, 308, 309
  pancreatic cyst, 370, 371
  pancreatic head, 338
  paraganglioma, 392, 393
  paraspinal/prevertebral tumor, 101
  partial volume artifact, 19
  perigastric lymph node enlargement, 163
  perivascular fat, 314, 316
  plaque and clot, 75
  pleural effusion, 103
  pulmonary artery emboli, 79
  sausage-shaped tumor, in esophagus, 126
  serous cystadenoma, 379
  situs inversus, 174
  subhepatic cyst, 248
  thickened bile duct wall, 280, 281
  tumor invasion, into portal vein, 262
  upstream pancreatic duct dilation, 332
  villous leison, duodenum, 199
  Whipple pancreaticoduodenectomy, 193
Consolidated lung, 105–106
Contrast resolution, 8–11
Courvoisier's sign, gallbladder, 245
CT. *See* Computed tomography (CT)
Cutaneous T-cell lymphoma, 364–366
Cystic lymphangioma, of colon, 445–448
Cystic neuroendocrine tumors, in pancreas, 359–360
Cysts
  bronchial, 94–96
  choledochal, 284
  duodenal pseudocyst (*see* Pseudocyst, duodenal)
  duplication
    duodenal pseudocyst, 207–210
    gastrointestinal tract, 135–136
  gallbladder, 244
  intramucosal cyst, of esophagus, 134
  mesenteric, 402–404
  pancreatic
    complex vessel relationships, 367–369
    polypoid structure, 370–372
    pseudocyst, 373–375
  todani choledochal, 284–286
Cytokeratin 7 immunostain, 92

D

DAVE Project, 198
DeBakey classification scheme, 76
Decision errors, 5
Detail resolution, 8
Diffuse cavernous rectal hemangioma, 442–444
Doppler endosonography
  mediastinum
    azygos vein, 40–41
    dorsal intercostal arteries, 42
  upper abdomen
    celiac artery variants, 49–51
    celiac ganglia, 52–53
    celiac vessels and superior mesenteric artery, 47–48
    hepatic veins, 42
    pelvis, 54
    portal vein, 43–44
    splenic vein and splenic artery, 45–46
Ducta EUS criteria, 308
Duodenal diverticula, 201–202
Duodenum
  ampullary carcinoma, 211–212
  cancer, 198–200
  duodenal diverticula, 201–202
  FAP, 213–214
  perforation by foreign body, 203–206
  periduodenal collaterals, 215–217
  primary duodenal non-Hodgkin's lymphoma, 218–221
  pseudocyst, 207–210
  transduodenal abscess drainage (*see also* Transduodenal abscess drainage)
    dilations to 12 mm, 228
    dimensions of abscess, 224
    Huibregtse needle knife, 225

Hurricane biliary balloon, 227
irrigated and cleaned abscess cavity, 229
pus exit from abscess, 226
Zollinger-Ellison syndrome, 230–233
Duplication cyst
duodenal pseudocyst, 207–210
gastrointestinal tract, 135–136
Dysphagia, 107–108

E
Endoscopic retrograde cholangiopancreatography (ERCP)
acute pancreatitis, 301
bile duct dilation, 344
bile duct stone, 271
cavernous transformation, portal vein, 264
chronic pancreatitis, 307
distal common bile duct stricture, 347
extrahepatic bile ducts, crenellation of, 277, 279
gallbladder carcinoma, 240
high-grade hilar stricture, 264
intrahepatic bile duct beading, 277, 279
pancreatic duct stone, 306, 307
Endoscopic ultrasound (EUS)
accessory spleens, 394, 395
acute pancreatitis, 301, 304–305
adrenal glands
anatomy and technique, 385–386
online resources, 386
ARM, 440–441
bile duct, 307
extrapancreatic portion, 301, 302
intrapancreatic segment, 301, 303
tumor, 280, 282
chronic pancreatitis, features of, 308
4-cm-diameter polyp, 431
colonic cystic lymphangioma, 445, 447, 448
colon, rectum and anus
anatomy, 415–418
flexible video-endoscopes, 419
forward-viewing endoscopes, 419
miniprobe catheters, 419
online resources, 420
preparation, 419
technique, 419–420
contrast resolution, 8–11
dilated cystic duct, 239
dilated main pancreatic duct, 308, 309
dilation of
extrahepatic biliary system, 265
right and left hepatic ducts, 265, 266
duodenal pseudocyst, 208
duodenum (*see also* Duodenum)
anatomy, 197
cancer, 198–200
duodenal diverticulum, 201–202
EUS probes, 197
online resorces, 198
technique, 197–198
fatty infiltration, of pancreas, 314, 315
with FNA. (*See* Fine-needle aspiration (FNA))
gallbladder carcinoma, 240, 242, 243
gallbladder with echogenic bile, 237, 239
hepatoduodenal ligament lymph node, 257
hepatomas, 253, 255
hypoechoic mass, 346
malignant rectal ulcer, 421
mesenteric cysts, 402–404
with MRI
pancreatic head tumor, 335
periportal lymph node, 335
mucinous cystic neoplasms, 376, 377
narcotic bile ducts, 275–276
non-Hodgkin's lymphoma, 219
omental cake, 405, 406
omentum, 398
pancreas (*see also* Pancreas)
anatomy, 298–300
online resources, 297, 298
radial/linear scanning echoendoscopes, 298
technique, 298
pancreatic cyst
appearance, 373, 375
with polypoid structure, 370–372
pancreatic duct, 265, 266
pancreatic mass, 326
papilla of Vater, 265, 267
paraganglioma, 392, 393
periportal lymph node, 258
PSC, 277, 278
serous cystadenoma, 379, 380
stomach
anatomy, 147, 148
EUS probes, 148
online resources, 149
patient preparation, 149
technique, 148–149
subcarinal lymph nodes, 428, 430
subhepatic cyst, 250
submucosal mass, in lower rectum, 435–437
textbooks and journals, 59
transduodenal abscess drainage
dilations to 12 mm, 228
dimensions of abscess, 224
Huibregtse needle knife, 225
Hurricane biliary balloon, 227
irrigated and cleaned abscess cavity, 229
pus exit from abscess, 226
Esophagogastroduodenoscopy
adenocarcinoma, 151
central umbilication, in gastric antrum, 188
granular cell tumor, of esophagus, 152
linitis plastica, 156
Esophagus. *See also* Mediastinum
bony spur, 24, 26
carcinosarcoma
barium esophagogram, 125
cystic degeneration, 127
exophytic nature, 128
polypoid nature, 126
sausage-shaped tumor, in CT scan, 126
tumor pseudopodia, 128

Esophagus (*cont.*)
esophageal duplication cyst, 135–136
esophageal intramucosal cyst, 134
esophageal leiomyomas, 137–139
muscularis mucosae, 130–131
examination of, 73–74
granular cell tumors, 132–133
intramucosal cyst, 134
intramural metastasis, esophageal cancer, 140–141
online resoursec, 72
recurrent esophageal cancer, 142–143
T1N1 esophageal cancer, 129
EUS. *See* Endoscopic ultrasound (EUS)
Extranodal marginal zone B-cell lymphomas. *See* Mucosa-associated lymphoid tissue (MALT) lymphoma

F
False-positive PET scan, 117–118
Familial adenomatous polyposis (FAP), 213–214. *See also* Gardner's syndrome
Fatty infiltration, of pancreas, 311–313
FigureSearch, 56
Fine-needle aspiration (FNA)
cystic neuroendocrine tumors, in pancreas, 359, 360
cytology
conventional processing, 65
pancreatic cancer, management of, 65
EUS-guided
adrenal glands, 387
hepatomas, 253, 256
metastatic cancer diagnosis, in pancreas, 348
peripancreatic lymph node, 287, 289
physaliphorous cells, of chordoma, 449, 450
pancreatic cystic lesions, 60–61
personalized tumor therapy, 62
Fluid in lesser sac, 400–401
Foreign body, duodenal perforation by, 203–206
Formalin-fixed paraffin-embedded (FFPE) specimens, 65

G
Gallbladder
carcinoma, 240–243
cholecystitis and cholelithiasis, 237–239
Courvoisier's sign, 245
cysts, 244
Heister valves, 246, 247
online resources, 235, 236
wall thickness, 235–236
Gardner's syndrome, 341–343
Gastric cancer
adenocarcinoma, 151
endoscopic ultrasound image, 152, 153
gastric wall thickening on CT, 152
incidence, 150
muscularis propria, 152
Gastric carcinoid, 179–181
Gastrointestinal stromal tumor (GISTs)
biopsy principles, 177–178
central ulceration, 168
incidence, 167
and interstitial cells of Cajal, 172–173
metastatic, 170–171
with situs inversus, 174–176
Glucose-avid mediastinal lymph nodes, 118
GoldMiner®, 58
Granular cell tumors, of esophagus, 132–133

H
Haggitt invasion levels, in polypoid carcinomas, 432
Heister valves, 246, 247
Helicobacter pylori, 159, 161
Hepatic veins
Doppler endosonography, 42
and portal vein, 260–261
Hepato-spleno-mesenteric trunk, 50–51
HIDA scan, 237, 238, 240, 277
Hounsfield units, 14
Hypoechoic cap, pancreatic orifices, 211, 212
Hypoechoic pancreas tumor calcification, 328
Hypoechoic tumor, 179, 180

I
Idiopathic acute pancreatitis, 396
Image perception research, 5
Image retrieval systems. *See* Medical image retrieval systems
iMedline®, 55
Infectious lesions, 387
Interrogation technique, 5
Interstitial cells of Cajal (ICCs), 172–173
Intramucosal cyst, of esophagus, 134
Intramural metastasis, esophageal cancer, 140–141
Isodense pancreatic cancer, 334–337
Isolated bile duct dilation, 265–267
Ivor-Lewis esophagectomy, 142

L
Large colon polyp, 431–432
Large peripheral hemangioma, calcifications in, 252
Large villous adenoma, with high-grade dysplasia, 433–434
Leather bottle, 154
Leiomyoma, esophageal, 130–131
Lesser sac, 399–401
Linear EUS endoscopes, 148
Linitis plastica
with bone metastases, 156–158
of stomach, 154–155
Liver
hemangiomas, 251–252
hepatic lymph nodes, 257–259
hepatic vein branches, 260–261

hepatomas, 253–256
online resources, 235, 236
portal vein
cavernous transformation of, 262–264
course of, 260, 261
subhepatic cyst growth, 248–250
Lymph node anatomy, 258
Lymphoma
biopsy, 85–86
recurrent Hodgkin's
hot spots, 87
Reed-Sternberg cells, 89
unimpressive subcarinal lymph node, 88

M
Magnetic resonance cholangiopancreatography (MRCP)
choledochal cysts, 284
common hepatic duct, filling defect in, 290
cystic duct stone, 237, 238
distal common bile duct abnormality, 237, 238
mucinous cystic neoplasms, 376, 377
pancreatic duct stone, 306
Magnetic resonance imaging (MRI)
hepatic duct displacement, 249
hepatic veins, 260, 261
hepatomas, 253, 254
liver lesions, 334, 337
melanoma, 442
metastatic lesions, 124
pancreatic head tumor, 335
periportal lymph node, 335
rectal cavernous hemangioma, 443, 444
Zollinger-Ellison syndrome, 230, 231
Malignant bile duct stricture, 280–283
Malignant invasion, pulmonary artery, 122–124
Mediastinum
anatomy, 71–72
azygos vein, 31–32
mediastinal lymph nodes, 33
thoracic duct, 29–30
aortic aneurysms, 74–75
aortic dissections, 76–77
biopsies, 73
bronchial carcinoid, 90–93
bronchial cysts, 94–96
centrally located primary lung lesions, 109–112
consolidated lung, 105–106
Doppler endosonography
azygos vein, 40–41
dorsal intercostal arteries, 42
dysphagia, 107–108
false-positive PET scan, 117–118
lung cancer restaging, 113–116
lymph node maps for, 73
malignant invasion, pulmonary artery, 122–124
mediastinal pseudocysts, 97–98
online resoursec, 72
paratracheal lymph node biopsy, 85–86
pericardial and pleural effusion, 103–104
plasmacytomas, 99–100
posterior mediastinal paravertebral mass, 101–102
pulmonary emboli, 78–82
recurrent Hodgkin's lymphoma
hot spots, 87
Reed-Sternberg cells, 89
unimpressive subcarinal lymph node, 88
right heart strain, 78–82
subcarinal lymph node biopsy, 83–84
triple cytology, lung cancer diagnosis, 119–121
Medical image retrieval systems
BioText, 55
FigureSearch, 56
iMedline®, 55
PubMed Central® (PMC), 55
Yale Image Finder, 57
Memorial Sloan Kettering Cancer Center, 199
Mesenteric cysts, 402–404
Metastatic gastrointestinal stromal tumor, 170–171
Micro RNAs (miRNA), 60–61
MRCP. *See* Magnetic resonance cholangiopancreatography (MRCP)
Mucinous cystic neoplasms, 376–378
Mucoceles, 134
Mucosa-associated lymphoid tissue (MALT) lymphoma
Ann Arbor staging system, 159
hematoxylin and eosin stain, 161
with local and distant lymph node involvement, 162–165
mucosal layer expansion, 160
spectrum of, 159
Myelolipoma, adrenal, 390–391

N
Narcotic bile ducts, 275–276
Neuroendocrine tumors, in pancreas
cystic, 359–360
metastatic carcinoid and symptomatic insulinoma, 355–358
Nonalcoholic fatty pancreas disease, 311
Non-Hodgkin's lymphoma
CT scan, 218
endoscopic ultrasound, 219
metastatic lesions, 220, 221

O
Omental cake, 405–408
Omentum, 398–399
Online resources, 2
adrenal incidentalomas, 386, 387
bile ducts, 235, 236
colon, rectum and anus, 420
duodenum, 198
gallbladder, 235, 236
liver, 235, 236
pancreas, 297, 298
stomach, 149

P
Pancreas
  acute pancreatitis, 301–305
  cancer
    and chronic pancreatitis, 329–331
    and Gardner's syndrome, 341–343
    isodense, 334–337
    missed, 344–347
    small, 332–333
    stage IV, 320–322
  chronic pancreatitis, 306–307
  development, in human embryos, 299
  dilated main pancreatic duct, 314–316
  fatty infiltration, 311–313
  hypodense area, 299, 300
  hypoechoic tumor calcifications, 328
  large pancreatic head, 338–340
  mucinous cystic neoplasm, 376–378
  mycosis fungoides, 364–366
  neuroendocrine tumors
    cystic, 359–360
    metastatic carcinoid and symptomatic insulinoma, 355–358
  ovarian cancer metastases, 348–350
  pancreatic parenchymal calcification, 308–310
  pancreatic tail mass, 326–327, 343
  primary pancreatic lymphoma, 361–363
  renal cancer metastases, 348
  serous cystadenoma, 379–380
  splenic and portal vein, 298
  T2 adenocarcinoma, 323–325
  vanishing pancreatic mass, 317–319
  ventral and dorsal pancreas, 299, 300
  Wallstent
    characteristic appearance of, 351–353
    FNA biopsies, 354
Pancreatic intraepithelial neoplasia, 376
Pancreatic rest
  cystic spaces, 188, 189
  echogenic foci, 190
  ectopic pancreas, 189
Pancreatic steatosis, 311
Pap stain, 92
Paraganglioma, 392–393
Paratracheal lymph node biopsy, 85–86
Parenchymal EUS criteria, 308
Paris staging system, 159
Partial volume artifacts, 18–21
Pelvis, 54
Perforations, in duodenal bulb, 203
Periampullary cancer, 213
Periampullary duodenal diverticula, 201–202
Pericardial and pleural effusion, 103–104
Periduodenal collaterals, 215–217
Periesophageal lymph node, 7
Perigastric abscess
  barium, stomach, 194, 195
  Whipple pancreaticoduodenectomy, 193
Perigastric lymphadenopathy, 165
Peritoneal carcinomatosis, 409–410
Pheocromocytomas, 387
Plasmacytomas, 99–100
Polypoid carcinomas, Haggitt invasion levels, 432
Positron emission tomography (PET)
  airspace disease, 119
  esophageal squamous cell carcinoma, 142
  GIST, 174–175
  glucose-avid mediastinal lymph nodes, 118
  Hodgkin's lymphoma, 87
  restaging of lung cancer, 114–116
  right hilar area, 428–430
  subcarinal lymph nodes, 428, 429
Power Doppler. *See also* Doppler endosonography
  aortic dissection, 82
  portal vein and collaterals, 320, 321
Primary pancreatic lymphoma, 361–363
Primary sclerosing cholangitis (PSC), 277–279
PSC. *See* Primary sclerosing cholangitis (PSC)
Pseudocyst, duodenal
  chronic pancreatitis, 210
  CT scan
    abdomen, 207
    collateral circulation, 208
    periduodenal mass, 209
  endoscopic ultrasound, 208
Pseudocysts, mediastinal, 97–98
PubMed Central® (PMC), 55
Pulmonary artery, malignant invasion of, 122–124
Pulmonary emboli, 78–82

R
Radiology centric image retrieval, 58
Rapid on-site evaluation (ROSE), 65
Recognition errors, 5
Rectal cancer
  EUS
    artifacts, 427
    vs. CT, 428
    deep wall invasion, 427
    early stage tumors, 427
    and MRI, 428
    neoadjuvant chemoradiation, 427
    nodal staging, 427–428
    recurrent cancer, 428
    staging of, 427
  T3N1 rectal carcinoma, 425–426
  T2N0-T3N1 stage, progression of, 421–424
Recurrent esophageal cancer, 142–143
Recurrent Hodgkin's lymphoma
  hot spots, 87
  Reed-Sternberg cells, 89
  unimpressive subcarinal lymph node, 88
Renal cancer, 348
Retroperitoneal carcinomatosis, 411–413
Reverberation artifacts, 16–17
Ring-down artifact, 16
Rosemont criteria, 308

S
Search errors, 5
Self-expandable metal stents (SEMSs), 351, 354
Seminal vesicles, 35–36
Serous cystadenoma (SCA), 379–380
Spectral Doppler signal
  azygos vein, 40
  celiac artery, 48
  lymph node, 257, 259
  portal venous system, 320, 322
Splenic artery, 45–46
Splenic vein thrombosis, 45
Sputum cytology, 119
Stanford classification, aortic dissection, 76, 77
Stomach
  gastric cancer, 150–153
  gastric carcinoid, 179–181
  gastric lipoma, 182–183
  gastrointestinal stromal tumor
    biopsy principles, 177–178
    central ulceration, 168
    incidence, 167
    and interstitial cells of Cajal, 172–173
    metastatic, 170–171
    with situs inversus, 174–176
  linitis plastica, 154–155
    with bone metastases, 156–158
  MALT
    Ann Arbor staging system, 159
    hematoxylin and eosin stain, 161
    with local and distant lymph node involvement, 162–165
    mucosal layer expansion, 160
    spectrum of, 159
  pancreatic rest, 188–190
  perigastric abscess, 193–195
  subepithelial gastric tumors, 166
  submucosal gastric pseudotumor, 191–192
  thickened gastric folds, 184–187
Stromal cells, 63–64
Subcarinal lymph node biopsy, 83–84
Subepithelial gastric tumors, 166
Submucosal gastric pseudotumor, 191–192
Superior mesenteric artery (SMA), 47

T
T2 adenocarcinoma, of pancreas, 323–325
Thyroid structure, 22–23
Thyroid transcription faction (TTF)-1 immunostain, 93
T1N1 esophageal cancer, 129
T3N1 rectal carcinoma, 425–426
Todani choledochal cyst, 284–286
Transabdominal ultrasound
  ascites, 396
  gallbladder carcinoma, 240
  liver lesion, 334, 336
Transduodenal abscess drainage
  CT scan
    compressing inferior vens cava, 223
    periduodenal abscess, 222
  endoscopic ultrasound
    dilations to 12 mm, 228
    dimensions of abscess, 224
    Huibregtse needle knife, 225
    Hurricane biliary balloon, 227
    irrigated and cleaned abscess cavity, 229
    pus exit from abscess, 226
Triple cytology, lung cancer diagnosis, 119–121
Type II choledochal cyst, 284–286

U
Ulcerated lesions, 150
Upper gastrointestinal barium study, of narrowing duodenum, 411, 412
Uterus, 39

V
Vagina, 37–38
Villous leison
  bulging of, in pancreatic duct, 213
  duodenal cancer, 199
Villous lesions, of distal common bile duct, 294–295

W
Wallstent
  characteristic appearance of, 351–353
  FNA biopsies, 354
Whipple pancreaticoduodenectomy, 193

Y
Yale Image Finder, 57
Yottalook™, 58

Z
Zollinger-Ellison syndrome, 179, 230–233

GPSR Compliance

The European Union's (EU) General Product Safety Regulation (GPSR) is a set of rules that requires consumer products to be safe and our obligations to ensure this.

If you have any concerns about our products, you can contact us on ProductSafety@springernature.com

In case Publisher is established outside the EU, the EU authorized representative is:

Springer Nature Customer Service Center GmbH
Europaplatz 3
69115 Heidelberg, Germany

Batch number: 10731049

Printed by Printforce, the Netherlands